Medical Care of the Liver Transplant Patient

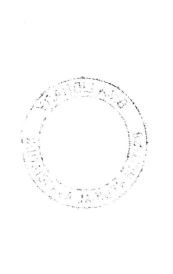

Medical Care of the Liver Transplant Patient

4th edition

Edited by

Pierre-Alain Clavien MD, PhD
Professor and Chairman
Department of Surgery
Swiss HPB (Hepato-Pancreato-Biliary) and Transplantation Center
University Hospital Zürich
Zürich, Switzerland

James F. Trotter MD
Professor of Medicine
Medical Director of Liver Transplantation
Baylor University Medical Center
Dallas, TX, USA

Associate Editor

Beat Müllhaupt MD
Head, Section of Hepatology
Division of Gastroenterology and Hepatology
University Hospital Zürich
Zürich, Switzerland

WILEY-BLACKWELL
A John Wiley & Sons, Ltd., Publication

Blackwell Publishing was acquired by John Wiley & Sons in February 2007. Blackwell's publishing program has been merged with Wiley's global Scientific, Technical and Medical business to form Wiley-Blackwell.

Registered office: John Wiley & Sons, Ltd, The Atrium, Southern Gate, Chichester, West Sussex, PO19 8SQ, UK

Editorial offices: 9600 Garsington Road, Oxford, OX4 2DQ, UK
The Atrium, Southern Gate, Chichester, West Sussex, PO19 8SQ, UK
111 River Street, Hoboken, NJ 07030-5774, USA

For details of our global editorial offices, for customer services and for information about how to apply for permission to reuse the copyright material in this book please see our website at www.wiley.com/wiley-blackwell

Library of Congress Cataloging-in-Publication Data

Medical care of the liver transplant patient / edited by Pierre-Alain
Clavien, James F. Trotter ; associate editor, Beat Müllhaupt. – 4th ed.
p. ; cm.
Includes bibliographical references and index.
ISBN-13: 978-1-4443-3591-0 (hardcover)
ISBN-10: 1-4443-3591-X
1. Liver–Transplantation. 2. Preoperative care. 3. Postoperative care. I. Clavien, Pierre-Alain. II. Trotter, James F.
[DNLM: 1. Liver Transplantation. 2. Patient Selection. 3. Perioperative Care. WI 770]
RD546.M375 2012
617.5'5620592–dc23

2011017804

A catalogue record for this book is available from the British Library.

Wiley also publishes its books in a variety of electronic formats. Some content that appears in print may not be available in electronic books.

Set in 9/11.5pt Sabon by Toppan Best-set Premedia Limited
Printed and bound in Singapore by Markono Print Media Pte Ltd

1 2012

Contents

Contributors

Juan G. Abraldes MD
Consultant
Liver Unit
Institut Clinic de Malalties Digestives i Metaboliques
Hospital Clinic, and University of Barcelona
Institut d'Investigacions Biomèdiques August Pi-Sunyer (IDIBAPS)
Ciber de Enfermedades Hepáticas y Digestivas (CIBERehd)
Barcelona, Spain

David Axelrod MD, MBA
Section of Solid Organ Transplant Surgery
Department of Surgery
Dartmouth-Hitchcock Medical Center
Lebanon, NH, USA

Markus Béchir MD
Consultant
Surgical Intensive Care Unit
University Hospital Zürich
Zürich, Switzerland

Beatrice Beck-Schimmer MD
Professor of Anesthesiology
Institute of Anesthesiology
University Hospital Zürich
Zürich, Switzerland

Thomas P. Beresford MD
Professor of Psychiatry
Department of Veterans Affairs Medical Center
Denver, CO, USA;
School of Medicine University of Colorado
Aurora, CO, USA

William Bernal MD, FRCP
Consultant Intensivist
Institute of Liver Studies
King's College Hospital
London, UK

Ulrich Beuers MD
Professor of gastroenterology and Hepatology
Head of Hepatology
Department of Gastroenterology and Hepatology
Academic Medical Center, University of Amsterdam
Amsterdam, The Netherlands

Jaime Bosch MD, PhD , FRCP
Chair of Medicine
Head, Hepatic Hemodynamic Laboratory
Liver Unit
Hospital Clinic IDIBAPS
University of Barcelona
Director, Biomedical Research Centre Network of Hepatic and Digestive Diseases (CIBERehd)
National Institute of Health Carlos III, Ministry of Science and Innovation Barcelona, Spain

Stefan Breitenstein MD
Clinical Assistant Professor
Department of Surgery
Swiss HPB (Hepato-Pancreato-Biliary) and Transplantation Center
University Hospital Zürich
Zürich, Switzerland

Robert S. Brown, Jr. MD, MPH
Frank Cardile Professor of Medicine
Center for Liver Diseases and Transplantation
Columbia University College of Physicians and Surgeons
New York, NY, USA

Jordi Bruix MD
Professor of Medicine BCLC group
BCLC group
Liver Unit
Hospital Clínic
Institut d'Investigacions
Biomèdiques August Pi-Sunyer (IDIBAPS)
Ciber de Enfermedades Hepáticas y Digestivas(CIBERehd)
University of Barcelona
Barcelona, Spain

Andrés Cárdenas MD, MMSc
GI Unit
Institut Clinic de Malalties Digestives i Metaboliques
Hospital Clinic, and University of Barcelona
Institut d'Investigacions Biomèdiques August Pi-Sunyer (IDIBAPS)
Ciber de Enfermedades Hepáticas y Digestivas (CIBERehd)
Barcelona, Spain

Natasha Chandok MD, MPH
Assistant Professor of Medicine
Division of Gastroenterology
Multi-Organ Transplant Program
University of Western Ontario
London, ON, Canada

Michael R. Charlton MB, BS, FRCP
Professor of Medicine
Head of Hepatobiliary Section
Medical Director Liver Transplantation
Division of Gastroenterology and Hepatology
Mayo Clinic
Mayo Clinic Transplant Center
Rochester, MN, USA

Abhideep Chaudhary MBBS, MS
Transplant Fellow
Thomas E. Starzl Transplantation Institute
University of Pittsburgh Medical Center
UPMC Montefiore
Pittsburgh, PA, USA

Srinath Chinnakotla MD
Associate Professor of Surgery and Pediatrics
University of Minnesota Medical School
Clinical Director of Pediatric Transplantation
University of Minnesota Amplatz Children's Hospital
Minneapolis, MN, USA

Pierre-Alain Clavien MD, PhD
Professor and Chairman
Department of Surgery
Swiss HPB (Hepato-Pancreato-Biliary) and Transplantation Center
University Hospital Zürich
Zürich, Switzerland

Audrey Coilly, MD
Consultant Hepatologist
Centre Hépato-Biliaire
AP-HP Hôpital Paul Brousse
and Univ. Paris-Sud Faculté de Médecine
Villejuif, France

Olivier de Rougemont MD
Research HPB and Transplant Fellow
Department of Surgery
Swiss HPB (Hepato-Pancreato-Biliary) and Transplantation Center
University Hospital Zürich
Zürich, Switzerland

Philipp Dutkowski MD
Professor of Surgery
Head Division of Transplantation Surgery
Department of Surgery
Swiss HPB (Hepato-Pancreato-Biliary) and Transplantation Center
University Hospital Zürich
Zürich, Switzerland

Ashraf Mohammad El-Badry MD
Clinical HPB and Transplant Fellow
Department of Surgery
Swiss HPB (Hepato-Pancreato-Biliary) and Transplantation Center
University Hospital Zürich
Zürich, Switzerland

Sylvie Euvrard MD
Consultant Physician
Department of Dermatology
Edouard Herriot Hospital Group
Hospices Civils de Lyon
Lyon, France

Michael B. Fallon MD
Professor of Medicine
Director, Division of Gastroenterology, Hepatology and Nutrition
University of Texas Health Science Center at Houston
Houston, TX, USA

Sheung Tat Fan MD, PhD
Sun Chieh Yeh Chair Professor of Surgery
Department of Surgery
The University of Hong Kong
Queen Mary Hospital
Hong Kong, China

Jay A. Fishman MD
Professor of Medicine
Harvard Medical School
Associate Director, MGH Transplant Program
Director, Transplant Infectious Disease and Compromised Host Program
Massachusetts General Hospital
Boston, MA, USA

Alejandro Forner MD
BCLC group
Liver Unit,
Hospital Clínic.
Institut d'Investigacions Biomèdiques August Pi-Sunyer (IDIBAPS)
Ciber de Enfermedades Hepáticas y Digestivas(CIBERehd)
University of Barcelona
Barcelona, Spain

Richard B. Freeman Jr MD
Allyn Professor and Chair
Department of Surgery
Dartmouth Medical School
Dartmouth Hitchcock Medical Center
Lebanon, NH, USA

Ed Gane MB, ChB, MD, FRACP
Professor
New Zealand Liver Transplant Unit
Auckland City Hospital
Auckland, New Zealand

Juan Carlos Garcia-Pagán MD, PhD
Senior Consultant in Hepatology
Liver Unit
Institut Clinic de Malalties Digestives i Metaboliques
Hospital Clinic, and University of Barcelona
Institut d'Investigacions Biomèdiques August
Pi-Sunyer (IDIBAPS)
Ciber de Enfermedades Hepáticas y Digestivas
(CIBERehd)
Barcelona, Spain

Andreas Geier MD
Consultant, Hepatologist
Division of Gastroenterology and Hepatology
Swiss HPB (Hepato-Pancreato-Biliary) Center
University Hospital Zürich
Zürich, Switzerland

Pere Ginès MD, PhD
Professor of Medicine
Chairman of Liver Unit
Institut Clinic de Malalties Digestives i Metaboliques
Hospital Clinic, and University of Barcelona
Institut d'Investigacions Biomèdiques August Pi-Sunyer (IDIBAPS)
Ciber de Enfermedades Hepáticas y Digestivas (CIBERehd)
Barcelona, Spain

Stevan A. Gonzalez MD, MS
Attending Physician, Division of Hepatology
Annette C. and Harold C. Simmons Transplant Institute
Baylor All Saints Medical Center
Fort Worth, TX, USA

Gregory J. Gores MD, FACP
Professor of Medicine
Division of Gastroenterology and Hepatology
The Miles and Shirley Fiterman Center for Digestive Diseases
Mayo Clinic College of Medicine
Rochester, MN, USA

Maureen M.J. Guichelaar MD, PhD
Consultant, Hepatology / Research collaborator
Mayo Clinic, Rochester MN, USA
Department of Gastroenterology and Hepatology
Medisch Spectrum Twente
Enschede, The Netherlands

Herman G.D. Hendriks MD, PhD
Consultant Anesthesiologist
Department of Anesthesiology
University Medical Center Groningen
University of Groningen
Groningen, The Netherlands

Michael A. Heneghan MD, MMedSc, FRCPI
Consultant Hepatologist
Institute of Liver Studies
King's College Hospital
London, UK

Abhinav Humar MD
Professor of Surgery
Transplant Surgery
Thomas E. Starzl Transplantation Institute
UPMC Montefiore
Pittsburgh, PA, USA

Jean Kanitakis MD
Professor of Medicine
Hospital Practitioner
Department of Dermatology
Edouard Herriot Hospital Group
Lyon, France

Goran Klintmalm MD, PhD, FACS
Chairman and Chief
Annette C. and Harold C. Simmons Transplant Institute
Baylor University Medical Center
Dallas, TX, USA

Mickaël Lesurtel MD, PhD
Swiss National Fund Professor
Department of Surgery
Swiss HPB (Hepato-Pancreato-Biliary) and Transplantation Center
University Hospital Zürich
Zürich, Switzerland

Ton Lisman PhD
Associate Professor of Experimental Surgery
Surgical Research Laboratory
Department of Surgery
University Medical Center Groningen
University of Groningen
Groningen, The Netherlands

Brandy Ries Lu MD
Sutter Pacific Medical Foundation
California Pacific Medical Center
Pediatric Gastroenterology and Hepatology
San Francisco, CA, USA

Victor I. Machicao MD
Associate Professor of Medicine
Medical Director of Liver Transplantation
Division of Gastroenterology, Hepatology and Nutrition
University of Texas Health Science Center at Houston
Houston, TX, USA

Howard C. Masuoka MD, PhD
Transplant Hepatology Fellow and Instructor
Division of Gastroenterology and Hepatology
The Miles and Shirley Fiterman Center for Digestive Diseases
Mayo Clinic College of Medicine
Rochester, MN, USA

Geoffrey W. McCaughan MBBS, PhD
Professor of Medicine
The AW Morrow Gastroenterology and Liver Centre
Royal Prince Alfred and the University of Sydney
The Centenary Research Institute
Sydney, NSW, Australia

Nicolas J. Mueller MD
Senior Staff Physician
Division of Infectious Diseases and Hospital Epidemiology
University Hospital Zürich
Zürich, Switzerland

Paolo Muiesan MD
Consultant Surgeon
Liver Transplantation and HPB Surgery
Liver Unit
Queen Elizabeth Hospital
Birmingham, UK

Beat Müllhaupt MD
Professor of Medicine
Head Section of Hepatology
Swiss HPB and Transplantation Centers
Division of Gastroenterology and Hepatology
University Hospital Zürich
Zürich, Switzerland

James Neuberger DM
Consultant Physician
Liver Unit
Queen Elizabeth Hospital
Birmingham, UK;
Associate Medical Director
Organ Donation and Transplantation
NHS Blood and Transplant
Bristol, UK

Kelvin Kwok-Chai Ng MS, PhD, FRCSEd (Gen)
Honorary Clinical Associate Professor
Department of Surgery
The University of Hong Kong
Queen Mary Hospital
Hong Kong, China

Sanna op den Dries BSc
Section of Hepatobiliary Surgery and Liver Transplantation
Department of Surgery
University Medical Center Groningen
University of Groningen
Groningen, The Netherlands

Marion G. Peters MD
Professor of Medicine
Chief of Hepatology Research
Division of Gastroenterology
University of California, San Francisco
San Francisco, CA, USA

Robert J. Porte MD, PhD, FEBS
Professor of Surgery
Head of Hepato-Pancreato-Biliary Surgery and Liver Transplantation
Department of Surgery
University Medical Center Groningen
University of Groningen
Groningen, The Netherlands

Marco Puglia MD, FRCPC
Assistant Professor
Department of Medicine
Division of Gastroenterology
McMaster University
Hamilton, ON, Canada

Maria Reig MD
BCLC group
Liver Unit
Hospital Clínic
Institut d'Investigacions Biomèdiques August Pi-Sunyer (IDIBAPS)
Ciber de Enfermedades Hepáticas y Digestivas(CIBERehd)
University of Barcelona
Barcelona, Spain

Eberhard L. Renner MD, FRCP(C)
Professor of Medicine
Director GI Transplantation
University Health Network
University of Toronto
Toronto, ON, Canada

Chiara Rocha MD
Resident in General Surgery
Liver Unit
Queen Elizabeth Hospital
Birmingham, UK

Charles B. Rosen MN
Professor of Surgery
Chair, Division of Transplantation Surgery
Mayo Clinic and Mayo Clinic College of Medicine
Rochester, MN, USA

Didier Samuel MD, PhD
Professor of Hepatology
Head of the Liver Unit and Liver ICU
Medical Director of the Liver Transplant Program Center
Hépato-Biliaire
AP-HP Hôpital Paul Brousse
Head of the Research Unit 785,
Univ. Paris-Sud and Inserm
Villejuif, France

Erik Schadde MD
Attending Surgeon
Department of Surgery
Swiss HPB (Hepato-Pancreato-Biliary) and Transplantation Center
University Hospital Zürich
Zürich, Switzerland

Nicole Siparsky MD
Section of Solid Organ Transplant Surgery
Department of Surgery
Dartmouth-Hitchcock Medical Center
Lebanon, NH, USA

Ronald J. Sokol MD
Professor and Vice Chair of Pediatrics
Chief, Section of Pediatric Gastroenterology, Hepatology and Nutrition
The Children's Hospital
Aurora, CO, USA

Peter G. Stock MD, PhD
Professor of Surgery
Department of Surgery
Division of Transplantation
University of California San Francisco
San Francisco, CA, USA

Laura Tariciotti MD
Specialist Registrar (Liver Surgery)
Liver Unit
Queen Elizabeth Hospital
Birmingham, UK

Lewis W. Teperman MD
Director of Transplantation
Vice-Chair of Surgery
NYU Langone Medical Center
The Mary Lea Johnson Richards Organ Transplant Center
Department of Surgery
New York, NY, USA

James F. Trotter MD
Professor of Medicine
Medical Director of Liver Transplantation
Baylor University Medical Center
Dallas, TX, USA

Robert C. Verdonk MD, PhD
Department of Gastroenterology and Hepatology
University Medical Center Groningen
University of Groningen
Groningen, The Netherlands

Kymberly D.S. Watt MD
Associate Professor of Medicine
Division of Gastroenterology/Hepatology
William J von Liebig Transplant Center
Mayo Clinic & Foundation
Rochester, MN, USA

Achim Weber MD
Assistant Professor of Molecular Pathology
Institute of Surgical Pathology
University of Zürich
Zürich, Switzerland

Aaron M. Winnick MD
Fellow, Transplant Surgery
NYU Langone Medical Center
The Mary Lea Johnson Richards Organ Transplant Center
Department of Surgery
New York, NY, USA

Preface

We are pleased to present the 4th edition of ***Medical Care of the Liver Transplant Patient***. The idea to produce such a book started in 1994 at Duke University Medical Center, NC, USA, where a new program for adult and pediatric liver transplantation was developed. The goals were to produce valuable information for any physicians dealing with liver transplantation either in training, established in one field of transplantation or for general praticioners dealing with these patients. Dr Paul Killenberg was the main architect of this project with Dr P-A Clavien, and participated very actively up to the first 3 editions of the book. In 2009, Paul Killenberg died suddenly from a cardio-vascular event, and we would like here to underline his major contributions to the filed of hepatology and this book. Logically, the job of co-editor was taken by James Trotter, who was already involved with the book from his time at Duke University.

Since the 3rd edition published in 2006, there have been a number of novel developments in the field of liver transplantation including, the search to solve the problem of organ shortening with the use of extended criteria donors and particularly donors after cardiac death (DCD), new approaches and indications regarding liver transplantation for malignancies, and the treatment of a variety of infectious diseases. A number of new authors were invited to update previous chapters or write new chapters.

The 4th edition of the book has been extensively revised with many new chapters and was subdivided in four parts covering management of potential transplant recipient (Part 1), donor issue and management in the peri-operative period (Part 2), chronic problems in the transplant recipients (Part 3), and pediatric liver transplantation (Part 4). As new features, we have included learning points for each chapter, and questions to enable the readers to test their understanding of the key information. Sixteen new chapters were added, namely for Part 1: Management of renal disease; Management of hepato-pulmonary syndrome and portal-pulmonary hypertension; Cholestatic and autoimmune liver disease; Cholangiocarcinoma; Rare indications (rare tumors, Budd Chiari, etc); HIV patients; for Part 2: Extended criteria donor; Donation after cardiac death (NHBD); Transmission of malignancies and infection through donor organs; Domino and split transplantation; Coagulation and blood transfusion management; Acute care after liver transplantation; Rejection and immunosuppression; for Part 3: Prevention and treatment of recurrent viral hepatitis; PTLD and other malignancies after liver transplantation; Sexual function and fertility after liver transplantation.

We are grateful to our many colleagues who have agreed to author chapters in this book. We are also grateful to our colleagues at Wiley-Blackwell, Jennifer Seward, Rebecca Huxley, and Kathy Syplywczak, whose interest in this project has been so very important. We would like to also express our greatest gratitude to Madeleine Meyer, from the Zurich office, who played a major role in coordinating and making this edition possible.

P-A Clavien
James Trotter
January 2012

PART ONE

Management of the Potential Transplant Recipient

1 Selection and evaluation of the recipient (including retransplantation)

Audrey Coilly[1,2] *and Didier Samuel*[1,3,4]
[1]AP-HP Hôpital Paul Brousse, Centre Hépato-Biliaire, Villejuif; [2]Univ. Paris-Sud, Faculté de Médecine, Paris; [3]Univ. Paris-Sud, UMR-S 785, Villejuif, Paris; and [4]Inserm, Unité 785, Villejuif, France

Key learning points

- Patients should be considered for liver transplantation if they have evidence of life-threatening complications of liver disease including cirrhosis and acute liver failure.
- Indications and contraindications perpetually change with regard to an organ shortage and medical improvements.
- Prioritization for transplantation is now determined by the Model of End Stage Liver Disease (MELD), which lists patients with the greatest risk of short-term mortality.
- At the liver center, a detailed evaluation of the recipient is performed to ensure that transplantation is indicated and feasible.
- Despite a high mortality comparing primary liver transplantation, retransplantation is the only therapy suitable for patients with loss of graft function.

Introduction

Selection and evaluation of a recipient for liver transplantation (LT) has become a great challenge, in the best interest of both the patient and society. Actually, limited organ availability and an increasing demand for organ transplantation has extended transplant waiting times and thus increased morbidity and mortality for potential recipients on waiting lists.

Patients should be referred to transplant centers when a life-threatening complication of liver disease occurs. A detailed medical evaluation is performed to ensure the feasibility of LT. Priority for transplantation has been determined by the MELD score, identifying patients with the highest estimated short-term mortality.

Selection of the recipient: why liver transplantation should be performed

Selection of the recipient is a main challenge for transplant physicians. LT is indicated in end-stage liver disease (ESLD). The most common indication in the adult is cirrhosis but the list of indications is growing. In contrast, the transplant community is currently faced with a major organ shortage; this has put extraordinary pressure on organ allocation programs. Since a successful outcome requires optimal patient

Medical Care of the Liver Transplant Patient, Fourth Edition. Edited by Pierre-Alain Clavien, James F. Trotter.

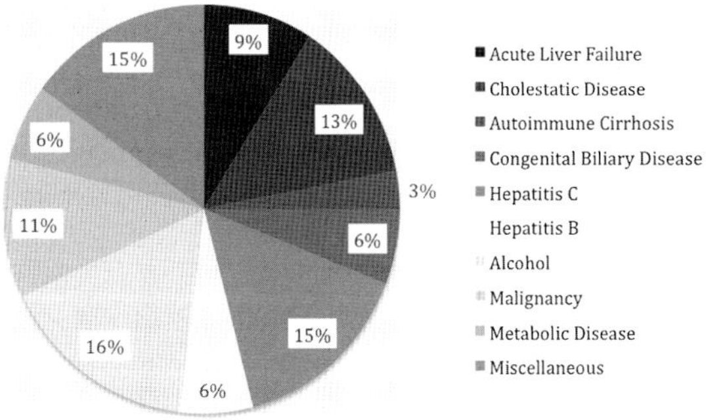

Figure 1.1 Indications for liver transplantation in Europe[38]

selection and timing, the issue of which patients to list for LT and when to transplant cirrhotic patients has generated great interest as well as considerable controversy.

Main indications for LT: complications of ESLD

LT should be considered in any patient with liver disease in whom the procedure would extend life expectancy beyond what the natural history of underlying liver disease would predict or in whom LT is likely to improve quality of life. Patients should be selected if expected survival in the absence of transplantation is 1 year or less, or if the patient has an unacceptable quality of life because of liver disease. Indications for LT in Europe are summarized in Figure 1.1.

Gastroesophageal variceal bleeding

Gastroesophageal varices are found in 30% of patients with compensated cirrhosis and 60% of patients with decompensated cirrhosis. Variceal bleeding usually does not occur until the Hepatic Venous Pression Gradient (HVPG) is above 12 mmHg. Each episode of bleeding carries a 20% mortality rate. If the varices are left untreated, after survival from the first episode, the rebleeding risk can be up to 70% within 1 year and is a major cause of death in patients with cirrhosis. Medical treatments are endoscopic variceal ligation and nonselective beta-blockers. Transjugular intrahepatic portosystemic shunt (TIPS) involves establishment of a direct pathway between the hepatic veins and the portal veins to decompress the portal venous hypertension that is the source of the patient's hemorrhage. The procedure is technically challenging, especially in critically ill patients, and has a mortality rate of 30–50% in the emergency setting, but has <90% effectiveness in controlling bleeding from gastroesophageal varices. LT remains the best way to decompress the portal system if other therapy has failed.[1]

Hepatic encephalopathy

Hepatic encephalopathy (HE) is a neuropsychiatric complication of cirrhosis in which clinical manifestations range from subtle personality changes and sleep disorder to coma. Although treatments have emerged, such as rifaximin to improve recurrence of HE,[2] LT remains the only effective therapy.

Ascites and hepatorenal syndrome

Refractory ascites occurs in 5–10% of cirrhotic patients and carries a mortality rate of >50% at 2 years. Patients are prone to develop gastrointestinal variceal bleeding, hepatorenal syndrome (HRS), spontaneous bacterial peritonitis (SBP) and HRS approximately 1 year after the development of ascites, reflecting the poor prognosis of patients with ascites. LT evaluation therefore should be instituted whenever refractory ascites develop.[3]

HRS is characterized by renal vasoconstriction in response to renal hypoperfusion from a low systemic effective circulating volume. The annual incidence of HRS in patients with cirrhosis and ascites is approximately 8%.[4] Two types of HRS are described. Type 1 HRS is characterized by a rapidly progressive impairment of the circulatory and renal functions associated with a very poor prognosis (median survival rate <2 weeks). Type 2 HRS is characterized by a steady impairment of the circulatory and renal function with a median survival rate of 6 months. LT should be considered as soon as a HRS is diagnosed.

Pulmonary complications

Hepatopulmonary syndrome (HPS) is found in 4–47% of patients with cirrhosis and is characterized by intrapulmonary vascular dilatations, especially in the basal parts of the lung. Liver injury and/or portal hypertension trigger the release of endothelin-l, TNF-alpha, cytokines and mediate vascular shear stress and release of nitric oxide and carbon monoxide, all contributing to intrapulmonary vasodilatation. This results in hypoxemia which may require oxygen therapy. Because it could reverse HPS, LT is the only curative treatment. HPS differs from portopulmonary hypertension (PPHTN) which occurs in 2–8% of patients with cirrhosis. Imbalance between vasodilating and vasoconstrictive agents may be responsible for misguided angiogenesis and pulmonary hypertension. It is associated with a higher risk for LT and increased post-transplantation mortality.

Specific indications for LT

Some indications for LT are specific and vary depending on the underlying liver disease.

Cholestatic diseases

Some criteria for primary biliary cirrhosis (PBC) are specific (see Chapter 10). As survival rate is considerably reduced when the bilirubin level is over 100 μmol/L for <1 year, this level is an indication of LT without any other complication. Uncontrolled and intolerable pruritus or major asthenia, even if isolated, are also indications for LT.

Primary sclerosing cholangitis (PSC) is a rare idiopathic cholestatic disease of unknown cause, characterized by a chronic fibrosing inflammation of the bile ducts (see Chapter 10). There is also an increased risk of cholangiocarcinoma, which is a difficult diagnosis with a prevalence over 30% after a 10-year disease course.[5] Specific indications for PSC are longstanding severe jaundice (bilirubin level over 100 μmol/L), cholestasis and pruritus not related to an acute episode of cholangitis, repeated episodes of cholangitis not controlled by antibiotics, and any suspicion of cholangiocarcinoma.

Autoimmune chronic hepatitis

Autoimmune chronic hepatitis is more common in young women. The clinical presentation of the disease is variable; classically it presents as active chronic hepatitis, but it may also present as established cirrhosis and in few cases as a fulminant course without chronic hepatic disease. A main characteristic of this disease is a good response to immunosuppressive treatment including steroids.[6]

LT is indicated in autoimmune hepatitis for clinical decompensation, despite long-term adequate immunosuppressive treatment, or in fulminant hepatic failure, in which immunosuppressive treatment is usually ineffective and potentially deleterious.

Viral hepatitis

Chronic viral hepatitis due to the hepatitis virus B, C and/or D is one of the most common causes of ESLD worldwide and a frequent diagnosis in patients referred to transplant centers. Viral recurrence after LT is a major issue and graft damage secondary to viral re-infection may lead to graft failure, retransplantation or death.

Alcoholic liver disease

Alcoholic cirrhosis is a common liver disease and a significant number of patients with alcoholic liver disease receive LT. Several centers have developed an evaluation process based on medical and psychiatric criteria to better determine patients who would benefit most from the procedure. Abstinence from alcohol of at least 6 months is usually required to evaluate the need and timing of LT and to obtain better control of alcoholism. This interval is neither a consensus nor an absolute requirement. The risk of recidivism is estimated to be between 15–40% depending on the series, which seems to be related to the duration of follow up after LT and the duration of abstinence before transplantation. Whichever the case, this remains controversial.[7]

Acute alcoholic hepatitis has been considered an absolute contraindication to liver transplantation on the grounds that patients with this disorder have been drinking recently and that a period of abstinence will allow many to recover. Unfortunately, many patients die during this interval. Patients who do not recover within the first 3 months of abstinence are unlikely to survive.[8] Consequently, liver transplantation centers face a dilemma when caring for a patient with alcoholism who has severe alcoholic hepatitis and whose condition deteriorates despite adherence to abstinence, nutritional support, corticosteroids, and other elements of medical management.[9]

Hepatobiliary malignancy

In certain cases, hepatobiliary malignancy is an indication for LT.

Hepatocellular carcinoma (HCC) is the commonest primary malignancy of the liver. LT is a suitable therapeutic option for early, unresectable HCC, particularly in the setting of chronic liver disease. The study by Mazzaferro in 1996 established LT as a viable treatment for HCC.[10] In this study, the "Milan criteria" were applied, achieving a 4-year survival rate similar to LT for benign disease. Since then various groups have attempted to expand these criteria[11] (see Chapter 11).

Cholangiocarcinoma (CCA) is the second most common cancer among the primary hepatic neoplasm, accounting for 5–20% of liver malignancies.[12] LT for CCA remains a controversial subject (see Chapter 12). A protocol combining neoadjuvant chemoradiation and LT was first used in patients with unresectable hilar CCA. Results have confirmed that this approach leads to significantly lower recurrence rates and higher long-term survival rates than other existing treatment modalities. Despite this, protocols to treat patients with CCA are not widespread, and are available at only a handful of transplant programs.

Other hepatobiliary malignancies may be successfully treated by LT, including without fibrolamellar carcinoma (without metastases), and hemangioendothelioma.

Classically, metastatic tumors of the liver have been considered a poor indication for LT, although some centers have performed this procedure associated with another therapy, such as chemotherapy and radiotherapy. In metastases from neuroendocrine tumors, liver transplantation could be indicated for patients with symptoms related to major hepatomegaly, hormone production, inavailability of effective therapeutic alternatives, diffuse metastases of the liver, slow-growing tumor and absence of extrahepatic disease.[13] Transplant offers the main advantage of a significant improvement of the quality of life in many patients, an alternative to palliative therapy and a possible cure in some patients.

Non-alcoholic fatty liver disease and non-alcoholic steatohepatitis

In the setting of the metabolic or insulin resistance syndrome (IRS), non-alcoholic fatty liver disease (NAFLD) and non-alcoholic steatohepatitis (NASH) are becoming increasingly common medical problems in the developed world. Patients with histological necrotic-inflammatory changes and/or fibrosis may progress to ESLD and require LT (see Chapter 9). It is likely that many potential LT candidates with NASH are excluded from LT due to co-morbid conditions related to IRS.

Fulminant hepatitis

Fulminant hepatitis is an emergency of LT.[14] Viruses (especially hepatitis viruses A and B), drugs, and toxic agents are the most common causes of fulminant hepatitis; its prevalence varies between countries. The prognosis is essentially determined by neurological status, but is also affected very rapidly by damage to other organs. LT has revolutionized the prognosis of fulminant hepatitis, increasing the survival rate from 10–20% (all causes combined) to 75–80% at 1 year and 70% at 5 years (see Chapter 16).

When to perform liver transplantation

The timing of LT is crucial. Physicians have to determine which patients have liver disease that will endanger their lives before life-threatening systemic complications occur. This consideration is balanced by the risk of surgery and immunosuppressive treatment of LT if it is performed too early.

The timing of LT has changed in recent years, reflecting the modification in the method of organ allocation. Up until 2002, a patient's position on the transplant list was determined by their time on the waiting list.[15] The MELD score was implemented for determining organ allocation in 2002 in the USA. This score is an algorithm based on objective measures comprising creatinine, bilirubin and international normalized ratio (INR). The MELD was developed initially to determine the short-term prognosis for patients undergoing TIPS.[16] It was considered to be highly accurate for predicting liver-related death. It was also regarded as a better system because it ignores waiting time and considers actual liver dysfunction.

Implementation of MELD led to an immediate reduction in liver transplant waiting list registrations for the first time in history of LT.[15] Moreover, the median waiting time to LT decreased.[17] In patients with MELD scores ≤14, the mortality rate with transplantation was found to be higher than that of patients with the same MELD score who had not undergone transplantation.[18] Consequently, a MELD score higher than 15 is now considered a valid indication of LT in patients with ESLD. In contrast to the clear benefit of accurately estimating mortality for those patients on the waiting list, MELD has not been found to be as useful in predicting mortality following

LT.[19] Mortality in the post-transplantation period is related not only to the degree of liver dysfunction prior to transplantation, but to other factors, such as donor characteristics, experience of the transplantation team, and random postoperative complications that cannot be predicted.

The MELD scoring system does have limitations. Not all candidates for LT suffer from diseases that carry an immediate mortality risk. These patients would not be well served by a priority system based solely on a mortality risk endpoint. Patients with HCC have relatively preserved synthetic function; they were not given priority in the early years of LT, which led to a high rate of death in these patients prior to LT. The MELD system offers a way to assign priority points for a diagnosis of HCC (see Chapter 11). Seventeen "exceptional diagnoses" have been identified to be underserved by the MELD score allocation system, including pulmonary complications of cirrhosis, hepatic encephalopathy, amyloidosis, and primary hyperoxaluria (Table 1.1). In these cases, extra points could be awarded to certain groups of patients as shown.[20]

Even if the MELD scoring system is well-recognized to be a revolution in the LT era, some studies have tried to improve the model, incorporating values as serum sodium (MELD-Na), and age (integrated MELD). Another example is ΔMELD, using a time-dependent analysis.[21] Some authors compared these models but the MELD score remains the only one used for organ allocation.[22]

Table 1.1 Exceptions to MELD score

Manifestations of cirrhosis
Ascites and hyponatremia
Gastrointestinal bleeding
Encephalopathy
Hepatopulmonary syndrome
Portopulmonary hypertension
Pruritus
Miscellaneous liver diseases
Budd–Chiari syndrome
Familial amyloidosis
Cystic fibrosis
Hereditary hemorrhagic telangiectasia
Polycystic liver disease
Primary hyperoxaluria
Recurrent cholangitis
Unusual metabolic disease
Malignancy
Cholangiocarcinoma and Hepatocellular carcinoma
Unusual tumors
Other
Small-for-size syndrome

Evaluating the recipient: Who shouldn't be transplanted?

Evaluation of the recipient aims to identify contraindications of surgery as well as the contraindications to taking long-term immunosuppressive treatment. This assessment is not consensual and should be discussed in each transplant center. The contraindications to LT are dynamic, ever-changing and vary among liver transplant centers, regarding local expertise. There is an expectation that those transplanted would have a survival probability of at least 50% at 5 years with a quality of life acceptable to the patient. Figure 1.2 shows a sample decision tree for selection and evaluation of an LT recipient.

Assessment of operability

The evaluation of the operability of the candidate requires a cardiovascular and respiratory assessment first.

To evaluate the cardiovascular risk, each patient should undergo an electrocardiogram and a transthoracic echocardiography to identify underlying heart disease. In patients with cirrhosis, increased cardiac output is described and the presence of latent cardiac dysfunction, which includes a combination of reduced cardiac contractility with systolic and diastolic dysfunction. Electrophysiological abnormalities are also noticed. This syndrome is termed "cirrhotic cardiomyopathy".[23] If the patient has multiple cardiovascular risk factors, a stress test should be carried out in order to reveal asymptomatic ischemic heart disease. A thallium stress test is now a minimally invasive and useful examination. In some cases, if coronary disease is suspected during the evaluation in high-risk patients, coronary angiography should be discussed.

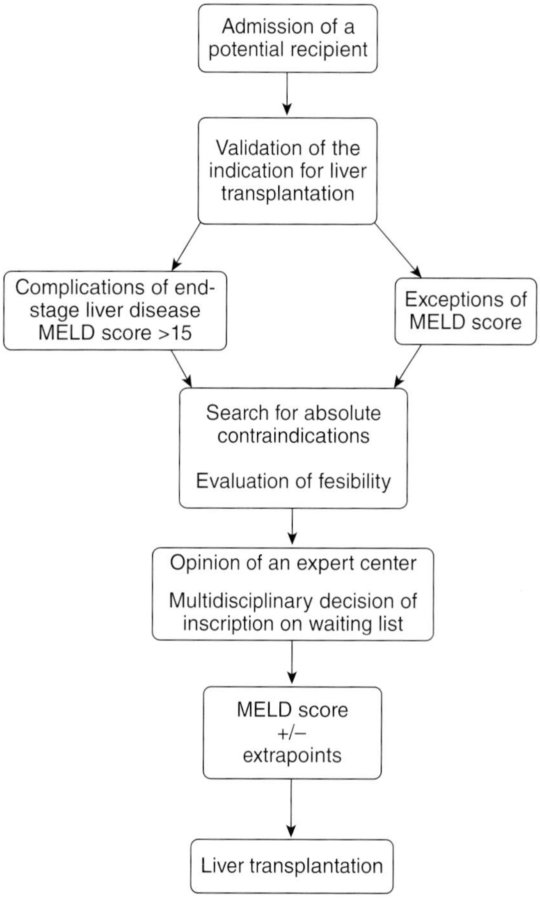

Figure 1.2 Proposed decision tree for selection and evaluation of LT recipient

To evaluate the respiratory risk, a lung function test and a chest X-ray are recommended to screen for lung disease related to cirrhosis or otherwise. When HPS or PPHTN are suspected, further investigation should be performed. The diagnosis of HPS is made by calculating the alveolar-arterial oxygen gradient and performing contrast echocardiography.

A diagnosis of PPHTN is made by performing echocardiography and right-heart catheterization when the systolic pulmonary artery pressure is higher than 30 mmHg on echocardiography.[24] PPHTN used to be an absolute contraindication to LT. The pre-LT management of patients with PPHTN requires early diagnosis and chronic therapy with pulmonary vasodilators such as intravenous epoprostenol to decrease pulmonary vascular resistance. Careful perioperative attention is imperative to avoid right ventricular failure from acutely elevated pulmonary artery pressure or sudden increases in right ventricular preload. With increased surgical and anesthetic expertise, PPHTN is no longer considered an absolute contraindication for LT[25](see Chapter 5).

An evaluation of renal function is essential. HRS, usually a reversible cause of renal failure, has to be differentiated from other causes of chronic kidney disease that are potentially nonreversible and mandate simultaneous liver–kidney transplantations. Estimated renal clearance could be hard to determine in patients with cirrhosis.[26] Performing inulin clearance and renal biopsies might help in the decision-making process. Chronic kidney disease patients with glomerular filtration rates of <30 ml/min, HRS patients requiring renal replacement therapy for >8–12 weeks, and patients with renal biopsy findings of >30% fibrosis and glomerulosclerosis would benefit from receiving both liver and kidney grafts.[27]

The general condition and nutritional status are sometimes difficult to assess in the patient with ESLD. Liver cirrhosis is associated with malnutrition. The clinical and biological parameters used may not apply in cases of severe hepatic insufficiency (body mass index, prealbumin etc.) More studies are needed to develop specific nutritional scores in cirrhosis.

Osteoporosis is also a common complication among patients with cirrhosis and may be detected by bone desitometry which can predict the risk of pathological fracture. An anesthesia consultation is mandatory at the end of this evaluation to assess operational risk. Human leukocyte antigen (HLA) typing and determination of blood group should be included in the general evaluation.

Anatomical evaluation

The surgeon must consider the type of vascularization of the recipient, mainly regarding the hepatic artery and portal system. The presence of shunts, which should be ligated during surgery, or the arcuate ligament are routinely sought. CT angiography of the liver is now performed in all recipients without contraindications. Hepatic arteriography has been largely replaced by CT angiography, but it is still indicated in cases of variant anatomy or previous hepatic surgery including LT.

In the past, portal vein thrombosis (PVT) was considered an absolute contraindication for LT. Thanks to improvement in medical care, surgical techniques and radiological interventions, PVT by itself can represent an indication for LT. Several studies showed that surgical thrombectomy, thromboendovenectomy with venous reconstruction, interposition of vein graft, porto-caval hemitransposition and radiological endovascular interventions can resolve venous obstruction in liver transplant recipients. Interestingly, PVT patients' rates of survival at 1 and 5 years after LT are equal.[28]

Infection screening

Patients with cirrhosis are prone to develop infections that could lead to the development of multiple organ failure and death.[29] Screening for latent infections is required in order to treat a potentially lethal infections before LT and to prevent an exacerbation after LT under immunosuppressive regimens.

A chest radiograph should be performed to identify indirect signs of bacterial or fungal lung infection, including tuberculosis. Some teams recommend conducting a skin test. The search for the tubercle bacillus is not required in the absence of risk factors and with a normal chest radiograph for others.

Examination by an otolaryngologist, and a stomatologist could be required with a nasofibroscopy, a stomatological sinus radiography and panoramic radiographs. Latent dental infection should be treated if possible before LT.

Serologic evaluation for aspergillosis, syphilis, and legionella is often recommended. Hepatitis B and C are systematically sought, even if it is not the cause motivating the transplant. Human immunodeficiency virus (HIV) infection has been considered until recently as a contraindication for LT due to the poor spontaneous prognosis of HIV infection. The advent of highly active antiretroviral drugs (HAART) was a therapeutic breakthrough, and the prognosis has been dramatically improved. The progression of chronic hepatitis B virus (HBV) and hepatitis C virus (HCV) seems more rapid in co-infected patients, and a high number of patients will develop life-threatening liver cirrhosis. Patients with a controlled HIV disease are now considered suitable candidates for LT[30] (see Chapter 14).

Serological tests of herpesviridae viruses (Epstein–Barr virus, cytomegalovirus, herpes simplex virus 1 and 2, varicella zoster virus, human herpes virus 6 and 8) are conducted to determine the potential risk of reactivation after LT.

Neoplasia screening

Cancer screening must take into account age, gender, and alcoholic and smoking status of the recipient. If an extrahepatic cancer is an absolute contraindication for LT, a past history of cancer already treated should not disqualify candidates for LT, in accordance, case by case with an oncologist to estimate the survival and risk of recurrence at 1 year, 5 years, and 10 years under long-term immunosuppressive treatment. Actually, the LT should be performed if the risk of recurrence is estimated to be <10%. More often, physicians require a waiting period of 5 years to exclude potential recurrence. This fact should be balanced by the severity of hepatic illness. Colorectal cancer screening is mandatory for any candidate older than 50. If a colonoscopy under general anesthesia is too risky, CT colonography may be an alternative, although its usefulness in cirrhotic patients with ascites has never been demonstrated. The search for pulmonary neoplasia, stomatology, and of the ear–nose–throat (ENT), esophageal and bladder regions is mandatory in cases of alcohol and smoking addiction. An ENT examination is associated with a nasofibroscopy, and an examination of the oral cavity and an upper gastrointestinal endoscopy are recommended.

All women should have regular gynecological care including Papanicolaou test (Pap smear) and mammogram if needed. In men older than 50, screening for prostate disease should be done, including the quantification of PSA and a vesico-prostatic ultrasound.

An examination of the skin is important but skin cancer rarely contraindicates LT.

Special screening for hepatic malignancy

Preoperative baseline metastatic work-up includes a bone scan and chest computed tomography (CT). Recently, a positron emission tomography (PET) scan also tends to be included because of the usefulness to find undetected malignancy and to avoid legal issues.

Social, psychiatric, and addiction assessment

It is important to search for social network problems, psychiatric illness, and addiction in order to evaluate the adherence of the recipient. In the case of hepatic encephalopathy, neuropsychological testing, CT brain scan, and electroencephalography could help to determine the reversibility of neuropsychiatric troubles. Drug or alcohol abuse is considered to be a contraindication to LT for many reasons: the risk of recidivism, risk of noncompliance, and risk of injury to the graft (see Chapter 6). A period of abstinence from alcohol for at least 6 months is generally a requirement though some teams currently criticize this rule. To date, other models should be defined to evaluate the risk of relapse, including a detailed psychiatric evaluation.

Stably abstinent, methadone-maintained opiate-dependent patients are generally good candidates for LT and show low relapse rates.[31] Current toxicology screening methods provide a positive result of screening for cannabinoids up to 2 months after the patient's last use. Patients who tested positive for marijuana had similar survival rates compared to those with negative test results. Whether patients who regularly use marijuana should be excluded from the waiting list remains a controversial issue.

Pre- and post-transplant smoking rates are high and cause significant morbidity and mortality by cardiovascular events or malignancies. Transplant teams should encourage smoking cessation treatments.

Age

The upper age limit for LT varies; the age of 65 is generally considered to be the upper limit but it has been successfully performed in patients as old as 70. The limit should be determined according to the patient's general medical condition and discussed within each transplant center.

Evaluating and selecting a good recipient for LT requires the collaboration of several specialists. The final decision should be made within each center by expert multidisciplinary staff, considering the benefits and risks for each recipient.

Retransplantation

After LT, graft loss still occurs in 10–20% of adults. The most frequent causes of irreversible graft damage are primary nonfunction, hepatic artery thrombosis, graft rejection and recurrent diseases. Liver retransplantation (re-LT) is the only therapy suitable for patients with loss of graft function after a primary liver transplantation but re-LT carries a high morbidity and mortality rate compared with LT. The 1-, 5-, and 10-year patient survival rates after retransplantation were 61%, 53.7%, and 50.1%, respectively. These percentages were significantly less than those after LT during the same period: 82.3%, 72.1%, and 66.9%. In some centers patients could receive three, four, or more transplants.

Although re-LT is inferior to initial LT, it is the only means of prolonging survival in the patients whose initial graft has failed, making it an important contribution to overall survival.[32]

Primary nonfunction

Primary nonfunction (PNF) is a postoperative condition characterized by absence of hepatic recovery due to various insults during harvesting, preservation or revascularization, unappreciated diseases in the donor, or accelerated rejection. Moderate steatosis of donor liver (30–60%) is associated with an increased incidence of PNF and re-LT rate. PNF, usually defined by the criteria of immediate graft failure with an elevated level of liver enzymes, scarce bile output, encephalopathy, and coagulopathy, is the main indication for re-LT.[33] The incidence is around 6%. In the setting of PNF, re-LT should be undertaken early, within the first 7 days of the primary LT. As shown by multiple studies, re-LT at an intermediate time interval (8–30 d) is associated with a worse prognosis.

Hepatic artery thrombosis

Hepatic artery thrombosis (HAT) after LT can cause significant morbidity or mortality and lead to liver failure or septic complications.[34,35] Allograft rejection is a possible cause of HAT. The incidence is near 3% (see Chapter 28).

Rejection

In the 1980s, acute hepatic allograft rejection occurred in approximately 80% of patients undergoing LT. Chronic rejection is always preceded by one or more episodes of acute rejection, and usually refractory to immunosuppressive therapy. Chronic rejection is an important cause of late graft failure. Despite improvement in immunosuppression therapy, the incidence is still 5% by tacrolimus-based immunosuppressive regimen (see Chapter 27).

Recurrent diseases

Hepatitis C

Approximately 20% or more of HCV-positive transplant recipients will develop allograft cirrhosis within 5 years after LT, and 10% of HCV-infected recipients will die or lose their allograft secondary to hepatitis C-associated allograft failure. The only solution is re-LT[36] but for HCV-positive transplant recipients, re-LT remains highly controversial: patients undergoing re-LT for recurrent HCV have a significantly shorter median survival than those patients undergoing re-LT for other reasons of graft loss (see Chapter 32).

Hepatitis B

The use of hepatitis B immunoglobulin and nucleoside analogues has reduced the risk of HBV recurrence and led to the improvement of patient and graft survival rates.

Other liver diseases

Primary biliary cirrhosis (PBC), primary sclerosing cholangitis (PSC), and autoimmune hepatitis have a recurrence rate of 20–30% within 5 years after liver transplantation (see Chapter 33).

Timing for retransplantation

There is no consensus among transplant physicians to define specific re-LT survival outcomes below which re-LT is to be avoided. Only the MELD scoring system for organ allocation provides an objective stratification of retransplant candidates based on severity of illness.

A reduction in short-term survival rate to <60% was observed in all re-LT patients with a MELD score over 25.[37] While mortality was increased in all groups with a concomitant rise in MELD score, patients with a score over 30 had a survival rate of 20–40%. Retransplantation may exhibit survival rates similar to primary transplant in select patients. It is more likely to be successful in healthier recipients with a lower MELD score.

The effect of allograft quality is exceedingly recognized as one of the important parameters that determine success of transplantation in general and re-LT in particular. More studies are needed to clearly define the parameters but older donors and a long, cold ischemia time (>8 hours) seem to be the key factors.

HCV used to be considered as an independent risk factor for higher mortality rate, but several studies have demonstrated that a reasonable rate of survival can be achieved following re-LT and no significant survival differences are observed between HCV-positive, cryptogenic, cholestatic, or alcoholic liver disease patients when adjusted for age and MELD scores.[38,39]

These data suggest that the selection of the recipient should integrate the severity of illness, the interval time since the primary LT and the graft quality more than the cause of retransplantation.

References

1. de Franchis R. Revising consensus in portal hypertension: report of the Baveno V consensus workshop on methodology of diagnosis and therapy in portal hypertension. J Hepatol 2010;53:762–8.
2. Bass NM, Mullen KD, Sanyal A, et al. Rifaximin treatment in hepatic encephalopathy. N Engl J Med 2010;362:1071–81.
3. Planas R, Montoliu S, Balleste B, et al. Natural history of patients hospitalized for management of cirrhotic ascites. Clin Gastroenterol Hepatol 2006;4:1385–94.
4. Gines A, Escorsell A, Gines P, et al. Incidence, predictive factors, and prognosis of the hepatorenal syndrome in cirrhosis with ascites. Gastroenterology 1993;105: 229–36.
5. LaRusso NF, Shneider BL, Black D, et al. Primary sclerosing cholangitis: summary of a workshop. Hepatology 2006;44:746–64.
6. Czaja AJ, Manns MP. Advances in the Diagnosis, Pathogenesis and Management of Autoimmune Hepatitis. Gastroenterology 2010;139:58–72.
7. Pfitzmann R, Schwenzer J, Rayes N, Seehofer D, Neuhaus R, Nussler NC. Long-term survival and predictors of relapse after orthotopic liver transplantation for alcoholic liver disease. Liver Transpl 2007;13: 197–205.
8. Mathurin P, Duchatelle V, Ramond MJ, et al. Survival and prognostic factors in patients with severe alcoholic hepatitis treated with prednisolone. Gastroenterology 1996;110:1847–53.

9. O'Shea RS, Dasarathy S, McCullough AJ. Alcoholic liver disease. Hepatology 2010;51:307–28.
10. Mazzaferro V, Regalia E, Doci R, et al. Liver transplantation for the treatment of small hepatocellular carcinomas in patients with cirrhosis. N Engl J Med 1996;334:693–9.
11. Duffy JP, Vardanian A, Benjamin E, et al. Liver transplantation criteria for hepatocellular carcinoma should be expanded: a 22-year experience with 467 patients at UCLA. Ann Surg 2007;246:502–9; discussion 9–11.
12. Khan SA, Davidson BR, Goldin R, et al. Guidelines for the diagnosis and treatment of cholangiocarcinoma: consensus document. Gut 2002;51(Suppl 6):VI1–9.
13. Hoti E, Adam R. Liver transplantation for primary and metastatic liver cancers. Transpl Int 2008;21:1107–17.
14. Hoofnagle JH, Carithers RL Jr, Shapiro C, Ascher N. Fulminant hepatic failure: summary of a workshop. Hepatology 1995;21:240–52.
15. Wiesner R, Edwards E, Freeman R, et al. Model for end-stage liver disease (MELD) and allocation of donor livers. Gastroenterology 2003;124:91–6.
16. Malinchoc M, Kamath PS, Gordon FD, Peine CJ, Rank J, ter Borg PC. A model to predict poor survival in patients undergoing transjugular intrahepatic portosystemic shunts. Hepatology 2000;31:864–71.
17. Wiesner R, Lake JR, Freeman RB, Gish RG. Model for end-stage liver disease (MELD) exception guidelines. Liver Transpl 2006;12:S85–7.
18. Merion RM, Schaubel DE, Dykstra DM, Freeman RB, Port FK, Wolfe RA. The survival benefit of liver transplantation. Am J Transplant 2005;5:307–13.
19. Habib S, Berk B, Chang CC, et al. MELD and prediction of post-liver transplantation survival. Liver Transpl 2006;12:440–7.
20. Freeman RB Jr, Gish RG, Harper A, et al. Model for end-stage liver disease (MELD) exception guidelines: results and recommendations from the MELD Exception Study Group and Conference (MESSAGE) for the approval of patients who need liver transplantation with diseases not considered by the standard MELD formula. Liver Transpl 2006;12:S128–36.
21. Merion RM, Wolfe RA, Dykstra DM, Leichtman AB, Gillespie B, Held PJ. Longitudinal assessment of mortality risk among candidates for liver transplantation. Liver Transpl 2003;9:12–18.
22. Biselli M, Gitto S, Gramenzi A, et al. Six score systems to evaluate candidates with advanced cirrhosis for orthotopic liver transplant: Which is the winner? Liver Transpl 2010;16:964–73.
23. Moller S, Henriksen JH. Cirrhotic cardiomyopathy. J Hepatol 2010;53:179–90.
24. Umeda N, Kamath PS. Hepatopulmonary syndrome and portopulmonary hypertension. Hepatol Res 2009;39:1020–2.
25. Fix OK, Bass NM, De Marco T, Merriman RB. Long-term follow-up of portopulmonary hypertension: effect of treatment with epoprostenol. Liver Transpl 2007;13:875–85.
26. Francoz C, Glotz D, Moreau R, Durand F. The evaluation of renal function and disease in patients with cirrhosis. J Hepatol 2010;52:605–13.
27. Eason JD, Gonwa TA, Davis CL, Sung RS, Gerber D, Bloom RD. Proceedings of Consensus Conference on Simultaneous Liver Kidney Transplantation (SLK). Am J Transplant 2008;8:2243–51.
28. Ponziani FR, Zocco MA, Campanale C, et al. Portal vein thrombosis: insight into physiopathology, diagnosis, and treatment. World J Gastroenterol 2010;16:143–55.
29. Gustot T, Durand F, Lebrec D, Vincent JL, Moreau R. Severe sepsis in cirrhosis. Hepatology 2009;50:2022–33.
30. Samuel D, Weber R, Stock P, Duclos-Vallee JC, Terrault N. Are HIV-infected patients candidates for liver transplantation? J Hepatol 2008;48:697–707.
31. Lucey MR, Weinrieb RM. Alcohol and substance abuse. Semin Liver Dis 2009;29:66–73.
32. Pfitzmann R, Benscheidt B, Langrehr JM, Schumacher G, Neuhaus R, Neuhaus P. Trends and experiences in liver retransplantation over 15 years. Liver Transpl 2007;13:248–57.
33. Lock JF, Schwabauer E, Martus P, et al. Early diagnosis of primary nonfunction and indication for reoperation after liver transplantation. Liver Transpl 2010;16:172–80.
34. Gunsar F, Rolando N, Pastacaldi S, et al. Late hepatic artery thrombosis after orthotopic liver transplantation. Liver Transpl 2003;9:605–11.
35. Bekker J, Ploem S, de Jong KP. Early hepatic artery thrombosis after liver transplantation: a systematic review of the incidence, outcome and risk factors. Am J Transplant 2009;9:746–57.
36. McCashland T, Watt K, Lyden E, et al. Retransplantation for hepatitis C: results of a U.S. multicenter retransplant study. Liver Transpl 2007;13:1246–53.
37. Watt KD, Lyden ER, McCashland TM. Poor survival after liver retransplantation: is hepatitis C to blame? Liver Transpl 2003;9:1019–24.
38. Carrión JA, Navasa M, Forns X. Retransplantation in patients with hepatitis C recurrence after liver transplantation. J Hepatol. 2010;53:962–70.
39. Adam R, McMaster P, O'Grady JG, et al. Evolution of liver transplantation in Europe: report of the European Liver Transplant Registry. Liver Transpl 2003;9:1231–43.

2 Monitoring the patient awaiting liver transplantation

Andreas Geier and Beat Müllhaupt
Swiss HPB (Hepato-Pancreato-Biliary) and Transplantation Centers, University Hospital Zürich, Zürich, Switzerland

Key learning points

- The recognition and prevention of complications in patients on the waiting list is crucial for successful transplantation.
- Prophylactic interventions in cirrhotic patients are indicated to prevent: 1) first variceal hemorrhage, 2) recurrent variceal bleeding, 3) infections in patients with gastrointestinal bleeding, 4) first spontaneous bacterial peritonitis in selected patients, and 5) recurrent spontaneous bacterial peritonitis in all patients.
- Regular follow-up examinations in patients on the waiting list are indicated in patients with: 1) hepatocellular cancer, 2) varices, and 3) portopulmonary and hepatopulmonary syndrome (HPS).
- Cancer screening is important in patients on the waiting list.

Introduction

Most stable patients on the waiting list can be managed as outpatients, with regular clinic visits at the transplant center and in close collaboration with the referring physicians. The frequency of visits is determined by the clinical condition, the current treatment regimen (e.g. treatment for hepatitis C) and by the requirements of the national transplant and allocation organization (the reassessment schedule required in the USA is listed in Table 2.1).

The most common complications of advanced liver disease, encountered in patients on the waiting list include refractory ascites, spontaneous bacterial peritonitis, hepatorenal syndrome (HRS), fluid and electrolyte disturbances, portal hypertensive bleedings, hepatic encephalopathy, hepatocellular carcinoma, malnutrition and progression of other medical diseases. In this chapter the different aspects in the care of patients on the waiting list will be reviewed. In addition, disease-specific aspects such as control of viral hepatitis and prevention of alcohol relapse will be covered in different chapters.

Refractory ascites

The appearance of ascites is the most common complication in patients with end-stage liver disease. Approximately 50% of patients with compensated cirrhosis will develop ascites over a 10-year period.[1] Development of ascites is associated with 50% mortality after 2 years. At the onset, ascites can usually be easily controlled with diuretics and salt restriction (see Chapter 3), but with worsening portal hypertension, the risk of developing refractory or treatment-resistant ascites increases. In this situation aggressive diuretic therapy places the patient at risk of developing renal failure, electrolyte disturbances, volume depletion and hepatic encephalopathy. Renal function and electrolytes therefore have to be monitored carefully and any deterioration of renal function should be fully investigated. If ascites can no longer be controlled with diuretics or the use of diuretics is associated with renal insufficiency and electrolyte disturbances, patients can either be treated with large-volume paracentesis with the use of plasma expanders or transjugular intrahepatic portosystemic

Medical Care of the Liver Transplant Patient, Fourth Edition. Edited by Pierre-Alain Clavien, James F. Trotter.

Table 2.1 MELD reassessment schedule*

Meld score	Status recertification	Laboratory value requirement
≥25	Every 7 days	No older than 48 hours
19–24	Every 1 month	No older than 7 days
11–18	Every 3 months	No older than 14 days
6–10	Every 12 months	No older than 30 days

*See: http://optn.transplant.hrsa.gov/PoliciesandBylaws2/policies/pdfs/policy_8.pdf

shunts (TIPS) (for details see Chapter 3). In patients undergoing therapeutic paracentesis the infusion of albumin (8 g/L of ascites drained) is crucial, to prevent the risk of developing circulatory dysfunction, which is associated with a shorter time until readmission and reduced survival.[2] After paracentesis patients should be treated with diuretics to prevent rapid fluid reaccumulation. TIPS placement was historically associated with a high rate of shunt stenosis and occlusion. The recent introduction of covered stents has significantly reduced this complication. It is generally recommended to regularly evaluate TIPS patency by duplex ultrasonography every 3 months in the first year and semi-annually thereafter.[3]

Spontaneous bacterial peritonitis

Spontaneous bacterial peritonitis (SBP) is characterized by the spontaneous infection of the ascitic fluid in the absence of any intra-abdominal source of infection. The diagnosis is established when there is a positive ascites culture and/or a polymorphonuclear cell (PMC) count ≥250 cells/mm^3. The SBP prevalence ranges between 10–30% in patients with ascites and is sufficiently common to justify a diagnostic paracentesis in every cirrhotic patient with ascites admitted to the hospital.[4] In addition, a paracentesis should be performed whenever there is clinical evidence for peritonitis (abdominal pain, rebound tenderness), clinical signs of infections (fever, leucocytosis, elevated CRP) and development of renal insufficiency, unclear clinical deterioration, and hepatic encephalopathy. This is especially true for patients on the liver transplant waiting list. Recent data even justify primary prophylaxis in the following clinical situations: 1) patients with an acute gastrointestinal hemorrhage, and 2) patients with advanced liver disease, each of which will be discussed in turn.

Patients with acute gastrointestinal hemorrhage

Patients with upper gastrointestinal bleeding in the presence or absence of ascites are at high risk for severe bacterial infections including SBP. A meta-analysis showed that antibiotic prophylaxis significantly improved survival in patients with gastrointestinal hemorrhage and led to a significant reduction in SBP incidence.[5] Therefore, antibiotic prophylaxis is recommended in all cirrhotic patients with upper gastrointestinal bleeding irrespective of the presence or absence of ascites. Although several antibiotic regimens are effective, the oral administration of norfloxacin (2 × 400 mg for 7 d) or ciprofloxacin (2 × 500 mg for 7 d) appear to be the first choice.[5] A recent study in patients with advanced cirrhosis (defined by at least two of the following: ascites, severe malnutrition, encephalopathy, or bilirubin level >3 mg/dl) showed that ceftriaxone IV is superior compared to norfloxacin orally[6] (Table 2.2).

Patients with advanced liver disease

In a recent double-blind, placebo-controlled trial, patients with low ascites protein levels (<15 g/L) and advanced liver failure (defined as Child–Pugh score ≥9 points with serum bilirubin level ≥3 mg/dl or impaired renal function (serum creatinine level ≥1.2 mg/dl, blood urea nitrogen level ≥25 mg/dl, or serum sodium level ≤130 mEq/L)) were randomized to receive either norfloxacin (400 mg/d) or placebo for 12 months.[7] Norfloxacin significantly improved the 3-month probability of survival as well as the 1-year probability of developing SBP and HRS. At 1 year the difference in survival was no longer significant. For patients with less advanced liver disease, primary prophylaxis cannot yet be recommended. Since most patients on the waiting list have or will develop advanced liver disease while waiting for a graft, this issue is of great importance and should be implemented as the above mentioned criteria are fulfilled (see Table 2.2).

Table 2.2 Prevention of complications in patients on the waiting list

Aim	First Choice Intervention	Alternative
1. Prevention of infections		
1.1. Acute variceal bleeding		
Compensated cirrhosis	Oral norfloxacin 2 × 400 mg for 7 days	Oral ciprofloxacin 2 × 500 mg for 7 days
Advanced cirrhosis*	Ceftriaxone 1 g for 7 days	
1.2. Primary prevention of SBP		
Compensated cirrhosis	Prophylaxis unnecessary	
Ascites protein <15 g/l + Advanced liver disease†	Oral norfloxacin 400 mg daily	
1.3. Secondary prevention of SBP	Norfloxacin 400 mg daily	Trimethoprim-sulfamethoxazole daily
2. Prevention of HRS in patients with SBP	Intravenous albumin (1.5 g/kg day 0 and 1 g/kg after 2 days)	
3. Prevention of variceal bleeding		
A. Primary prophylaxis		
3.1. Small varices and low risk for bleeding†	Propranolol or nadolol‡ optional	
3.2. Small varices and high risk for bleeding	Propranolol or nadolol‡ recommended	
3.3. At least medium sized varices	Propranolol or nadolol‡ recommended	
3.4. At least medium sized varices No red wale markings	Band ligation in patients intolerant or contraindications to beta-blockers	
B. Secondary prophylaxis		
High risk for treatment failure§	Consider early TIPS (<72 h)	
Other patients	Band ligation in combination with propranolol or nadolol	
Failure of secondary prophylaxis	Rescue TIPS	

*Defined by at least two of the following: ascites, severe malnutrition, encephalopathy, or bilirubin >3 mg/dl.
†defined as: Child–Pugh score ≥9 points with serum bilirubin level ≥3 mg/dl or impaired renal function (serum creatinine level ≥1.2 mg/dl, blood urea nitrogen level ≥25 mg/dl), or serum sodium level ≤130 mEq/L.
‡Stepwise increase in dose until 25% reduction in heart rate.
§Child–Pugh C patients or Child–Pugh B patients with active bleeding at the time of the diagnostic endoscopy

Secondary prophylaxis

In patients with a previous episode of SBP, the 1-year probability for a recurrent SBP ranges between 40–70%. In patients with a previous history of SBP, the continuous administration of norfloxacin (400 mg/d) significantly reduced the 1-year probability of SBP from 68% in the placebo group to 20% in norfloxacin group.[8] Secondary long-term prophylaxis is therefore recommended for all patients with a history of a previous SBP (Table 2.2).

Treatment of SBP

Empiric antibiotic treatment has to be started when the PMC count is >250/mm^3 and SBP is suspected. Currently intravenous treatment with a third-generation cephalosporin (e.g. cefotaxime 2 g every 8–12 h, ceftriaxone 1 g/24 h for 5–7 d) is recommended.[9] Therapy needs to be modified according to the culture results. SBP resolves in approximately 90% of patients. The most important predictor of survival is the development of renal insufficiency. The administration of albumin (1.5 g/kg at diagnosis and 1 g/kg at day 3) is able to prevent the development of renal insufficiency and reduces the mortality rate from 30% to 10% (Table 2.2).[9]

Renal failure, fluid, and electrolyte disturbances

The management of renal failure in patients with liver cirrhosis will be extensively discussed in Chapter 4.

Patients with end-stage liver disease are at an increased risk to develop renal failure, either spontaneously (HRS) or due to iatrogenic interventions (diuretics, nephrotoxic drugs). Patients with advanced cirrhosis and ascites are at the highest risk. Renal vasoconstriction associated with advanced liver disease leads to severe renal vasoconstriction and functional renal insufficiency. This occurs in up to 10% of patients with advanced liver disease and even more frequently in patients on the waiting list. HRS can only be diagnosed after other nonfunctional causes of renal failure have been excluded, including obstruction, volume depletion, glomerulonephritis, acute tubular necrosis and drug-induced nephrotoxicity. There should be no improvement in kidney function despite stopping all diuretics for at least 2 days and expanding the volume with albumin 1 g/kg/d up to a maximum of 100 g/d.[10]

The prognosis of patients with HRS is poor, with a median survival of only 15 d in patients with Type I and 150 d in patients with Type II. Until recently there was no effective therapy apart from liver transplantation, but fortunately this has changed in recent years (see Chapter 4). The use of a vasoconstrictor drug, mostly terlipressin, often in combination with volume expansion with albumin, is effective in about 40–50% of patients.[11] The response to treatment increases the probability that the patients with HRS survive long enough to undergo transplantation, and there is some evidence that the improvement of renal function reduces post-transplantation morbidity and mortality.[12]

Hemodialysis or venovenous hemofiltration has been used as a bridge to transplantation and it might be useful in patients who fail to respond to medical treatment.

Patients with advanced liver disease and portal hypertension have a decreased effective arterial blood volume with activation of the renin–angiotensin–aldosterone system, the sympathetic nervous system, and an increased secretion of antidiuretic hormones. The activation of these counteracting regulatory mechanisms leads to renal vasoconstriction. In this situation the renal perfusion is dependent upon prostaglandin-mediated vasodilatation. Nonsteroidal anti-inflammatory drugs (NSAIDs), which inhibit prostaglandin synthesis, may lead to a further decrease in renal blood flow and may precipitate acute renal failure, therefore they should be avoided in patients with end-stage liver disease. In addition, all potentially nephrotoxic drugs should be used with caution and overtreatment with diuretics should be avoided. It is generally recommended that diuretics be stopped if the serum creatinine level is >150 μmol/L and serum urea is >8 μmol/L. Several studies have clearly shown that pre-transplant renal function significantly impacts on post-transplant survival.

The most common electrolyte abnormality in patients with advanced liver cirrhosis is hyponatremia defined as a serum sodium level <130 mmol/L. This occurs as a consequence of impaired free water clearance by the kidney due to a non-osmotic hypersecretion of antidiuretic hormone (ADH) or due to hypovolemia, mostly related to diuretic therapy.[9] Whereas in the former ascites is common, this is usually lacking in the latter. Impaired free water clearance occurs several months after the onset of sodium retention and ascites formation, and therefore represents a late event in the course of decompensated liver disease. Hyponatremia indicates a poor prognosis and for some authors is an important predictor of survival. It has been proposed to incorporate sodium in the MELD score, however this remains controversial. As long as the serum sodium level remains >125 mmol/L, no specific prophylactic measures are required. If the serum sodium concentration falls to <125 mmol/L, diuretics should be withheld and free water restriction instituted, although there is no data-supported specific threshold for initiating fluid restriction (1000 ml/24 h).[13] Fluid restriction will lead in only a minority of patients to an increase in serum sodium, but may be effective in preventing further decrease.[9] There is some evidence that albumin might lead to an increase in serum sodium.[9] It is important to remember that attempts to rapidly correct hyponatremia with hypertonic saline can lead to more complications than the hyponatremia itself.[13] In some countries

Table 2.3 Recommended follow-up examinations for patients on the waiting list

Complication	Examination	Time interval
Esophageal varices	Esophagogastroduodenoscopy (EGD)	Screening EGD, when cirrhosis is diagnosed No varices at screening EGD, repeat EGD every 2–3 years Small varices at screening, repeat EGD every 1–2 years Decompensated cirrhosis, repeat EGD every year
PPHTN	Echocardiography	12 months, if baseline examination normal 6 months, if RV pressure at baseline 35–50 mmHg
HPS	Pulse oxymetry in sitting position	6–12 months: arterial blood gas analysis, if $SpO_2 < 97\%$. If $PaO_2 < 70$ mmHg, then perform echocardiography
	Alternative: Arterial blood gas analysis in sitting position	6–12 months: If $PaO_2 < 70$ mmHg, then perform echocardiography
Known HCC	Abdominal CT or MRI	Every 3 months
Cancer screening		
HCC	Abdominal ultrasound	Every 3 months
	Alternative: Abdominal CT or MRI	Every 6 months
CCA	CA 19-9 and MR or CT	Every 12 months
Colon cancer in PSC patients	colonoscopy	Every 12 months

CCA: cholangiocarcinoma, CT: computed tomography, EGD: Esophagogastroduodenoscopy, HCC: hepatocellular carcinoma, HPS: hepatopulmonary syndrome, MRI: magnetic resonance imaging, PPHTN: portopulmonary hypertension

vaptans (tolvaptan, conivaptan) are already licensed for the treatment of severe hyponatremia (<125 mmol/L).[9]

Finally it is important to remember that hyponatremia has been associated with an increased morbidity after liver transplantation, especially neurologic complications, and in some studies also with reduced survival.[9]

Portal hypertensive bleeding

The management of portal hypertensive bleeding is extensively covered in Chapter 3. In this section only the prophylactic measures relevant for patient management on the waiting list will be reviewed.

Several studies have been published regarding the result of upper gastrointestinal endoscopy in patients being evaluated for liver transplantation. Overall 66–85% of these patients had varices and 16–46% presented with large (Grade III–IV) varices. It is therefore generally accepted that at the time of listing all patients should undergo an esophagogastroduodenoscopy (EGD). In the rare patients where no varices are found, EGD should be repeated in 2–3 years and in patients with small varices who do not undergo some kind of primary prophylaxis, EGD should be repeated every 1–2 years. In patients with decompensated cirrhosis, EGD should be repeated at yearly intervals[14] (Table 2.3).

Prevention of first variceal bleed (primary prophylaxis)

The high mortality rate of a first variceal bleeding episode justifies the development of prophylactic regimens to prevent the development of and bleeding from varices.

Noncardioselective beta-blockers such as propranolol and nadolol have been the mainstay of primary prevention. In cirrhotic patients with esophageal varices, both propranolol and nadolol have been shown to reduce the risk of an initial bleeding episode by 40–50%, while there was a trend of reducing mortality.[15] It is customary to adjust the dose of beta-blockers until a 25% fall of the heart rate is achieved. About 30% of patients will not respond to beta-blockers with a reduction in HVPG, despite adequate dosing. Moreover, beta-blockers may cause side effects such as fatigue and impotence, which may impair compliance, especially in younger males, or may be contraindicated.

In patients with medium to large varices, the equal effectiveness of band ligation compared to beta-blockers in the prevention of a first bleeding is well documented, whereas no differences in survival were observed.[16] In patients with low risk (no red wale markings) small varices and well-preserved liver function, the use of nonselective beta-blockers is optional,[17] however, in patients with small varices and high-risk signs for bleeding, the use of beta-blockers for the primary prevention of variceal bleeding is clearly recommended.[18]

Whether carvedilol (6.25–12.5 mg), which proved to be superior compared to band ligation in a recent randomized, controlled trial,[19] will replace the nonselective beta-blockers, remains to be seen.

Currently, the following scheme can be recommended for primary prophylaxis of variceal hemorrhage:[18]

1. Patients at low risk for bleeding and small varices: nonselective beta-blockers are optional

2. Patients at high risk for bleeding and small varices: nonselective beta-blockers are recommended.

3. In patients with at least medium-sized esophageal varices and/or red color signs, nonselective beta-blockers (propranolol or nadolol) should be given. Start at a low dose, if necessary, and increase the dose step by step until a reduction of resting heart rate by 25% is reached, but not lower than 50–55 bpm. Band ligation can be considered equally effective.

4. In patients with esophageal varices who do not tolerate or have contraindications to beta-blockers, endoscopic band ligation is indicated (Table 2.2).

Secondary prevention of variceal bleeding

About 60% of patients surviving an acute variceal hemorrhage will develop a recurrent bleeding within the first year.[20] Clinical predictors of early recurrence include severity of the initial hemorrhage and the underlying liver disease, impaired renal function, and encephalopathy. Endoscopic features include active bleeding at the time of endoscopy, large varices, and stigmata of a recent hemorrhage. There is a strong correlation between the severity of portal hypertension and the survival rate as well as the rebleeding risk. This high rebleeding rate with its associated morbidity and mortality justifies the implementation of a secondary prevention program.

Current guidelines recommend the use of nonselective beta-blockers and band ligation in combination, since a recent meta-analysis revealed that the combination is superior compared to either intervention alone regarding the rebleeding rate, whereas no difference in survival was observed[21] (Table 2.2).

In cases with rebleeding despite secondary prophylaxis with beta-blockers and band ligation, TIPS is currently considered by most clinicians to be an effective bridge to transplantation. Meta-analysis of 11 trials comparing TIPS with endoscopic treatment found a lower rebleeding rate in patients with TIPS placement,[22] however TIPS was associated with a higher incidence of encephalopathy, and no difference was found regarding overall survival. Additionally, the long-term use of TIPS is limited by the frequent shunt occlusion. During the first year, 50–70% of TIPS occlude and as a consequence 20% of these patients develop rebleeding.[23] The recent introduction of covered TIPS significantly reduced the shunt occlusion rate as well as the rebleeding rate.

In patients at high risk for treatment failure (Child–Pugh C patients or Child–Pugh B patients with active bleeding at the time of the diagnostic endoscopy), the current recommendations for the prevention of rebleeding might be challenged by a recent study, which suggests that in this patient population early (within 72 h) TIPS placement is associated with a significant reduction of treatment failure and improved survival.[24] The following recommendations can therefore be made:

1. Consider early TIPS in patients at high risk for treatment failure

2. Use secondary prophylaxis with nonselective beta-blocker and band ligation for all other patients

3. Use rescue TIPS for patients failing secondary prophylaxis with beta-blocker and band ligation.

Hepatic encephalopathy

Some degree of clinically obvious hepatic encephalopathy (HE) is found in one-third of patients with end-stage liver disease.[25] It is important to remember that the diagnosis of hepatic encephalopathy is a diagnosis of exclusion. Other etiologies such as intracranial space-occupying lesions, vascular events and other metabolic disorders should be excluded. Ammonia levels are widely scattered in patients with liver cirrhosis and individual values are a poor predictor of the degree of encephalopathy. In spite of the limitations, ammonia levels are sometimes useful, when there is uncertainty if a liver disease is the cause of an encephalopatic episode. The changes of ammonia levels should, however, not be considered as an indicator of therapeutic benefit. Improvement of the mental status is the sole therapeutic endpoint. It is also important to remember that blood samples should be processed promptly (on ice) and arterial measurement is preferable, as arteriovenous differences can be observed.

The severity of HE is most commonly graded according to the West Haven criteria (Box 2.1). Mostly, changes in the mental status are caused by a precipitating event. Therefore as soon as deterioration in the mental status is recognized, a search for a precipitating event should be immediately started. Among the factors are:

Box 2.1 West Haven criteria for semiquantitative grading of mental state

Grade 1:	Lack of awareness Euphoria or anxiety Shortened attention span
Grade 2:	Lethargy or apathy Minimal disorientation for time or place Subtle personality change Inappropriate behaviors Impaired performance of subtraction
Grade 3:	Somnolence to semi-stupor, but responsive to verbal stimuli Confusion Gross disorientation
Grade 4:	Coma (unresponsive to verbal or noxious stimuli)

- **Renal and electrolyte abnormalities:** including uremia, hypokalemia (favors the entry of ammonia into the brain) and dehydration
- **Gastrointestinal bleeding:** increases the nitrogen load in the gut
- **Infection:** cultures, especially from ascites to exclude spontaneous bacterial peritonitis, are important
- **Use of benzodiazepines or other sedatives:** sometimes even urinary screening is necessary to exclude their presence
- **Excessive dietary proteins or constipation:** increase the nitrogen load in the gut
- **Worsening liver function:** for example in portal vein thrombosis
- **Noncompliance with medications**.

Development of acute HE is associated with a poor prognosis. In a recent study the 1- and 3-year survival rates were only 42% and 23%, respectively.[26]

The mainstay of therapy centers on correcting the precipitating event. Depending on the level of consciousness, intubation has to be considered to prevent aspiration. In these patients a nasogastric tube should be placed and treatment with non-absorbable disaccharides, such as lactulose or lactilol, should be started.[27] In cooperative patients this can be given by mouth; the usual starting dose is 20 ml 3–4 times daily with the aim of achieving 2–4 soft bowel movements per day.

Recently the use of rifaximin, a non-absorbable antibiotic, in a dose of 1200 mg/d, is becoming increasingly popular, because it is well tolerated and seems to be more efficacious than lactulose.[28] In addition, in a large well-designed study, it was shown that rifaximin is clearly superior in preventing a HE recurrence and reduced the hospitalization rate due to HE recurrence.[29] Other therapeutic interventions such as L-ornithine-L-aspartate, sodium benzoate, and branched chain amino acids are less well established.[30]

For years, protein restriction used to be an integral part of the treatment algorithms for patients with HE. It is important to avoid long-term protein restriction to prevent worsening of the nutritional status and in a recent study it could be clearly shown that protein restriction had no beneficial effect in cirrhotic patients with hepatic encephalopathy.[31] It is important to remember that sedatives should be avoided in patients with a history of HE.

PPHTN and HPS

Portopulmonary hypertension (PPHTN) and HPS will be extensively discussed in Chapter 5.

The detection of PPHTN before liver transplantation is crucial, because the presence of PPHTN of any severity increases the perioperative and long-term risk of liver transplantation.[32] If moderate to severe PPHTN is confirmed, treatment with specific pulmonary vasodilators should be instituted (see Chapter 5). Although rare, PPHTN can develop after the initial evaluation for liver transplantation.[33] In another study, PPHTN was diagnosed in 65% of patients only in the operating room prior to transplantation.[32] These data clearly suggest that regular echocardiographic examinations of liver transplant candidates on the waiting list are mandatory, although the optimal screening frequency remains to be determined. The echocardiography should be repeated annually in patients with normal echocardiographic findings at initial evaluation and in patients with an RV systolic pressure between 35–50 mmHg it should be repeated every 6 months (Table 2.3).[33]

HPS

HPS is a serious complication that should be diagnosed before liver transplantation. Medical management has so far been disappointing and therefore liver transplantation has been increasingly advocated as the treatment of choice for patients with HPS.[34] It is currently recommended that all patients, undergoing a work-up for liver transplantation, should be screened for HPS (Table 2.3). Hypoxemia is the prerequisite for the diagnosis of HPS, therefore every diagnostic approach should begin with the documentation of hypoxemia in the sitting position and at rest. The routine measurement of arterial blood gases has been advocated in all liver transplant candidates. Considering the prevalence of HPS this would lead to a large number of unnecessary arterial blood gas analyses. For this reason, a recent study evaluated the usefulness of pulse oxymetry for the detection of arterial hypoxemia in liver transplant candidates.[35] In this study all patients with a $SpO_2 \geq 97\%$ had a $PaO_2 \geq 65$ mmHg, therefore no patient with severe or very severe HPS was missed (see later). On the other hand, by restricting the arterial blood gas analysis to patients with an O_2 saturation of <97%, only 32% needed arterial blood gas analysis, and a high sensitivity of 96% and an acceptable specificity to identify hypoxemic patients (75%) were maintained. If hypoxemia is established the diagnosis of HPS should be confirmed by echocardiography or lung perfusion scanning. Only patients with severe (PaO_2 50–59 mmHg) or very severe HPS ($PaO_2 < 50$ mmHg) should be considered for liver transplantation.[36] Because the mortality rate for patients with HPS and $PaO_2 < 50$ mmHg is very high,[37] it has been recommended that these patients be evaluated on a case-by-case basis.[38] The allocation of MELD exception points is guided by the severity of hypoxemia. It is important that all these patients have an arterial blood gas analysis carried out while in the sitting position on a 3-monthly basis for further documentation of disease progression.

In patients with no evidence of HPS at the time of listing, a SpO_2 in the sitting position should be obtained every 3 months.[38]

Cancer development

Hepatocellular carcinoma

Hepatocellular carcinoma (HCC) may be the indication for liver transplantation or may develop de novo while patients are on the waiting list.

Follow up of patients with known HCC

In patients listed for liver transplantation with an HCC fulfilling the Milan criteria, an abdominal CT or MRI should be carried out every 3 months to assess local tumor progression (Table 2.3). The criteria used for delisting patients vary from country to country. The contraindications to transplantation that are accepted by most centers include: 1) tumor spread outside of the liver, and 2) invasion of the portal vein, hepatic vein, or hepatic artery.

No strong recommendation can be given with regard to size and number of nodules. Some consider a solitary tumor >5 cm, more than three lesions or three lesions with one of three exceeding 3 cm in maximum diameter as an indication for delisting,[39] whereas others are less strict.[40] Furthermore, there is no consensus about how to handle the suggestive, but inconclusive findings of new tumors of radiologic reports and what confirmatory criteria should be used to accept uncontrolled progression.

Most centers are reluctant to observe patients with HCC on the waiting list without using any kind of neoadjuvant therapy to prevent tumor progression, although evidence from randomized controlled trials is still lacking. The options include chemoembolization, percutaneous ablative therapies such as ethanol injection and radiofrequency ablation, as well as surgical resection.

Transarterial chemoembolization is the most widely used option. It is known that hepatic arterial obstruction preceded by the selective injection of chemotherapy suspended in lipiodol induces extensive tumor necrosis in the majority of patients and that this translates into a delayed occurrence of vascular invasion and improved survival.[41] In a recent study the drop-out rate from the waiting list of patients with HCC treated with chemoembolization was 15%,[39] which is lower than the 25% drop-out rate reported by Llovet et al. in his study, where no chemoembolization was employed.[42] This might be explained by differences in staging and listing or by the use of chemoembolization prior to liver transplantation.

Percutaneous ablation has been used more frequently in recent years to bridge patients with HCC to transplantation. Surgical resection can also be used as a bridge to liver transplantation in cirrhotic patients with mild portal hypertension and preserved liver function. Their risk of postoperative liver failure has to be balanced against the risk of delisting them while waiting and a clear benefit will be reached only when the waiting time is long enough. A recent Markov analysis of liver resection or percutaneous ablation as adjuvant therapies while waiting for liver transplantation concluded that surgical resection provides a moderate gain in life expectancy and is cost effective if waiting time exceeds 1 year, but for shorter waiting times, only percutaneous treatment provides a relative survival advantage.[43]

Screening of patients without HCC at time of listing
The main risk factors for the development of HCC are the presence of cirrhosis, male sex, and chronic viral infection, therefore patients on the waiting list are a high-risk population for the development of HCC. Despite this fact, little is known about the de novo HCC development in liver transplant candidates listed for transplantation. A recent study investigated de novo development of HCC and analyzed the different screening methods in 100 patients transplanted for end-stage liver disease with no HCC at the time of listing.[44] These patients were followed with 3-monthly ultrasound (US) and alphafetoprotein (AFP) measurements as well as 6-monthly triphasic computed tomography (CT). HCC was detected in the explanted livers from 20 patients: six were incidental findings, whereas 14 were detected during follow up. None of the HCC cases was detected because of AFP elevations; 12 were detected by US and 14 by CT. Only one tumor was found to measure >5 cm at the time of transplantation; this tumor was understaged by the imaging method and was also found in the only patient who developed a recurrence in the post-transplant follow up. All tumors developed after a waiting time of 1–757 d, therefore not all tumors were truly de novo HCC – some must have been already present at the time of listing but were not detected. Nevertheless a screening US every 3 months and a CT every 6 months seems reasonable, considering the high rate of HCC development in this patient group (Table 2.3). The role of the AFP for the detection of HCC is less clear.

Cholangiocarcinoma

Primary sclerosing cholangitis (PSC) is a chronic liver disease characterized by inflammation, destruction and fibrosis of intra- as well as extrahepatic bile ducts, which eventually results in biliary cirrhosis. Cholangiocarcinoma (CCA) is a well-recognized complication of PSC. The reported frequency in studies describing the natural history ranged from 6–11%, whereas it was as high as 7–36% in patients undergoing liver transplantation.

The occurrence of CCA is unpredictable and is often difficult to diagnose. In a substantial number of patients CCA is either the initial symptom or develops within the first 2 years after the diagnosis of PSC. Liver transplantation is only a viable option for a highly selected group of patients with early-stage CCA. The outcome is improved by using preoperative radiation and chemotherapy, and ensuring the absence of metastases.[45] The issue of how patients with PSC should be screened while on the waiting list is still unresolved, however screening would be important, because if the tumor is detected in its early stages, when it is still confined to the biliary tree, transplantation still offers the best chance for a cure.

Although firm data regarding screening are lacking, the American and European guideline on PSC recommends yearly determination of CA 19–9 (cut-off 20 U/ml) and a cross-sectional imaging study on a yearly basis.[46,47] In addition, in the case of any rapid and progressive stricture formation with dilatation of the proximal bile duct, a superimposed CCA should be suspected. Repeated endoscopic retrograde cholangio-pancreatography (ERCP) with brush cytology is indicated in this situation and the use of fluorescent in situ hybridization (FISH) showing polysomy might increase the diagnostic yield.[48]

Other cancers

The most common extrahepatic cancer in PSC patients with ulcerative colitis is colon cancer. These patients should undergo yearly colonoscopy while awaiting liver transplantation[47] (Table 2.3).

Progression of other medical diseases

Diabetes mellitus

Patients with established diabetes mellitus will need careful monitoring to ensure that the blood glucose level is within acceptable limits. If necessary, insulin treatment should be initiated.

Hypertension

Patients with arterial hypertension will need to be monitored to ensure that blood pressure is optimally controlled. If there are any cardiac abnormalities at screening, ECG and echocardiography should be repeated at 6-monthly intervals.

Preventing further liver damage

Patients with end-stage liver disease have an increased risk of developing fatal hepatic failure, when they develop superimposed hepatitis A.[49] The vaccine is clearly more effective in patients with compensated liver cirrhosis (seroconversion rate 98%) compared with patients with decompensated disease (66%).[50] Therefore all patients with chronic liver disease should be vaccinated against hepatitis A as early as possible in the course of their disease. According to few data available, hepatitis B superinfection in patients with chronic liver disease may also take a more severe course. In addition, in patients without immunity against hepatitis B, the risk of developing de novo hepatitis B infection after liver transplantation ranges between 1–3.5%.[51] It is, however, clear that the antibody response after active immunization in these patients is significantly lower (20–40%).[51] A recent study using an accelerated schedule with a higher HBs-Ag dose (40 µg) showed promising results, achieving an overall response in 62% of patients studied.[52] Therefore, all patients on the liver transplant waiting list without pre-existing chronic hepatitis B or pre-existing immunity should be vaccinated, although the best immunization strategy is not yet defined.

All potentially hepatotoxic drugs should be avoided, and medications that increase the risk of gastrointestinal bleeding or renal insufficiency (aminosalicylic acid, NSAIDs, antiplatelet drugs) should be completely omitted.

Malnutrition

Malnutrition is common in patients with chronic liver disease awaiting transplantation and is a potentially reversible risk factor for mortality subsequent to liver transplantation.[53] A prospective randomized, controlled trial examined the effect of pretransplant nutritional supplementation on the outcome of patients undergoing liver transplantation. Supplementation did not affect outcome, even though the number of patients who died was higher in the control group (seven deaths before and two deaths after transplant) compared to the supplemented group (two deaths before and three deaths after transplant). There was no overall difference in survival.[54] The study, however, was not adequately powered to detect a 10% difference in survival. Although an improvement of perioperative mortality or complication rate by preoperative tube feeding or oral nutritional supplements has not yet been unequivocally proven, it is in general recommended that 35–40 kcal/kg/d and 1.2–1.5 g of protein/kg of dry body weight should be provided.[55] Patients with end-stage liver disease waiting for a liver transplant should take daily multivitamin and other supplements as needed. Fat-soluble vitamins should be given if a specific deficit is present.

Temporary suspension from waiting list

Patients may temporarily be inactivated on the waiting list for several reasons and reactivated as soon as the temporary problem is resolved. The most common reasons for temporary suspension are intercurrent infections and variceal bleeding.

Disease-specific aspects of the pretransplantation management of patients with viral hepatitis (Chapter 8), hepatocellular carcinoma (Chapter 11), alcoholic liver disease (Chapter 6), autoimmune diseases (Chapter 10), metabolic diseases (Chapter 9), and fulminant hepatic failure (Chapter 16) are extensively covered elsewhere.

Abbreviations

CCA: cholangiocarcinoma, HCC: hepatocellular carcinoma, HE: hepatic encephalopathy, HPS: hepatopulmonary syndrome, HRS: hepatorenal syndrome, PPHTN: portopulmonary hypertension, PSC: primary sclerosing cholangitis, SBP: spontaneous bacterial peritonitis.

References

1. Fernandez-Esparrach G, Sanchez-Fueyo A, Gines P, et al. A prognostic model for predicting survival in cirrhosis with ascites. J Hepatol 2001;34:46–52.
2. Gines A, Fernandez-Esparrach G, Monescillo A, et al. Randomized trial comparing albumin, dextran 70, and polygeline in cirrhotic patients with ascites treated by paracentesis. Gastroenterology 1996;111: 1002–10.
3. Rössle M, Siegerstetter V, Euringer W, et al. The use of a polytetrafluoroethylene-covered stent graft for transjugular intrahepatic portosystemic shunt (TIPS): Long-term follow-up of 100 patients. Acta Radiologica 2006;47:660–6.
4. Rimola A, Garcia-Tsao G, Navasa M, et al. Diagnosis, treatment and prophylaxis of spontaneous bacterial peritonitis: a consensus document. International Ascites Club. J Hepatol 2000;32:142–53.
5. Bernard B, Grange JD, Khac EN, Amiot X, Opolon P, Poynard T. Antibiotic prophylaxis for the prevention of bacterial infections in cirrhotic patients with gastrointestinal bleeding: a meta-analysis. Hepatology 1999;29:1655–61.
6. Fernández J, del Arbol LR, Gómez C, et al. Norfloxacin vs ceftriaxone in the prophylaxis of infections in patients with advanced cirrhosis and hemorrhage. Gastroenterology [doi: DOI: 10.1053/j.gastro.2006.07.010]. 2006;131:1049–56.
7. Fernández J, Navasa M, Planas R, et al. Primary prophylaxis of spontaneous bacterial peritonitis delays hepatorenal syndrome and improves survival in cirrhosis. Gastroenterology [doi: DOI: 10.1053/j.gastro.2007.06.065]. 2007;133:818–24.
8. Gines P, Rimola A, Planas R, et al. Norfloxacin prevents spontaneous bacterial peritonitis recurrence in cirrhosis: results of a double-blind, placebo-controlled trial. Hepatology 1990;12(4 Pt 1):716–24.
9. Ginès P, Angeli P, Lenz K, et al. EASL clinical practice guidelines on the management of ascites, spontaneous bacterial peritonitis, and hepatorenal syndrome in cirrhosis. J Hepatol [doi: DOI: 10.1016/j.jhep.2010.05.004]. 2010;53:397–417.
10. Salerno F, Gerbes A, Ginès P, Wong F, Arroyo V. Diagnosis, prevention and treatment of hepatorenal syndrome in cirrhosis. Gut 2007;56:1310–8.
11. Ginès P, Schrier RW. Renal failure in cirrhosis. N Engl J Med 2009;361:1279–90.
12. Restuccia T, Ortega R, Guevara M, et al. Effects of treatment of hepatorenal syndrome before transplantation on posttransplantation outcome. A case-control study. J Hepatol 2004;40:140–6.
13. Runyon BA. Management of adult patients with ascites due to cirrhosis: An update. Hepatology 2009;49: 2087–107.
14. Garcia-Tsao G, Sanyal AJ, Grace ND, Carey W. Prevention and management of gastroesophageal varices and variceal hemorrhage in cirrhosis. Hepatology 2007;46:922–38.
15. D'Amico G, Pagliaro L, Bosch J. Pharmacological treatment of portal hypertension: an evidence based approach. Semin Liver Dis 1999;19:475–505.
16. Gluud LL, Klingenberg S, Nikolova D, Gluud C. Banding ligation versus beta-blockers as primary prophylaxis in esophageal varices: Systematic Review of Randomized Trials. Am J Gastroenterol 2007;102: 2842–8.
17. Merkel C, Marin R, Angeli P, et al. A placebo-controlled clinical trial of nadolol in the prophylaxis of growth of small esophageal varices in cirrhosis. Gastroenterology [doi: DOI: 10.1053/j.gastro.2004.05.004]. 2004;127: 476–84.
18. Garcia-Tsao G, Bosch J. Management of varices and variceal hemorrhage in cirrhosis. N Engl J Med 2010;362:823–32.
19. Tripathi D, Ferguson JW, Kochar N, et al. Randomized controlled trial of carvedilol versus variceal band liga-

tion for the prevention of the first variceal bleed. Hepatology 2009;50:825–33.
20. Bosch J, Garcia-Pagan J. Prevention of variceal bleeding. Lancet 2003;361:952–4.
21. Gonzalez R, Zamora J, Gomez-Camarero J, Molinero L-M, Bañares R, Albillos A. Meta-analysis: combination endoscopic and drug therapy to prevent variceal rebleeding in cirrhosis. Ann Intern Med 2008;149: 109–22.
22. Papatheodoridis G, Goulis J, Leandro G, Patch D, Burroughs A. Transjugular intrahepatic portosystemic shunt compared with endoscopic treatment for prevention of variceal rebleeding. Hepatology 1999;30:612–22.
23. Casado M, Bosch J, Garcia-Pagan J, Bru C, Banares R, Bandi J. Clinical events after transjugular intrahepatic portosystemic shunt: corrolation with hemodynamic findings. Gastroenterology 1998;114:1296–303.
24. García-Pagán JC, Caca K, Bureau C, et al. Early use of TIPS in patients with cirrhosis and variceal bleeding. N Engl J Med 2010;362:2370–9.
25. Lizardi-Cervera J, Almeda P, Guevara L, Uribe M. Hepatic encephalopathy: a review. Ann Hepatol 2003;2:122–30.
26. Bustamante J, Rimola A, Ventura PJ, et al. Prognostic significance of hepatic encephalopathy in patients with cirrhosis. J Hepatol 1999;30:890–5.
27. Sharma BC, Sharma P, Agrawal A, Sarin SK. Secondary prophylaxis of hepatic encephalopathy: an open-label randomized controlled trial of lactulose versus placebo. Gastroenterology [doi: DOI: 10.1053/j.gastro.2009.05.056]. 2009;137:885–91.
28. Maclayton DO, Eaton-Maxwell A. Rifaximin for treatment of hepatic encephalopathy. Ann Pharmacother 2009;43:77–84.
29. Bass NM, Mullen KD, Sanyal A, et al. Rifaximin treatment in hepatic encephalopathy. N Engl J Med 2010;362:1071–81.
30. Bajaj JS. Review article: the modern management of hepatic encephalopathy. Alim Pharmacol Ther 2010;31:537–47.
31. Córdoba J, López-Hellín J, Planas M, et al. Normal protein diet for episodic hepatic encephalopathy: results of a randomized study. J Hepatol [doi: DOI: 10.1016/j.jhep.2004.03.023]. 2004;41:38–43.
32. Krowka MJ, Plevak DJ, Findlay JY, Rosen CB, Wiesner RH, Krom RA. Pulmonary hemodynamics and perioperative cardiopulmonary-related mortality in patients with portopulmonary hypertension undergoing liver transplantation. Liver Transpl 2000;6:443–50.
33. Minder S, Fischler M, Muellhaupt B, et al. Intravenous iloprost bridging to orthotopic liver transplantation in portopulmonary hypertension. Eur Respir J 2004;24:703–7.
34. Rodríguez-Roisin R, Krowka MJ. Hepatopulmonary syndrome – a liver-induced lung vascular disorder. N Engl J Med 2008;358:2378–87.
35. Abrams GA, Sanders MK, Fallon MB. Utility of pulse oximetry in the detection of arterial hypoxemia in liver transplant candidates. Liver Transpl 2002;8: 391–6.
36. Fallon MB, Mulligan DC, Gish RG, Krowka MJ.Model for end-stage liver disease (MELD) exception for hepatopulmonary syndrome. Liver Transplant 2006;12: S105–7.
37. Arguedas MR, Abrams GA, Krowka MJ, Fallon MB. Prospective evaluation of outcomes and predictors of mortality in patients with hepatopulmonary syndrome undergoing liver transplantation. Hepatology 2003;37:192–7.
38. Pastor CM, Schiffer E. Therapy insight: hepatopulmonary syndrome and orthotopic liver transplantation. Nat Clin Pract Gastroenterol Hepatol 2007;4:614–21.
39. Maddala YK, Stadheim L, Andrews JC, et al. Drop-out rates of patients with hepatocellular cancer listed for liver transplantation: Outcome with chemoembolization. Liver Transpl 2004;10:449–55.
40. Millonig G, Graziadei IW, Freund MC, et al. Response to preoperative chemoembolization correlates with outcome after liver transplantation in patients with hepatocellular carcinoma. Liver Transpl 2007;13: 272–9.
41. Llovet JM, Real MI, Montaña X, et al. Arterial embolisation or chemoembolisation versus symptomatic treatment in patients with unresectable hepatocellular carcinoma: a randomised controlled trial. Lancet [doi: DOI: 10.1016/S0140-6736(02)08649-X]. 2002;359: 1734–9.
42. Llovet JM, Fuster J, Bruix J. Intention-to-treat analysis of surgical treatment for early hepatocellular carcinoma: resection versus transplantation. Hepatology 1999;30:1434–40.
43. Llovet JM, Mas X, Aponte JJ, et al. Cost effectiveness of adjuvant therapy for hepatocellular carcinoma during the waiting list for liver transplantation. Gut 2002;50:123–8.
44. Van Thiel DH, Yong S, Li SD, Kennedy M, Brems J. The development of de novo hepatocellular carcinoma in patients on a liver transplant list: Frequency, size, and assessment of current screening methods. Liver Transpl 2004;10:631–7.
45. Rosen CB, Heimbach JK, Gores GJ. Surgery for cholangiocarcinoma: the role of liver transplantation. HPB (Oxford). 2008;10:186–9.
46. Chapman R, Fevery J, Kalloo A, et al. Diagnosis and management of primary sclerosing cholangitis. Hepatology 2010;51:660–78.

47. European Association for the Study of the L. EASL Clinical Practice Guidelines: Management of cholestatic liver diseases. J Hepatol [doi: DOI: 10.1016/j.jhep.2009.04.009]. 2009;51:237–67.
48. Barr Fritcher EG, Kipp BR, Halling KC, et al. A multivariable model using advanced cytologic methods for the evaluation of indeterminate pancreatobiliary strictures. Gastroenterology [doi: DOI: 10.1053/j.gastro.2009.02.040]. 2009;136:2180–6.
49. Keeffe EB. Acute hepatitis A and B in patients with chronic liver disease: prevention through vaccination. Am J Med [doi: DOI: 10.1016/j.amjmed.2005.07.013]. 2005;118(Suppl):21–7.
50. Arguedas MR, Johnson A, Eloubeidi MA, Fallon MB. Immunogenicity of hepatitis A vaccination in decompensated cirrhotic patients. Hepatology 2001;34: 28–31.
51. Castells L, Esteban R. Hepatitis B vaccination in liver transplant candidates. Eur J Gastroenterol Hepatol 2001;13:359–61.
52. Domínguez M, Bárcena R, García M, López-Sanroman A, Nuño J. Vaccination against hepatitis B virus in cirrhotic patients on liver transplant waiting list. Liver Transpl 2000;6:440–2.
53. Alberino F, Gatta A, Amodio P, et al. Nutrition and survival in patients with liver cirrhosis. Nutrition. [doi: DOI: 10.1016/S0899-9007(01)00521-4]. 2001;17: 445–50.
54. Le Cornu KA, McKiernan FJ, Kapadia SA, Neuberger JM. A prospective randomized study of preoperative nutritional supplementation in patients awaiting elective orthotopic liver transplantation. Transplantation 2000;69:1364–9.
55. Plauth M, Cabré E, Riggio O, et al. ESPEN Guidelines on Enteral Nutrition: Liver disease. Clinical Nutrition [doi: DOI: 10.1016/j.clnu.2006.01.018]. 2006;25:285–94.

3 Management of portal hypertension

Juan Carlos Garcia-Pagan, Juan G. Abraldes and Jaime Bosch
Hepatic Hemodynamic Laboratory, Liver Unit, Institut d'Investigacions Biomediques August Pi i Sunyer (IDIBAPS), University of Barcelona, Spain; and Centro de Investigación Biomédica en Red de Enfermedades Hepáticas y Digestivas (Ciberehd)

Key learning points

- Patients with moderate to large varices as well as patients with small varices with red signs or with advanced liver failure (Child–Pugh C) should be considered for preventive therapy with a nonselective beta-blocker.
- Patients with moderate to large varices with contraindications to or who cannot tolerate beta-blockers should be offered endoscopic band ligation. Band ligation might be used as first-choice treatment in patients with moderate to large varices depending on the patient's preferences and local resources.
- The best approach for acute variceal bleeding is the combined use of a vasoactive drug, started from admission (or even during transferral to hospital) and an endoscopic procedure. Transjugular intrahepatic portosystemic shunts (TIPS) should be used as a rescue procedure when medical and endoscopic therapies fail. Patients bleeding from gastric varices may require an earlier decision for TIPS.
- Patients with acute variceal bleeding and a high risk of treatment failure benefit from an early decision for TIPS.
- All patients surviving a bleeding episode should receive specific therapy to prevent rebleeding. Nonselective beta-blockers +/− 5-isosorbide mononitrate (IMN), endoscopic band ligation (EBL) or both should be used for prevention of recurrent bleeding. Combination of beta-blockers +/− IMN and EBL may be the best treatment.

Introduction

The relevance of portal hypertensive syndrome is due to the frequency and severity of its complications, which represent the first cause of hospital admission, death and liver transplantation in patients with cirrhosis. Portal hypertension is a frequent clinical syndrome, defined by a pathologic increase in the portal venous pressure. This increases the pressure gradient between the portal vein and the inferior vena cava (portal perfusion pressure of the liver or portal pressure gradient) above normal levels (1–5 mmHg.) When the portal pressure gradient rises above 10 mmHg, complications of portal hypertension may arise. This pressure threshold defines clinically significant portal hypertension (CSPH). Values of portal pressure gradient between 5–9 mmHg correspond to pre-clinical portal hypertension.[1] Portal hypertension can arise from any condition interfering with blood flow at any level within the portal system. According to the anatomic location of the obstacle to blood flow the causes of portal hypertension can be classified as pre-hepatic (involving the splenic, mesenteric or portal vein), intra-hepatic (liver diseases) and post-hepatic (diseases blocking the hepatic venous outflow). Cirrhosis of the liver is by far the most common cause of portal hypertension in the world, followed by hepatic schistosomiasis. All other causes account for <10% of the cases ("noncirrhotic portal hypertension").

Medical Care of the Liver Transplant Patient, Fourth Edition. Edited by Pierre-Alain Clavien, James F. Trotter.

In cirrhosis, an increase in vascular resistance to portal blood flow at the hepatic microcirculation is the initial factor leading to portal hypertension. Contrary to what was traditionally thought, this increased hepatic vascular resistance is not only a mechanical consequence of the hepatic architectural distortion caused by fibrosis, nodule formation, sinusoidal remodelling and vascular occlusion characteristic of cirrhosis, but there is also a dynamic component due to the active contraction of portal/septal myofibroblasts, activated hepatic stellate cells and vascular smooth muscle cells in portal venules, which is due to an imbalance between increased vasoconstrictor stimuli in the presence of impaired vasorelaxating mechanisms.[2] In the cirrhotic liver there is an increase in the activity of several endogenous vasoconstrictors such as endothelin, leukotrienes or thromboxane A_2 among others[2] and a reduced nitric oxide bioavailability due to both decreased release by endothelial nitric oxide synthase (eNOS) and increased scavenging by enhanced oxidative stress.[2]

Reducing intrahepatic resistance is a strategy to reduce portal pressure. This can be achieved by improving the architectural abnormalities, using drugs or cell therapy to prevent/reverse sinusoidal remodelling and fibrogenesis or by specific treatments for the underlying liver disease. In addition, the increased hepatic vascular tone of the cirrhotic liver can be reduced by improving intrahepatic nitric oxide (NO) availability, increasing its production by nitric oxide synthase (NOS) and by preventing its scavenging using anti-oxidant-based therapies. Other potential approaches are the inhibition of the vasoconstrictor system COX-1/TXA2 pathway or increasing hydrogen sulfide (H_2S). The increased resistance can also be reduced bypassing the liver using portal-systemic shunt surgery or TIPS.

A second factor contributing to portal hypertension is an increased blood flow through the portal venous system due to splanchnic arteriolar vasodilatation. Splanchnic vasodilation is likely to be multifactorial. The more important are local vasoactive factors produced by the vascular endothelium, such as NO, prostacyclin and carbon monoxide. Endocannabinoids and glucagon have also been shown to play a role. In addition, active angiogenesis driven by vascular endothelial growth factor (VEGF) and platelet-derived growth factor (PDGF) is involved in the development and maintenance of the hyperdynamic splanchnic circulation of portal hypertension. Splanchnic hyperemia contributes to aggravate the increase in portal pressure and explains why portal hypertension persists despite the establishment of an extensive network of portalsystemic collaterals that may divert more than 80% of the portal blood flow. The increased portal venous inflow can be corrected pharmacologically by means of splanchnic vasoconstrictors such as vasopressin and its derivatives, somatostatin and its analogues and nonselective beta-adrenergic blockers.

Splanchnic vasodilatation is accompanied by increased cardiac index and hypervolemia, representing the hyperkinetic circulatory syndrome associated with portal hypertension. An expanded blood volume is necessary to maintain the hyperdynamic circulation, which provides a rationale for the use of low-sodium diet and spironolactone to attenuate the hyperkinetic syndrome and the portal pressure elevation in patients with cirrhosis.

Combined pharmacologic therapy attempts to enhance the reduction of portal pressure by associating vasoconstrictive drugs, which act by decreasing portal blood inflow, and vasodilators, which reduce the intrahepatic vascular resistance.[1]

Diagnosis of cirrhotic portal hypertension

Hepatic venous pressure gradient measurement

Measurement of hepatic venous pressure gradient (HVPG) at hepatic vein catheterisation is the preferred technique to estimate portal pressure in cirrhosis. Although it is easy and simple to perform, accurate measurements require specific training.[1] HVPG has been proven to add prognostic information in many settings, including compensated cirrhosis, acute variceal bleeding and patients awaiting liver transplantation, however as previously mentioned, not all patients with increased HVPG have varices. Patients with clinically significant portal hypertension (CSPH) are at high risk of varices and should undergo endoscopic screening.

Endoscopy

Upper gastrointestinal endoscopy is mandatory in patients with cirrhosis in whom portal hypertension is suspected. It allows the assessment of the presence and size of esophageal and gastric varices, the presence of red signs in the variceal wall and the presence and severity of portal hypertensive gastropathy. The use of conscious sedation markedly increases the patients' compliance to the procedure.

Endoscopic videocapsule

Recently, endoscopic videocapsule has been suggested to be a more tolerable way to detect the presence of esophageal varices. Capsule endoscopy has been shown to allow a correct identification of varices in 80% of cases.; in one of these studies capsule endoscopy correctly identified red wale marks.[3] It may not, however, be as good in assessing variceal size and it may have poor accuracy in identifying portal hypertensive gastropathy and gastric varices, therefore, it cannot be currently recommended as the routine screening method for gastroesophageal varices.

Non-invasive tests

Several laboratory and radiologic parameters have been used to predict the presence of portal hypertension and/or gastroesophageal varices with variable success.

Clinical signs and laboratory findings

The presence of splenomegaly, or spleen size, is the clinical sign more often reported in studies on non-invasive prediction of portal hypertension and esophageal varices. Platelet count, and a platelet count to spleen diameter ratio above 909, has been suggested to be useful in selecting patients with a high risk of developing large esophageal varices, however the diagnostic value of platelet count in compensated cirrhosis is not good enough to avoid endoscopy.[4] The cut-offs for platelet count vary across studies, indicating low specificity. In addition, in viral cirrhosis platelet count can decrease independently from the development of portal hypertension. Fibrotest, a panel of blood tests, has also been applied to the diagnosis of portal hypertension and of gastroesophageal varices, however the negative predictive value is not sufficient to allow an accurate diagnosis or exclusion of portal hypertension and/or gastroesophageal varices.[4]

Liver stiffness (FibroScan®)

Several studies have evaluated the possible role of transient elastography (*FibroScan*®), a noninvasive method for assessing liver fibrosis, in estimating the severity of portal hypertension or predicting the presence of esophageal varices. The majority of these studies were carried out on hepatitis C patients. According with current evidence, finding of a liver stiffness value ≤13.6 kPa would discard and values ≥21 kPa would substantiate with a reasonable accuracy the absence or presence of CSPH, respectively. There is, however, a significant proportion of patients with compensated liver disease (around 40% in some series) who have liver stiffness values that fall in the grey zone between both cut-off values. Additionally, although there is an excellent correlation between liver stiffness and HVPG for values <10–12 mmHg, there is no linear correlation between liver stiffness and HVPG values higher than that, probably because structural abnormalities within the liver (e.g. fibrosis) are not the only mechanism promoting portal hypertension, which is also determined by the magnitude of porto-collateral blood flow and changes in hepatic vascular tone (which are not reflected by the fibroscan).[5] Although liver stiffness may classify around 60% of compensated cirrhotic patients as having or not CSPH, it is not useful to estimate HVPG. In addition, it is important to recognize that different circumstances such as hepatic congestion, steatosis, inflammation and cholestasis may influence the value of liver stiffness without any relation with HVPG changes.

In a large series of patients with hepatitis C virus recurrence after liver transplantation, a liver stiffness value ≥8.74 kPa had a sensitivity and specificity of 90% and 81% for the diagnosis of portal hypertension (HVPG ≥6 mmHg)[6] and therefore elastography was very useful in classifying this group of patients. Although an overall good correlation between liver stiffness and HVPG was also shown in this group, when only patients with a HVPG >10 mmHg were considered the correlation was not so good. Initial studies suggested that liver stiffness might be used to select those patients likely to have large varices and requiring screening endoscopy.[1] This has not been confirmed and is not surprising because although increased portal pressure is a requirement for the formation of varices, in itself the magnitude of the portal pressure elevation does not correlate with either the presence or size of varices. Therefore, liver stiffness measurement cannot obviate the need of endoscopy to screen varices in those patients in the grey zone or with a liver stiffness value above the threshold for CSPH.

MR elastography is a novel method proposed to evaluate liver stiffness. The measurement is obtained by synchronizing motion-sensitive imaging sequences with the application of acoustic waves in tissue media. Preliminary results support its practicability in predicting the stage of fibrosis in patients with chronic liver disease.

Imaging techniques

Ultrasonography (US)/color-Doppler–US (CDUS) is the preferred initial examination in patients with suspected portal hypertension. US can detect signs of portal hypertension such as splenomegaly, presence of portocollateral vessels, and ascites, and complement this information with data on liver dimension, echotexture and margins, which can suggest underlying cirrhosis. Among the US parameters, spleen length is the strongest independent predictive marker of esophageal varices. Increased portal vein diameter (above 13 mm) and reduced portal vein velocity (maximal and mean velocimetry of portal vein flow, respectively <20 cm/s and <10–12 cm/s) are also signs of portal hypertension. These variables, however, do not show a satisfactory predictive accuracy in independent sets of patients, probably due to the high interobserver and intraobserver variability.

CT scan and magnetic resonance imaging allow good visualization of the portal venous system, and both techniques permit the diagnosis of esophageal varices. The technical complexity and cost of these techniques, however, makes unlikely their use for the screening of gastroesophageal varices in cirrhosis.

Clinical scenarios for treatment

The treatment of portal hypertension takes place in different scenarios, which go from the asymptomatic patient who has never bled from varices, to the treatment of the acute variceal bleeding episode and the prevention of recurrent bleeding. The main difference between these scenarios is that natural history and prognosis are very different from one to another.

Patients without varices

Variceal bleeding is the last step in a chain of events initiated by an increase in portal pressure, followed by the development and progressive dilation of varices until these finally rupture and bleed. Once portal pressure increases above a critical threshold value complications of portal hypertension can appear. Varices do not develop until the HVPG increases above 10 mmHg. It has been estimated that varices are present in about 30–40% of compensated patients at the time of diagnosis, and in 60% of decompensated patients. In cirrhotic patients without varices at first endoscopy the annual incidence of new varices is 5–10%. In patients without varices on initial endoscopy, a second (follow-up) evaluation should be performed after 2–3 years.[7]

An HVPG over 10 mmHg is the strongest predictor for the development of varices.[8] Once developed, varices usually increase in size from small to large before they eventually rupture and bleed. The reported rate of progression is heterogeneous (5–30% per year). The factor that has been most consistently associated with variceal progression is liver failure, as assessed by Child–Pugh class.[7] Other factors include alcoholic etiology of cirrhosis and presence of red wale markings at the varices.

Nonselective beta-adrenergic blockers were proposed for the prevention of the development of varices. Unfortunately, in a large randomized study, the rate of development of esophageal varices or variceal hemorrhage did not differ but adverse events were more frequent in patients treated with the nonselective beta-blocker timolol than with placebo. Therefore, beta-adrenergic blockers cannot be recommended for the prevention of the development of esophageal varices. A different approach to avoid development of EV is to prevent the progression of cirrhosis (i.e. abstinence in alcoholics, antivirals in viral cirrhosis, weight loss in NASH, corticosteroids in autoimmune hepatitis, phlebotomies in hemochromatosis, and copper chelators in Wilson's disease). Two examples support this approach. First, alcohol abstinence has been demonstrated to decrease the incidence of complications of cirrhosis and portal hypertension, resulting in prolonged survival. Second, it has been shown that cirrhotic patients with a sustained virologic response, after interferon therapy, had a lower probability of clinical decompensation during follow up, including variceal bleeding. It is worth noting that interferon treatment has been effective in reducing portal pressure,[9] which is the driving force for EV formation. Additionally, studies in experimental models of portal hypertension have shown that blockade of the vascular endothelial growth factor (VEGF) signalling cascade is highly effective in reducing the formation of collaterals, but no study has explored this clinically.

Prevention of first bleeding

The yearly incidence of first variceal bleeding in cirrhotic patients is estimated at 4%, but when medium to large varices are present, this risk increases to 15%.[4] Patients with "large" varices (>5 mm in diameter) and patients with small varices but with red color signs or in a Child–Pugh class C are those at a high risk of variceal bleeding and therefore in these patients profilaxis of first bleeding is mandatory. In the remaining patients with small varices (Child–Pugh A–B and/or without red signs), the decision to initiate treatment at this time, or wait until follow-up endoscopies show the increase in variceal size should be taken according to the preferences of the patient.

Variceal bleeding occurs when the HVPG exceeds a critical threshold of 12 mmHg.[10] Conversely, a marked reduction in the risk of bleeding has been observed when a substantial reduction of the HVPG (<12 mmHg or by >20% of baseline levels) could be achieved.[10] Nonselective beta-blockers (NSBBs; propranolol or nadolol) decrease HVPG and this is the rationale to use them in the prevention of bleeding. Indeed, these drugs have been shown to reduce the risk of first variceal bleeding from 24% to 15% after a median follow up of 2 years. Mortality was also reduced (from 27% to 23%) although this did not reach statistical significance. NSBBs do not protect all patients from variceal bleeding due to noncompliance, inadequate dosing, or lack of hemodynamic response. One approach to this clinical problem has been to perform a baseline HVPG measurement and repeat the measurement after 1–3 months, thereby identifying "nonresponders". Recently, the acute hemodynamic response to intravenous propranolol, administered during a baseline HVPG study, has been also shown to effectively stratify patients with a reduction in HVPG ≥10% of baseline as acute hemodynamic responders and with a lower risk of first bleeding on NSBB treatment. This strategy allows responders and nonresponders to NSBBs to be determined following a single procedure. Addition of isosorbide 5-mononitrate (ISMN) significantly increases the reduction of HVPG achieved with beta-adrenergic blockers and it was suggested that a greater clinical efficacy occurs in primary prophylaxis with the combination of nadolol + isosorbide mononitrate over nadolol alone. A large double-blind, placebo-controlled study, however, failed to confirm these results and the use of this combination drug therapy is not recommended for primary prophylaxis. A drawback of nonselective beta-blockers is the fact that around 25% of cirrhotic patients may have either contraindications or cannot tolerate these drugs.

EBL is effective in preventing first variceal bleeding in patients with medium to large varices. There is no agreement on how frequently the varices should be ligated in the initial course of eradication, the interval varying from 1 to 4 weeks.

A recent trial evaluated the effectiveness and complications of EBL every 2 weeks vs every 2 months. This trial included patients with and without previous bleeding, though most patients were treated for primary prophylaxis.[9] The 2-month interval scheme obtained a higher total eradication rate and lower recurrence rate, thus, although admittedly weak, current evidence favors monthly intervals. This might not apply to prophylaxis of recurrent bleeding (in which the risk of rebleeding is maximal in the first few weeks) where a 1–2-week interval might be more appropriate. Once the varices are eradicated, follow-up endoscopies should be performed at 1–3 months and every 6 months thereafter, and varices should be re-eradicated upon recurrence. This is in marked contrast with prophylaxis with beta-blockers, in which no follow-up endoscopies are needed.

EBL has been compared to beta-blockers as a first-line option for primary prophylaxis. Meta-analysis of these trials shows an advantage of EBL over beta-adrenergic blockers in terms of prevention of first bleeding, but without differences in mortality.[11] These results, however, have several problems. When reviewing the results of those trials that adequately specified the method used for the allocation to the different treatment arms or those with the longest follow up (at least 20 months) no significant differences in first bleeding rates or in mortality was found.[12] In these comparing studies, NSBBs had a higher number of side effects than EBL, however most reported side effects related to beta-blockers (hypotension, tiredness, breathlessness, poor memory, and insomnia) were easily managed by adjusting the dose or discontinuing the medication. Additionally, hospital admission was not required and no fatalities were observed.[11] In contrast, side effects related to EBL included 12 treatment-related bleeding episodes and one esophageal perforation. In most cases, these complications required hospitalization and blood transfusion and resulted in three deaths out of 292 treated patients (1%), thus, severity and impact of side effects is different in the EBL than in the beta-blocker-treated groups. Because of the portal pressure reducing the effect of beta-blockers, they are not only beneficial in decreasing variceal bleeding, but may also attenuate the development of other complications of portal hypertension such as ascites, hepatorenal syndrome or bleeding related to portal hypertensive gastropathy. EBL does not modify portal pressure and therefore has no potential to modify other complications of portal hypertension. According with all these data, both NSBBs and EBL could be used. Taking into consideration all the above it is the current authors' recommendation to use NSBBs as the first treatment option, offering EBL to those patients with contraindications or who cannot tolerate beta-blockers. The recommendation is more clear in patients with small varices, where NSBBs are the recommended therapy. There is no scientific evidence to support that this approach to esophageal varices may be different in patients who are candidates for liver transplantation. Indeed, the only randomized trial comparing both alternatives suggested that both are similarly effective in reducing the incidence of variceal bleeding, but EBL can be complicated by fatal bleeding and is more expensive.[13]

A recent multicenter randomized, controlled trial (RCT)[14] compared carvedilol (a drug that has been shown to produce a higher reduction in portal pressure than NSBBs) vs EBL in the prevention of first bleeding. This study showed significantly lower bleeding rates in the group treated with carvedilol (9% vs 21% in those receiving EBL), but without significant differences in mortality. Carvedilol may be a promising pharmacologic agent to be further tested in primary prophylaxis.

Prevention of recurrent bleeding from esophageal varices

Patients surviving a first episode of variceal bleeding have a risk of >60% of experiencing recurrent hemorrhage within 2 years from the index episode. Because of this, all patients surviving variceal bleeding should receive active treatments for the prevention of rebleeding.[11] Available treatments for preventing variceal rebleeding include pharmacologic therapy, endoscopic therapy, TIPS, and surgical shunting.

Pharmacologic therapy

Several meta-analyses have consistently found a marked benefit of beta-blockers showing a reduction in rebleeding rate (from 63% to 42%), in overall mortality (from 27% to 20%) and in bleeding-related mortality.[11]

The combination of propranolol or nadolol plus IMN enhances the reduction of portal pressure induced by NSBBs. There is only one published study comparing IMN associated with propranolol vs propranolol alone in the prevention of rebleeding. The study showed a significant benefit of the pharmacologic association. The association of propranolol/nadolol and ISMN has been compared to EBL in four studies. A meta-analysis of the four studies does not show significant differences between both treatments in preventing rebleeding or in mortality. The association of beta-blockers and IMN seems to be the best pharmacologic approach to prevent rebleeding.

EBL is clearly superior to sclerotherapy, due to less frequent and severe complications, thus EBL is at present the endoscopic treatment of choice. Variceal eradication is achieved with a lower number of EBL sessions than with sclerotherapy, but EBL is associated with a higher rate of recurrence of varices. There is no benefit and it is probably harmful to add sclerotherapy to EBL and therefore this combination should not be recommended.

Two RCTs have shown that adding beta-blockers to EBL reduces the risk of rebleeding and variceal recurrence, suggesting that if EBL is used, it should be used in association with beta-blockers. In addition, the combination of the two best strategies for prevention of rebleeding (EBL and the combination of beta-blockers + isosorbide-5-mononitrate) has been evaluated. Indeed, two recent randomized clinical trials evaluated whether EBL may improve the efficacy of the combined administration of nadolol plus ISMN. Both studies showed that adding EBL to nadolol plus ISMN is superior to nadolol plus ISMN alone in preventing variceal rebleeding without significant differences in mortality. Although in both studies there was a trend, no significant differences in bleeding from any cause (due to a greater number of ulcer-related bleedings in the treatment arm including EBL) were found.[15,16] Therefore, a combination of EBL and drug therapy (beta-blocker preferably in association with isosorbide-5-mononitrate) may be the first option in preventing recurrent bleeding. Patients who rebleed despite combined treatment with EBL and drug therapy, especially if experiencing a major rebleeding episode, require a derivative procedure (a TIPS or a surgical shunt).

TIPS has been compared with surgical shunts in two RCTs (an 8 mm portocaval H-graft shunt in one, and distal splenorenal shunt (DSRS) in the second).[17,18] The first study favored surgical shunts, which showed a significantly lower rebleeding rate and a lower incidence of the composite endpoint of rebleeding, shunt thrombosis, deaths, and need for transplant compared with TIPS. There was no difference in mortality. The second and larger trial[18] showed no significant differences in rebleeding rate (5.5% in the DSRS group, and 9% in the TIPS group), incidence of hepatic encephalopathy, liver transplantation, or mortality. There was a significantly higher reintervention rate in the TIPS group (82%), which used bare stents, than in the DSRS group (11%). The obstruction and reintervention rates, however, can be markedly decreased with the use of polytetrafluoroethylene (PTFE)-covered stents.[19] Although both alternatives can be used depending on expertise, TIPS using PTFE-covered stents seems to be the best treatment option as a rescue therapy for failures of medical and endoscopic treatment.

HVPG-guided therapy in the prevention of rebleeding

Pharmacologic (or spontaneous) reduction of HVPG to <12 mmHg or by ≥20% of the baseline value (HVPG responders) decreases dramatically the risk of rebleeding and significantly reduces mortality.[10] The rebleeding risk in the group of responders is as low as that achieved using surgical shunts or TIPS. As a consequence, adding further treatment (i.e. band ligation) in this group is unlikely to enhance efficacy, but may increase severe side effects. On the other hand, current data does not support that patients with an insufficient hemodynamic response to pharmacologic therapy (nonresponders) would benefit from shifting to or adding EBL.[15] Probably more effective and aggressive therapies are needed to reduce the high rebleeding risk of HVPG nonresponders. Until more data is available HVPG-guided therapy should only be used in the setting of clinical research.

Acute bleeding episode

Ruptured esophageal varices cause 70% of all upper gastrointestinal bleeding episodes in patients with portal hypertension, thus in any cirrhotic patient with acute upper gastrointestinal bleeding, a variceal origin should be suspected. Diagnosis is established at emergency endoscopy based on observing one of the following:

1. Active bleeding from a varix (observation of blood spurting or oozing from the varix) (approximately 20% of patients)
2. White nipple or clot adherent to a varix
3. Presence of varices without other potential sources of bleeding.

Endoscopy should always be performed within 12 hours of admission (preferably within 6 hours).

Treatment of acute variceal bleeding

Acute variceal bleeding should be managed in an intensive care setting by a team of experienced medical staff, including well-trained nurses, clinical hepatologists, endoscopists, interventional radiologists, and surgeons. Lack of these facilities demands immediate referral. Decision-making should follow the guidelines set up in a written protocol developed to optimize the resources of each centre. Initial therapy is aimed at correcting hypovolemic shock, preventing complications associated with gastrointestinal bleeding, and achieving hemostasis at the bleeding site. Figure 3.1 shows how acute bleeding from ruptured oesophageal varices can be managed effectively.

General management

The general management of the bleeding patient is aimed at correcting hypovolemic shock (with

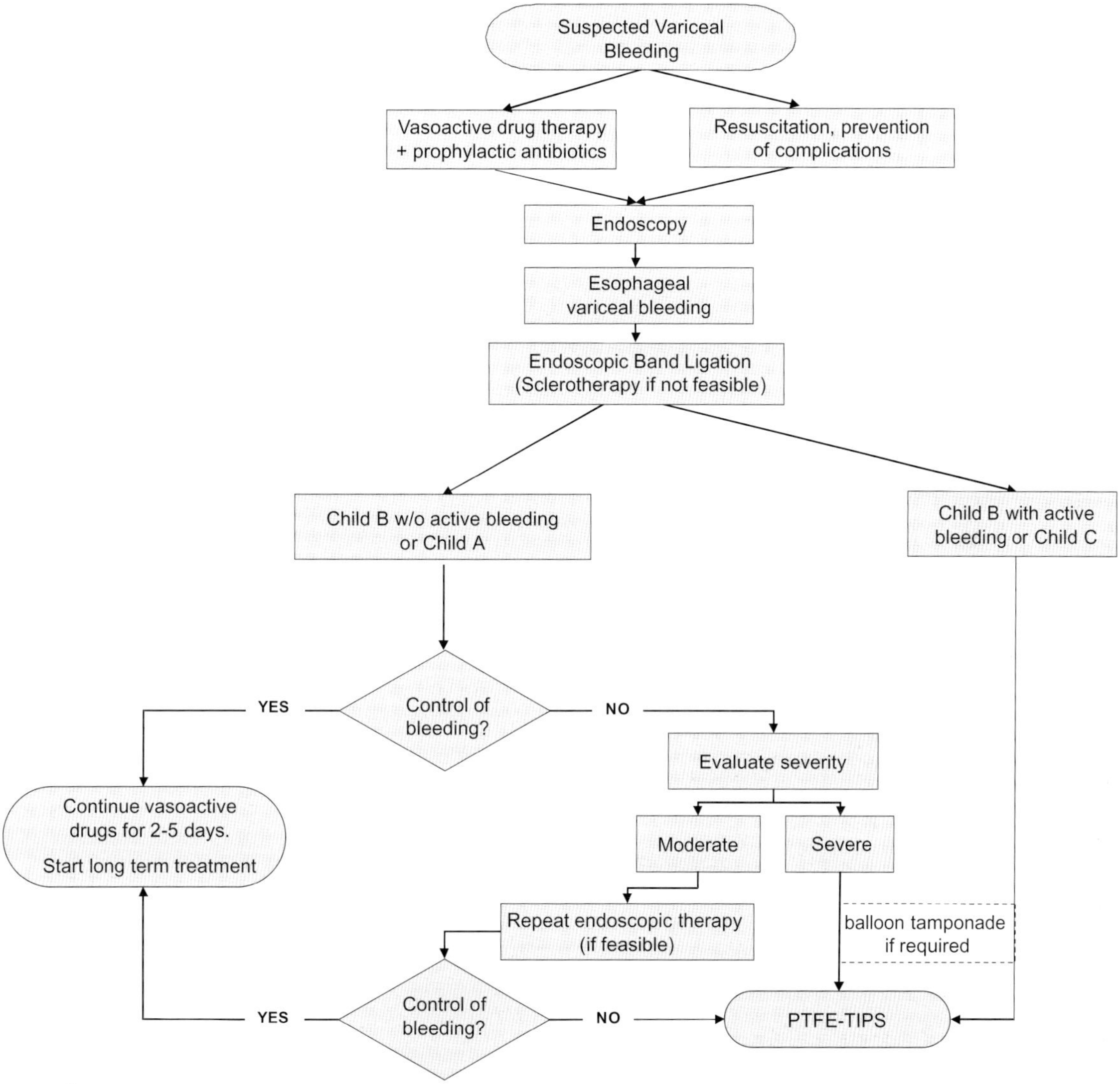

Figure 3.1 Algorithm of the management of acute bleeding from ruptured oesophageal varices

judicious volume replacement and transfusion) and at preventing complications associated with gastrointestinal bleeding (bacterial infections, hepatic decompensation, renal failure), which are independent of the cause of the hemorrhage. Initial resuscitation is aimed at restoring an appropriate delivery of oxygen to the tissues. The airway should be immediately secured, especially in encephalopatic patients, since the patient is at risk of bronchial aspiration of gastric content and blood. This risk is further exacerbated by endoscopic procedures. Endothracheal intubation is mandatory if there is any concern about the safety of the airway.

Blood volume replacement should be initiated as soon as possible with plasma expanders, aiming at maintaining systolic blood pressure around 100 mmHg. Avoiding prolonged hypotension is particularly important to prevent infection and renal failure, which are associated with increased risk of rebleeding and death. Blood transfusion should aim at maintaining the hematocrit at 0.21–0.24 (Hb 7–8 g/L),[7] except in patients with rapid ongoing bleeding or with ischemic heart disease.

The role of platelet transfusion or fresh–frozen plasma administration has not been assessed appropriately. Additionally, although the post-hoc analysis of an RCT suggested that the addition of recombinant activated factor VII (rFVIIa) aimed to normalize the coagulative defect of cirrhotic patients and improved the results of the standard treatment with drugs + EBL in patients with moderate and advanced liver failure (stages B and C of the Child–Pugh classification), these findings were not confirmed in a trial specifically designed to test this issue in a high-risk population (defined in this study as patients with active bleeding at endoscopy and a Child–Pugh score ≥8 points.) Therefore, according to these data, rFVII is not currently recommended in the management of acute variceal bleeding.

The use of prophylactic antibiotics has been shown to reduce both the risk of rebleeding and mortality, and therefore antibiotics should be given to all patients from admission. Quinolones are frequently used due to their easy administration and low cost. In high-risk patients (with hypovolemic shock, ascites, jaundice, or malnutrition) i.v. ceftriaxone has been shown to be superior to oral norfloxacin.

Specific therapy for control of bleeding

Initial therapy for acute variceal bleeding is based on the combination of vasoactive drugs with endoscopic therapy. The rationale for that comes from a number of RCTs demonstrating that early administration of a vasoactive drug facilitates endoscopy and improves control of bleeding and 5-day rebleeding. Vice versa, the association of endoscopic therapy also improves the efficacy of vasoactive treatment.

Pharmacologic therapy

The current recommendation is to start vasoactive drug therapy early (ideally during the transferral or arrival to hospital, even if active bleeding is only suspected). The selection of the drug depends on the local resources. Terlipressin should be the first choice if available, since it is the only drug that has been shown to improve survival. Somatostatin and somatostatin analogues (octreotide or vapreotide) are second choice. If these drugs are not available vasopressin plus transdermal nitroglycerin is an acceptable option. The optimal duration of drug therapy is not well established. The current recommendation is to maintain the drug for 2–5 days.

Terlipressin is a long-acting triglycyl lysine derivative of vasopressin that is used at a dose of 2 mg/4 hours for the first 48 hours, and it may be maintained for up to 5 days at a dose of 1 mg/4 hours to prevent rebleeding. The most common side effect of this drug is abdominal pain. Serious side effects such as peripheral or myocardial ischemia occur in <3% of patients.

Somatostatin is empirically used as an initial bolus of 250 μg followed by a 250 μg/h infusion that is maintained until the achievement of a 24-hour bleed-free period. The bolus injection can be repeated up to three times in the first hour if bleeding is uncontrolled. Therapy may be further maintained for up to 5 days to prevent early rebleeding. Major side effects with somatostatin are rare. Minor side effects, such as nausea, vomiting and hyperglycemia occur in up 30% of patients. The use of higher doses (500 μg/h) causes a greater fall in HVPG and translates into increased clinical efficacy and lower mortality in the subset of patients with more difficult bleedings (those with active bleeding at emergency endoscopy).

Octreotide is a somatostatin analogue with a longer half-life. This, however, is not associated with longer hemodynamic effects. The optimal doses are not well determined. It is usually given as an initial bolus of 50 μg, followed by an infusion of 25 or 50 μg/h. As with somatostatin, therapy can be maintained for 5 days to prevent early rebleeding. The safety profile of octreotide is close to that of somatostatin. The efficacy of octreotide as a single therapy for variceal bleeding is controversial. However, RCTs using octreotide after sclerotherapy have shown a significant benefit in terms of reducing early rebleeding.

Endoscopic therapy

Both sclerotherapy and band ligation (EBL) have been shown to be effective in the control of acute variceal bleeding, however current evidence shows that EBL is better than sclerotherapy in the initial control of bleeding, and is associated with less adverse events and improved mortality. Additionally, sclerotherapy, but not EBL, may increase portal pressure, therefore EBL is the endoscopic therapy of choice in acute variceal bleeding, though injection sclerotherapy is acceptable if band ligation is not available or technically difficult. Endoscopic therapy should be performed soon after initial resuscitation, when the patient is stable and bleeding has ceased or slowed.

Rescue therapies: tamponade, surgery, and TIPS

In 10–20% of patients variceal bleeding is unresponsive to initial endoscopic and/or pharmacologic treatment. If bleeding is mild and the patient is stable a second endoscopic therapy might be attempted. If this fails, or bleeding is severe, the patient should be offered a derivative treatment, before clinical status further deteriorates. Balloon tamponade achieves hemostasis in 60–90% of variceal bleedings but should only be used in the case of a massive bleeding, for a short period of time (<24 hours) as a temporal "bridge" until definite treatment is instituted. Bleeding recurs after deflation in over half of the cases and severe complications are common. A recent report suggested that the use of esophageal covered stents might achieve hemostasis in most patients with refractory bleeding,[20] with the advantage over tamponade of less severe complications despite longer periods of treatment. Adequately designed trials should confirm these findings.

Both TIPS and surgical shunts are extremely effective in controlling variceal bleeding (the control rate approaches 95%), but due to worsening of liver function and encephalopathy the mortality rate remains high. TIPS is the first-choice therapy, since most patients requiring rescue treatment have advanced liver disease with unacceptable surgical risk. Rarely, if ever, a patient with a Child–Pugh score over 13 will survive TIPS; this clearly indicates that some patients do not benefit from TIPS in this setting.

Targeting therapy to risk stratification

Current recommendations for the treatment of acute variceal bleeding are applied homogenously to all cirrhotic patients without considering special characteristics that may influence the outcome of these treatments. As previously mentioned, despite the application of these gold-standard treatments, 10–15% of cirrhotic patients still have treatment failure and a high mortality rate even with the use of rescue TIPS. Two recent studies that use early treatment with TIPS (in most cases within 24 hours from admission) in high-risk patients, identified by an HVPG >20 mmHg or by clinical data (Child C or Child B patients with active variceal bleeding), had significantly less treatment failure and lower mortality rates than patients undergoing standard therapy using TIPS as a rescue therapy for failures. These data strongly recommend that in high-risk patients more aggressive therapies such as the early use of PTFE–TIPS could be the treatment of choice.

Gastric varices

Gastric varices are the source of 5–10% of all upper digestive bleeding episodes in patients with cirrhosis. Type 1 gastric varices (GOV 1) are an extension of esophageal varices along the lesser curvature of the stomach, and their management is the same as for esophageal varices. Isolated gastric varices (IGV 1) and fundal gastroesophageal varices (GOV 2) are those that present differential features. When cases of IGV 1 are due to isolated splenic vein thrombosis, splenectomy is curative treatment. In acute bleeding from gastric varices, the initial treatment is similar to that for esophageal variceal bleeding, including the administration of a vasoactive drug and endoscopic variceal obturation (EVO) with N-butyl-cyanoacrylate, isobutyl-2-cyanoacrylate (bucrylate) or thrombin. N-butyl-2-cyanoacrylate (Histoacryl) is a tissue adhesive that polymerizes on contact with blood, resulting in a firm "cast" of the varix. Complications of the technique include thromboembolism of cyanoacrylate, inadvertent adhesion of the injector to the varix and deep mucosal ulceration when the cast falls out 3–5 days later. In experienced hands this technique has shown efficacy for acute GV bleeding, although only three small RCTs have been performed and each suffers with the limitation of including patients with both fundal varices and GOV. Moreover, concerns have been raised about rebleeding rates even if the varices can be initially obliterated.

TIPS is very effective in the treatment of bleeding gastric varices, with >90% success rate for initial hemostasis and a very low rebleeding rate. A recent trial has shown that it is more effective than glue injection in preventing rebleeding.[21] Derivative and devascularization surgery are also effective, but with limited applicability in advanced cirrhosis. Another approach is the retrograde intravascular obliteration of spontaneous spleno-renal shunts (B-RTO) that are frequently present in patients with large fundal varices. B-RTO is a procedure that has emerged from South-East Asia for the treatment of fundal varices associated with a splenorenal shunt. The technique involves retrograde cannulation of the left renal vein via the jugular or femoral vein under fluoroscopic guidance, followed by balloon occlusion and injection of sclerosant to obliterate the splenorenal shunt and fundal varices. Initial, uncontrolled studies suggested that B-RTO was an effective treatment for fundal varices, however the real safety and efficay of this technique is not yet clear and more studies are needed before establishing the actual role of this technique in the management of fundal varices.

The current authors' recommendation is to start treatment with a vasoactive drug. If bleeding is not controlled and if an expert endoscopist is available, variceal obturation might be attempted. In cases of massive bleeding or after failure of previous therapies, TIPS (or surgical shunt in Child A patients) is mandatory. A second attempt at endoscopic therapy should never be allowed in these patients.

Portal hypertensive gastropathy

Portal hypertensive gastropathy (PHG) is a macroscopic finding of a characteristic mosaic-like pattern of the gastric mucosa ("mild" PHG), red-point lesions, cherry red spots, and/or black–brown spots ("severe" PHG). These lesions, however, are not entirely specific, i.e. can occur in the absence of portal hypertension. In PHG there is marked dilatation of the vasculature of the gastric mucosa and submucosa, together with an increased blood flow and tendency to decreased acid secretion. The overall prevalence of PHG in patients with cirrhosis strongly correlates with the severity of the disease and ranges between 11% and 80%. The incidence of acute bleeding is low (<3% at 3 years) with a mortality rate of 12.5%, while the incidence of chronic bleeding is 10–15% at 3 years. In acute bleeding from PHG beta-adrenergic blockers, somatostatin, octreotide, vassopressin, terlipressin and estrogens have been proposed based on their ability to decrease gastric perfusion in this condition. Only one uncontrolled study so far, however, has evaluated one of these drugs (somatostatin) in acute bleeding from PHG. Hemostasis was achieved in all patients. Nonselective beta-blockers effectively decrease chronic bleeding from PHG.[22]

Special issues in liver transplantation

Impact of previous derivative procedures on liver trasplant

In evaluating the impact of previous decompressive surgical shunts or TIPS on liver transplantation, it has been suggested that by reducing portal hypertension they might have a favorable impact in the course of intervention by lowering intraoperative blood loss and shortening the duration of surgery associated to liver transplantation. It should be noted, however, that previous laparotomy and/or manipulation of the vessels in the hepatic hilum by increasing the difficulty of the hepatectomy may negatively influence all these parameters. Several studies have evaluated these issues with contradictory results although current evidence supports that portosystemic derivative surgery involving the hepatic hilum has a negative impact on liver transplantation as evidenced by high blood loss and mortality and therefore should be avoided in potential liver transplant candidates. By contrast, surgical shunts not compromising the hepatic hilum such as splenorenal or mesocaval shunts or TIPS do not have a bad impact on liver transplantation – they may even facilitate the surgical procedure in some studies, and therefore these derivative techniques should be preferred[23].

Development of portal vein thrombosis

The development of portal vein thrombosis (PVT) is a significant milestone in the natural history of cirrhosis with an annual incidence of 16%. It is associated with worsening liver function, ascites, and the occurrence of gastroesophageal variceal bleeding. On the other hand, PVT increases morbidity and mortality associated with liver transplant and may even contraindicate it.[24] Factors associated with increased risk of PVT are a portal blood flow velocity of <15 cm/s at US–Doppler evaluation and the presence of prothrombotic disorders. No randomized trials have been conducted to establish the best management of these patientsTherapeutic decisions must be established on a case-by-case basis.

Acknowledgments

We thank Ms Clara Esteva for expert secretarial support.

Supported in part by grants from the Ministerio de Educación y Ciencia (SAF-07/61298), and from Instituto de Salud Carlos III (FIS 06/0623 and 05/0519). Ciberehd is funded by Instituto de Salud Carlos III.

References

1. Bosch J, Berzigotti A, Garcia-Pagan JC, Abraldes JG. The management of portal hypertension: rational basis, available treatments and future options. J Hepatol 2008;48(Suppl 1):S68–92.
2. Rodriguez-Vilarrupla A, Fernandez M, Bosch J, Garcia-Pagan JC. Current concepts on the pathophysiology of portal hypertension. Ann Hepatol 2007;6:28–36.
3. Eisen GM, Eliakim R, Zaman A, et al. The accuracy of PillCam ESO capsule endoscopy versus conventional upper endoscopy for the diagnosis of esophageal varices: a prospective three-center pilot study. Endoscopy 2006;38:31–5.
4. De Franchis R. Non-invasive (and minimally invasive) diagnosis of oesophageal varices. J Hepatol 2008 Oct;49:520–7.
5. Vizzutti F, Arena U, Romanelli RG, et al. Liver stiffness measurement predicts severe portal hypertension in patients with HCV-related cirrhosis. Hepatology 2007;45:1290–7.
6. Carrion JA, Navasa M, Bosch J, Bruguera M, Gilabert R, Forns X. Transient elastography for diagnosis of advanced fibrosis and portal hypertension in patients with hepatitis C recurrence after liver transplantation. Liver Transpl 2006;12:1791–8.
7. de Franchis R. Evolving Consensus in Portal Hypertension Report of the Baveno IV Consensus Workshop on methodology of diagnosis and therapy in portal hypertension. J Hepatol 2005;43:167–76.
8. Groszmann RJ, Garcia-Tsao G, Bosch J, et al. Beta-blockers to prevent gastroesophageal varices in patients with cirrhosis. N Engl J Med 2005;353:2254–61.
9. Yoshida H, Mamada Y, Taniai N, et al. A randomized control trial of bi-monthly versus bi-weekly endoscopic variceal ligation of esophageal varices. Am J Gastroenterol 2005;100:2005–9.
10. D'Amico G, Garcia-Pagan JC, Luca A, Bosch J. Hepatic vein pressure gradient reduction and prevention of variceal bleeding in cirrhosis: a systematic review. Gastroenterology 2006;131:1611–24.
11. Garcia-Pagan JC, De Gottardi A, Bosch J. Review article: the modern management of portal hypertension – primary and secondary prophylaxis of variceal bleeding in cirrhotic patients. Aliment Pharmacol Ther 2008;28:503–22.
12. Gluud LL, Klingenberg S, Nikolova D, Gluud C. Banding ligation versus beta-blockers as primary prophylaxis in esophageal varices: systematic review of randomized trials. Am J Gastroenterol 2007; 102:2842–8.
13. Norberto L, Polese L, Cillo U, et al. A randomized study comparing ligation with propranolol for primary prophylaxis of variceal bleeding in candidates for liver transplantation. Liver Transpl 2007;13: 1262.
14. Tripathi D, Ferguson JW, Kochar N, et al. Randomized controlled trial of carvedilol versus variceal band ligation for the prevention of the first variceal bleed. Hepatology 2009;50:825–33.
15. Garcia-Pagan JC, Villanueva C, Albillos A, et al. Nadolol plus isosorbide mononitrate alone or associated with band ligation in the prevention of recurrent bleeding: A multicenter randomized controlled trial. Gut 2009;58:1045–6.
16. Lo GH, Chen WC, Chan HH, et al. A randomized, controlled trial of banding ligation plus drug therapy versus drug therapy alone in the prevention of esophageal variceal rebleeding. J Gastroenterol Hepatol 2009;24:982–7.
17. Rosemurgy AS, Serafini FM, Zweibel BR, et al. Transjugular intrahepatic portosystemic shunt vs. small-diameter prosthetic H-graft portacaval shunt: extended follow-up of an expanded randomized prospective trial. J Gastrointest Surg 2000;4:589–97.
18. Henderson JM, Boyer TD, Kutner MH, Rikkers L, Jeffers L, Abu-Elmagd K. DSRS vs TIPS for refractory variceal bleeding: a prospective randomized controlled trial. Hepatology 2004;40(Suppl 1):725A.
19. Bureau C, Garcia-Pagan JC, Otal P, et al. Improved clinical outcome using polytetrafluoroethylene-coated stents for tips: Results of a randomized study. Gastroenterology 2004;126:469–75.

20. Hubmann R, Bodlaj G, Czompo M, et al. The use of self-expanding metal stents to treat acute esophageal variceal bleeding. Endoscopy 2006;38:896–901.
21. Lo GH, Liang HL, Chen WC, et al. A prospective, randomized controlled trial of transjugular intrahepatic portosystemic shunt versus cyanoacrylate injection in the prevention of gastric variceal rebleeding. Endoscopy 2007;39:679–85.
22. Perez-Ayuso RM, Pique JM, Bosch J, et al. Propranolol in prevention of recurrent bleeding from severe portal hypertensive gastropathy in cirrhosis. Lancet 1991;337: 1431–4.
23. Dell'Era A, Grande L, Barros-Schelotto P, et al. Impact of prior portosystemic shunt procedures on outcome of liver transplantation. Surgery 2005;137:620–5.
24. Yerdel MA, Gunson B, Mirza D, et al. Portal vein thrombosis in adults undergoing liver transplantation: risk factors, screening, management, and outcome. Transplantation 2000;69:1873–81.

4 Management of renal disease in the liver transplant candidate

Andrés Cárdenas[1] *and Pere Ginès*[2]

[1]Gastrointestinal Unit and [2]Liver Unit, Institut Clinic de Malalties Digestives i Metaboliques, Hospital Clinic, and University of Barcelona, Institut d'Investigacions Biomèdiques August Pi-Sunyer (IDIBAPS), Ciber de Enfermedades Hepáticas y Digestivas (CIBEREHD), Barcelona, Spain

Key learning points

- The estimation of glomerular filtration rate (GFR) is difficult and overestimated in cirrhotics by calculations using serum creatinine.
- The causes of renal failure in cirrhotics include infections, hypovolemia, intrinsic disease, hepatorenal syndrome, drugs, or a combination of these.
- The most effective therapy for pre-transplant management of hepatorenal syndrome is intravenous albumin with vasoconstrictors.
- The number of simultaneous liver–kidney transplants (SLKs) is increasing and appropriate candidates have the following features: end-stage renal disease or GFR <30 ml/min and proteinuria >3 g/d or a requirement for dialysis for >6 weeks.

Introduction

Patients with advanced cirrhosis awaiting liver transplantation are prone to several complications including fluid retention, gastrointestinal hemorrhage, hepatic encephalopathy and renal failure. Renal failure is perhaps one of the most challenging complications of cirrhosis and an important risk factor for liver transplantation. Patients with cirrhosis and renal failure have increased morbidity and mortality while awaiting transplantation and have more complications and reduced survival after transplantation as compared to patients without renal failure.[1–3] Serum creatinine, the most common marker of renal function, is one of the variables included in the Model for End-stage Liver Disease (MELD) score.[4] The score, a reliable predictor of survival in patients with cirrhosis, is currently used as an allocation model for determining patient priority for orthotopic liver transplantation (OLT) in the USA and other countries.[4,5] Serum creatinine before OLT is an important predictor of post-liver transplant survival.[2,3,6]

There are multiple etiologies of renal failure in patients with cirrhosis, thus the proper diagnosis, prevention, and therapy of the different causes of renal dysfunction in the pre-transplant period are of paramount importance in providing care for liver transplant candidates. This chapter will discuss the definitions of renal failure in cirrhosis, the diagnostic approach and management of renal dysfunction in the liver transplant candidate.

Definition of renal failure in cirrhosis

The diagnosis of renal failure in patients with cirrhosis is defined when serum creatinine increases to

Medical Care of the Liver Transplant Patient, Fourth Edition. Edited by Pierre-Alain Clavien, James F. Trotter.

>1.5 mg/dl, which corresponds to a GFR of approximately 30 ml/min.[7] Although serum creatinine is a prognostic marker in cirrhosis, it has limitations as a marker of GFR in most patients with advanced liver disease.[8] Serum creatinine may overestimate GFR mainly due either to decreased creatinine production or reduced muscle mass. It is considered that baseline serum creatinine <1.5 mg/dl does not necessarily exclude renal dysfunction.[9–11] Creatinine clearance is slightly better for estimating GFR than serum creatinine concentration but still overestimates GFR by 50%, more so in those with a low GFR.[11] That said there is no data to indicate that creatinine clearance is better or preferred as a marker of GFR in patients with cirrhosis. In addition, creatinine clearance is difficult to perform because it depends on the adequate collection of urine volume over 24 hours, which in many cases is inadequate, especially in oliguric patients.[11,12] The estimation of GFR with the Cockcroft and Modification of Diet in Renal Disease (MDRD) equations are based on serum creatinine and therefore have not been shown to be very useful in cirrhosis.[13,14] A large study of 1447 patients awaiting liver transplantation revealed that only 65–70% of estimates (Cockcroft and MDRD) were within 30% of the measured GFR using I^{125}-iothalamate clearance.[15] In the study, the precision of the MDRD in estimating GFR was lower than that reported for MDRD estimation of GFR in other disease states. Estimation of GFR with these equations is therefore not considered better than measurement of serum creatinine concentration in patients awaiting liver transplantation.

The gold standard for measuring GFR in cirrhosis relies on clearance techniques of exogenous markers.[8] Measurement of GFR allows the precise estimation of GFR, which helps to classify patients with chronic kidney disease according to categories previously defined by the National Kidney Foundation.[16] Inulin has been the most widely used marker as it is completely filtered by the glomerulus without being secreted, synthesized, or metabolized by the ducts. After an intravenous infusion and at a stable concentration in healthy subjects, the amount filtered equals the amount excreted in urine. Disadvantages to using this method are that it is very cumbersome, expensive and not available in all settings.[8] Other markers such as radiolabeled compounds (51Cr-EDTA, 99mTc-DPTA and 125I-iothalamate) or iohexol/iothalamate are useful, but they are expensive, expose the patient to radiation if used repeatedly, and they have not been specifically or adequately studied in cirrhosis.

The main limitation of using serum creatinine as a marker of renal function may require that the current definition undergo reassessment. New proposed criteria including the acute kidney injury and chronic kidney disease definitions may be useful in patients with cirrhosis but this needs to be properly studied.[16,17] Given the above, serum creatinine concentration is still considered the method of choice to estimate GFR in cirrhosis in clinical practice. Although a single measurement of serum creatinine alone is probably inadequate for identifying and/or quantifying either acute or chronic renal disease in cirrhosis, repeated measurements over time may be useful in indicating variations of GFR in clinical practice.

Causes of renal failure in cirrhosis

There are several causes of renal failure in cirrhosis due to a variety of clinical conditions (Box 4.1). These etiologies can be classified as: 1) renal failure associated with infections, 2) hypovolemia-related renal failure, 3) hepatorenal syndrome (HRS), 4) renal failure due to intrinsic renal diseases, and 5) drug-induced renal failure. According to a recent analysis of 562 hospitalized patients with cirrhosis and renal failure, the most frequent cause of renal failure in cirrhosis was that associated with bacterial infections (46%), followed by hypovolemia-induced renal failure (32%), HRS (13%), parenchymal nephropathy (9%), mixed causes (8%), drug-induced renal failure (7.5%), and other causes (2%) (Figure 4.1).[18] Patients with intrinsic renal disease had a 73% survival rate at 3 months followed by a 46% survival rate in those with hypovolemia-related renal failure. Those with renal failure associated with infections and HRS, which had had the lowest 3-month probability, had survival rates of 31% and 15%, respectively[18] (Figure 4.2).

Since management of renal failure in cirrhotic patients varies according to the underlying cause, it is essential to establish the underlying etiology of renal failure before considering further management. There are no specific tests that secure the diagnosis of the different types of renal failure in cirrhosis; in most cases a detailed clinical history, physical examination

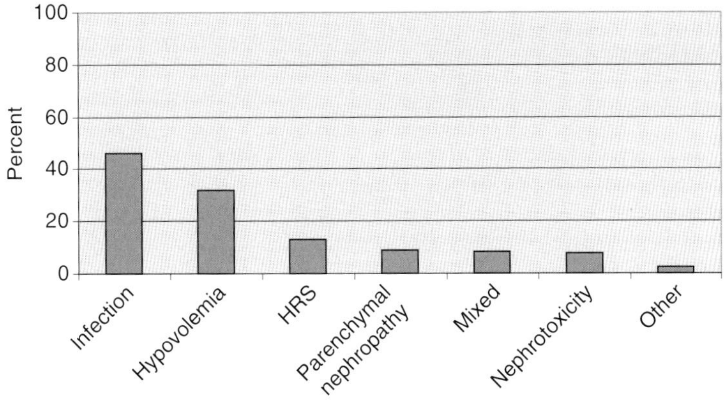

Figure 4.1 Causes of renal failure in a cohort of 562 patients with cirrhosis. The most frequent cause of renal failure due to: bacterial infections (46%), hypovolemia-induced renal failure (32%), hepatorenal syndrome (HRS) (13%), parenchymal nephropathy (9%), mixed causes (8%), drug-induced renal failure (7.5%), and other causes (2%). From Martin-Llahi M, Guevara M, Torre A, et al. Prognostic importance of the cause of renal failure in patients with cirrhosis. Gastroenterology 2011;140:488–96. *Patients with infection-related renal failure are considered to have HRS based on new criteria for the definition of HRS

Box 4.1 Main causes of renal failure in patients with cirrhosis

Infections
- Spontaneous bacterial peritonitis
- Spontaneous bacteremia
- Urinary tract infection, pneumonia, skin infections

Hypovolemia-induced renal failure
- Shock
- Vomiting, diarrhea
- Gastrointestinal bleeding
- Diuretic induced

Hepatorenal syndrome

Intrinsic renal diseases
- Glomerulopathies – IgA nephropathy, membranous nephropathy, membranoproliferative glomerulonephritis, polyarteritis nodosa, cryoglobulinemia due to viral hepatitis, hepatic disease or alcohol

Drug-induced renal failure
- Hemodynamically induced – nonsteroidal anti-inflammatory agents, ACE inhibitors, angiotensin receptor blockers
- Acute tubular necrosis – aminoglycosides, amphotericin B
- Acute interstitial nephritis – penicillin, rifampin and sulfonamides

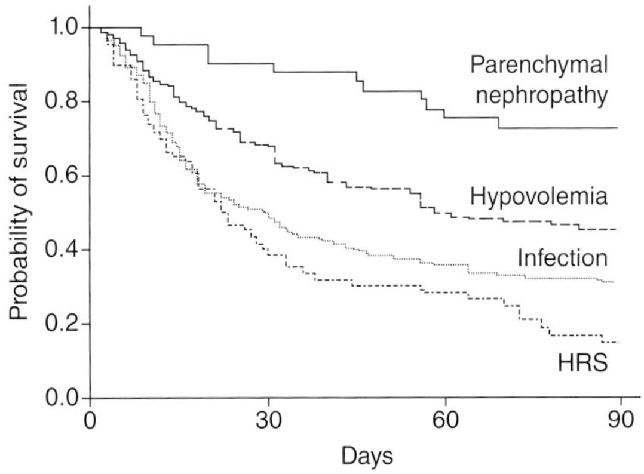

Figure 4.2 Survival of patients with renal failure and cirrhosis according to etiology of kidney disease. Patients with intrinsic renal disease had a 73% survival at 3 months followed by a 46% survival in those with hypovolemia-related renal failure. Those with renal failure associated with infections and HRS which had had the lowest 3-month probability at 31% and 15%, respectively. From Martin-Llahi M, Guevara M, Torre A, et al. Prognostic importance of the cause of renal failure in patients with cirrhosis. Gastroenterology 2011;140:488–96

Box 4.2 Evaluation of patients with cirrhosis and renal failure

Complete history
- Infections/sepsis
- NSAID use, high doses of diuretics or other nephrotoxic drugs
- Gastrointestinal bleeding
- Diabetes, hypertension
- Urinary tract obstruction

Physical examination
- Volume status
- Hemodynamics
- Signs of infection or gastrointestinal bleeding

Laboratory data
- Serum creatinine, electrolytes, liver tests
- Routine urine analysis, urine electrolytes, sediment
- 24-hour urine volume, sodium, protein, creatinine
- Culture – ascites, blood, urine

Renal ultrasound/Doppler

and assessment of renal function with thorough evaluation of urine and serum electrolytes will suffice for establishing the cause (Box 4.2). Renal ultrasonography needs to be performed in order to rule out the existence of abnormalities in renal structure suggestive of chronic kidney disease or urinary tract obstruction. The data on urine biomarkers and renal biopsy in the assessment of renal failure in cirrhosis is limited and therefore cannot be routinely recommended in the workup of renal failure in cirrhosis.[19,20] The differential diagnosis of renal failure is described later.

Infections

As discussed earlier, this is the most common cause of renal failure in cirrhosis. The pathogenesis seems to be related to an impairment of the systemic arterial vasodilation present in cirrhosis due to bacterial products, cytokines or vasoactive mediators that appear in relation with the infection.[21] This occurs mainly in patients who develop spontaneous bacterial peritonitis (SBP) and spontaneous bacteremia, but may occur with any bacterial infection.[18,22] Bacterial infections in patients with cirrhosis are common and it is estimated that they are present at admission or during hospitalization in 20–60% of patients.[18,22,23] Of these, most are secondary to SBP; other common causes are urinary tract infection, pneumonia and bacteremia,[22,23] which are due to both Gram-negative bacteria and aerobic Gram-positive bacteria.[24] Bacterial infections significantly increase the mortality rate in patients with cirrhosis. A pooled analysis of 178 studies estimated that the overall mortality rate of infected patients with cirrhosis was 38%.[25] The same analysis concluded that the mortality rate in those with SBP was 43.7% and in those with bacteremia (1437 patients), the mortality was 42.2%.[25]

In any patient with cirrhosis who develops renal failure while awaiting OLT, the presence of a bacterial infection should be thoroughly sought after. It is important to take into account that signs and symptoms of early bacterial infection may be vague or even absent in some patients with cirrhosis. Moreover, it is not uncommon that in hospitalized patients renal failure is detected before symptoms of infection become clinically evident. Therefore, objective signs of infection should be sought in all patients with cirrhosis and renal failure. The mandatory work-up consists of a complete blood cell count, liver chemistries, polymorphonuclear cell count in a sample of ascitic fluid, ascitic fluid cultures, urine sediment and culture, abdominal ultrasound, chest x-ray and blood cultures.[26]

Hypovolemia

Another type of renal failure that may occur in cirrhosis is pre-renal renal failure. This type of renal dysfunction is related to a reduction in intravascular volume leading to a fall in renal plasma flow and GFR. The main causes of hypovolemia are gastrointestinal bleeding and overdiuresis due to excessive diuretic treatment followed by gastrointestinal fluid losses due to vomiting and/or diarrhea. If renal failure is secondary to volume depletion, renal function rapidly improves after elimination of the precipitating cause and plasma volume expansion. In hypovolemia-induced renal failure the major mechanism responsible for renal hypoperfusion is a reduction in intravascular volume, which may lead to acute tubular necrosis (ATN) if left untreated.[1,26]

The clinical assessment of significant volume losses begins with measurement of blood pressure and pulse. Patients need to be thoroughly questioned about gastrointestinal bleeding, and physical examination should include a rectal examination to rule out melena or bright red blood per rectum, if gastrointestinal bleeding is suspected. Additionally, if patients were taking diuretics, the type and doses need to be checked. Data from patients with cirrhosis and gastrointestinal bleeding indicate that an important reduction in blood volume (in most cases associated to hypovolemic shock) is required to induce renal failure.[27] Therefore it is unlikely that small reductions in blood volume could lead to renal failure. This suggests that specific measures to assess blood volume status, such as measurement of central venous pressure, are not required in all patients with renal failure unless there is significant history of volume losses.

Intrinsic renal diseases

Most intrinsic renal diseases are related to common etiologic factors of cirrhosis, including chronic hepatitis B or C infection or alcoholic liver disease, and encompass kidney diseases secondary to the deposition of circulating immunocomplexes in the glomeruli. The most common in hepatitis C are membranoproliferative glomerulonephritis, membranous glomerulonephritis and focal segmental glomerular sclerosis.[28] Membranous nephropathy is commonly encountered in patients with hepatitis B and IgA nephropathy patients with alcoholic cirrhosis.[28] In some patients, the glomerular deposits are mild and do not affect kidney function, whereas in other patients they are so severe that glomerular function is disrupted, GFR decreases and renal failure develops.

In patients with cirrhosis and renal failure due to intrinsic renal diseases, there is usually proteinuria or hematuria. Intrinsic renal disease is considered if there is either proteinuria >500 mg/24 hours, abnormal urine sediment with >50 red cells per high-power field, or abnormal renal ultrasound findings in the absence of other causes of renal failure.[26] Although criteria for this definition are very specific they lack sensitivity and thus need to be properly studied. The role of kidney biopsy in the evaluation of renal failure in cirrhosis is a matter of debate in some transplant centers because findings demonstrating glomerulosclerosis or significant fibrosis in the renal parenchyma may require the patient receive a SLK as patients with significant findings have a high risk of developing renal insufficiency in the post-transplant period due to nephrotoxicity from calcineurin inhibitors and other medication.[20] Limited data indicates that in transvenous renal biopsies in patients with hematuria or proteinuria, various types of lesions may be present. In one retrospective study of 65 patients, renal biopsy showed that glomerular, vascular, and tubulointerstitial changes in 77%, 69% and 94% of cases, respectively.[29] Fibrous endarteritis was the most common renal vascular lesion and pathologic changes to different structures were frequently combined. Nonetheless the study did not address the outcome of these patients before or after OLT. There were no reported complications of transvenous renal biopsy.[29] Another report of 44 liver transplant candidates with renal failure of undetermined etiology who underwent percutaneous renal biopsy revealed that IgA nephropathy and ATN were the most common findings, however there was more than one pathologic finding (i.e. interstitial fibrosis, glomerular sclerosis, or membranoproliferative disease) in 64% of patients.[30] A disturbing finding was the development of serious complications (mainly bleeding) requiring intervention in 18% of patients. Therefore the role of renal biopsy in patients awaiting OLT still needs be studied, taking into account the potential of simultaneous kidney allocation for this group of liver transplant candidates. Current recommendations from the International Liver Transplantation Society state that given the lack of data in this setting, renal biopsy cannot be recommended to allocate kidneys for SLK.[20]

Hepatorenal syndrome

HRS is a pre-renal renal failure without any identifiable kidney pathology that occurs in patients with advanced cirrhosis.[31,32] Owing to the lack of specific diagnostic markers, the diagnosis of HRS is currently made using criteria to exclude other causes of renal failure that can occur in cirrhosis (Box 4.3). HRS is commonly seen in patients awaiting OLT and remains one of the most challenging complications of cirrhosis to manage. There are two types of HRS: in Type 1 HRS renal function deteriorates rapidly with an increase in serum creatinine to a level higher than 2.5 mg/dl in less than 2 weeks. This type of HRS is associated with a very poor prognosis without treatment, with a median survival time of only 2

Box 4.3 Diagnostic criteria of hepatorenal syndrome in cirrhosis*

Cirrhosis with ascites

Serum creatinine >1.5 mg/dl (133 μmol/L)

No improvement of serum creatinine (decrease to a level lower than 1.5 mg/dl (133 μmol/L) (after at least 2 days off diuretics and volume expansion with albumin (1 g/kg body weight up to a maximum of 100 g/d)

Absence of shock

No current or recent treatment with nephrotoxic drugs

Absence of signs of parenchymal renal disease, as suggested by proteinuria (>500 mg/d) or hematuria (>50 red blood cells per high power field), and/or abnormal

Renal ultrasound

*From Salerno F, Gerbes A, Wong F, et al. Diagnosis, prevention and treatment of the hepatorenal syndrome in cirrhosis. A consensus workshop of the international ascites club. Gut 2007; 56:1310–8.

weeks if left untreated. In Type 2 HRS there is a steady impairment of renal function and serum creatinine levels usually range between 1.5–2.5 mg/dl. Patients with Type 2 HRS have a median survival time of 6 months if not transplanted. Patients with Type 2 HRS may go on to develop Type 1 HRS, either due to progression of disease or triggering factors such as bacterial infections. HRS can be prevented in the setting of SBP by giving iv albumin (1.5 g/kg body weight at diagnosis and 1 g/kg 48 hours later) or by the administration of norfloxacin in patients with advanced cirrhosis and low protein concentration in the ascitic fluid.[33,34] Although differential diagnosis between HRS and ATN remains difficult and the presence of granular casts may be observed in the urine sediments of both HRS and ATN, if renal tubular cells are seen this favors the diagnosis of ATN.[26]

Drug use

Drug nephrotoxicity in patients with cirrhosis occurs due to medications that cause hemodynamic changes, ATN, and/or acute interstitial nephritis (AIN).[35,36] Hemodynamically mediated renal failure is mainly caused by nonsteroidal antinflammatory drugs (NSAIDs) and diuretics.These drugs alter the equilibrium between vasodilator and vasoconstrictor factors in the renal circulation. NSAIDs inhibit the enzymes cycloxygenase-1 and -2, which are responsible for prostaglandin synthesis. Prostaglandins are important renal vasodilators that contribute significantly to maintaining normal renal perfusion. The risk of developing renal failure due to NSAID administration is higher in patients with cirrhosis and ascites, and increased activity of the vasoconstrictor systems.[35,36] Renal failure after NSAID use is followed by a rapid improvement of the GFR to pretreatment values after cessation of the drug in most cases. Diuretic-induced renal failure is usually moderate and reversible after diuretic withdrawal and is related to an imbalance between the fluid loss from the intravascular space caused by diuretic treatment and the passage of fluid from the peritoneal compartment to the general circulation. Drug-induced ATN occurs mainly due to the use of aminoglycosides, amphotericin B, or vancomycin. Owing to this increased risk of nephrotoxicity and the existence of other effective antibiotics (i.e third-generation cephalosporins) treatment with the above mentioned antibiotics should be avoided in patients with chronic liver disease. Finally, AIN may occur due to use of antibiotics such as penicillin, Rifampin and sulfonamides. In drug-induced AIN there is an inflammatory component that affects the renal tubules and interstitium and occurs as a hypersensitivity reaction to medications. In most cases renal failure will return to normal function after discontinuation of the offending agent.

Management

Successful management of patients with renal failure depends on the prompt recognition of renal failure and of its underlying cause. In general, patients with severe acute renal failure awaiting liver transplantation should be admitted to a monitored unit, where an appropriate work-up and therapy can be performed.[26,32] If there are any complications such as associated bacterial infections or gastrointestinal bleeding or shock these should be promptly identified and treated. In most cases third-generation cephalosporins are the initial treatment of choice for suspected bacterial infections while awaiting cultures.[32] Patients with renal failure and severe sepsis may have associated relative adrenal insufficiency and may benefit from hydrocortisone administration, however more studies are needed in this area before recommending steroids in patients with advanced cirrhosis.[37,38] Patients with renal failure due to hypovolemia usually respond to volume repletion and therapy for gastrointestinal bleeding, if present. Those with intrinsic renal disease and chronic kidney disease may be managed as outpatients along with a nephrologist. As mentioned earlier, those with drug-induced renal disease will experience improved renal function upon discontinuation of the toxic drug. Patients with renal failure that requires therapy for large volume ascites or edema should not be treated with spironolactone or furosemide. These patients benefit from large-volume paracentesis and administration of albumin (8 g/L ascites removed) if necessary.[32] Although cirrhotic patients rarely develop renal failure after contrast media for radiologic studies, they should undergo standard prophylactic measures such as saline hydration and monitoring of renal function after the procedure.

Patients with hepatorenal syndrome

The main objective of the management of patients with HRS awaiting liver transplantation is reversing renal failure in order to provide a successful bridge to OLT so that suitable candidates can undergo transplantation without renal failure. Thus, all efforts should be made to improve renal function in order to obtain a better outcome after transplantation. The best available therapy for HRS other than OLT, is the use splanchnic vasoconstrictors plus albumin. Other modalities such as transjugular intrahepatic portosystemic shunts (TIPS), renal replacement therapy and albumin dialysis may be useful in some patients, but data on these approaches is very limited.

Vasoconstrictors

The administration of vasoconstrictors is the best medical therapy currently available for the management of HRS. The rationale of this therapy is to improve circulatory function by causing vasoconstriction of the extremely dilated splanchnic arterial bed, which subsequently improves arterial underfilling, reduces the activity of the endogenous vasoconstrictor systems, and increases renal perfusion. The available vasoconstrictors used in HRS are vasopressin analogues (terlipressin) and alpha-adrenergic agonists (noradrenaline or midodrine), which act on V1 vasopressin receptors and alpha-1 adrenergic receptors, respectively, which are present in vascular smooth muscle cells. In most studies, vasoconstrictors have been given in combination with intravenous (IV) albumin to further improve the arterial underfilling. Most of the published data comes from the use of IV terlipressin for Type 1 HRS.[39–51] Initial noncontrolled studies showed a response rate of 60–75%.[39–42] Results from two recent randomized, controlled studies and systematic reviews indicate that treatment with terlipressin together with albumin is associated with marked improvement of renal function in approximately 40–50% of patients[47–51] (Figure 4.3). Although there are no dose–efficacy studies, treatment is usually started with 0.5–1 mg/4–6 hours IV, and the dose is increased up to a maximum of

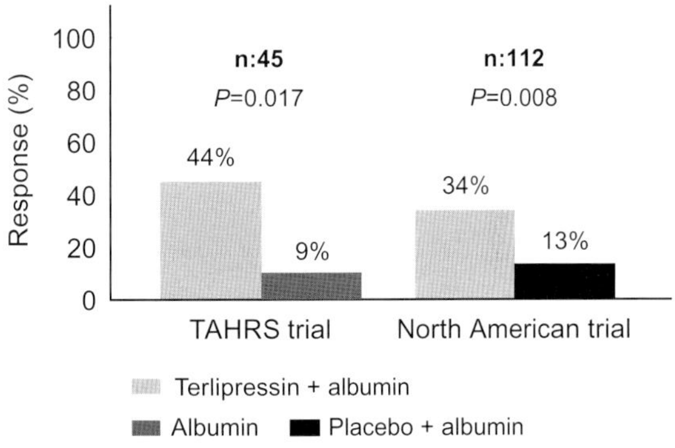

Figure 4.3 Data from two recent multicenter, randomized, controlled studies in patients with HRS receiving terlipressin and albumin. In the North American trial reversal of HRS was achieved in 34% in the terlipressin group vs 13% in the placebo group ($P = 0.008$). In the Terlipressin and Albumin for Hepatorenal Syndrome Study (TAHRS) trial, improvement of renal function occurred in 44% in the terlipressin group compared to 9% in the albumin alone group ($P < 0.05$). Adapted from Sanyal A, Boyer T, Garcia-Tsao G, et al. A prospective, randomized, double blind, placebo-controlled trial of terlipressin for type 1 hepatorenal syndrome (HRS). Gastroenterology 2008;134:1360–8, and Martin-Llahi M, Pepin MN, Guevara G, et al. Terlipressin and albumin vs albumin in patients with cirrhosis and hepatorenal syndrome: a randomized study. Gastroenterology 2008;134:1352–9)

2 mg/4–6 hours after 2 days if there is no response to therapy as defined by a reduction of serum creatinine >25% of pre-treatment values. Response to therapy is considered when there is marked reduction of the high serum creatinine levels, at least below 1.5 mg/dl, which is usually associated with increased urine output and improvement of hyponatremia. The incidence of ischemic side effects requiring the discontinuation of treatment is of approximately 10%. Some patients may develop transient pulmonary edema during the first few days of therapy. The two randomized studies described previously[47,48] have shown that the overall population of patients treated with terlipressin and albumin do not have an improved survival rate compared to that of patients treated with albumin alone. Both studies, however, showed that responders in terms of improvement of renal function after therapy had a significant (but moderate) increase in survival compared to nonresponders. In one study, patients who responded to therapy had a 3-month probability of survival of 58% vs 15% in those who did not respond to therapy (median survival >90 d vs 13 d, respectively, $P = 0.03$).[48] That said, the improvement in survival is subtle, meaning that responders still have a high risk of death while awaiting transplantation and therefore they should continue as priority candidates although their MELD score may decrease after therapy because of reduction in serum creatinine concentration. Factors associated with poor response include a bilirubin level ≥10 mg/dl, no increase in mean arterial pressure >5 mmHg or lack of a drop in serum creatinine >0.5 mg/dl at day 3 of therapy.[52] Alpha-adrenergic agonists (noradrenaline, midodrine) represent an attractive alternative to terlipressin because of low cost, wide availability, and apparently similar efficacy compared with that of terlipressin.[46,53–55] The information on the efficacy and side effects of alpha-adrenergic agonists in patients with Type 1 HRS is still very limited.

There is limited data on use of vasoconstrictors plus albumin for patients with Type 2 HRS. Data from uncontrolled studies suggest that they are effective in decreasing serum creatinine levels in these patients. In two controlled studies, patients with Type 2 HRS who received terlipressin plus albumin had a response between 67% and 88%, however few were treated with this strategy in both studies (n = 13) and therefore more controlled studies are needed in order to better define the role of vasoconstrictors plus albumin in the management of Type 2 HRS.[46,48]

Transjugular intrahepatic portosystemic shunts (TIPS)

Two uncontrolled studies indicate that TIPS may improve GFR as well as reduce the activity of the renin–angiotensin–aldosterone system and the sympathetic nervous system in approximately 60% of patients with Type 1 HRS.[56,57] A limitation of these studies is that they included patients with moderately severe liver failure and excluded those with a history of hepatic encephalopathy, Child–Pugh scores ≥12 or serum bilirubin >5 mg/dl. The applicability of TIPS in patients with Type 1 HRS is low because TIPS is considered contraindicated in patients with features of severe liver failure, which are common findings in the setting of Type 1 HRS. The use of TIPS in Type 2 HRS may improve renal function and reduce the risk of progression to Type 1 HRS, but these data would require confirmation in specifically designed studies.[58]

Renal replacement therapy and other dialysis methods

Renal replacement therapy (RRT), mainly hemodialysis, has been used in the management of patients with Type 1 HRS, especially in patients who are candidates for liver transplantation, in an attempt to maintain patients alive until liver transplantation is performed or spontaneous improvement in renal function occurs.[59] Unfortunately, the potential beneficial effect of this approach has not been demonstrated. Most patients develop side effects during RRT that include severe arterial hypotension, bleeding, and infections that may contribute to death during treatment. Additionally, indications for RRT (severe fluid overload, acidosis or hyperkalemia) are uncommon in Type 1 HRS, at least in the early stages. Other methods such as the use of the molecular readsorbent recirculating system (MARS), an alternative of dialysis that clears albumin-bound substances, including vasodilators, is promising but more data is needed in order to consider it as a therapeutic device for HRS.[60] The results of a recent study using another extracorporeal liver support system, Prometheus, suggests that this system may improve survival in patients with Type 1 HRS,[61] however these results require confirmation in larger studies.

Liver transplantation

OLT is the treatment of choice for patients with cirrhosis and HRS, either Type 1 or Type 2. A main limiting factor in LT for Type 1 HRS, however, is the high mortality rate in the waiting list due to the combination of short survival expectancy and prolonged waiting times in many transplant centers. This limitation can be overcome by assigning these patients a high priority for transplantation. The short survival rate of patients with Type 2 HRS (median 6 months) should also be taken into account when these patients are assessed for OLT. Although there is limited data, pharmacologic treatment of HRS before transplantation may improve outcome after transplantation.[62] In patients who respond to therapy with a fall in serum creatinine values, the subsequent decrease in the MELD score should not change the decision to perform liver transplantation since the prognosis after recovering from Type 1 HRS is still poor. Since cyclosporine and tacrolimus treatment may contribute to renal impairment postoperatively, these drugs should be not be given until renal function is within normal limits. Steroids, mycophenolate mofetil and IL-2 receptor antibodies (i.e. basilximab, daclizumab) should preferably be used until diuresis and improvement of renal function is observed, usually 5–7 days after transplantation.[20]

Management strategies when considering OLT in patients with HRS include OLT alone, SLK transplantation, OLT followed by kidney transplantation and reversal of HRS followed by OLT. Patients with HRS who undergo OLT alone usually require more days in the intensive care unit and longer hospitalizations compared to patients without HRS. Moreover, RRT requirements are high during the first weeks after LT, but decline thereafter, yet 10% of patients may need RRT after 6 weeks.[3,63] The long-term outcome for these patients is similar to that of patients without HRS.[3] Another approach that has been advocated for patients with HRS is SLK. Current criteria for SLK include established end-stage renal disease and dialysis, GFR <30 ml/min and proteinuria >3 g/d with 24-hour urine protein/creatinine ratio >3, and/or acute kidney injury and a requirement for dialysis for more than 6 weeks.[20] After the introduction of the MELD score system for organ allocation in the USA there has been an increase in the use of SLK for patients with cirrhosis and renal failure, which has been associated with a decline in survival after SLK compared to preceding years.[64–66] Moreover, the outcome of patients with HRS treated with SLK is not better than that of patients with HRS treated with LT alone.[64] In addition, this approach uses kidneys that could be used for patients with chronic renal failure without liver disease, who have prolonged waiting times for renal transplantation. All these factors, together with the fact that renal function in HRS patients usually recovers after LT alone, suggest that SLK is not a good approach for the management of patients with HRS. The only exception may be that of patients with HRS who meet the earlier mentioned criteria for SLK.[20,66] Performance of OLT alone followed by kidney transplantation, if necessary, has been advocated by some centers. With this approach, kidney transplantation is performed in patients who undergo LT for HRS and require RRT for more than 60 days after LT. Data on this approach is limited to only one study and thus more studies are needed in order to consider this strategy acceptable.[67] Finally, treatment of HRS with vasoconstrictors plus albumin while the patient is on the waiting list followed by LT is another approach commonly used in Europe. Since pre-transplant renal failure is an independent risk factor for both the short-term and long-term post-transplantation patient and graft survival, all effort should be made to improve renal function in order to obtain a better outcome after transplantation.[2] The reversal of both Types 1 and 2 HRS before transplantation may help patients not only to reach transplantation, but also to avoid the relatively high morbidity and mortality after LT characteristic of HRS. In a small study, therapy for patients with Type 1 HRS with terlipressin before LT led to excellent 3-year survival rates compared with those without HRS.[62] Data is however limited with regard to post-transplant outcomes; MELD scores may decrease with therapy and patients may experience side effects in 10% of cases, therefore more studies and a longer follow-up period are still needed to determine whether pre-OLT therapy for HRS actually will translate into better post-LT outcomes.

Summary

Renal failure is a common complication in patients with advanced cirrhosis awaiting transplantation. The most common causes include infection, hypovolemia, parenchymal diseases, HRS and drug-induced renal failure. Patients with cirrhosis develop renal failure due to a variety of clinical conditions, including gastrointestinal bleeding (with or without hypovolemic shock), diuretic therapy, bacterial infections (with or without septic shock), administration of certain types of drugs, particularly nonsteroidal anti-inflammatory drugs (NSAIDs), and intrinsic renal diseases, particularly glomerulonephritis associated with hepatitis B or C infection or alcoholic liver disease. An appropriate and extensive work-up of patients should be performed in order to establish the cause of renal failure before starting specific therapy. Successful treatment of renal failure with currently available therapies such as vasoconstrictors for HRS allows normalization of renal function in nearly 40% of patients before they reach transplantation, which likely benefits patients and may help improve the outcome after transplantation.

Acknowledgments

Part of the research reported in this article was funded by grants EC 07/90077 and FIS PI080126 from the Instituto de Salud Carlos III. CIBERHED is funded by the Instituto de Salud Carlos III.

Conflict of interest

Dr Andres Cárdenas is a consultant for Otsuka Pharmaceuticals and has been a consultant for Orphan Therapeutics and GlaxoSmithKline.

Dr Pere Ginès has been a consultant for Otsuka Pharmaceuticals and Orphan Therapeutics.

References

1. Ginès P, Cárdenas A, Schrier RW. Liver disease and the kidney. In: Schrier RW, editor. Diseases of the Kidney and Urinary Tract. 8th ed. Philadelphia: Lippincott Williams & Wilkins, 2007:2179–205.
2. Nair S, Verma S, Thuluvath PJ. Pretransplant renal function predicts survival in patients undergoing orthotopic liver transplantation. Hepatology 2002;35:1179–85.
3. Gonwa TA, Klintmalm GB, Levy M, Jennings LS, Goldstein RM, Husberg BS. Impact of pretransplant renal function on survival after liver transplantation. Transplantation 1995;59:361–5.
4. Wiesner R, Edwards E, Freeman R, et al. Model for end-stage liver disease (MELD) and allocation of donor livers. Gastroenterology 2003;124:91–6.
5. Kamath PS, Kim WR. The Model for End-stage Liver Disease (MELD). Hepatology 2007;45:797–805.
6. Weismuller TJ, Prokein J, Becker T, et al. Prediction of survival after liver transplantation by pre-transplant parameters. Scand J Gastroenterol 2008;43:736–46.
7. Salerno F, Gerbes A, Wong F, et al. Diagnosis, prevention and treatment of the hepatorenal syndrome in cirrhosis. A consensus workshop of the international ascites club. Gut 2007;56:1310–8.
8. Francoz C, Glotz D, Moreau R, Durand F. The evaluation of renal function and disease in patients with cirrhosis. J Hepatol 2010;52:605–13.
9. Sherman DS, Fish DN, Teitelbaum I. Assessing renal function in cirrhotic patients: problems and pitfalls. Am J Kidney Dis 2003;41:269–78.
10. Papadakis MA, Arieff AI. Unpredictability of clinical evaluation of renal function in cirrhosis. Prospective study. Am J Med 1987;82:945–52.
11. Caregaro L, Menon F, Angeli P, et al. Limitations of serum creatinine level and creatinine clearance as filtration markers in cirrhosis. Arch Int Med 1994;154:201–5.
12. Proulx NL, Akbari A, Garg AX, Rostom A, Jaffey J, Clark HD. Measured creatinine clearance from timed urine collections substantially overestimates glomerular filtration rate in patients with liver cirrhosis: a systematic review and individual patient meta-analysis. Nephrol Dial Transplant 2005;20:1617–22
13. Cockcroft DW, Gault MH. Prediction of creatinine clearance from serum creatinine. Nephron 1976;16:31–41.
14. Levey AS, Bosch JP, Lewis JB, Greene T, Rogers N, Roth D. A more accurate method to estimate glomerular filtration rate from serum creatinine: a new prediction equation. Modification of Diet in Renal Disease Study Group. Ann Int Med 1999;130:461–70.
15. Gonwa TA, Jennings L, Mai ML, Stark PC, Levey AS, Klintmalm GB. Estimation of glomerular filtration rates before and after orthotopic liver transplantation: evaluation of current equations. Liver Transplant 2004;10:301–9.
16. National Kidney Foundation. K/DOQI clinical practice guidelines for chronic kidney disease: evaluation,

classification and stratification. Am J Kidney Dis 2002;39(Suppl 1):S1–266.
17. Mehta RL, Kellum JA, Shah SV, et al. Acute Kidney Injury Network: report of an initiative to improve outcomes in acute kidney injury. Crit Care 2007;11:R31.
18. Martin-Llahi M, Guevara M, Torre A, et al. Prognostic importance of the cause of renal failure in patients with cirrhosis. Gastroenterology 2011;140:488–96.
19. Waikar SS, Bonventre JV. Biomarkers for the diagnosis of acute kidney injury. Nephron Clin Pract 2008;109: c192–7.
20. Charlton MR, Wall WJ, Ojo AO, et al. Report of the first international liver transplantation society expert panel consensus conference on renal insufficiency in liver transplantation. Liver Transpl 2009;15:S1–34.
21. Tandon P, Garcia-Tsao G. Bacterial infections, sepsis, and multiorgan failure in cirrhosis. Semin Liver Dis 2008;28:26–42.
22. Fasolato S, Angeli P, Dallagnese L, et al. Renal failure and bacterial infections in patients with cirrhosis: epidemiology and clinical features. Hepatology 2007; 45:223–9.
23. Fernández J, Navasa M, Gómez J, et al. Bacterial infections in cirrhosis: epidemiological changes with invasive procedures and norfloxacin prophylaxis. Hepatology 2002;35:140–8.
24. Acevedo J, Fernandez J, Castro M, et al. Current recommended empirical antibiotic therapy in patients with cirrhosis and bacterial infection. J Hepatol 2009;50:6A.
25. Arvaniti V, D'Amico G, Fede G, et al. Infections in patients with cirrhosis increase mortality 4-fold and should be used in determining prognosis. Gastroenterology 2010;139:1246–56.
26. Ginès P, Schrier RW. Renal failure in cirrhosis. N Engl J Med. 2009;361:1279–90.
27. Cárdenas A, Ginès P, Uriz J, et al. Renal failure after upper gastrointestinal bleeding in cirrhosis: incidence, clinical course, predictive factors, and short-term prognosis. Hepatology 2001;34:671–6.
28. Lhotta K. Beyond hepatorenal syndrome: glomerulonephritis in patients with liver disease. Semin Nephrol 2002;22:302–8.
29. Trawalé JM, Paradis V, Rautou PE, et al. The spectrum of renal lesions in patients with cirrhosis: a clinicopathological study. Liver Int. 2010;30:725–32.
30. Wadei HM, Geiger XJ, Cortese C, et al. Kidney allocation to liver transplant candidates with renal failure of undetermined etiology: role of percutaneous renal biopsy. Am J Transplant 2008;8:2618–26.
31. Salerno F, Gerbes A, Wong F, et al. Diagnosis, prevention and treatment of the hepatorenal syndrome in cirrhosis. A consensus workshop of the international ascites club. Gut 2007;56:1310–8.
32. Ginès P, Angeli P, Lenz K, et al. EASL Clinical Practice Guidelines. Management of ascites, spontaneous bacterial peritonitis and hepatorenal syndrome in cirrhosis. J Hepatol 2010;53:397–417.
33. Sort P, Navasa M, Arroyo V, et al. Effect of intravenous albumin on renal impairment and mortality in patients with cirrhosis and spontaneous bacterial peritonitis. N Engl J Med 1999;341:403–9.
34. Fernández J, Navasa M, Planas R, et al. Primary prophylaxis of spontaneous bacterial peritonitis delays hepatorenal syndrome and improves survival in cirrhosis. Gastroenterology 2007;133:818–24.
35. Salerno F, Badalamenti S. Drug induced renal failure in cirrhosis. In: Ginès P, Arroyo V, Rodes J, Schrier R, editors. Ascites and Renal Dysfunction in Liver Disease. 2nd ed. Oxford: Blackwell Publishing; 2005:372–82.
36. Pannu N, Nadim MK. An overview of drug-induced acute kidney injury. Crit Care Med 2008;36(Suppl): S216–23.
37. Tsai MH, Peng YS, Chen YC, et al. Adrenal insufficiency in patients with cirrhosis, severe sepsis and septic shock. Hepatology 2006;43:673–81.
38. Fernández J, Escorsell A, Zabalza M, et al. Adrenal insufficiency in patients with cirrosis and septic shock: Effect of treatment with hydrocortisone on survival. Hepatology 2006;44:1288–95.
39. Uriz J, Ginès P, Cardenas A, et al. Terlipressin plus albumin infusion: an effective and safe therapy of hepatorenal syndrome. J Hepatol 2000;33:43–8.
40. Moreau R, Durand F, Poynard T, et al. Terlipressin in patients with cirrhosis and type 1 hepatorenal syndrome: a retrospective multicenter study. Gastroenterology 2002;122:923–30.
41. Ortega R, Ginès P, Uriz J, et al. Terlipressin therapy with and without albumin for patients with hepatorenal syndrome. Efficacy and outcome. Hepatology 2002;36: 941–8.
42. Halimi C, Bonnard P, Bernard B. Effect of terlipressin (Glypressin) on hepatorenal syndrome in cirrhotic patients: results of a multicentre pilot study. Eur J Gastroenterol Hepatol 2002;14:153–8.
43. Solanki P, Chawla A, Garg R, et al. Beneficial effects of terlipressin in hepatorenal syndrome: a prospective, randomized placebo-controlled clinical trial. J Gastroenterol Hepatol 2003;18:152–6.
44. Neri S, Pulvirenti D, Malaguarnera M, et al. Terlipressin and albumin in patients with cirrhosis and type I hepatorenal syndrome. Dig Dis Sci 2008;53:830–5.
45. Triantos CK, Samonakis D, Thalheimer U, et al. Terlipressin therapy for renal failure in cirrhosis. Eur J Gastroenterol Hepatol 2010;22:481–6.
46. Alessandria C, Ottobrelli A, Debernardi-Venon W, et al. Noradrenalin vs terlipressin in patients with

hepatorenal syndrome: a prospective, randomized, unblinded, pilot study. J Hepatol 2007;47:499–505.
47. Sanyal A, Boyer T, Garcia-Tsao G, et al. A prospective, randomized, double blind, placebo-controlled trial of terlipressin for type 1 hepatorenal syndrome (HRS). Gastroenterology 2008;134:1360–8.
48. Martin-Llahi M, Pepin MN, Guevara G, et al. Terlipressin and albumin vs albumin in patients with cirrhosis and hepatorenal syndrome: a randomized study. Gastroenterology 2008;134:1352–9.
49. Gluud LL, Christensen K, Christensen E, Krag A. Systematic review of randomized trials on vasoconstrictor drugs for hepatorenal syndrome. Hepatology 2010;51:576–84.
50. Fabrizi F, Dixit V, Martin P. Meta-analysis: terlipressin therapy for the hepatorenal syndrome. Aliment Pharmacol Ther 2006;24:935–44.
51. Sagi SV, Mittal S, Kasturi KS, Sood GK. Terlipressin therapy for reversal of type 1 hepatorenal syndrome: a meta-analysis of randomized controlled trials. J Gastroenterol Hepatol 2010;25:880–5.
52. Nazar A, Pereira GH, Guevara M, et al. Predictors of response to therapy with terlipressin and albumin in patients with cirrhosis and type 1 hepatorenal syndrome. Hepatology 2010;51:219–26.
53. Angeli P, Volpin R, Gerunda G, et al. Reversal of type 1 hepatorenal syndrome with the administration of midodrine and octreotide. Hepatology 1999,29: 1690–7.
54. Wong F, Pantea L, Sniderman K. Midodrine, octreotide, albumin, and TIPS in selected patients with cirrhosis and type 1 hepatorenal syndrome. Hepatology 2004;40:55–64.
55. Duvoux C, Zanditenas D, Hezode C, et al. Effects of noradrenaline and albumin in patients with type 1 hepatorenal syndrome: a pilot study. Hepatology 2002;36: 374–80.
56. Brensing KA, Textor J, Perz J, et al. Long term outcome after transjugular intrahepatic portosystemic stent-shunt in non-transplant cirrhotics with hepatorenal syndrome: a phase II study. Gut 2000;47:288–95.
57. Guevara M, Ginès P, Bandi JC, et al. Transjugular intrahepatic portosystemic shunt in hepatorenal syndrome: effects on renal function and vasoactive systems. Hepatology 1998;28:416–22.
58. Ginès P, Uriz J, Calahorra B, et al. Transjugular intrahepatic portosystemic shunting versus paracentesis plus albumin for refractory ascites in cirrhosis. Gastroenterology 2002;123:1839–47
59. Wong LP, Blackley MP, Andreoni KA, et al. Survival of liver transplant candidates with acute renal failure receiving renal replacement therapy. Kidney Int 2005;68:362–70.
60. Bañares R, Nevens F, Larsen FS, et al. Extracorporeal liver support with the molecular adsorbent recirculating system (MARS) in patients with acute-on-chronic liver failure (AOCLF). The RELIEF Trial. J Hepatol 2010;52:1184A.
61. Rifai K, Kribben A, Gerken G, et al. Extracorporeal liver support by fractionated plasma separation and adsorption (Prometheus®) in patients with acute-on-chronic liver failure (Helios study): a prospective randomized controlled multicenter study. J Hepatol 2010;52:6A.
62. Restuccia T, Ortega R, Guevara M, et al. Effects of treatment of hepatorenal syndrome before transplantation on posttransplantation outcome. A case–control study. J Hepatol 2004;40:140–6.
63. Ruiz R, Kunitake H, Wilkinson AH, et al. Long-term analysis of combined liver and kidney transplantation at a single center. Arch Surg 2006;141:735–42.
64. Jeyarajah DR, Gonwa TA, McBride M, et al. Hepatorenal syndrome: combined liver kidney transplants versus isolated liver transplant. Transplantation 1997;64: 1760–5.
65. Locke JE, Warren DS, Singer AL, et al. Declining outcomes in simultaneous liver–kidney transplantation in the MELD era: ineffective usage of renal allografts. Transplantation 2008;85:935–42.
66. Eason JD, Gonwa TA, Davis CL, et al. Proceedings of Consensus Conference on Simultaneous Liver Kidney Transplantation (SLK). Am J Transplant 2008;8: 2243–51.
67. Ruiz R, Barri YM, Jennings LW, et al. Hepatorenal syndrome: a proposal for kidney after liver transplantation (KALT). Liver Transpl 2007;13:838–43.

5 Management of hepatopulmonary syndrome and portopulmonary hypertension

Victor I. Machicao and Michael B. Fallon

Division of Gastroenterology, Hepatology and Nutrition, Department of Internal Medicine, University of Texas Health Science Center at Houston, Houston, TX, USA

Key learning points

- It is important to be aware of the effects of hepatopulmonary syndrome (HPS) and portopulmonary hypertension (PPHTN) on the survival of cirrhotic patients.
- Pulse oximetry and contrast-enhanced transthoracic echocardiography play a key role in diagnostic screening for HPS in liver transplant candidates.
- Transthoracic Doppler echocardiography is an important tool for use in screening PPHTN in liver transplant candidates, requiring confirmation with right heart catheterization.
- It is important to know when liver transplantation can be carried out on patients with HPS and PPHTN, and to know the indications for the MELD exception for both conditions.

Hepatopulmonary syndrome

Hepatopulmonary syndrome (HPS) is characterized by an oxygenation defect induced by pulmonary vascular dilatation in the setting of liver disease. This syndrome is recognized in as many as 15–30% of patients with cirrhosis, and mortality in cirrhotics is significantly increased relative to cirrhotic patients without HPS. HPS may also present in patients in the absence of documentedcirrhosis or portal hypertension, for example, HPS has been associated with other chronic, and even acute liver conditions such as acute viral and hypoxic hepatitis. Liver transplantation (LT) is currently the only proven effective therapy for HPS, and it should be considered when severe hypoxemia is present.

The oxygenation defect in HPS is defined as an alveolar-arterial gradient ≥15 mmHg while breathing room air, or ≥20 mmHg in individuals 65 or older.[1] The presence of pulmonary vascular dilatation is documented by positive findings on contrast-enhanced transthoracic echocardiography (CE-TTE) and may be confirmed by abnormal uptake in the brain (>6%) with ^{99m}Tc-macroaggregated albumin radionuclide lung perfusion scan (MAA scan). A particular problem is that HPS may occur in patients with other cardiopulmonary conditions associated with hypoxemia and contribute significantly to gas exchange abnormalities in these patients.

Natural history

The natural history of HPS is incompletely characterized and derives largely from observational studies at large transplant centers, in which, deleterious effects on quality of life and survival have been well

Medical Care of the Liver Transplant Patient, Fourth Edition. Edited by Pierre-Alain Clavien, James F. Trotter.

described.[2] In patients with moderate to severe HPS with well-preserved hepatic synthetic function, the presence of HPS has been associated with poor outcomes.[2,3] In studies where CE-TTE has been done in cohorts of cirrhotic patients awaiting LT, 40–50% were found to have detectable intrapulmonary shunting but the majority are not hypoxemic, suggesting that mild intrapulmonary vasodilatation, insufficient to alter gas exchange, is common in cirrhotics.[4] The prevalence of HPS as previously defined, including mild stages, is approximately 15–30% in LT candidates.[5] The majority of HPS patients develop progressive intrapulmonary vasodilatation and worsening gas exchange over time, and spontaneous improvement is rare.[3] In one small cohort study of HPS patients, partial pressure of oxygen (PaO_2) declined in 85% of patients over time with an average decline of 5 mmHg per year.[3]

Mortality appears to be significantly increased in patients with HPS relative to unaffected cirrhotic patients.[3,5] Two single-center cohort studies and one prospective multi-center cohort study have evaluated the natural history and prognosis of HPS in cirrhotics. In the prospective single-center study, 111 patients with cirrhosis were evaluated, of whom 20 had HPS. The median survival rate was 4.8 and 35.2 months for patients with HPS and those without HPS who did not undergo LT, respectively.[5] Mortality remained higher in those with HPS after adjusting for the severity of liver disease. In patients with HPS, mortality largely resulted from complications of liver disease or portal hypertension, and correlated with the degree of hypoxemia. The second retrospective single-center study examined 61 patients with cirrhosis and HPS, 37 of whom did not undergo LT. Patients with HPS who did not undergo LT (n = 37) had a median survival of 24 months and a 5-year survival of 23%. In contrast, those without HPS who did not undergo LT (n = 47) had a median survival of 87 months and a 5-year survival of 63%.[3] It should, however, be noted that a subset of the HPS group not undergoing surgery were excluded from LT due to co-morbidities that may have influenced survival. Finally, in the prospective multi-center cohort study, mortality was doubled in cirrhotic patients with HPS being evaluated for LT compared to nonHPS cirrhotics (adjusted hazard ratio of 2.41) and was independent of age, MELD and co-morbidities.[2] Together, these data support that mortality in patients with cirrhosis not undergoing LT is significantly increased in those with HPS relative to those without HPS, and that the degree of hypoxemia and severity of hepatic dysfunction adversely influence outcome. Additional investigation is needed to precisely characterize the natural history of HPS and to define specific factors influencing mortality and LT candidacy in cirrhotics.

Diagnosis of HPS

The majority of patients with HPS are either asymptomatic or develop the insidious onset of dyspnea. Dyspnea while standing (platypnea) and hypoxemia exacerbated in the upright position (orthodeoxia) are characteristic but not pathognomonic features present in 25% of patients with HPS. Both of these clinical features are attributed to the predominance of the vasodilatation in the lung bases and the increased blood flow through these regions when assuming the upright position. Spider angioma, digital clubbing and cyanosis, are seen in advanced HPS, but are not specific. Significant sleep-time oxygen desaturation also appears to occur commonly in patients with HPS, even in patients with mild hypoxemia while awake.[6]

In potential LT candidates, regardless of the presence of symptoms, screening is important and cost effective. In this special population, it is particularly important to diagnose and characterize the severity of HPS early in the transplant evaluation process, given that the presence of this disorder may influence transplant candidacy, potential treatment before and after LT, and listing priority. However, there is currently significant variability in routine pre-transplant screening for cardiopulmonary disease between transplant centers. In addition, the spectrum of oxygenation abnormalities in HPS ranges from mild increases in the alveolar–arterial gradient to profound hypoxemia, so the target group for screening during LT evaluation is not clearly defined. In 2004, the European Respiratory Society Task Force proposed a classification of the severity of HPS, which is applicable to LT selection. This classification is based on the degree of hypoxemia on arterial blood gas separating patients in four categories according to severity: mild ($PaO_2 \geq 80$ mmHg), moderate ($PaO_2 \geq 60$ to <80 mmHg), severe ($PaO_2 \geq 50$ to <60 mmHg), and very severe ($PaO_2 < 50$ mmHg)[1].

From a practical standpoint, detecting all HPS patients with a resting $PaO_2 < 70$ mmHg during LT evaluation is a reasonable goal standard to identify patients who qualify for or may sufficiently deteriorate over a short time frame to be eligible for Model of End-stage Liver Disease (MELD) exception criteria. A cost-effective approach to identify clinically important HPS in LT candidates is to screen all patients with pulse oximetry to detect hypoxemia, and CE-TTE to detect intrapulmonary vasodilatation. Pulse oximetry was found to be an effective technique to screen for hypoxemia ($PaO_2 < 70$ mmHg) in patients with cirrhosis in a large prospective study of 200 LT candidates.[7] Using a pulse oximetry threshold value of ≤94% is highly sensitive and specific in detecting all HPS patients with a PaO_2 of <60 mmHg, and resulted in arterial blood gas testing in only 9% of the cohort. A more recent prospective study, using a pulse oximetry threshold value of <96% was highly sensitive (100%) and specific (88%) in detecting all HPS patients with a PaO_2 of <70 mmHg, and resulted in arterial blood gas testing in only 14% of the cohort.[8] CE-TTE is the most sensitive test to detect intrapulmonary vasodilatation, and has the additional advantage of commonly distinguishing intracardiac from intrapulmonary shunting and screening additionally for pulmonary hypertension. Agitated saline is the contrast agent used for CE-TTE. Delayed appearance of the microbubbles in the left cardiac chambers 3–6 cardiac cycles after administration is considered a positive test.[4] Immediate visualization of injected contrast in the left atrium indicates intracardiac right-to-left shunting.

If pulse oximetry reveals a value ≥96% and CE-TTE shows no intrapulmonary vasodilatation, then HPS is not present and patients may be re-evaluated in the future if symptoms develop. If oximetry is ≥96% and CE-TTE shows intrapulmonary vasodilatation, then yearly pulse oximetry surveillance to detect development of hypoxemia is undertaken. If oximetry is <96% and intrapulmonary vasodilatation is absent, then evaluation for other causes of hypoxemia is appropriate. If oximetry is <96% and CE-TTE shows intrapulmonary vasodilatation, then clinically significant HPS is likely and arterial blood gas and further testing are indicated to define the severity of HPS and exclude intrinsic cardiopulmonary disease, ascites or hepatic hydrothorax. If additional testing is negative and the PaO_2 is ≤60 mmHg, then a diagnosis of severe HPS warrants MELD exception in LT candidates. If HPS is less severe ($PaO_2 > 60$ mmHg), then interval arterial blood gas determinations to assess for progression are reasonable. If both hypoxemia and a positive CE-TTE are identified in the presence of significant intrinsic cardiopulmonary disease or fluid retention, then the severity of HPS may be difficult to gauge. In this setting, the MAA scan may be useful to define the contribution of HPS to the abnormal gas exchange.[9] In the MAA scan, macroaggregated albumin particles 20 µm in size are injected intravenously, which in normal circumstances are trapped in the pulmonary capillaries. In HPS patients these particles escape through abnormal capillaries and lodge in downstream capillary beds such as the brain, kidneys, liver, or spleen. Quantitative imaging of the brain allows the calculation of a shunt fraction. A positive MAA scan in the setting of coexisting intrinsic lung disease and hypoxemia suggests that HPS is a significant contributor to gas exchange abnormalities and may improve after LT. The shunt fraction can also be used to quantify intrapulmonary shunting.[4,9] Figure 5.1 summarizes our proposed algorithm for the screening for HPS in LT candidates.

Treatment of HPS

Currently, LT is the only effective treatment for patients with HPS.[10] In the largest single-center series, patients with HPS had a 5-year survival rate of 76% after LT, a rate comparable to patients without HPS.[3] There has been substantial evidence to support LT as an effective therapy for HPS, resulting in complete resolution or significant improvement in gas exchange in over 85% of patients. However, the length of time to normalization of arterial hypoxemia after transplantation is variable and may take longer than 1 year. A single prospective study has assessed the severity of HPS as a predictor of post-LT outcome in a cohort of 24 patients with HPS (overall mortality rate 29%). Post-LT mortality was significantly higher in severe HPS ($PaO_2 < 60$ mmHg), and was in part attributable to the development of unusual postoperative complications recognized in HPS patients, including pulmonary hypertension, cerebral embolic hemorrhages, and immediate postoperative hypoxemia requiring prolonged mechanical ventilation. The strongest predictor of mortality was a preoperative PaO_2 of ≤50 mmHg alone or in combination with a MAA scan shunt fraction ≥20%, in which case mortality was approximately 60%.[11] Two smaller

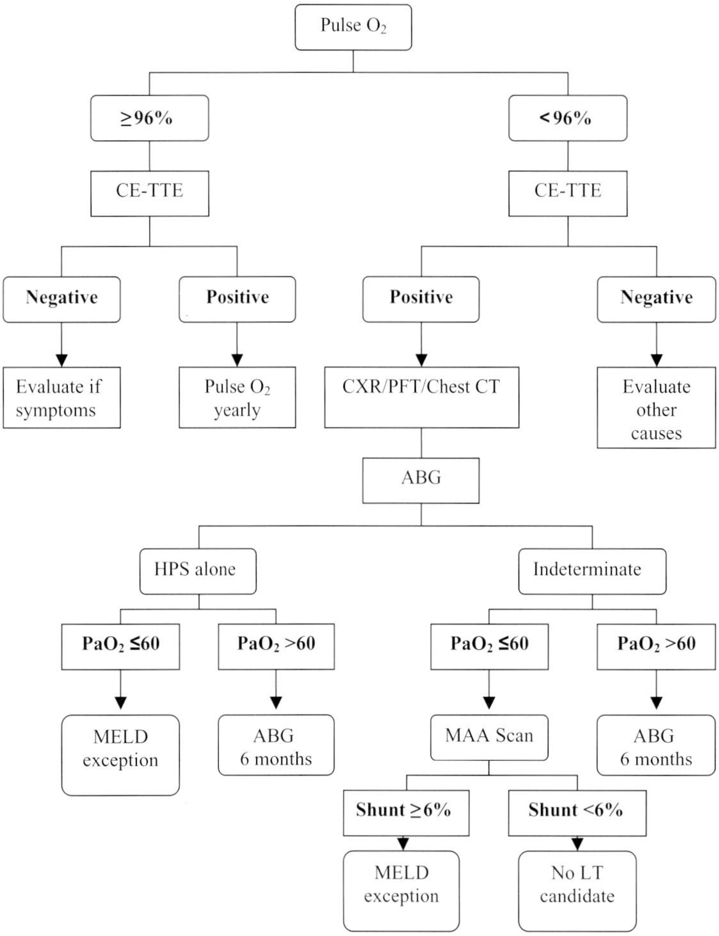

Figure 5.1 Screening and treatment for HPS in LT candidates. ABG: arterial blood gas; CE-TTE: contrast-enhanced transthoracic echocardiography; CXR: chest-x-ray; PFT: pulmonary function test; PaO_2: partial pressure of oxygen; MAA scan: 99mTc-macroaggregated albumin lung perfusion scan

prospective studies and three retrospective studies have also found increased postoperative mortality in severe HPS patients ranging from 21–50%. In contrast, a recent single-center study has found no increase in mortality after LT in HPS patients relative to nonHPS patients.[12] Based on this information the role of LT for patients with very severe HPS ($PaO_2 < 50$) remains under question. However, severity of preoperative hypoxemia and underlying liver disease appear to be factors that increase mortality.

No clearly effective medical therapy for HPS is available. Somatostatin, almitrine, indomethacin, inhaled nitric oxide, garlic preparation, aspirin, beta-blockers, and plasma exchange have all been tried without clear benefit. Two recent small case series have evaluated the effects of pentoxifylline in HPS. In one study, there was significant improvement in gas exchange and in the other the medication was poorly tolerated and gas exchange was unchanged.[13] Eight case reports have evaluated the effects of transjugular intrahepatic portosystemic shunt (TIPS) on HPS, however, the limited available data do not provide support for its use as a palliative strategy. In all patients with severe hypoxemia ($PaO_2 < 60$ mmHg) at rest or with exertion, the administration of supplemental oxygen is appropriate, based on the concept that the effect of chronic hypoxemia itself may contribute to mortality in HPS.[2] The efficacy and cost–benefit comparison for this regimen, however, have not been properly studied. The role of coil embolization during pulmonary angiography of large arteriovenous communications in the pulmonary circulation is limited since they are infrequently seen.

MELD exception and management after LT

The observations that HPS increases mortality without LT and that post-LT outcomes are worse in cases of severe HPS has led to the policy in US centers of assigning MELD exception points in the presence of severe hypoxemia ($PaO_2 < 60$) in order to facilitate LT and improve the outcome. In 2007, the United Network for Organ Sharing (UNOS)-sponsored MELD Exception Study Group (MESSAGE) recommended the assignment of a MELD score of 22 for the initial UNOS application of HPS patients meeting the criteria of severe hypoxemia. If the candidate's PaO_2 stays below 60 mmHg, he or she receives a 10% increase every 3 months. While significant data is available to support priority for patients with severe HPS,[2] a recent report using the UNOS data from the Scientific Registry of Transplant Recipients (SRTR) has found a significant pre-LT survival benefit advantage in patients receiving MELD exception for HPS compared with standard LT candidates.[14] It is important, however, to recognize the limitations of the UNOS data including lack of information on cardiopulmonary parameters, causes of death or relationships between outcome and oxygenation. In addition, no uniform HPS screening protocol is used across transplant centers. Most importantly, the current UNOS policy appears to have been successful in preventing HPS progression and increasing survival compared to findings of prior studies.

An area of debate concerning the current MELD exception policy for HPS includes the definition of a degree of severity of HPS at which LT should no longer be considered. Based on previously mentioned mortality data,[11] LT has been discouraged in patients with a preoperative PaO_2 of ≤50 mmHg, but there is no UNOS support for such a recommendation. Subjects with severe HPS who also have a minimal response to 100% inhaled oxygen ($PaO_2 < 100$ mmHg) might be expected to have poor oxygenation during the postoperative period, but this is a weak mortality predictor.[11] No study has addressed whether specific complications of cirrhosis (such as bleeding or spontaneous bacterial peritonitis) or rapid changes in hepatic synthetic function influence oxygenation in cirrhotic patients with HPS. Expanded prospective studies are needed to characterize the factors that influence post-LT outcomes in patients with severe HPS. Therefore, more information on oxygenation changes and on factors that influence HPS progression and outcome are needed to optimize allocation of MELD exception points and post-LT survival. Finally, a definition of such a cutoff should take into account the presence of co-morbidities since they may adversely influence the outcome during the often prolonged recovery phase following LT.

In patients with HPS who have undergone LT, the perioperative period may present particular clinical challenges. Worsening hypoxemia may occur in the early postoperative period and should be anticipated. Innovative approaches such as frequent body positioning or inhaled nitric oxide may be useful in improving gas exchange during this period. Since many patients with severe HPS who recover slowly have prolonged intensive care unit stays and unique postoperative complications, meticulous critical care, with particular attention to preventing infection, is an important goal. In the current authors' experience, two additional clinical considerations frequently arise in patients with severe hypoxemia in the early postoperative period. The first one is the continued use of aggressive diuresis to treat hypoxemia due to HPS after having accounted for perioperative fluid accumulation and shifts. In this situation, pre-renal azotemia and thickened respiratory secretions with the development of mucus plugging have occurred and may prolong intensive care unit stays. A second common scenario is the continuation of mechanical ventilation for hypoxemia, related to persistent intrapulmonary vasodilatation, in HPS patients otherwise recovering well after LT. Early extubation and administration of maximal oxygen concentrations may decrease complications related to prolonged ventilation and intensive care unit stays in these patients.

Portopulmonary hypertension

The association between pulmonary arterial hypertension and portal hypertension was originally described by Mantz and Craige in 1951. More recently, portal hypertension has been recognized as a common secondary cause of pulmonary arterial hypertension. Portopulmonary hypertension (PPHTN) is a specific entity characterized by pulmonary hypertension in association with portal hypertension, with or without advanced liver disease.

PPHTN has been defined by the European Respiratory Society Task Force in 2004 as a mean pulmonary arterial pressure (mPAP) of >25 mmHg at rest, or >30 mmHg during exercise; a mean pulmonary artery occlusion pressure (mPAOP) of <15 mmHg; and an elevated pulmonary vascular resistance (PVR) of >240 dyn/s/cm^{-5} occurring in the setting of portal hypertension.[1] This definition is consistent with the diagnostic criteria for pulmonary arterial hypertension as defined by the World Health Organization. Therefore, mild to moderate elevation in mPAP without pulmonary vascular remodeling (normal PVR), which is seen in up to 20% of cirrhotics with portal hypertension and results from increased cardiac output or blood volume, is not included in this definition. The presence of portal hypertension may be manifested by esophageal or gastric varices, thrombocytopenia, splenomegaly, or portosystemic shunts, and can be confirmed by hemodynamic measurements. Cirrhosis itself is not necessary for the development of PPHTN, as prehepatic portal hypertension may also be associated with the development of PPHTN without cirrhosis.

The severity of PPHTN is graded according to the elevation in mPAP in three categories: mild or early (mPAP >25 and <35 mmHg), moderate (mPAP ≥ 35 and <45 mmHg), and severe (mPAP ≥ 45 mmHg). Patients with moderate and severe PPHTN (mPAP ≥ 35 mmHg) appear to have higher operative mortality and are targeted for medical therapy.[15]

Epidemiology and natural history

PPHTN occurs most commonly in patients with cirrhosis of any etiology and portal hypertension, but it is also seen in portal hypertension without cirrhosis. This observation supports the concept that portal hypertension is the predisposing condition. An autopsy study performed almost 30 years ago, revealed pathologic features of pulmonary hypertension in 0.73% of cirrhotics as compared with 0.13% of those without cirrhosis. Several retrospective series in patients referred for LT have found a prevalence of PPHTN of 6–16%.[10] The high prevalence found in LT candidates by some authors, however, may be related to the use of echocardiography for PPHTN diagnosis, without right heart catheterization for confirmation. The most comprehensive study diagnosing PPHTN in LT candidates with right heart catheterization found a prevalence of 6%.[16]

Generally, the diagnosis of PPHTN is made on average 4–7 years after the recognition of portal hypertension. Although there are no definitive clinical predictors of PPHTN in patients with portal hypertension, a recent multicenter study has found that female sex and a diagnosis of autoimmune hepatitis increase the risk for developing PPHTN between patients with portal hypertension, and a lower risk is seen in patients with hepatitis C as the etiology of liver disease.[17] A single study has identified a higher prevalence of PPHTN in patients with cirrhosis complicated by refractory ascites. Otherwise, the prevalence and severity of PPHTN do not appear to correlate with the degree of hepatic synthetic dysfunction or the severity of portal hypertension. The placement of a portosystemic shunt does not seem to increase the risk of PPHTN.

PPHTN may be complicated by the development of progressive right ventricular dysfunction and eventual cor pulmonale as well as by the complications inherent to the cirrhosis and portal hypertension. Survival in pulmonary hypertension correlates with the severity of right-sided cardiac dysfunction, as assessed by the degree of elevation in the right-sided cardiac pressures and the degree of decline in cardiac output. The cardiac index appears to be the most significant prognostic variable. The survival rate in patients with PPHTN is poor, with a reported mortality rate of 15–50% at 1 year and 50–70% at 5 years.[15,18] The survival rate in PPHTN also appears to be worse than in primary pulmonary hypertension (PPH) and correlates with the presence and severity of cirrhosis.[18] This association may be explained in part by the exacerbation of portal hypertension caused by elevated right-sided cardiac pressure. Causes of mortality in PPHTN are equally related to the progression of liver cirrhosis and pulmonary hypertension with right-sided heart failure.

Diagnosis of PPHTN

Dyspnea on exertion is the most common symptom upon diagnosis in patients with PPHTN. Fatigue, orthopnea, chest pain, peripheral edema, syncope, and dyspnea at rest may develop as the disease progresses. Initial symptoms of PPHTN are subtle and many patients may be asymptomatic.[16] Elevated jugular venous pressure, a loud pulmonic component of the second heart sound, a systolic murmur resulting from tricuspid regurgitation, and lower extremity edema are common features of PPH but their frequency in PPHTN are not well defined. Therefore, patients with portal hypertension and dyspnea require a thorough cardiopulmonary evaluation. Similarly, patients with portal hypertension undergoing LT evaluation should be carefully screened for the presence of PPHTN, since they may be asymptomatic. Other causes of dyspnea in patients with cirrhosis and portal hypertension, including intrinsic lung disease, HPS, muscle wasting, ascites, hepatic hydrothorax, and deconditioning should be considered when the diagnosis of PPHTN is entertained. In addition, other causes of elevated pulmonary pressures and/or right heart failure, including left ventricular dysfunction, volume overload, and chronic obstructive lung disease, may present with clinical features similar to those of PPHTN.

Radiographic findings are generally subtle, but in advanced cases a prominent main pulmonary artery or cardiomegaly due to prominent right cardiac chambers may be appreciated. Electrocardiographic abnormalities seen in patients with pulmonary hypertension may also be present in PPHTN, and consist of right atrial enlargement, right ventricular hypertrophy, right axis deviation, and/or right bundle branch block. Pulmonary function tests commonly show reduced lung volumes, forced vital capacity, and diffusing capacity for carbon monoxide. Gas exchange abnormalities are generally mild and less severe than in HPS. An increased alveolar-arterial gradient with mild hypoxemia and hypocarbia may be seen, particularly in severe disease. A recent small retrospective analysis documented nocturnal oxygen desaturation in patients with moderate to severe PPHTN, which was unrelated to lung function or sleep apnea, suggesting the need for overnight screening and oxygen supplementation in those patients with moderate to severe PPHTN.[19]

Because patients with PPHTN may be asymptomatic and the diagnostic utility of various clinical features is low, the diagnosis requires a high index of suspicion. In general, in patients not being evaluated for liver transplantation, the presence of "compatible" symptoms and signs, in the absence other cardiopulmonary disease signals the need for screening for PPHTN. In all patients being evaluated for LT, regardless of signs or symptoms, screening is warranted because the presence of PPHTN may influence transplant candidacy.[20] Transthoracic Doppler echocardiography (TDE) is the best noninvasive screening study to detect PPHTN. This study allows the estimation of the right ventricular systolic pressure (RVSP) using the Bernoulli's equation, based on the interrogation of the velocity of the tricuspid regurgitant jet, when present, and an assumed right atrial pressure. In the absence of significant pulmonary artery stenosis, pulmonary artery systolic pressure is extrapolated from this measurement. Therefore, the estimated RVSP correlates well with the systolic pulmonary artery pressure and allows a valid estimation of the mPAP. TDE may also show pulmonic insufficiency, right ventricular hypertrophy, dilatation and dysfunction, and right atrial enlargement in patients with PPHTN. Left-sided valvular abnormalities or left ventricular dysfunction make PPHTN much less likely. Significant left atrial enlargement may also imply chronically increased left ventricular end-diastolic pressure. An additional advantage of TDE is that screening for HPS and PPHTN can be accomplished at the same time if combined with intravenous contrast injection.

Several studies have evaluated the utility of estimated RVSP measurements in the diagnosis of PPHTN. A retrospective analysis showed that an estimated RVSP of >50 mmHg identified essentially all patients who should proceed to right-heart catheterization. A prospective study of LT candidates who underwent TDE and cardiac catheterization measurements revealed sensitivity and specificity of 100% and 96%, respectively, and positive and negative predictive values of 59% and 100%, respectively. The prevalence of elevated estimated RVSP in LT candidates has been estimated to be around 18%.[16] The precise methods for estimating RVSP, however, are not standardized between centers and impact the operating characteristics of TDE screening. Variability in the assumptions and measurements that are necessary to calculate RVSP may contribute substantially to the performance of TDE as an adequate screening test and to institutional differences in the threshold value for suspecting PPHTN. The most common causes for a false-positive TDE are elevated pulmonary venous pressures due to the hyperdynamic circulatory state of cirrhosis and volume overload.[16]

In general, either an estimated RVSP of >40–50 mmHg or the presence of right ventricular abnormalities are sensitive criteria for PPHTN. Most importantly, the absence of both findings effectively rules out significant PPHTN at that evaluation, therefore TDE is the screening test of choice for LT candidates. Patients listed for LT without evidence of PPHTN, should undergo TDE annually. Those patients with documented PPHTN may require closer follow up with TDE every 6 months, however no study has validated these time intervals for wide recommendation. A proposed algorithm for the screening of PPHTN in transplant candidates is depicted in Figure 5.2.

Right-heart catheterization is required for the definitive diagnosis of PPHTN. Patients with suggestive TDE findings should undergo right-heart catheterization to confirm elevated mPAP and to exclude pulmonary venous hypertension. Direct measurement of pulmonary artery pressures, including mPAP, mPAOP, cardiac output, and calculation of systemic and PVR should be done. Responsiveness to a number of vasodilator agents, most frequently nitric oxide and/or epoprostenol, may be measured in those with confirmed PPHTN in an effort to predict a favorable response to long-term vasodilator therapy. Although up to 50% of patients with PPHTN have an acute response to vasodilators, the utility of this finding in predicting long-term response or outcomes is not established.

The performance of right-sided cardiac catheterization also allows accurate classification of patients with chronic liver disease and elevated estimated RVSP in into one of three categories.[1] First, up to

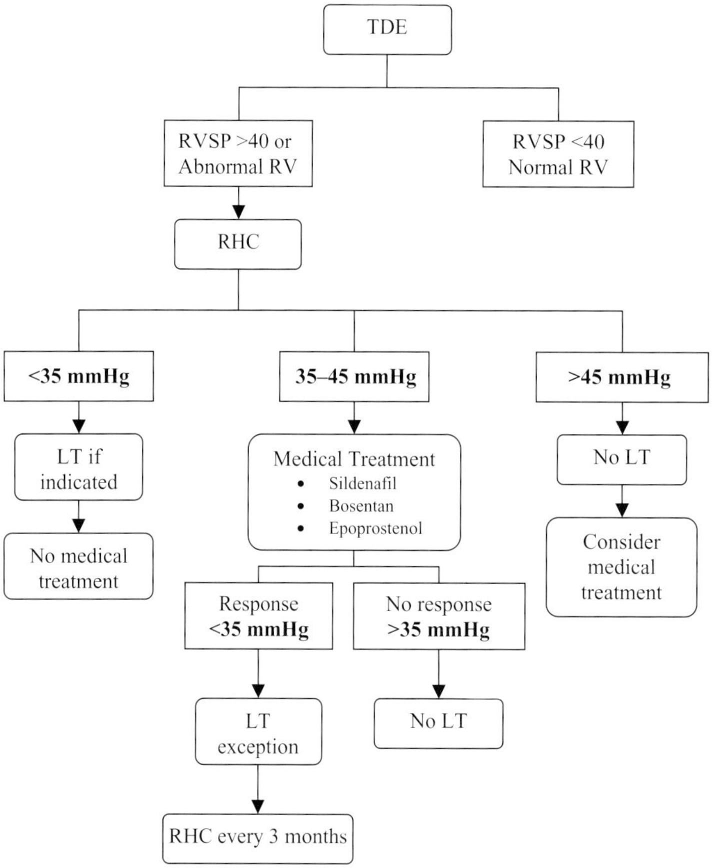

Figure 5.2 Screening and treatment for PPHTN in LT candidates. TDE: transthoracic Doppler echocardiography; RVSP: right ventricular systolic pressure; RV: right ventricle; LT: liver transplantation; RHC: right-heart catheterization

50% of patients with elevated RVSP have the hemodynamic features of PPHTN with markedly increased mPAP, PVR and cardiac output. Second, up to 20% of patients with an elevated RVSP have a pure hyperdynamic circulatory state on cardiac catheterization, characterized by increased cardiac output, with a mild elevation in mPAP, usually <35 mmHg. In this group there is a mild decrease in the PVR and mPAOP, consistent with a passive distention of pulmonary vessels. Finally, a third group comprising up to 25% of those with elevated RVSP have increased pulmonary venous volume. This group is characterized by an increase in volume and/or pressure increase due to a limitation in pulmonary blood flow to the left atrium because of left ventricular dysfunction. This results in a severe increase in the mPAOP, with a moderate increase in mPAP. This third hemodynamic presentation is more commonly seen in alcoholic cirrhosis, familial amyloidosis and liver–kidney failure patients.

Treatment

There are no consensus guidelines for the treatment of PPHTN. No study has demonstrated that medical therapy alone for PPHTN improves survival, although combined medical therapy and LT has the potential to improve outcomes in selected patients and should be studied in clinical trials.[20] Medical treatment for PPHTN is based largely on experience in PPH. The treatment of patients with mild PPHTN (mPAP <35 mmHg) remains controversial. Most of these patients have symptomatic cirrhosis but no symptoms attributable to PPHTN and LT outcomes do not appear to be influenced by the presence of PPHTN.[18] This group of patients has not been formally studied in a prospective fashion, and therefore no solid treatment recommendations are available. On the contrary, patients with moderate to severe PPHTN appear to have significantly increased mortality after LT and may benefit from treatment directed toward lowering mPAP and PVR, and improving symptoms.[15]

Oral anticoagulation, a common intervention in patients with PPH, is not recommended in PPHTN because of the potentially increased risk of bleeding in the presence of thrombocytopenia, coagulopathy, and varices. This concern, however, is based on anecdotal experience and no studies have addressed the role of anticoagulation in patients with PPHTN. Diuretics are often required to control fluid retention in cirrhosis and portal hypertension, and also for the symptomatic control of right-sided heart failure due to PPHTN. However, diuretics should be used carefully in PPHTN, as intravascular volume depletion may critically reduce the cardiac output by decreasing right ventricular preload.

Treatment with vasodilators is the mainstay of therapy and can reverse the vasoconstriction associated with PPH, but may have less or little effect on the fibrotic and proliferative remodeling changes present in PPHTN. In PPH, the administration of calcium channel blockers improves cardiac hemodynamics due to its vasodilator effect, but they are not recommended in PPHTN due to the potential for increasing the hepatic venous pressure gradient. The use of beta-adrenergic blockers in patients with PPHTN remains a controversial issue. Beta-blockers are commonly used in patients with portal hypertension with large esophageal or gastric varices for both primary and secondary prophylaxis of variceal bleeding. In a single short-term study in patients with moderate to severe PPHTN, the use of beta-blockers was associated with significant worsening of exercise capacity and pulmonary hemodynamics.[21] Discontinuation of beta-blockers improved cardiac output with no change on mPAP, resulting in a net decrease on PVR. Based on these findings, the use of beta-blockers in patients with moderate to severe PPHTN needs to be carefully considered. An alternative option for bleeding prophylaxis in this group of patients is the use of endoscopic variceal banding.

Epoprostenol is a potent pulmonary and systemic vasodilator and platelet aggregation inhibitor that results in clinical improvement and increased survival in PPH, and is useful as a bridge to lung transplantation. Several studies and case reports using continuous epoprostenol infusion in PPHTN support its role in improving pulmonary hemodynamics and exercise capacity.[22] No randomized, controlled trial, however, has been performed in PPHTN. Recent case series of patients with moderate to severe PPHTN who had a significant reduction in mPAP when treated with intravenous epoprostenol, and subsequently underwent a successful LT, have been reported.[22] A survival advantage has not been documented with such an approach and reversibility of PPHTN was not clearly established. Complications of intravenous epoprostenol remain an important limiting factor, including central venous catheter thrombosis, infection, and infusion pump failure. Patients may also develop profound thrombocytopenia and splenomegaly, although most frequently without clinical significance. Two newer prostacyclin analogs – treprostinil, given as an intravenous or subcutaneous infusion and iloprost, given by inhalation, are easier to administer and may be equally useful to improve pulmonary hemodynamics in PPHTN.[23,24]

Endothelin receptor antagonists are a newer class of orally administered agents used in PPH, which may also be useful in patients with PPHTN. Bosentan is a dual nonselective endothelin receptor antagonist that blocks both the endothelin A and B receptors, mitigating the vasoconstrictor effect of endothelin-1. Several case reports and small series have described its use in PPHTN to improve pulmonary hemodynamics,[23] however this agent may increase liver enzymes and bilirubin in up to 10% of patients, by inhibiting hepatocyte bile acid transport, and may lower systemic blood pressure. The safety of this agent in advanced cirrhosis is not fully established. Ambrisentan is a selective endothelin receptor A antagonist that also appears to be effective and well tolerated in PPH, but its role on PPHTN remains undefined.

Finally, recent case series support a role for sildenafil, a phosphodiesterase-5 inhibitor, in PPHTN management. In patients with PPHTN, sildenafil improves cardiac output and decreases pulmonary artery pressures and PVR without serious adverse effects.[25] There are concerns, however, regarding potential exacerbation of portal hypertension associated with its use. The safety and efficacy of these newer agents, alone or in combination, has not been studied in randomized, controlled studies for PPHTN.

LT may be beneficial in highly selected patients with PPHTN, although its use and efficacy remain controversial. Based on retrospective and clinical experience, severe PPHTN (mPAP >45 mmHg) is a contraindication to transplantation due to a perioperative mortality rate of 40% and lack of reversibility of pulmonary hypertension.[20] Patients with mild PPHTN (mean pulmonary artery pressure <35 mmHg) appear to have no increased risk of perioperative cardiopulmonary mortality after LT, although long-term outcomes have not been reported. Recent case series have reported favorable short-term outcomes after LT in patients with moderate PPHTN who respond to medical therapy achieving a mPAP <35 mmHg,[10,15] however, the percentage of patients with PPHTN who improve significantly to undergo LT and how often PPHTN reverses in this situation is not well defined.

Recently, UNOS recommended the assignment of a MELD score of 22 for the initial UNOS application of PPHTN patients meeting the following criteria: elevated initial mPAP and PVR levels, documentation of vasodilator treatment, and post-treatment mPAP <35 mmHg and PVR <400 dyn/s/cm^{-5}. The MELD score may be increased by 10% every 3 months requiring documentation by cardiac catheterization of the already mentioned hemodynamic measurements. Although case reports have demonstrated a successful outcome after combination lung–liver or heart–lung–liver transplantation, limited organ availability and the technical challenges limit the feasibility of such approaches for PPHTN.

Abbreviations

CE-TTE: contrast-enhanced transthoracic echocardiography, HPS: hepatopulmonary syndrome, LT: liver transplantation, MAA scan: ^{99m}Tc-macroaggregated albumin lung perfusion scan, MELD: Model for End-stage Liver Disease, mPAOP: mean pulmonary artery occlusion pressure, mPAP: mean pulmonary artery pressure, PaO_2: partial pressure of oxygen, PPHTN: portopulmonary hypertension, PVR: pulmonary vascular resistance, PPH: primary pulmonary hypertension, RVSP: right ventricular systolic pressure, TDE: transthoracic Doppler echocardiography, UNOS: United Network for Organ Sharing.

References

1. Rodriguez-Roisin R, Krowka MJ, Herve P, Fallon MB. ERS Task Force Pulmonary-Hepatic Vascular Disorders Scientific Committee. Pulmonary-Hepatic Vascular Disorders (PHD). Eur Respir J 2004;24:861–80.
2. Fallon MB, Krowka MJ, Brown RS, et al. Impact of hepatopulmonary syndrome on quality of life and survival in liver transplant candidates. Gastroenterology 2008;135:1168–75.
3. Swanson KL, Wiesner RH, Krowka MJ. Natural history of hepatopulmonary syndrome: Impact of liver transplantation. Hepatology 2005;41:1122–9.

4. Abrams GA, Jaffe CC, Hoffer PB, Binder HJ, Fallon MB. Diagnostic utility of contrast echocardiography and lung perfusion scan in patients with hepatopulmonary syndrome. Gastroenterology 1995;109:1283–8.
5. Schenk P, Schöniger-Hekele M, Fuhrmann V, Madl C, Silberhumer G, Muller C. Prognostic significance of the hepatopulmonary syndrome in patients with cirrhosis. Gastroenterology. 2003;125:1042–52.
6. Palma DT, Phillips GM, Arguedas MR, Harding SM, Fallon MB. Oxygen desaturation during sleep in hepatopulmonary syndrome. Hepatology 2008;47: 1257–63.
7. Abrams GA, Sanders MK, Fallon MB. Utility of pulse oximetry in the detection of arterial hypoxemia in liver transplant candidates. Liver Transpl 2002;8:391–6.
8. Arguedas M, Singh H, Faulk D, Fallon MB. Utility of pulse oximetry screening for hepatopulmonary syndrome. Clin Gastroenterol Hepatol 2007;5:749–54.
9. Abrams GA, Nanda NC, Dubovsky EV, Krowka MJ, Fallon MB. Use of macroaggregated albumin lung perfusion scan to diagnose hepatopulmonary syndrome: a new approach. Gastroenterology 1998;114:305–10.
10. Krowka MJ, Mandell MS, Ramsay MA, et al. Hepatopulmonary syndrome and portopulmonary hypertension: a report of the multicenter liver transplant database. Liver Transpl 2004;10:174–82.
11. Arguedas MR, Abrams GA, Krowka MJ, Fallon MB. Prospective evaluation of outcomes and predictors of mortality in patients with hepatopulmonary syndrome undergoing liver transplantation. Hepatology 2003; 37:192–7.
12. Gupta S, Castel H, Rao RV, et al. Improved survival after liver transplantation in patients with hepatopulmonary syndrome. Am J Transplant 2009;10:354–63.
13. Tanikella R, Philips GM, Faulk DK, Kawut SM, Fallon MB. Pilot study of pentoxifylline in hepatopulmonary syndrome. Liver Transpl 2008;14:1199–203.
14. Sulieman BM, Hunsicker LG, Katz DA, Voigt MD. OPTN policy regarding prioritization of patients with hepatopulmonary syndrome: does it provide equitable organ allocation? Am J Transplant 2008;8:954–64.
15. Swanson KL, Wiesner RH, Nyberg SL, Rosen CB, Krowka MJ. Survival in portopulmonary hypertension: Mayo Clinic experience categorized by treatment subgroups. Am J Transplant 2008;8:2445–53.
16. Colle IO, Moreau R, Godinho E, et al. Diagnosis of portopulmonary hypertension in candidates for liver transplantation: a prospective study. Hepatology 2003; 37:401–9.
17. Kawut SM, Krowka MJ, Trotter JF, et al. Clinical risk factors for portopulmonary hypertension. Hepatology 2008;48:196–203.
18. Kawut SM, Taichman DB, Ahya VN, et al. Hemodynamics and survival of patients with portopulmonary hypertension. Liver Transpl 2005;11: 1107–11.
19. Halank M, Langner S, Kolditz M, Miehlke S, Höffken G. Nocturnal oxygen desaturation is a frequent complication in portopulmonary hypertension. Z Gastroenterol 2008;46:1260–5.
20. Krowka MJ, Plevak DJ, Findlay JY, Rosen CB, Wiesner RH, Krom RA. Pulmonary hemodynamics and perioperative cardiopulmonary-related mortality in patients with portopulmonary hypertension undergoing liver transplantation. Liver Transpl 2000;6:443–50.
21. Provencher S, Herve P, Jais X, et al. Deleterious effects of beta-blockers on exercise capacity and hemodynamics in patients with portopulmonary hypertension. Gastroenterology 2006;130:120–6.
22. Fix OK, Bass NM, De Marco T, Merriman RB. Long-term follow-up of portopulmonary hypertension: effect of treatment with epoprostenol. Liver Transpl 2007;13:875–85.
23. Hoeper MM, Seyfarth HJ, Hoeffken G, et al. Experience with inhaled iloprost and bosentan in portopulmonary hypertension. Eur Respir J 2007;30:1096–102.
24. Melgosa MT, Ricci GL, García-Pagan JC, et al. Acute and long-term effects of inhaled iloprost in portopulmonary hypertension. Liver Transpl 2010;16:348–56.
25. Reichenberger F, Voswinckel R, Steveling E, et al. Sildenafil treatment for portopulmonary hypertension. Eur Respir J 2006;28:563–7.

6 Psychiatric and substance abuse evaluation of the potential liver transplant recipient

Thomas P. Beresford

Department of Veterans Affairs Medical Center, Denver, CO, and School of Medicine University of Colorado, Aurora, CO, USA

Key learning points

- The sources of clinical history include the patient and a required, corroborating third person.
- The examination will cover both the basic and complex principles of cognition.
- An alcohol/substance use diagnosis must be made, differentiating dependence vs abuse, and primary alcohol dependence vs polysubstance dependence.
- The patient's ambivalence to following recommendations in primary alcohol use disorders must be assessed.
- There are various methods to use to measure social stability, a necessary determinant.
- Vaillant's factors for assessing abstinence prognosis can help to determine the patient's compliance with recommendations given to them.

Clinical art and science in candidate evaluation

A computer-based search of the medical literature on the topic of this chapter yields a series of relatively recent review publications that discuss evaluation,[1–5] all of them encyclopedic in their approach, presenting many lists of possible psychiatric phenomena that the liver transplant team may encounter and should attend to. The lists contradict each other on some points and they refer most often to cross-section studies and to naturalistic outcome studies as their scientific base. The phrase "controlled clinical trial," or its analogues, is conspicuously absent and most of the reference lists fall well short of a comprehensive record of the available literature on the topic.

Were the novice, or even the experienced, evaluator of liver transplant candidates to base the clinical interview on the information in these articles, it would be as if on a sailboat with lots of canvas and no rudder, changing direction with the force of one or another breeze of clinical fashion. This is not to criticize encyclopedic reviews since comprehensiveness is their aim; rather it is to say that the actual process of a clinical evaluation requires less the approach of the encyclopedist and more that of the physician applying the art and science of medicine, both at the same time. Put simply, what does the evaluating psychiatrist actually *do* when the patient, and in this case a family member or significant other person, walks in the door, and how do they go about doing it? This chapter aims at answering that question in as clear a manner as possible and with reference to the encyclopedias as necessary. If the medical professionals who read this chapter come away with a clinical sense of how to approach an often difficult task, it will have accomplished its primary goal.

Medical Care of the Liver Transplant Patient, Fourth Edition. Edited by Pierre-Alain Clavien, James F. Trotter.

The description will focus principally on alcohol dependence (AD) since this is by far the most frequent of the psychiatric disorders that present to the liver teams and because it best illustrates the approach to other substance use disorders. The discussion will consider two general areas: 1) diagnosis, including particularly relevant points in the history and examination, and 2) prognosis, in some ways the most difficult part of the evaluation and yet the most pressing where allocating the precious resource of a liver graft is concerned.

Format and setting

With two specific changes derived from the experience of providing psychiatric evaluations in this setting, the standard medical history format continues to serve both patient and clinician well. It is the format most familiar across medical and health disciplines and it is that in use by most large health care systems, such as the US Department of Veterans Affairs, that require a central approval based on clinical assessments done locally. The clinical document begins by listing identifying data and occasions the first change in standard format.

Patient and Other Third Party

Traditionally, the clinical history derives from the patient himself and identifies only that person. In the setting of liver transplant, however, candidates present with a high frequency of lifetime alcohol or drug abuse, and current diagnostic manuals list both as psychiatric disorders.[6,7] The presence of a third party, usually a spouse or significant other person who knows and frequently sees the patient, constitutes an absolute requirement. Until the spouse or significant other attends the evaluation in person with both psychiatrist and patient present, the evaluation remains incomplete. The identifying data then includes mention of the third person, as in "John Jones is a 47-year-old male accompanied by his wife, Sally Jones, aged 39 years."

The absolute requirement of a third party serves three purposes 1) corroboration, 2) gauging social stability, 3) establishing the drug use setting, each of which will be discussed in turn.

Corroboration

Through the course of the interview, the evaluator can gather information from the candidate and then turn to a third party and say "Does this match your recollection?" For example, when proceeding through a list of alcohol withdrawal symptoms, a patient may describe only rare tremor while the spouse remarks, "His hands shook every morning."

Social stability

The spouse or other third party functions as the key individual in pre- and post-liver graft care, as discussed in further detail later. Their participation in the interview allows assessment of how stable and knowledgeable that social setting is for a graft recipient who will likely ever after require attention to immunosuppressant medication.

Alcohol/drug use setting

It is not uncommon for patient–other dyads to share pathologic alcohol or other drug-use activities. Evaluating this concern generally fits best when the interviewer goes over alcohol and drug use questions with the patient, includes third party corroboration questions, and then can easily extend them to include the use patterns of the third party. In most cases a screen instrument, such as the CAGE or T-ACE[8,9] screening questions for alcohol asked of the significant other, will introduce the topic along with general questions on nicotine and other drug use in the home setting. Screen questions eliciting a positive response allow the evaluator to follow up with more clinical detail as well as to include the candidate for corroboration as a participant in the home environment. Since the third party will serve as the primary distress warning indicator of a return to pathologic behavior after transplant, that person's own health and capabilities become a critical part of the assessment. At the same time, this process allows all three – patient, third party, and the evaluator as a representative of the transplant team – to build an alliance in the interest of the patient's health.

Clinically, the above requirement assumes a viable transplant candidate in an outpatient setting. What about the alcoholic or other patient who presents in fulminant hepatic failure in the medical intensive care unit, possibly comatose, and with no hope of leaving the hospital without a liver graft? The same requirement applies: the home setting will serve as the patient's primary safety net and requires a careful assessment. Interviews with as many adults as possible who live in that setting yield the best picture of ongoing clinical safety and the soundest basis for proceeding to transplant in the likelihood of extended abstinence from alcohol.

Patient's cognition

By definition, liver transplant candidates present in various stages of hepatic failure. Some may be well compensated and stable on medical treatment while others may arrive in coma or suffering other forms of mental incapacitation due to liver failure. Whether known as delirium,[6,7] confusion state, cognitive impairment, or any of the other terms used historically, the result is a loss of one or more of the cognitive components needed to think properly, recall a personal history accurately, make informed decisions, and carry out future plans in a reliable manner. Optimally, and in the candidate's best interest, the interview should take place with the patient in the best clinical state in the setting of hepatic insufficiency or failure. In the great majority of cases, this indicates an *outpatient* visit. Most inpatient hospitalizations occur when the liver disease has worsened; some clinicians request evaluation in hospital in the interest of getting it done, but this will not yield the best information if a delirium is present.

In an outpatient setting, with the transplant candidate in their best state of health, the evaluator can follow the Identifying Data and Chief Complaint – in this case, the request for liver transplant – with an assessment of the patient's cognitive state. Asking the patient the following questions offers another obvious possibility:

"Are you thinking clearly today?"
"Are you clear headed today?"
"Are you thinking like your old self today?"

Another variation on this theme introduces the issue:

"You appear to have some jaundice, today."
"How is your thinking doing?"

The patient answers and the interviewer can turn to the third party and ask, "Does he/she seem his/her usual self today or do you see a change in thinking ability?" Generally patient and significant other perceive changes concurrently but sometimes the third party may pick them up when the patient is too confused or slowed mentally to do so. Most often, the corroborating party mentions a worsening of forgetfulness, especially in recalling recent events or plans. Referred to in cognitive science as working memory, this impairment often presents as a subtle change in recall that may not be obvious in routine medical encounters that do not look for it. In outpatient cases, the patient often appears cognitively clear and their third party agrees. If the patient and corroborator say that the patient's cognition seems to be functioning normally, the evaluator may defer the cognitive examination for a few minutes, adding "Later in the interview I will ask you some questions that will let me know how your thinking is today," most often providing an appropriate transition to the history of the present illness in well-compensated liver cases.

Although more frequent in hospital settings, any time either the patient or the third party note changes in mentation, or if the interviewer notices the patient is having difficulty with attention and engagement in the conversation, a careful cognitive examination is best performed at the *beginning of the interview.* If the candidate suffers from cognitive incapacity, he or she may not provide accurate historical data simply because of memory retrieval, concentration, or other problems. As discussed extensively in neuropsychiatric texts, standard cognition assessment is best considered in two forms: basic and complex.[10]

The Mini-Mental State Exam (MMSE[11]), in widest use for cognitive screening, has been standardized by age and offers a reasonable tool for assessing basic cognition. It does not address complex cognitive functions. In the present author's experience with liver transplant candidates, the MMSE does not offer a sufficient clinical test of short term, or working, memory defined here clinically as the ability to record new memory information and then retrieve it 5 minutes later. Asking the patient to register (repeat out loud) four unrelated words, rather than the MMSE's three, and then asking the patient to recall them after 5 minutes by the clock, rather than after the MMSE's minute or two of varying elapsed time, offers a better window into the candidate's new memory capabilities. A patient who can recall 3 or 4 of the words after 5 minutes can usually give a more reliable history than one who can recall only 2, 1, or none. Impaired working memory performance often indicates a subtle "subclinical" hepatic encephalopathy that often will improve with adding or increasing lactulose treatment, for example.

The Frontal Assessment Battery (FAB[12]) allows a standardized, scored evaluation of complex cognition. It contains tasks that address motivation, judgment, and planning – all referring to frontal lobe functions and mediated by the fronto-subcortical tracts. Used in its standard fashion, the examiner should have a printed or electronic copy before him/her and give the standard directions to the patient. The resulting additive score can then be used in a formula that accounts for normal age-related changes. Probably more important clinically, responses to the specific FAB tasks can give specific information on present complex cortical abilities in areas such as judgment, memory, level of involvement, and executive/planning.

Another standardized instrument, the Verbal Trails B (VTB[10]) test, a spoken form of the original written Trails B test, recognizes the often subtle changes in complex cognition brought on by early hepatic encephalopathy. The interviewer can introduce the VTB at the bedside or office by saying, "I am going to give you a pattern and I would like you to follow the pattern as far as you can go with it. The pattern is "1-A, 2-B . . . What comes next?" With encouragement but not prompting, the patient continues the sequence of alternating numbers and letters. A normal response is set at proceeding through "13-M" or further with no errors in the space of 1 minute. A below-normal response usually indicates difficulties in the frontal lobe functions mediated through the dorso-lateral pre-frontal cortex that are needed to plan and execute tasks, such as taking medications properly.

A bedside/clinic test of judgment provides a functional window into the orbito-frontal cortex and its state of health. "I am going to give you a situation and I want you to tell me what you would do in that situation. You are feeling well, you go to a movie, and you are sitting in a crowded movie theater watching the movie. You are the first one to see a fire break out in the theater. What would you do?" This standard question asks the patient to attend not only to the fire danger but also to the danger of panic in the theater. An acceptable response is "Inform the theater management that there is a fire" because it: 1) implies understanding of the panic danger, and provides an option for action against the fire while taking the panic danger into account. A frequent answer that may imply orbito-frontal compromise is: "Yell FIRE!," an option that does not account for the panic danger. The interviewer can follow up with "What might happen if you did that?" and listen for the secondary danger. If the patient says "It might cause a panic," the interviewer then asks for other action options, "What could you do instead?," listening for viable alternatives.

In clinical practice, the present author includes these, as well as a description of motivation that sustains active attention throughout the interview. This last is an indication of the third major complex cognitive ability, one mediated by the anterior cingulate cortex of the frontal lobe. Attention to these and the basic cognitive functions allow an assessment of: 1) the reliability of the patient's clinical history, 2) the patient's abilities to judge, plan and manage pre-transplant care in working with the liver team, and 3) baseline cognitive functions that may often be impaired in post-transplant deliria that may go unrecognized owing to their subtlety.

When careful examination raises concern about a candidate's cognitive ability, one question every transplant team asks is "Are the changes permanent?," since few teams will provide liver grafting for demented patients. In the vast majority of candidates, it is important to consider changes of this nature as most likely indications of delirium – a temporary loss due to pathophysiologic causes from the liver failure – will reverse with transplant. Improvement in the cognitive functions themselves, with lactulose or, in some cases with methylphenidate before transplant, provides clinical evidence of a reversible delirium. True dementias, on the other hand, present with gradual lessening of cognitive abilities that do not reverse with these agents and indicate the necessity of an extensive dementia evaluation. Wernicke–Korsakoff's syndrome, also known as Alcohol Amnestic Syndrome, characterized by a profound working memory deficit in the setting of generally normal cognition – especially of normal registration whereby a patient can recall seven or more random order digits spoken as a series by the examiner – indicates a trial of thiamine and the B-complex vitamins in an effort to demonstrate acceptable improvement prior to a liver graft procedure.

History of present illness

The history of present illness (HPI) is the work horse of the clinical evaluation and takes up the greatest part of the hour required for a capable assessment in experienced hands. Its specific sections in the liver transplant evaluation include the history and course of the: 1) liver disease, 2) alcohol use, 3) other drug use including nicotine, 4) psychiatric disorders and conditions, and 5) social stability.

Liver history

The psychiatric interviewer need not go into extensive detail that repeats the work of the hepatologists. A productive use of the first few minutes of history taking, however, includes meeting the patient and their significant other person on the common ground of concern about the liver disease. This builds a clinical alliance while giving the interviewer useful data. For example, the question "When did you first learn about your liver problem?" provides a beginning point in understanding the course of events. Some report that their liver disease was first discovered from routine laboratory tests well before any symptoms. Others note that they were unaware of any conditions until the onset of a decompensation such as from acute alcoholic hepatitis. In the latter condition some follow-up studies describe a window of approximately 18 months between the first alcoholic hepatitis flare and the onset of more rapid compensation from cirrhosis. In other cases, however, alcoholic hepatitis may be more pathophysiologically aggressive and lead to more immediate transplant consideration. If the conclusion of the transplant team's evaluation is to refer the patient for alcoholism treatment, for example, it is important to know where the patient might be in this relative time window of stable mental and physical functioning.

Bearing on the alcohol use history itself, discussing the medical condition offers a useful point at which to ask "Did your physician or any other caregiver think you should stop alcohol use at that time?" Use of a substance despite clear physical health consequences is one of the hallmarks of any addictive disorder. The course of giving up alcohol or substance use may often take many months and include repetitive warnings from health care givers. On the other hand, a patient who minimizes the stated concerns of physicians and others about alcohol or drug use, with clear evidence to the contrary as in clinical records, may suggest an unresolved ambivalence with respect to stopping use.

Assessing a history of prior confusion rounds out this section. This includes asking about bleeding episodes that included confusion, any periods of confusion that occurred spontaneously, and treatment for liver-related confusion such as lactulose. The corroborating other person often provides useful information on this topic since the patient may not remember all or part of a confusion episode. Prior occurrences, generally caused by the clinical or subclinical delirium due to the liver disease referred to as hepatic encephalopathy, signal that cognitive impairment has occurred in the past and that it continues to be an important focus in the present assessment. In alcoholic cases, for example, confusion is sometimes wrongly misinterpreted as alcohol intoxication. A significant other person in the patient's life who can differentiate the two will be an asset in continuing post-transplant care.

Last use

One way of transitioning from this part of the history into the next often more sensitive section on substance use is to ask the general question "When was your last use of alcohol or substances of any kind?" The clinician may then record the patient's recollection of last use and seek corroboration from the patient's significant other person. This further introduces the third person's role in the interview, and gives it a normal, matter of fact, tone that most third persons find helpful in being able to describe the patient's drinking openly and honestly. It also introduces the focus on drinking and other drug use.

Alcohol use history

Clinically, two general concepts guide the use assessment of alcohol and other addictive drugs. First, the interviewer is assessing an addiction, or addictive disorder and alcoholism is a form of this phenomenon. Alcoholism, defined more specifically below as "alcohol dependence" (AD), is second in prevalence only to nicotine addiction in the general population and is the most frequent disorder for which persons seek liver transplantation.

Second, AD and other forms of substance dependence are clinical diagnoses of specific behaviors, rather than quantifications of amounts and frequencies of use. An easily available source, the American Psychiatric Association's *Diagnostic and Statistical Manual of Mental Disorders: DSM-IV-TR*, Fourth Edition,[7] outlines the phenomena common to all addictive disorders. Further, experience in assessing liver transplant candidates suggests using the medical model of addictive disorders as disease states. Other models – such as moral choice, habit and reinforcement, or learned behavior – may make up useful discussions in other arenas but these have far less support from empirical data and offer very limited clinical utility. An empirically based medical model focuses on diagnosis and prognosis.

Making a diagnosis

The diagnosis of AD, and those of the other drug dependencies, requires specific evidence of phenomena in three clinical domains: physiologic dependence, including 1) tolerance and withdrawal, 2) loss of control of alcohol use, which is often erroneously referred to as "craving," and 3) decline in either physical or social functioning, or both. Of the seven dependence criteria listed in DSM-IV-TR,[7] for example, two refer to physical dependence, two to the Loss of Control phenomenon, and three to social or physical impairment. For our purpose, however, the three large symptom domains offer an easier way of remembering and assessing relevant symptoms in the clinic.

Physiologic dependence: Tolerance and withdrawal

Tolerance refers to the ability of the central nervous system (CNS) to approximate normal functioning in the presence of ever-increasing doses of ethyl alcohol or any other CNS substance. Clinically, the person reports needing more alcohol to get the same effect once noticed at a much lower dose earlier in the natural history of drinking. To assess this, the physician must establish a baseline effect that has changed over time. This necessitates careful attention to the details of the drinking history.

One useful approach may be to ask the patient what the effect of alcohol was when drinking alcohol alone was first commenced. Results include such things as nausea, feeling high, or other unique descriptors that the patient can provide: what they noticed after one or two standard alcoholic drinks. A standard drink, each containing roughly 3–4 oz of ethyl alcohol may be approximately defined as a 12 oz can or bottle of beer, 6 oz glass of table wine, or 1.5 oz shot of whiskey or other spirits.

After establishing a baseline, for example "in high school I got high after one or two cans of beer, the interviewer may then ask how many standard drinks the person notices achieved the same effect at the time when their drinking was at its greatest. Formal DSM-IV-TR criteria require a 50 percent increase. In the case of alcohol, most will describe a doubling or more of the amount used for an initial effect. Many AD patients will describe amounts several times greater than those drunk in the state naïve to alcohol, such as "I wouldn't notice anything until after I drank a six pack." This signals that the CNS has adapted to heavy alcohol use, that is, reached a tolerance.

Alcohol withdrawal

Defined clinically as an excessive activity of the sympathetic nervous system triggered by a rapid decline in alcohol blood level, withdrawal symptoms accompany tolerance in the great majority of individuals. In those who report no withdrawal symptoms despite a history of clear tolerance to alcohol, the clinician must ask whether the patient is drinking in the morning before withdrawal symptoms manifest themselves, or is regularly taking some other CNS depressant, such as a benzodiazepine or an anticholinergic agent that covers withdrawal symptoms, especially in the morning. On rare occasions, the physician will encounter patients who have little or no withdrawal symptoms despite clear tolerance development; although relatively infrequent, this recognized clinical phenomenon appears most likely due to a genetically based constitutional invulnerability to withdrawal.

Since ethanol is a CNS depressant, its quick removal triggers CNS hyperactivity both centrally, as for example expressed by a subjective sense of jitteriness or impending disaster (anxiety), and peripherally through the symptoms of sympathetic nervous system discharge. Box 6.1 lists acute withdrawal symptoms that patient's commonly report.

Box 6.1 Patient-reported symptoms of early alcohol withdrawal

Anxiety	Palpitations (tachycardia)
Tremor	Rapid breathing
Nausea and vomiting	Low-grade fever
Sweating	High blood pressure

Of note is that neither headache nor blackout are symptoms of alcohol withdrawal. The former, a component of "hangover," often may have to do with fluid shifts in the brain, and the latter is a state-dependent amnesia. Later occurrences, however, such as generalized grand mal seizures on or after the first day of withdrawal and the delirium tremens (DTs) occurring after the third day make up the most severe and most dangerous withdrawal phenomena. The DTs, characterized by: 1) confusion, 2) usually visual or tactile hallucinations, and 3) extreme rises and vital signs, such as malignant hypertension or tachycardia, presents a true medical emergency and often results in hospitalization. Again, however, because of the affected person's confusion during the DTs, the patient may not appreciate the significance of a hospitalization for withdrawal. The corroborating third party is again useful in this instance.

Loss of control phenomenon

Assessment Lost of control (LOC) is the essence of any addiction and certainly of AD, and refers to the inability of the AD person to predict with any degree of certainty how much they will imbibe from one drinking episode to the next. Clinically, once the drinking episode starts, the alcohol-dependent person will be unable to stop in the middle of the drinking/use bout without a very great struggle. Useful questions at interview include the phrasing presented in Box 6.2.

While the phrasing may seem indirect, the word structure allies both interviewer and patient in looking at one phenomenon – the patient's experience – rather than an implied adversarial setting in which the interviewer is examining the patient, as if under a microscope. Experience suggests that an allying approach gains much more detailed and more useful information.

At the same time, it is important to distinguish the LOC phenomenon from "craving." The former has to do with the inability to stop drinking once started. Craving, classically defined, refers to the episodic and often intense desire or compulsion to drink or use in an alcohol- or drug-free state between bouts of use. It may also be confused with the search for alcohol to treat withdrawal symptoms. The distinction can be made accurately in the clinical setting by paying attention to what occurs during episodes of use and what occurs between them. LOC during use is a hallmark of addiction while craving between use episodes appears to be a much more complex phenomenon involving brain/environment interactions.

Box 6.2 Assessing loss of control

Statements to make:

"Some people tell me they notice these things when they drink and I would like to know if you've ever noticed them"

"Some find it very hard to stop drinking once they start. They feel that they are 'off to the races' where drinking is concerned"

"Some people find themselves drinking more than they wanted to or had planned to"

"Some people notice that they try to make rules to control their drinking"

Social or physical decline

The combination of physical addiction and LOC usually results in a patient's expending a large portion of time and effort to sustain heavy drinking or to manage or recover from its effects. To assess this, the clinician asks whether drinking has become a problem with respect to family relationships, legal status, work, friendships, or physical health. The physician will be especially attuned to the last of these since the physical illness sequelae of AD and other drug dependencies often result in frequent clinical visits and hospitalizations. The family relationships, however, usually offer the most sensitive indications of social difficulties due to alcohol or drug use. A change in work status is usually one of the last indicators of social difficulty since income provides the basis for continued use.

AD may be reliably diagnosed when evidence in all three domains presents. The DSM-IV-TR diagnostic criteria do not require evidence in all three domains and therefore cast a somewhat wider diagnostic net. While either approach is defensible, the physician will do well to use both concurrently. The present author generally takes the more conservative approach, especially in the setting of life-threatening illness for which there is only one treatment alternative, as in the case of liver or other solid organ transplantation.

Gauging a prognosis

When liver transplant teams ask for psychiatric expertise in evaluating liver graft candidates, they ask primarily for the candidate's prognosis: Will this person "waste" a liver graft with a return to uncontrolled alcohol or other drug use?

Post-transplant risk

From a physical perspective, the risk of graft injury or loss from a return to drinking emanates from two sources principally. The first entails alcohol injury to the new liver graft, a relatively rare occurrence that hepatologic knowledge cannot predict at present. Only about 15% of heavy drinkers acquire potentially fatal cirrhosis to begin with and the mechanisms that trigger the process in some, but not in most other heavy-drinking individuals, remain unknown. The second risk to graft injury is much more frequent, and more ominous: graft rejection due to an inattention to post-transplant immune-suppression. Behaviorally, a return to uncontrolled drinking carries a high risk of non-adherence to the medicine regimen. Missing even a few doses in a twice-daily regimen can lead to a graft rejection reaction that the patient may not notice until its late stages, potentially irreversible and fatal by that time. This factor, mentioned here in the context of alcohol use, applies to *any* psychoactive agent used in an uncontrolled setting that may affect memory, planning, and judgment functions in the brain.

Both risks – direct alcohol liver injury, and graft rejection reaction – are real and worth mentioning in the psychiatric interview since they provide candidate and significant other with an important perspective on life following transplant. The present writer brings them up near the end of the interview and usually in the context of: 1) focusing the previous diagnostic and prognostic information on the risks of life after transplant, and 2) justifying the readiness of the significant other to alert the transplant team to any drinking or other concerning behavior that might have occurred.

Positive vs negative How, then, to go about the task of assessing the prognosis for alcohol-/drug-free living post-transplant?[13] While each individual patient and their social network provide unique considerations, a series of general factors, gleaned mostly from research on nontransplant populations of alcohol- or drug-dependent persons, offer useful windows on prognosis. In the great majority of cases these include: 1) the substance use diagnosis, 2) an understanding of the patient's ambivalence towards continuing use, 3) measures of the candidate's social stability, and 4) a series of four empirically based factors that Vaillant[14] found in prospective research studies.[15] In addition, candidates with a co-occurring diagnosis of a major psychiatric disorder require: 1) an evaluation of psychoactive medication response to the primary disorder and 2) a medication adherence history in addition to the factors already mentioned.

Some liver teams focus more on what they see as negative prognostic predictors – those that predict a return to drinking or use – rather than positive factors such as those that predict continued abstinence as mentioned earlier. The negative factors often include mention of: 1) alcohol or other drug use in the past 6 months – the infamous "Six Month Rule" that has not been borne out in prospective research, and 2) counting previous "recidivist" episodes, a term that calls to mind criminal incarceration and punishment, rather than a remitting/relapsing medical condition. At the same time, many teams, and outcome reports in the literature, often ignore one of the primary indicators of relapse – the presence or absence of polydrug dependence, a phenomenon described separately or in clinical subtyping of AD presentations as described later. While negative factors, such as evidence of current drinking in the setting of AD, come into play in the evaluation, focus on the positive factors at present offers a sound approach, if one that indicates the need for further empirical research in transplant populations as its basis.

Diagnosis is prognosis The diagnostic procedure described in detail earlier provides the basis for important prognostic distinctions bearing on post-transplant abstinence. One of the most common, and surprisingly least referred to in the published studies on candidate evaluation, is the distinction between AD history as a primary dependence and AD as part of a polysubstance-dependence history.

AD typology and polydrug dependence AD affects as many as 7–10% of persons in the USA. In a great majority of cases it involves alcohol as the primary, and often only, drug of sustained abuse. Research reports refer to this as Type 1 alcohol dependence. By contrast polydrug dependence – that is, addiction to two or more substances, not including nicotine, that may include alcohol as one of the dependence substances – affects about 0.5% of persons in the USA. Viewed from the perspective of alcoholism research, this group refers to Type 2 alcohol dependence. Although the distinction between the two clinical groups and their abstinence prognoses has been known for many years,[15] remarkably few programs take this distinction into account. For example, transplant programs that separate the two demonstrate high rates of abstinence in the primary AD (Type 1) group after transplant while those that do not make this distinction often report much lower abstinence rates. Prior research on nontransplant samples demonstrates that the much more common primary AD persons will enjoy a better prognosis than the polydrug-dependent group.[14] Table 6.1 summarizes the distinctions between the two in brief form.

Further evidence for the usefulness of this distinction in transplant candidate selection comes from a recently published long-term, prospective study on the outcome histories of liver transplant recipients from one center with respect to return to alcohol use.[16] Of five post-liver transplant groups whose "trajectories" were separated by careful statistical analysis, the group that had the most frequent and most severe relapses was that whose members reported the most frequent pre-transplant history of abusing multiple substances. While the authors did not report on specific drug dependency diagnostic criteria for any of their groups, their data suggests that this group most resembles the polydrug abuse, or Type 2 AD, population.

Table 6.1 Alcohol dependence vs polydrug dependence (alcoholism Types 1 and 2)

Primary alcohol dependence	Polydrug dependence
• 7–10% of US population • Alcohol primary dependence • Normal childhood • No conduct disorder (CD) • Regular use: teens, twenties • No personality diagnosis • Natural remission: 30%/year • With treatment: 45%/year	• 0.5% of US population • Polysubstance dependence • Deprivation/abuse • CD symptoms: before age 15 • Polydrug dependency: teens • Adult personality disorder • Natural remission: 10%/year • With treatment: 10%/year

Practically speaking, the psychiatrist must evaluate AD type as a clinical guide to prognosis. While the Six Month Rule has little justification for use in Type 1 AD,[17] a history of recent use of *any* dependent drug – including alcohol – in a Type 2 AD person constitutes an ominous finding. Empirical data on the polydrug group suggests that continuous, stable abstinence comes only after the emotional growth of many years, often in the person's late 30s or early 40s.[14] In a person with Type 2 AD, demonstration of a corroborated, sustained, stable abstinence from both drugs *and* alcohol for a significant period of time – often measured by one or more years rather than by months – affords the liver transplant team the confidence to proceed in providing a scarce resource for which clinical need far exceeds the liver graft supply.

Abuse rather than dependence When diagnosing AD or other drug dependence, it is important to establish whether the LOC phenomenon exists in each case. Its absence, even in the face of a clear history of tolerance or alcohol-related social or physical problems for example, strongly suggests the lesser diagnosis of alcohol abuse (AA). In a clinical series previously reported[15] about 10% of those applying for a liver transplant for alcoholic cirrhosis did not meet dependence criteria but could clearly be considered in the abuse category. Abuse generally suggests that the behavioral process of moving towards LOC and dependence appears to be in place but that the clinical line into dependence has not been crossed. Even though a lesser diagnosis, therefore, it still indicates asking the patient to cease all alcohol use. In that case, two phenomena often occur: 1) the person achieves and maintains abstinence without a struggle, and 2) the risk of relapse over the long term appears considerably lower. Generally speaking, AA offers a much better prognosis with respect to natural course than does AD. While the lesser diagnosis requires better definition, especially in the setting of transplant candidates, it is a generally more optimistic diagnosis to make.

Behavioral vs hepatic diagnosis A significant portion of those candidates referred to as "alcoholic" will not merit the AD diagnosis. Some time ago a hepatologist colleague and the present author compared notes.[15] Only about 75% of those with a tissue diagnosis of alcoholic liver disease fit the behavioral AD diagnosis. Conversely, only about 80% of those referred as "alcoholics" met the AD diagnosis. Of the remaining 20%, half fit the AA diagnosis and half did not merit either. This was especially true of women who, because of a well-known gender-specific vulnerability to alcoholic liver disease, may injure the liver without ever reaching AD. This limited overlap emphasizes the need for diagnostic precision, especially in the behavioral realm, rather than deny a life-saving procedure on the basis of diagnosed alcoholic hepatitis alone.

Assessing ambivalence and continuing LOC risk Clinically, longitudinal studies of abstinence make it clear that once the control of drinking behavior departs, it does not return in the great majority of cases.[14] Once lost, controlled alcohol or drug use cannot be re-learned or re-constituted. In this sense a diagnosis of dependence signals a permanent condition – including a permanent risk of uncontrolled drinking or use. This has a critical bearing on life after liver transplant since it suggests that any alcohol use will remain, always, a high-risk behavior in the setting of both a new organ and continuing twice daily use of immunosuppressive agents. Even brief noncompliance with the immunosuppressive medicines can result in the rejection reaction and death. One component of the interview, therefore, requires review of this risk with the patient and third party. Poor understanding, or ambivalent acceptance, of post-transplant drinking/use risk in a patient with normal cognition, may indicate an unresolved ambivalence toward AD itself and therefore the need for alcohol or other drug-focused behavioral treatment. This can be followed by a return for re-evaluation, prior to transplant.

Social stability

This assessment tests the foundation upon which ongoing medical adherence and favorable prognosis are built. While several social stability scales exist, the simplest comes from the work of Strauss and Bacon,[18] who found that the presence of any two of four social factors predicted clinic appointment compliance among AD persons. These factors included: 1) being married, 2) not living alone, 3) stable employment for 3 years, and 4) a stable residence for 2 years. Viewed teleologically, falling below the cut point suggests, but does not establish, the likelihood of insufficient social resources, such as social isolation and homelessness, that raise the likelihood of both drinking relapse and medical noncompliance. When present, the specialized involvement of a treatment clinic program aimed at increasing social resources offers the best next step towards return to the liver team for re-evaluation.

Vaillant's four prognostic factors

In the best available prospective, longitudinal study of AD prognosis, Vaillant's 8-year study noted four operating factors, any two or more of which, when present, predicted long-term sobriety – defined as 2 years or more in his study – while one or none indicated a return to drinking within 1 year.[14] A proper prognosis evaluation includes them.

1. *Structured time* Because AD-style drinking requires a lot of time and effort, newly abstinent persons often encounter considerable "dead" or unstructured time that can itself foster a relapse. Structuring that time corrects this concern and is a frequent ingredient in specialized clinic and self-help group (such as Alcoholics Anonymous) formats. Any setting that fills time with productive and engaging activity – that the person's "heart is in" – fits the need. At interview, a brief assessment of how the candidate spends their days addresses whether they engage in active projects that involve other people, or live an isolated existence such as in filling the time with endless television viewing.

2. *Rehabilitation relationship* Sustained, heavy drinking or drug use serves to isolate the person from others and to create the need in those who come into social contact – such as family members – to "fix" the drinking or use. Direct intervention – such as telling the person not to drink or use – generally results in an interpersonal struggle that works against continued abstinence. Rather, abstinence sets the stage for proper boundaries between person and social network. In brief, the family, a clinic, and a self-help network communicate the same approach to the person: "You can stay but the drinking has to go." Assessing the extent to which the significant other person present at the liver transplant evaluation interview understands: 1) that they cannot control the

patient's drinking or use, and 2) that they are ready to inform the transplant team when any return to use occurs or appears likely to, is a necessity.

This can be done by asking "Is it clear to you that neither you nor I have any control over [the candidate's] drinking?" and, "What would you do if, many months after transplant, you suspected that [the candidate] was drinking?" The proper answer to the first question is "Yes" and to the second, "Call the transplant team" as well as to mobilize any local caregivers, such as a specialized treatment clinic. When the significant other person does not indicate their own limits, further education on the topic is in order. Most third parties who do not apprehend the need to call for help in a dangerous situation involving alcohol or drug use find relief in a review of whom to call and when, then and there in the interview.

3. Sources of hope or self-esteem Regretful thoughts about having hurt others during drinking days frequently return to most alcohol-dependent people during abstinence periods. Ruminating on them has the effect of lowering hope and self-confidence and thereby promoting a return to drinking or use: "I am a terrible person, I may as well drink." In assessing prognosis, the interviewer inquires after mechanisms that help a person through such periods. These include hope for the future: "What keeps you going in life?" and "What do you look forward to?" – and sources of accomplishment or self-esteem: "What helps you to feel good about yourself?" "What gives you a sense of usefulness or accomplishment?" The evaluator may also note "Most people run into regrets about their drinking days. Does this happen to you?" If the answer is positive, the evaluator may go on to ask: "What helps you get past regretful thoughts without drinking?" For some it may be religious beliefs; for others the "higher power" without religion as AA describes it, and for others a concentration on items of hope and accomplishment, such as "another day behind me without drinking." Clinically, the absence of forces that counterbalance regretful ruminations presents an ominous sign and one indicating further specialized treatment focus.

4. A negative behavioral reinforcer In other words "Is there something very painful that will happen to you, without doubt, the very next time you drink alcohol?" Very few circumstances meet these criteria; severe pancreatic pain and the disulfiram–ethanol reaction qualify and are the most frequently encountered. Liver failure and impending transplant do not fulfill the criteria because of their subtlety and lack of predictability on each occasion. While the others of Vaillant's factors can be considered positive changes in the path to sustained abstinence, this is the only negative one and is generally the least frequently encountered in the liver transplant setting.

Summing-up prognosis

While none of the factors listed under the prognosis section may individually offer absolute certainty in respect to sustained abstinence in each individual case, their combination of variables offers a prognostic pattern – the process of clinical art – that appears useful. Our early algorithm,[19] for example, predicted high rates of abstinence in AD liver transplant recipients who present a series of good prognostic factors and that appears to have been put into practice in many if not most US programs. With further experience, the individual factors might be summed clinically in Box 6.3. The reader will notice that the prognosis factors listed there can be addressed and re-evaluated longitudinally. While this offers liver transplant teams the best option in moving forward clinically, sometimes the clinical presentation does not allow it, as when a patient's acute liver decompensation indicates transplantation as the only viable option for leaving hospital. In that situation, the evaluator addresses as many of the earlier mentioned factors as possible, including communication with the patient and family, and presents the clinical data in the discussion with the liver transplant team wherein the various sets of data can be considered and a consensus reached.

Other psychiatric assessment

The foregoing discussion relates to the great majority of persons with alcohol or substance use histories referred for liver transplantation who do not have other pre-existing psychiatric conditions. One critically important feature of this patient group recalls that AD can mimic all of the major psychiatric

Box 6.3 Addressing prognostic factors before transplant

Physical diagnosis

Cognitive impairment: lactulose or other treatment and re-evaluate

Substance use diagnosis

Type 1 dependence: proceed to further prognostic evaluation

Type 2 dependence: verify either lengthy sustained abstinence and the "maturing out" process or verify continued effective treatment as for example in methadone maintenance for opiate dependence

Abuse: verify cessation and abstinence and proceed to transplant

No diagnosis: proceed to transplant

Substance use prognosis:

Unresolved ambivalence toward use: focused treatment on this aspect of abstinence; re-evaluate in 3–6 months

Unstable social adjustment: establish viable social resources; 3–6-month follow-up re-assessment

One or none of Vaillant's Factors: focused treatment referral; 3–6-month follow-up re-assessment

disorders including major depressive disorder, bipolar disorder, psychosis, several anxiety disorders, and obsessive compulsive disorder, as well as other entities such as sleep discontinuity and anorexia. These and others can be assessed through a series of standard screening questions that will not appear here. When addressing them, the evaluator must keep one truly important factor in mind: other psychiatric disorders cannot be established with certainty during periods of heavy drinking and, to some extent, during periods of other drug use. Diagnostic clarity for the listed psychiatric disorders requires *evidence during abstinence periods*, generally exceeding 1 month. Failing to observe this may lead to misdiagnosis and utilization of treatments, most often psychoactive medications, gratuitously.

Summary

Liver transplantation remains the only successful treatment for liver failure at the present moment, although new developments in genetic engineering and hepatocellular growth may someday replace allograft procedures. The current author and others' recent work has suggested that some of the immunosuppressants or their analogues may have a role to play in treating alcohol use disorders.[20] In proceeding to allocate liver grafts that preserve lives, transplant teams have acted fairly and compassionately in considering patients with AD and have done so empirically in the best traditions of clinical medicine.[13] The foregoing review raises many questions that deserve to be addressed at this intersection of medical, surgical, and psychiatric knowledge, including the currently unresolved areas of precision in evaluating polysubstance-dependent persons and the ambivalence concerns in the primary AD setting, not to mention unresolved issues involving post-transplant care. This field has the opportunity to grow in these important areas that will derive knowledge widely applicable in other settings and conditions from which many more than the transplant recipient population will benefit.

References

1. Surman OS, Cosimi AB, DiMartini A. Psychiatric care of patients undergoing organ transplantation. Transplantation 2009;87:1753–61.
2. Heinrich TW, Marcangelo M. Psychiatric issues in solid organ transplantation. Harv Rev Psychiatry 2009;17: 398–406.
3. Kotlyar DS, Burke A, Campbell MS, Weinrieb RM. A critical review of candidacy for orthotopic liver transplantation in alcoholic liver disease. Am J Gastroenterol 2008;103:734–43; quiz 44.
4. DiMartini A, Crone C, Fireman M, Dew MA. Psychiatric aspects of organ transplantation in critical care. Crit Care Clin 2008;24:949–81, x.
5. McCallum S, Masterton G. Liver transplantation for alcoholic liver disease: a systematic review of psychosocial selection criteria. Alcohol Alcohol 2006;41: 358–63.
6. WHO. International Classification of Diseases, Tenth Revision, Clinical Modification (ICD-10-CM). 2010.
7. APA. Diagnostic and Statistical Manual Of Mental Disorders: DSM-IV-TR. 2000.
8. Beresford TP, Blow FC, Hill E, Singer K, Lucey MR. Comparison of CAGE questionnaire and computer-assisted laboratory profiles in screening for covert alcoholism. Lancet 1990;336:482–5.

9. Sokol RJ, Martier SS, Ager JW. The T-ACE questions: practical prenatal detection of risk-drinking. Am J Obstet Gynecol 1989;160:863–8; discussion 8–70.
10. Arciniegas DB, Beresford TP. Neuropsychiatry, an Introductory Text. Cambridge: Cambridge University Press; 2001.
11. Folstein MF, Robins LN, Helzer JE. The Mini-Mental State Examination. Arch Gen Psychiatry 1983;40:812.
12. Dubois B, Slachevsky A, Litvan I, Pillon B. The FAB: a Frontal Assessment Battery at bedside. Neurology 2000;55:1621–6.
13. Beresford TP. Probabilities of relapse and abstinence among liver transplant recipients. Liver Transpl 2006; 12:705–6.
14. Vaillant GE. The Natural History of Alcoholism, Revisited. Cambridge, MA: Harvard University Press; 1995.
15. Lucey M, Merion RM, Beresford TP. Liver Transplantation and the Alcoholic Patient. Cambridge: Cambridge University Press; 1994.
16. Dimartini A, Dew MA, Day N, et al. Trajectories of alcohol consumption following liver transplantation. Am J Transplant 2010;10:2305–12.
17. DiMartini A, Day N, Dew MA, et al. Alcohol consumption patterns and predictors of use following liver transplantation for alcoholic liver disease. Liver Transpl 2006;12:813–20.
18. Straus R, Bacon SD. Alcoholism and social stability; a study of occupational integration in 2,023 male clinic patients. Q J Stud Alcohol 1951;12:231–60.
19. Beresford TP, Turcotte JG, Merion R, et al. A rational approach to liver transplantation for the alcoholic patient. Psychosomatics 1990;31:241–54.
20. Beresford HF, Deitrich R, Beresford TP. Cyclosporine-A discourages ethanol intake in C57bl/6j mice: a preliminary study. J Stud Alcohol 2005;66:658–62.

7 Organ allocation in liver transplantation: ethics, organ supply, and evidence-based practice

Nicole Siparsky, David Axelrod and Richard B. Freeman
Section of Solid Organ Transplant Surgery, Department of Surgery, Dartmouth-Hitchcock Medical Center, Lebanon, NH, USA

Key learning points
- Liver organ allocation and distribution should be viewed as the application of ethical principles to the management of a scarce, life-saving resource.
- Individual justice can be equated to individual need for liver transplantation (LT). Defining need for LT requires objective definitions such as mortality risk.
- Overall results for any liver allocation policy should account for both patients receiving the organ and those who remain on the list. Measuring the overall outcome for all candidates for liver transplant, regardless of whether an organ is received, is termed "survival benefit."
- Since the quality of a liver graft influences liver transplant results, allocation and distribution systems should take donor characteristics into account.
- Liver allocation and distribution policies can only meet ethical principles if they are transparent. This requires objective, comprehensive, patient-specific data and robust, analytic, constructive, criticisms over time.

Introduction

The fundamental limitation facing organ transplantation is the overwhelming disparity between the supply of usable donor organs and the demand by patients with end-stage organ failure who would benefit. The distribution and allocation of scarce life-saving resources is a classic problem facing biomedical ethicists and an ongoing challenge for regulatory authorities. Design of ethical organ allocation systems requires policymakers to balance three competing ethical principles: justice, equity, and utility. Their challenge is to develop a transparent method that incorporates these principles in an efficient system that is acceptable to potential donors and recipients. In this chapter, we will briefly outline how these three ethical principles bear on specific aspects of LT, distinguish between distribution and allocation, and compare specific distribution and allocation policies that are currently employed for deceased donor livers.

Ethical principles

Justice is the lawful and moral maintenance of what is right for a person, or what is due to a person. This principle includes both distributive justice, or distributing a resource fairly throughout a given population, and compensatory justice, which is the belief that an injured person should receive a benefit proportional to a loss. In transplantation, distributive justice guides organ allocation and distribution polices (Table 7.1). Using distributive justice as a metric, the allocation

Medical Care of the Liver Transplant Patient, Fourth Edition. Edited by Pierre-Alain Clavien, James F. Trotter.

Table 7.1 Applying ethics to system of organ transplantation

Ethical principal	Definition	Application to transplant allocation
Justice	Lawful or moral approach to decision making	Justice demands that allocation systems distribute organs according to objective, uniformly applied rules
Equity	Similar treatment of individuals without regard to cause of illness or other factors	Allocation systems should be based on severity of disease rather than type of diagnosis. Patients with similar risk of death should have similar access to transplant
Utility	Available resources are used for the greatest good for the greatest number of people	Organ allocation systems should prioritize patients most likely to benefit from transplant as defined by incremental life-years from transplant gained compared to waiting list survival

and distribution systems should ensure that each patient on the waiting list receives a fair chance at transplantation. Application of compensatory justice suggests that, in cases where the recipient has agreed to accept higher risks, such as choosing to accept an organ with higher likelihood of failure, he or she should receive some advantage, such as improved access to the higher risk organs. For example, in the USA, patients agreeing to accept a kidney with a higher risk of graft failure are given higher priority for these organs (see later).

Applying justice within the organ allocation system requires balancing reasonable competing demands between individual recipients. For example, individuals with early-stage hepatocellular cancer (HCC) have the best chance for cure when they receive a timely liver transplant. These patients would be systemically disadvantaged under an allocation system where the risk of dying from liver disease drives priority for organs since many would die from cancer progression prior to transplantation. Conversely, if patients with HCC are given too much priority for liver grafts, patients with low-stage cancers who could undergo alternative treatments would be transplanted, resulting in less access and higher waiting list mortality rates for patients with other diagnoses.

Access to re-transplantation also offers challenges to the principals of distributive and compensatory justice. As recurrence of hepatitis C after liver transplant becomes more prevalent, there are increasing numbers of patients seeking second liver transplants, even as the list of patients waiting for their first liver grows. While retransplantation offers the only opportunity for survival for these patients, outcomes are often not as good as for primary liver transplants.[1] Another interpretation of distributive justice would suggest that patients receiving a first liver transplant should get a better chance as they have not had access to the organ supply. Patients who receive a graft from an older donor, which is associated with a higher rate of recurrence, may be entitled to retransplantation under a system of compensatory justice despite the fact that retransplantation for hepatitis C generally results in a poorer outcome. In a system with a constrained supply of resources, designing just allocation and distribution policies requires the constant assessment of the benefit of directing organs to one class of individuals in a specific population against the potential for compromising access for the entire population.

Utility is the principle that directs policymakers to achieve the maximal benefits from a limited resource (e.g. supply of donor organs) for the population under consideration. Often in transplantation, utility has been defined as survival after transplant.

If an attempt were made to maximize post-transplant survival, the organ distribution and allocation policy would rank patients in order of likelihood of achieving the best results after transplantation. This measure of utility, however, only addresses the outcome of the patients receiving the transplant and does not account for those candidates who remain on the list or who do not receive the transplant.

More recently, transplant benefit, defined as the incremental life expectancy of a patient receiving a transplant compared with a patient who remains on the waiting list, has been suggested as a better measure of utility because it accounts for the entire population being served by the allocation and distribution system.[2]

The advantage of a system that emphasizes net transplant benefit is that it balances the risk of death on the waiting list with the opportunity for post-transplant survival. This approach would tend to reduce the use of organs for patients who are least likely to do well after transplant (those too sick to survive) and those least likely to survive longer with a transplant than without (those too healthy at the time of transplant).

Equity in medical practice is achieved when patients with similar expected degrees of illness and similar expected outcomes have comparable access to treatment. In organ allocation and distribution considerations, equity requires that patients are placed on the waiting list with the same degree of illness and that patients likely to have comparable amounts of transplant benefit have a similar probability of receiving an organ offer. Equity here necessitates that the waiting list criteria are developed, the prioritization system be consistent and transparent, and that organs are broadly distributed in attempt to equalize the probability of an organ offer.

Inequities in the USA in all three of these areas are well recognized. For example, the US system allows patients to enroll simultaneously on the waiting list in multiple regions, which allows patients with means (primarily private health insurance) to seek care in a region with a shorter list or higher availability of organs. This results in earlier transplantation at a less risky stage of their liver disease.[3]

The principle of equity in transplant access can be challenged due to factors beyond the allocation system. For example, there is evidence that referring providers perceive that patients with alcohol-related liver disease are less deserving of a liver transplant and, consequently, are less likely to refer patients even though there is ample evidence that outcomes are equivalent for these patients compared with those with non-alcohol-related liver disease etiologies.[4] Moreover, recurrence rates for hepatitis C after LT are at least as frequent as alcohol-related recurrence. Equity would argue that patients with alcoholic liver disease should have the same opportunity for transplant as patients suffering from non-alcohol-related liver diseases as the overall survival benefit does not differ between the two.

The ethical principles underlying organ allocation and distribution sometimes provide conflicting directions for policymakers. Design of the allocation system requires a balance of these principles, appreciation for political and geographic realities, and the availability of adequate data infrastructures to optimize the benefit derived from the scarce pool of available donated organs.

Distribution and allocation

It is useful to distinguish between organ distribution and organ allocation to appreciate the complexities in applying the ethical principles outlined earlier. Organ distribution defines the population of recipients who are eligible to receive a donated organ. Organ allocation is the system by which the organ distribution population is prioritized to receive a given organ. In the USA, the Organ Procurement and Transplantation Network (OPTN) defines the organ distribution units. OPTN polices specify that organs are distributed first to patients waiting at transplant centers within the donation service area (DSA) from which the donor was identified. DSAs are geographic areas over which organ procurement organizations provide organ donation services. In general, a DSA includes multiple donor hospitals and usually one or more transplant centers (Figure 7.1A). If no patient within the donor's DSA accepts the organ offer, the liver is then offered to patients waiting at centers within that DSA's OPTN region (Figure 7.1B). There are 11 OPTN regions in the USA, all of which contain several DSAs. Finally, if no candidate accepts the organ within the region, the organ is offered across the entire nation, representing the largest distribution unit.

Other areas of the world have distribution units based on national borders, other internal geographic or politically defined units, or in some cases, over several countries. For example, in Europe, Eurotransplant represents a distribution unit that covers six countries. Distribution units are defined along national borders and then over the entire Eurotransplant region. In other examples, the smallest distribution unit is based on administrative governmental subunits such as the Canton in

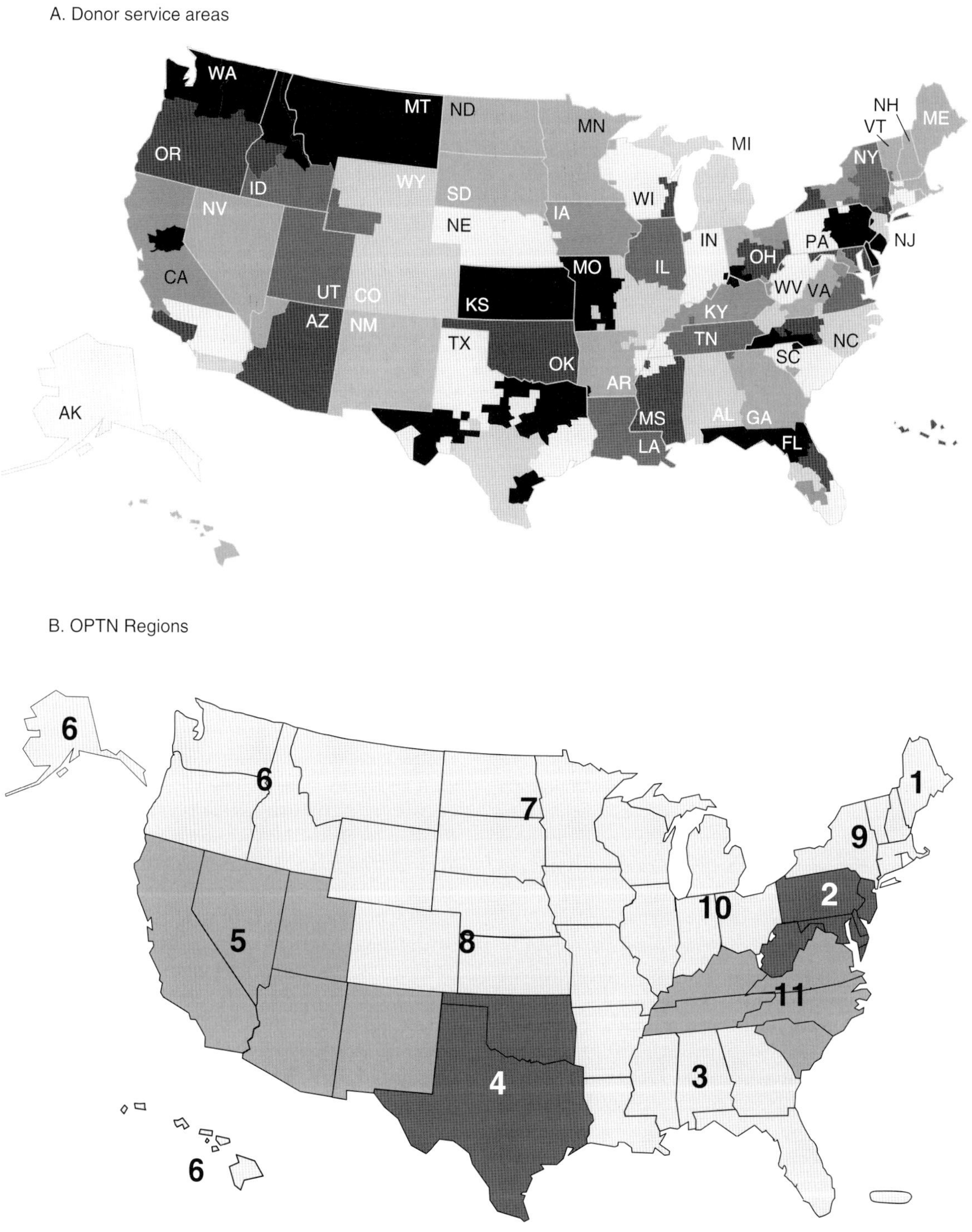

Figure 7.1 (A) US donor service regions; (B) OPTN regions

Switzerland or individual territories in Spain. Interestingly, almost uniformly around the world, these distribution units are based on political or administrative boundaries instead of specifying areas prospectively designed for optimal distribution of organs among waiting candidates. Adherence to these established boundaries persists despite many studies documenting heterogeneous distributions of candidates and donors.[5,6]

In other instances, the donor distribution unit is defined as a transplant center. This situation is referred to as center-based distribution since the population of candidates eligible to receive a given graft is represented by a single center's waiting list. For example, in the UK, in non-emergent cases, a liver graft is distributed first to a transplant center, wherein a responsible transplant surgeon then identifies a recipient based upon donor and recipient factors and center practice.[7] Each center is assigned to a donor area, which is adjusted regularly to reflect the transplant activity and number of donors in the region. However, the geographic unit does not reflect the size of the center's waiting list or severity of the candidate disease. One benefit to such a system is that it allows the surgeon to select optimal candidates from his or her own center to receive a marginal donor or a split-liver transplant (SLT). Some of the best results for SLT recipients have been where the surgeon carefully selects both recipients based on their size and severity of illness.[8] Center-based allocation may have some benefits in allowing surgeon judgment to determine the best possible recipient for non-ideal donor organs.

Organ allocation is defined as the method for ranking the eligible candidates within a defined distribution unit. In the past, candidates for LT were prioritized within distribution units using waiting time on the list. With experience it became clear that an allocation system based on waiting time results in significant discrepancies based on income and insurance status (patients with means are more likely to be placed on the list earlier in their disease and thus accrue more waiting time), and systematically disadvantages patients with greater severity of illness at the time of presentation (patients who are more ill with no waiting time are not likely to supersede a less an ill patient with less severe disease but more accrued waiting time).

In 1997, US liver allocation policies had to be revised to prioritize patients using severity-of-disease metrics. Initially, location of care (home, hospital, ICU) was initially used as a surrogate for severity of disease. Unfortunately it soon became clear that location of care was more a reflection of physician behavior than an intrinsic characteristic of the patient's disease state. Later allocation policy employed the Child–Turcotte–Pugh score to measure disease severity. This metric was limited by the subjective nature of some of the variables and it imposed a categorization of patients into broad classes of patients with a ceiling effect.[9]

The limitations recognized in these allocation systems compelled researchers to look for more accurate and objective measures of need for liver transplant. This led to the adoption of waiting mortality risk as a reasonable way to prioritize waiting candidates. In 2002, policymakers in the USA chose the Model for End-stage Liver Disease (MELD)[10] to rank patients on the waiting list. This mathematical model defines the risk of death for patients with chronic liver disease relatively consistently using three laboratory values: international normalized ratio (INR), total bilirubin (TBili), and creatinine (Cr). By using these simple, readily available variables that are intrinsic to the patient, more objective and difficult to manipulate, and that are not subject to behavioral biases, individual justice of the system and equity were more easily and transparently measured and understood.

Unique in the development and application of the MELD model for liver allocation was the prospective validation of this model, to be sure it consistently predicted 3-month mortality risk for waiting liver patients with a variety of disease etiologies.[11] These studies documented that, for liver transplant candidates, the MELD score was a very good, but not perfect, model to determine who would survive to transplant and who would die. Even though the results consistently showed that the MELD score was highly predictive for patients with hepatic synthetic dysfunction, policymakers recognized at the outset that there may be additional factors that could improve the MELD score's applicability to all patients and the MELD-based allocation system would require specific accommodations for certain diagnoses such as hepatocellular carcinoma or recently hepatopulmonary syndrome.[12] Of note, despite initial concern that a "sickest first" system would decrease post-transplant survival, the change to a MELD-based allocation has not worsened liver transplant outcomes.[13]

The application of the MELD system to organ allocation has assisted in the development of objective limits to help identify patients who are "too sick" or "too well" for transplant. Merion and colleagues examined whether the survival benefit for LT varied based on MELD score.[14] Candidates with low MELD scores (<15) had a lower risk of death without a transplant than those who underwent transplantation. This implies that the surgical, donor, and immunosuppressive risks for recipients with these low mortality risks exceed the mortality risk associated with their liver disease alone. Conversely, despite the higher operative risk for patients with high MELD scores, the survival benefit conferred by a successful liver transplant was present even for those with the greatest severity of illness. In more recent studies in which the quality of the donor organ is taken into account, patients with mild liver disease defined by a MELD score <15 incur more risk than benefit from LT with almost any organ type and this risk is escalated when an organ with higher risks for graft failure is used. In contrast, for patients with more severe liver disease and higher MELD scores, using higher risk grafts confers survival benefit since the risk of dying without the transplant is so much greater for these patients.[12]

Internationally, the MELD score has been incorporated into many liver allocation plans and is widely acknowledged as improving transparency and allowing for development of metrics to better evaluate the systems' efficacy. For example, in Europe, Eurotransplant has adopted a MELD score-based organ allocation system, and others are evaluating modifications.

Optimizing the allocation system: improving MELD

One approach to improving a MELD-based allocation system has been to improve the accuracy, and thereby the transparency, of the MELD score for predicting mortality by adding additional laboratory variables. Hyponatremia is commonly associated with ascites, hepatorenal syndrome, and an increased mortality rate. Based on these clinical observations, several investigators have suggested that including serum sodium in the calculation of mortality risk may improve a model's predictive accuracy,[15] especially for those patients with otherwise lower MELD scores.[16]

The OPTN database is currently collecting serum sodium values for waitlisted candidates to prospectively assess this factor in the USA. Others have also suggested scores that factor in serum sodium, such as the iMELD (age, serum sodium, and MELD composite score),[17] MESO index (MELD score, serum sodium),[18] and the United Kingdom End-stage Liver Disease (UKELD) score.[19] The UKELD score appears to be more accurate than MELD score for predicting short-term mortality from liver disease for patients in the UK.[20]

Another approach aimed at standardizing MELD variables, has been to examine the laboratory tests themselves. First, the international pro-thrombin normalized ratio (INR) currently in clinical use was developed for monitoring anticoagulant therapy and was never validated as an accurate measure of the coagulopathy associated with liver disease since cirrhosis impacts coagulation in numerous ways. Moreover, inter-laboratory variability in INR can result in alteration of the MELD score by as much as 11 or 12 MELD points, dramatically affecting a candidate's position on the waiting list.[21] Investigators in Italy have developed a "liver INR" to overcome these limitations.[22]

Medication effects on INR, such as Coumadin therapy, may also affect the MELD score. Other assessments of coagulation, however, have not yet been validated. The MELD-XI, a composite score calculated using serum creatinine and serum bilirubin but excluding INR, has been proposed for patients on anticoagulation therapy.[23] Others have reassessed the coefficients in the MELD equation to update the relative weights assigned to the laboratory values. A number of studies suggest that patients with worse renal function enjoy less survival benefit and have worse outcomes when compared to MELD-matched counterparts. As such, they advocate for a change in the weight of creatinine in the MELD score. Such a change has been modeled by Sharma et al., who described an "updated MELD" score using the same components (INR, TBili, Cr) weighted differently to reflect a current waiting list mortality model. In their study, the "updated MELD score" assigns a *lower* weight to creatinine and INR and a higher weight to bilirubin, which resulted in a more accurate prediction of the current waiting list mortality.[24] Some have expressed concern for the accuracy of some blood test assays in cases where the bilirubin or creatinine exceed normal ranges.[25]

Other modified scores have been suggested to account for issues that may influence patient mortality, such as the rapidity of clinical decline, also known as delta MELD (Δ MELD), which is simply the difference between MELD scores calculated at two separate times. However, Bambha et al. demonstrated the limited value of Δ MELD in predicting patient survival using a model that incorporated data from the UNOS registry from 1990 to 1999. They found that Δ MELD was predictive of death only within 4 days of death, thereby limiting its value in liver allocation.[26]

Some experts feel that the patient's gender should be included in the equation because, at similar serum creatinine values, women usually have lower glomerular filtration rates when compared to men (MELD Modified-by-Gender score).[27] In a retrospective analysis of the UNOS registry from 2002 to 2006, Moylan et al. provided evidence that the use of serum creatinine does produce a gender bias. These investigators demonstrated that women were more likely to die on the waiting list after a MELD-based allocation system was adopted. In this study, women also had a shorter time to death while waiting compared to their male counterparts,[28] presumably because women on the waiting list had more severe liver disease than men with the same MELD score.

The extent of the impact of the creatinine on a MELD-based allocation system has been well documented. In 2007, the OPTN reported a dramatic rise in the number of combined liver and kidney transplants performed in the USA related to the fact that more patients with severe renal insufficiency reach the top of the waiting list than previously.[29] A number of groups have published algorithms that include renal biopsy,[30] GFR measurement, and dialysis duration[31] to try to better select patients whose renal failure is likely to recover with LT from those with more fixed renal disease. Recent consensus guidelines have been promulgated to assist in the determination of the need for simultaneous liver–kidney transplant.[32]

As indicated earlier, prioritization of patients with HCC requires consideration of principles of both justice and equity. Patients with early-stage HCC have better survival rates with liver transplantation than can be achieved with resection alone,[33–35] however most patients with HCC present with relatively mild intrinsic liver disease and thus have a relatively low risk of dying in the near term from chronic liver disease. Prioritizing these patients for donor organs using a mortality risk index based solely on hepatic function would rank them below the majority of waiting candidates. Such a scheme would fail to deliver organ offers in a timely manner, which would result in the cancer progressing beyond the favorable, earlier stages. In such a system, many patients with HCC would be forced to drop off of the waiting list. Most liver transplant experts recognize the Milan criteria[36] as defining a favorable stage for LT. Ample documentation exists that patients with HCC meeting the Milan criteria have LT results that are comparable with patients who do not have malignant liver disease. The US liver allocation policymakers recognized that patients with HCC meeting the Milan criteria should be eligible for priority on the waiting list greater than what would be allowed by their intrinsic MELD score alone. Consequently, the US allocation system arbitrarily assigns patients with HCC meeting Milan criteria a MELD score of 22 in an effort to equate the risk of dropping off the list due to HCC tumor progression with the risk of dying that is borne by patients with chronic liver disease without HCC.

The Milan criteria have been challenged in single-center series that suggest that some patients with HCC advanced beyond the Milan criteria may have outcomes similar to patients meeting the Milan criteria after liver transplant. Investigators have developed several other selection methods such as total tumor volume and AFP.[37] The University of California at San Francisco (UCSF) group has advocated expanding the HCC criteria for which increased priority is assigned and have proposed this: tumor size ≤6.5 cm or up to three tumors, none larger than 4.5 cm and the sum of the diameters <8 cm defines liver transplant candidates who have excellent survival rates after transplantation. Other studies, however, have documented inferior 5-year survival rates in patients falling outside the Milan criteria: 70%, 63%, and 34% (for patients within Milan criteria, patients within UCSF but outside of Milan criteria, and patients outside both UCSF and Milan criteria, respectively).[38]

The Metroticket method for estimating survival after LT for HCC equates the number and size of HCC nodules with 5-year survival rates. Using this concept, the "rule of sevens" (seven as the sum of the size of the largest tumor (in cm) and the number of tumors), the Metroticket investigators observed nearly equivalent survival at 5 years for patients within the Milan criteria and patients falling within the rule of sevens (76% vs 71%, respectively). However, patients with microvascular invasion were more common in the group with HCC beyond the Milan criteria and this subset fared far worse 5 years after liver transplant (patient survival rate 33%).[39]

Allowing an increased priority for patients with HCC advanced beyond the Milan criteria may be acceptable in terms of individual justice since these patients have no other hope for cure. However, such a policy may violate the principals of utility, equity, and distributive justice by further disadvantaging other candidates on the waiting list and could reduce overall transplant benefit from the available organs. The potential effects of transplanting patients with advanced HCC have been estimated by Volk and Marrero using Markov model techniques.[40] Their models estimated that allowing patients with HCC meeting the UCSF criteria would likely result in a 44% increased risk for dying on the list for the candidates without HCC and MELD scores >20. Since there is a large variation in the distribution of MELD scores for waiting candidates among the US regions, allowing more patients beyond Milan criteria to receive extra priority would have differing effects in different areas around the country, depending on the relative numbers of candidates and donors.

There are other conditions for which mortality risk due to liver disease does not appropriately define the need for LT, including hepatopulmonary syndrome, familial amyloidosis, and metabolic liver diseases.[41] For these patients, poor quality of life and/or ongoing non-hepatic end-organ disease is a more accurate measure of liver transplant need. Additionally in these cases, by the time the liver disease has progressed, the concomitant end-organ disease may be irreversible. Recently, the OPTN has determined that patients with hepatopulonary syndrome or amyloidosis can be granted additional priority if they meet strict guidelines. There are many other conditions for which LT has been suggested as an effective treatment. Some of these conditions manifest mostly as deteriorations in quality of life rather than progressing to increased risk of death (e.g. polycystic liver disease). In these cases, it is difficult to equate the risk of quality of life deterioration with the risk of death, making it difficult to justify granting additional priority to these conditions beyond others associated with a high risk of death. At the present time, the US system employs a regional peer-review process to assess individual requests for increased priority on the list for patients with conditions where mortality risk is not an applicable prioritization endpoint.

Ultimately and ideally, endpoints other than mortality risk can, and should, be developed to define the need for liver transplant for the more rare conditions that are not necessarily life threatening in the near term. An international consensus conference addressed these conditions and suggested that a much more rigorous data collection effort be undertaken so that need for liver transplant endpoints similar to risk of death or risk of HCC progression could be developed. The goal of these efforts should be to better equate the progression of these conditions with the mortality risk so that patients with differing indications for liver transplant can be treated with justice and equity without impacting utility.

Distribution and allocation of organs from expanded donor pool

The growing disparity between the deceased donor organ supply and demand has refocused attention on the use of less-than-ideal liver allografts. In the past, many of these higher risk donor (HRD) livers were not utilized due to fear of poor outcomes, such as: initial poor graft function, primary graft nonfunction, postoperative complications, and decreased patient or graft survival. More recently, however, to address the ongoing waiting list mortality, transplant centers have increased the use of these livers in selected patients with promising results. Consequently, to better estimate the risk and benefit of using HRD grafts, and to assess their place in organ allocation and distribution, investigators have been intensely focused on charactering the factors that predict successful outcome with these so-called "marginal", expanded criteria, or HRD livers.

Expanding the donor pool: the kidney experience

The study of HRDs has a counterpart in the field of kidney transplantation. In 2001, members of the transplant community met in Crystal City, Virginia, to develop guidelines to maximize the use of deceased donor organs, particularly those recovered from donors >60 years of age where the discard rate of kidneys was almost 50%. The conferees estimated that the increased utilization of such kidneys could increase the donor pool by 38%.[42] To more accurately define the characteristics for these expanded-criteria kidney donors, the Scientific Registry of Transplant Recipients (SRTR) developed a set donor risk factors that defined a relative risk of kidney graft failure of >1.7. The donor risk factors are as follows: 1) history of hypertension, 2) stroke as the cause of death, and 3) a pre-procurement creatinine level >1.5 mg/dl. The 1-year graft survival for extended criteria donor (ECD) kidneys was 82% vs 89% for standard criteria donor kidney transplants performed during the same time interval.

Policymakers used the conclusions from the Crystal City conference to develop an allocation policy for these kidneys in which a waiting candidate could, with informed consent, choose to indicate that he or she is willing to accept a kidney from an ECD.[43] Subsequent studies suggested that all adult diabetic kidney transplant candidates, and all other adult kidney transplant candidates over the age of 40 who were likely to wait on the list for more than 3.5 years, would benefit from receiving one of these ECD kidneys.[44]

The original ECD criteria for kidney donors impose an arbitrary and dichotomous distinction of donor quality and therefore do not always accurately define the likelihood for success, and, importantly, do not apply to liver donors. More recently, Feng et al. addressed this gap by describing a continuous scale, the donor risk index (DRI), which estimated the relative risk of *liver* graft failure based on the following factors: 1) donor age >70, 2) African–American race, 3) reduced donor height, 4) cerebrovascular accident as the cause of donor death, 5) donation after cardiac death (DCD), 6) split graft, and 7) cold ischemia time >8 hours.[45] The DRI suffers from several limitations, and, for this reason, it has not been incorporated into an allocation or distribution policy. Factors such as liver steatosis and transmissible donor infections are not included in the DRI but can affect the risk associated with a donor liver and should be considered if graft quality is to be incorporated into such policies. Unlike the kidney ECD system, it is difficult to conceive of a separate waiting list or consent process for higher risk donor livers, since there is ample evidence that even the highest risk liver transplant candidates are likely to attain a survival benefit when allocated an HRD liver.

Schaubel et al. utilized data from the SRTR from 2001 to 2005 and found that patients with a MELD score ≥20 experienced a statistically significant reduction in the relative risk of death with transplantation compared with no transplant, even when a very high-DRI liver was used. Conversely, patients with low MELD scores had increased relative risks of death with the transplant, indicating that these low-risk patients may actually be harmed when the higher risk, high-DRI liver is transplanted into them.[14] These trends for poorer overall survival for patients with low MELD scores who receive higher risk grafts have been confirmed in other single-center[46] and national database[47] studies.

Future liver allocation and distribution systems will likely limit HRD liver graft availability for lower risk candidates and widen access to higher risk candidates since it is clear that very ill patients with high MELD scores receive much more benefit than lower risk candidates. A more extensive discussion of ECDs or HRDs is included in Chapters 17, 18 and 19.

Several allocation approaches have attempted to better match grafts and candidates by risk characteristics to "optimize" outcomes. One example is the D-MELD score, which used donor age (a component of the DRI) and MELD.[48] In this study the authors identified combinations of donor age and recipient MELD scores that were associated with better outcomes. These authors did not, however, account for overall survival benefit and did not assess whether an allocation system based on D-MELD would improve overall survival benefit. Other, more complicated proposals where donor and recipient factors have been combined to predict post-transplant outcome have been published, but these have failed to account for the survival benefit consideration.

Using sophisticated modeling programs, extensive effort has been made to assess the potential effects of using a combination of donor and recipient variables to define survival benefit. The OPTN is currently evaluating various scenarios to prioritize liver transplant candidates. For example, a calculation made at the time of an organ offer could incorporate the transplant benefit, donor variables, and candidate variables.[19] Such a score could be applied over any, or all, organ distribution units.

Split-liver transplantation

Distribution and allocation of liver segments split either during, or immediately after, retrieval remains controversial. Several European distribution systems have promoted splitting all appropriate grafts and have achieved improvement in utility as a result of the ability to provide liver transplants to more than one recipient per donor organ. Estimates in improved life-years saved by a national policy that would require splitting of suitable donor livers with segments II and III being distributed to a pediatric candidate and the remaining segments to an adult, indicate a gain in total life-years for the system, even though there may be a slight increase in technical complications under such a policy.[49] A more recent single-center report documented results for splitting donor livers for two adult recipients, where one partial liver graft was allocated according to a MELD-based ranking system and the other liver graft was transplanted into a second candidate irrespective of his or her place on the waiting list. For each potential split, the predicted graft-to-recipient weight ratio (GRWR) for the graft allocated based on MELD score had to be more than 1. Of the 22 grafts assigned by MELD, 13 and the remaining seven were assigned using a GRWR of >0.7.[50] The patient and graft survival rates were 90% and 86%, respectively. The fact that a large proportion of the splits ultimately did not get allocated to the higher MELD candidates (nine out of 22 donors) indicates that donor and patient selection in a center-based system may be important for achieving these excellent results.

Carving out a center-based allocation system to potentially encourage more splitting of liver donors is controversial in the USA. Other areas of the world, however, have been able to overcome these difficulties by employing experienced donor teams adept at the technical aspects and educating recipient teams to be willing to accept these grafts. Alternative allocation systems have been proposed to increase the utilization of split livers, particularly in the case where an organ appropriate for splitting is initially allocated to an adult.[51] The possibility of jumping over potentially more ill candidates with higher mortality risks on the waiting list just to enable two smaller sized, but less ill, individuals to receive split-liver grafts remains a difficult ethical challenge. Balancing individual justice and population utility are both in play.

Joining distribution with allocation

As discussed earlier, the ethical principles of organ allocation apply across both organ distribution and organ allocation polices. The goal of current allocation policy is to rank candidates in order of need, with patients thought to receive the most benefit ranked with highest priority. Based on the data indicating that patients with MELD scores <15 have a higher mortality risk if they receive a transplant compared with continuing to wait on the list, the US organ allocation system manipulated the organ distribution units and allocation system within the units to try to increase the probability of transplanting patients with the most to gain.[52] This policy, informally known as "Share 15," was created to address the need for sharing of livers more broadly for patients at higher risk of mortality while at the same time directing fewer organs to patients who are not likely to benefit from transplantation. Share 15 mandates that livers are offered regionally if there are no waitlisted patients within a DSA with a MELD score >15 so that organs are directed primarily to candidates most likely to benefit with less regard to distribution unit boundaries. Many have raised concern that widening organ distribution units and the resultant increases in organ travel distances may increase ischemic times and negatively affect graft function after transplant. To address this concern, Mangus et al. examined their center's experience with organs imported from other OPTN regions. These investigators did not observe a difference in initial graft function, early graft loss, or intraoperative death for the recipients of imported grafts compared with recipients of grafts from their local DSA.[53] These data suggest that wider organ sharing in the USA does not necessarily result in poorer outcomes. Such findings may support policymakers' efforts to change distribution units to more efficiently direct liver grafts to candidates most likely to benefit regardless of their geographic location. However, this challenge is extremely complex since deceased donor potential is not evenly distributed across the geography and waiting lists are extremely variable in terms of candidate numbers and severity of disease. Moreover, the donor and waiting list densities are not matched to each other. Increasing distribution units in some areas will enhance organ availability for the more needy patients but, in other instances, will also serve to combine already higher density waiting lists with each other without a coincidental increase in the number of available organs, thereby perturbing distributive justice and limiting utility of the system.[54]

Summary

Organ distribution and allocation policies and practice must take the ethical principles of justice, utility, and equity into account. The donor resource is so constrained that no one ethical principle can be dominant; trying to improve one aspect can negatively impact the others. In the past, donor distribution units have been based mostly on geographic or administrative/political boundaries with little consideration for optimizing donor organ distribution or survival benefit of LT. It is well recognized that donor livers are not all uniform in quality and that selecting new distribution units and/or methods to prioritize candidates must increasingly account for the variations in risks that the deceased donor pool carry. Future policy developments are likely to put more emphasis on optimizing overall survival benefit, rather than just focusing on post-transplant survival. To do so, policymakers will increasingly be compelled to accommodate the well-recognized variations in donor quality since justice, utility, and equity are influenced by the distribution of, and prioritization for, higher risk donor organs. Unfortunately, current models for estimating survival after LT remain relatively inaccurate and are too imprecise on which to base organ distribution or allocation policy. Much more research based on objectively defined patient and donor variables will be necessary to move these efforts forward.

References

1. Watt KD, Pedersen RA, Kremers WK, Heimbach JK, Charlton MR. Evolution of causes and risk factors for mortality post-liver transplant: results of the NIDDK long-term follow-up study. Am J Transplant 2010;10:1420–7.
2. Merion RM, Schaubel DE, Dykstra DM, Freeman RB, Port FK, Wolfe RA. The survival benefit of liver transplantation. Am J Transplant 2005;2:307–13.
3. Merion RM, Guidinger MK, Newmann JM, Ellison MD, Port FK, Wolfe RA. Prevalence and outcomes of multiple-listing for cadaveric kidney and liver transplantation. Am J Transplant 2004;4:94–100.
4. Perut V, Conti F, Scatton O, Soubrane O, Calmus Y, Vidal-Trecan G. Might physicians be restricting access to liver transplantation for patients with alcoholic liver disease? J Hepatol 2009;51:707–14.
5. Trotter JF, Osgood MJ. MELD scores of liver transplant recipients according to size of waiting list: impact of organ allocation and patient outcomes. JAMA 2004;291:1871–4.
6. Hayashi PH, Axelrod DA, Galanko J, Salvalaggio PR, Schnitzler M. Regional differences in deceased donor liver transplantation and their implications for organ utilization and allocation. Clin Transplant 2011;25: 156–63.
7. Neuberger J, Gimson A, Davies M, et al. Selection of patients for liver transplantation and allocation of donated livers in the UK. Gut 2008;57:252–7.
8. Rogiers X, Sieders E. Split-liver transplantation: an underused resource in liver transplantation. Transplantation 2008;86:493–9.
9. Freeman RB, Wiesner RH, Harper A, et al. The New Liver Allocation System: moving towards evidence-based transplantation policy. Liver Transplant 2002;8:851–8.
10. Kamath PS, Wiesner RH, Malinchoc M, et al. A model to predict survival in patients with end-stage liver disease. Hepatology 2001;33:464–70.
11. Wiesner RH, Edwards EB, Freeman RB, et al. Model for end stage liver disease (MELD) and allocation of donor livers. Gastroenterology 2003;124:91–6.
12. Schaubel, Sima CS, Goodrich NP, Feng S, Merion RM. The survival benefit of decreased donor liver transplantation as a function of candidate disease severity and donor quality. Am J Transplant 2008;8:419–25.
13. Freeman RB, Harper A, Edwards EB. Liver outcomes under the model for end-stage liver disease and pediatric

end-stage liver disease. Curr Opin Organ Transplant 2005;10:90–4.
14. Schaubel DE, Guidinger MK, Biggins SW, et al. Survival benefit-based deceased-donor liver allocation. Am J Transplant 2009;9:970–81.
15. Biggins, SW, Kim WR, Terrault NA, et al. Evidence-based incorporation of serum sodium concentration into MELD. Gastroenterology 2006;130:1652–60.
16. Heuman DM, Abou-Assi SG, Habib A, et al. Persistent ascites and low serum sodium identify patients with cirrhosis and low MELD scores who are at high risk for early death. Hepatology 2004;40:802–10.
17. Luca A, Angermayr B, Bertolini G, et al. An integrated MELD model including serum sodium and age improves the prediction of early mortality in patients with cirrhosis. Liver Transpl 2007;13: 1174–80.
18. Lu XH, Liu HB, Wang Y, Wang BY, Song M, Sun MJ. Validation of model for end-stage liver disease score to serum sodium ratio index as a prognostic predictor in patients with cirrhosis. J Gastroenterol Hepatol 2009;24:1547–53.
19. Lewsey JD, Dawwas M, Copley LP, Gimson A, Van der Meulen JH. Developing a prognostic model for 90-day mortality after liver transplantation based on pretransplant recipient factors. Transplantation 2006;82: 898–907.
20. Young AL, Rajagenashan R, Asthana S, et al. The value of MELD and sodium in assessing potential liver transplant recipients in the United Kingdom. Transpl Int 2007;20:331–7.
21. Porte RJ, Lisman T, Tripodi A, Caldwell SH, Trotter JF. The international normalized ratio (INR) in the MELD score: Problems and solutions; the Coagulation in Liver Disease Study Group. Am J Transplant 2010;10: 1349–53.
22. Tripodi A, Chantarangkul V, Primignani M, et al. The international normalized ratio calibrated for cirrhosis (INR(liver)) normalizes prothrombin time results for model for end-stage liver disease calculation. Hepatology 2007;46:520–7.
23. Heuman DM, Mihas AA, Habib A, et al. MELD-XI: a rational approach to "sickest first" liver transplantation in cirrhotic patients requiring anticoagulant therapy. Liver Transpl 2007;13:30–7.
24. Sharma P, Schaubel DE, Sima CS, Merion RM, Lok AS. Re-weighting the model for end-stage liver disease score components. Gastroenterology 2008;135:1575–81.
25. Cholongitas E, Marelli L, Kerry A, et al. Different methods of creatinine measurement significantly affect MELD scores. Liver Transpl 2007;13:523–9.
26. Bambha K, Kim WR, Kremers WK, et al. Predicting survival among patients listed for liver transplantation: an assessment of serial MELD measurements. Am J Transplantation 2004;4:1798–1804.
27. Cholongitas E, Marelli L, Kerry A, et al. Female liver transplant recipients with the same GFR as male recipients have lower MELD scores – a systematic bias. Am J Transplant 2007;7:685–92.
28. Moylan CA, Brady CW, Johnson JL, et al. Disparities in liver transplantation before and after introduction of the MELD score. JAMA 2008;300: 2371–8.
29. Davis CL, Feng S, Sung R, et al. Simultaneous liver–kidney transplantation: evaluation to decision making. Am J Transplant 2007;7:1702–9.
30. Tanriover B, Mejia A, Weinstein J, et al. Analysis of kidney function and biopsy results in liver failure patients with renal dysfunction: a new look to combined liver kidney allocation in the post-MELD era. Transplantation 2008;86:1548–53.
31. Ruiz R, Jennings LW, Kim P, et al. Indications for combined liver and kidney transplantation: propositions after a 23-yr experience. Clin Transplant 2010; 24:807–11.
32. Charlton MR, Wall WJ, Ojo AO, et al. Report of the first international liver transplantation society expert panel consensus conference on renal insufficiency in liver transplantation. International Liver Transplantation Society Expert Panel. Liver Transpl 2009;15:S1–34.
33. Llovet JM, Fuster J, Bruix J. Intention to treat analysis of surgical treatment for early hepatocellular carcinoma: resection versus transplantation. Hepatology 1999;30:1434–40.
34. Figueras J, Jaurrieta E, Valls C, et al. Resection or transplantation for hepatocellular carcinoma in cirrhotic patients: outcomes based on indicated treatment strategy. J Am Coll Surg 2000;190:580–7.
35. Hemming AW, Cattral MS, Reed AI, et al. Liver Transplantation for hepatocellular carcinoma. Ann Surg 2001;233:652–9.
36. Mazzaferro V, Regalia E, Doci R, et al. Liver transplantation for the treatment of small hepatocellular carcinomas in patients with cirrhosis. N Engl J Med 1996;334:693–9.
37. Toso C, Asthana S, Bigam DL, Shapiro AM, Kneteman NM. Reassessing selection criteria prior to liver transplantation for hepatocellular carcinoma utilizing the scientific registry of transplant recipients database. Hepatology 2008;49:832–8.
38. Decaens T, Roudot-Thoraval F, Hadni-Bresson S, et al. Impact of UCSF criteria according to pre- and post-OLT tumor features: analysis of 479 patients listed for HCC with a short waiting time. Liver Transpl 2006;12: 1761–9.
39. Mazzaferro V, Llovet JM, Miceli R, et al. for the Metroticket Investigator Study Group. Predicting sur-

vival after liver transplantation in patients with hepatocellular carcinoma beyond the Milan criteria: a retrospective, exploratory analysis. Lancet Oncol 2009; 10:35–43.
40. Volk M, Marrero JA. Liver transplantation for hepatocellular carcinoma: who benefits and who is harmed? Gastroenterology 2008;134:1612–14.
41. Freeman RB, Gish RG, Harper A, et al. Model for end stage liver disease (MELD exception guidelines: Results and recommendations from the MELD exception study group and conference (MESSAGE) for the approval of patients who need liver transplantation with diseases not considered by the standard MELD formula. Liver Transplantation 2006;12(Suppl 3):S128–36.
42. Metzger RA, Delmonico FL, Feng S, et al. Expanded criteria donors for kidney transplantation. Am J Transplant 2003;3(Suppl 4):114–25.
43. See http://optn.transplant.hrsa.gov/policiesAndBylaws/policies.asp for ECD kidney allocation policy (accessed May 20, 2010)
44. Merion RM, Ashby VB, Wolfe RA, et al. Deceased-donor characteristics and the survival benefit of kidney transplantation. JAMA 2005;294:2726–33.
45. Feng S, Goodrich NP, Bragg-Gresham JL, et al. Characteristics associated with liver graft failure: the concept of a donor risk index. Am J Transplant 2006;6:783–90.
46. Bonney GK, Aldersley MA, Asthana S, et al. Donor risk index and MELD interactions in predicting long-term graft survival: a single-centre experience. Transplantation 2009;87:1858–63.
47. Volk ML, Lok AS, Pelletier SJ, Ubel PA, Hayward RA. Impact of the model for end-stage liver disease allocation policy on the use of high-risk organs for liver transplantation. Gastroenterology 2008;135: 1568–74.
48. Halldorson JB, Bakthavatsalam R, Fix O, Reyes JD, Perkins JD. D-MELD, a simple predictor of post liver transplant mortality for optimization of donor/recipient matching. Am J Transplant 2009;9:318–26.
49. Merion RM, Rush SH, Zinsser DM, Goodrich N, Freeman RB, Wolfe RA. Predicted lifetimes for adult and pediatric split liver versus adult whole liver transplant recipients. Am J Transplant 2004;4: 1792–7.
50. Cescon M, Grazi GL, Ravaioli M, et al. Conventional split liver transplantation for two adult recipients: a recent experience in a single European center. Transplantation 2009;88:1117–22.
51. Emond JC, Freeman RB Jr, Renz JF, Yersiz H, Rogiers X, Busuttil RW. Optimizing the use of donated cadaver livers: analysis and policy development to increase the application of split-liver transplantation. Liver Transpl 2002;8:863–72.
52. For a full description of current OPTN policies see: http://www.optn.org/PoliciesandBylaws/policies/docs/policy_8.doc
53. Mangus RS, Fridell JA, Vianna RM, et al. No difference in clinical transplant outcomes for local and important liver allografts. Liver Transpl 2009;15:640–7.
54. Freeman RB, Harper AM, Edwards EB. Redrawing organ distribution boundaries: Results of a computer simulated analysis for liver transplantation. Liver Transpl 2002;8:659–66.

8

Viral hepatitis and transplantation

Geoffrey W. McCaughan
AW Morrow Gastroenterology and Liver Centre, Royal Prince Alfred and the University of Sydney, Centenary Research Institute, Sydney, NSW, Australia

Key learning points

- Hepatitis B virus (HBV) recurrence post liver transplantation is now <5% with excellent outcomes.
- Hepatitus C virus (HCV) recurrence post-transplant can be prevented if the patient is rendered polymerase chain reaction (PCR) negative pre transplant.
- Progressive HCV allograft injury is strongly associated with increasing donor age.
- Pulse corticosteroid use in HCV patients should be avoided.
- HCV antiviral therapy has only modest success in the post-transplant setting but if successful leads to improved outcomes.

Burden of disease

The major reasons for liver transplantation in the context of viral hepatitis is in the setting of chronic hepatitis B or chronic hepatitis C infection. It is estimated over 350 million people worldwide are chronically infected with hepatitis B and it is estimated that approximately 20% will develop the complications of cirrhosis or hepatocellular cancer.[1] Both these conditions are well-recognized indications for liver transplantation. Hepatocellular cancer is the third most common solid cancer worldwide. In the western world, it is the most rapidly increasing cancer in Europe, the USA and Australia.[2]

Similarly to hepatitis B, chronic hepatitis C is associated with infection in over 200 million people worldwide.[3] Developments of progressive disease are similar to hepatitis B, with approximately 20% developing cirrhosis and complications of end-stage liver disease with a cumulative incident rate of 3–4% of hepatocellular cancer in these patients.

For both hepatitis B and C, there is emerging data that the introduction of antiviral therapies in the early stages of disease is associated with decreased risk of cirrhosis, liver failure and hepatocellular cancer.[4,5] Despite this, the logistics of delivering these therapies worldwide are considerable. Furthermore, antiviral therapies in hepatitis C infection are only successful in 50% of cases, thus the vast majority of patients coming to transplantation with chronic hepatitis C have already failed antiviral therapy. It is anticipated that the burden of end-stage liver disease and cancer related to chronic HCV infection will only increase over the 10–20 years. There is evidence, however, for a decrease in the use of liver transplantation in chronic hepatitis B infection since the introduction of antiviral therapy, suggesting that the burden of disease certainly in the western world and the need for liver transplantation in this situation is decreasing. This may be due to the successful control of viral replication and improved outcomes of the complications of end-stage disease.

Indications for liver transplantation: chronic hepatitis B and hepatitis C infection

Indications for liver transplantation for chronic hepatitis B and hepatitis C are the presence of hepatic

Medical Care of the Liver Transplant Patient, Fourth Edition. Edited by Pierre-Alain Clavien, James F. Trotter.

decompensation in a patient with cirrhosis or the development of HCC with or without decompensation. The indications for liver transplantation in the setting of HCC are discussed in a separate chapter (see Chapter 11). Furthermore the indications for transplantation in fulminant hepatitis are discussed in Chapter 16.

It is generally thought that patients should be listed for liver transplantation for chronic hepatitis B or chronic hepatitis C cirrhosis once there are single clinical features such as uncontrolled ascites, recurrent/persistent encephalopathy or persistent gastrointestinal bleeding despite therapeutic interventions. This usually means that the patient has a Child–Pugh score of ≥10. More recently, the introduction of the Model for End-stage Liver Disease (MELD) scoring system has become a much more evidence-based means of listing patients for transplantation. The MELD score is a severity score with predictive mortality in patients with chronic liver disease and applies well to chronic hepatitis B and C. Recent data suggests that the benefit of liver transplantation tends to come in with a MELD score of around 15–17 and thus it seems reasonable, in the absence of uncontrollable symptoms, that the MELD score alone can be used for listing of liver transplantation.[6] Other general indications for liver transplantation are applicable to chronic hepatitis B and C infection (see Chapter 1 and Box 8.1).

It should be realized, however, that an indication for liver transplantation for chronic hepatitis B often involves patients who are having flares of their active disease. Although these can often be controlled with early antiviral therapy there exist a group of patients who do progress despite control of viremia. These patients have a serum bilirubin >120 μmol for late onset, elevated renal function (creatinine >200 μmol/L), and detectable HBV DNA in sera. The combination of all of these invariably leads to progression of liver failure and death despite antiviral therapy and transplantation should be considered in these patients earlier rather than later.[7]

Box 8.1 Early predictors of need for liver transplant in an acute "flare" of chronic HBV infection[7]

Serum bilirubin >120 μmol/L
Serum creatinine >200 μmol/L
Detectable HBV DNA

Pre-transplantation antiviral therapy

Hepatitis B infection

Studies have shown that active HBV replication before orthotopic liver transplantation is the major risk factor for disease recurrence, thus therapeutic strategies to reduce or eliminate hepatitis B viral replication prior to liver transplantation are a priority. In patients with cirrhosis or cirrhosis and portal hypertension with HCC, interferon-based therapies have limited efficacy and may be associated with severe sepsis and worsening of hepatic failure. Over the last 15 years, the availability of several nucleoside and/or nucleotide analogs have significantly changed the management of end-stage liver disease due to hepatitis B. These drugs inhibit HBV DNA polymerase activity by binding to its active site but do not eradicate HBsAg because of persistence of HBV cccDNA within hepatocytes. These agents will be discussed later.

Lamivudine

Lamivudine has been extensively studied in the situation of liver transplantation. It is well-tolerated in patients with decompensated cirrhosis and results in undetectable DNA in approximately 70% of patients within 2–3 months. It is clear that such therapy improves the Child–Pugh Score and decreases the need for hospital admissions for complications such as ascites, subcutaneous bacterial peritonitis and encephalopathy. These observations led to a series of papers that showed that lamivudine could stabilize patients on the waiting list, allowing them to proceed to transplantation with negative HBV DNA and thus minimal chance of disease recurrence.[8] However as mentioned earlier, there are certain patients who may progress despite the antiviral efficacy of this drug.

This agent however is limited by the emergence of lamivudine resistance due to one or more mutations in the polymerase gene. These mutations are detected in approximately 20–30% of patients after 1 year of therapy and in up to 70% of patients within 5 years. It is well documented that the onset of lamivudine resistance in patients with cirrhosis leads to

Table 8.1 Recommendations of approaches to resistance when using anti-HBV agents[10]

Primary agent	Secondary agent
Lamivudine resistance	Add in adefovir
	Add in or replace with tenofovir
	Do not use entecavir
Adefovir resistance	Replace with entecavir (provided no lamivudine resistance exists)
	Replace with tenofovir
Entecavir resistance	Replace with tenofovir
Tenofovir resistance	None as yet?

worsening liver disease and can result in flares that are associated with mortality,[9] thus lamivudine would only be currently indicated in the situation where agents such as entecavir and tenofovir (see Table 8.1) were not available.

Adefovir

This agent, a nucleotide analog was shown to be effective as monotherapy in patients with mild forms of chronic hepatitis B. At the dose of 10 mg/d, however, it is mainly used in a setting of hepatic decompensation as an add-on therapy in patients who develop lamivudine resistance. It is not recommended that such patients switch from lamivudine to adefovir as this is associated with adefovir resistance (30% at 3 years).[10]

The combination of lamivudine and adefovir, however, is associated with minimal adefovir resistance and may control active viral replication, even in decompensated patients. It should be recognized that adefovir at 10 mg/d is a rather weak agent; its ability to induce clinical improvement in such situations is often slow and many patients fail to improve clinically to avoid liver transplantation. Despite this, several patients do go to liver transplantation with lamivudine resistance on a combination of lamivudine and adefovir therapy.

Entecavir and tenofovir

These two new agents have very potent HBV antiviral activity. They control HBV viral replication in the vast majority of patients with cirrhosis and both are associated with little resistance in previously untreated patients. A choice between them as primary therapy in patients with hepatic decompensation is not clear. There is evidence that both these drugs may reverse hepatic decompensation in the absence of lamivudine resistance.[8,11] It should be noted that a single case of lactic acidosis associated with entecavir therapy in the setting of decompensated disease has been reported.[12] Furthermore, a recent report suggests that entecavir may not be as useful as lamivudine in the setting of a hepatic flare and decompensation,[13] however this was not a controlled trial and the follow up regarding lamivudine resistance was not addressed. It is likely that the experience with entecavir in this setting simply reflects the type of patients previously reported who fail lamuvudine therapy despite control of viral load.[7] Entecavir should not be used in patients with previous lamivudine exposure or resistance as resistance to entecavir has been observed in such patients (50% at 3 years). Patients with lamivudine resistance are often now treated with tenofovir and increasingly patients in this situation will go to transplantation on lamivudine and tenofovir, or tenofovir monotherapy.

In summary, in the past many patients without lamivudine resistance went on to liver transplantation on lamivudine monotherapy. Today such patients may go to transplantation on tenofovir or entecavir monotherapy. Lamivudine-resistant patients are usually on lamivudine and adefovir/tenofovir combination therapy, although some may be on tenofovir alone. As mentioned earlier, patients with chronic HBV who still require transplantation despite these therapies fall into two groups: 1) those with HCC, and 2) those who present with such severe decompensation they can't be rescued with these therapies despite virologic control.

Chronic hepatitis C infection

Interferon–ribavirin-based therapies for chronic hepatitis C infection usually exclude patients with cirrhosis and portal hypertension and certainly patients with hepatic decompensation with Child–Pugh scores ≥10. There have been attempts to treat the latter with disastrous outcomes. There are a number of patients who proceed to liver transplantation with portal hypertension and HCC that may be suitable for antiviral therapy and are candidates for viral eradication in the pre-transplant period. These patients are however difficult to treat and caution should be given when using interferon-based therapies in such patients. Patients should certainly have bacterial prophylaxis with agents such as norfloxacin and preferably have eradicated significant esophageal varices before starting therapy. Furthermore, their nutritional intake should be maximized as interferon-based therapies are catabolic and often lead to falling albumin, which may precipitate ascites and further hepatic decompensation.

There are several studies with small numbers of patients that have been modestly successful in viral eradication in such settings;[14] this particularly applies to non-genotype 1 patients where SVR can be achieved on the intention-to-treat basis in up to 20–30% of patients. It should be noted, however that in genotype 1 patients, this is more likely to be in the 10–15% range. Despite these relatively low numbers it is thought that therapies might be worthwhile in patients with MELD scores <18 and no evidence of hepatic decompensation such as ascites or encephalopathy because the potential benefit of a true SVR in the pre-transplant setting has shown to be associated with the prevention of HCV recurrence in the post-transplant setting. It should be realized however that some patients who are on antiviral therapy and who are PCR negative at the time of transplantation (hence haven't yet established a true SVR) may relapse post transplant. It is recommend that the so-called "LADR" approach to use of pegylated interferon and ribavirin be used regarding dosing in these patients, i.e. starting at half doses of pegylated interferon and half doses of ribavirin and increasing over the first 2–4 weeks depending on tolerability regarding symptoms and cytopenias.[13]

Post liver transplant

Hepatitis B infection

The major issue here is that of HBV recurrence and this should be monitored for by testing for HBsAg and HBV DNA on a regular basis once the perioperative phase has passed. By the mid-1990s it had been recognized that administration of high-dose intravenous anti-HBsAg immunoglobulin (HBIG) could result in a reduction in the incidence of chronic hepatitis B infection post liver transplantation, particularly in DNA-negative and e-antigen-negative patients.[15] The use of HBIG requires the monitoring of anti-HBsAg, usually monthly, before each HBIG injection. The titres required to prevent HBV recurrence are not clear but if HBIG monotherapy was used (which is now not recommended) then levels of >100 IU/L are generally required. Following the introduction of lamivudine, several studies investigated the continuation of lamivudine monotherapy in the absence of HBIg to prevent viral replication.[16] Although this was moderately successful, there was re-infection in up to 50% of patients particularly who were HBV DNA positive at the time of transplant. Breakthroughs of HBV with lamivudine-resistant mutations were common and there was significant mortality when this occurred. One of the exceptions to this was the use of lamivudine monoprophylaxis in Asian recipients who received live donors from hepatitis B surface antigen negative but anti-HBs-positive donors.[12] These patients developed peak anti-HBs titres within 3 months after transplantation that exceeded 100 IU/ml and the HBV reaction in recipients was only 8%. It is almost certain that this antibody was produced by functional lymphocytes transferred from the donor to the recipient, suggesting the possibility of adoptive transfer of immunity from the liver graft.

Lamivudine monotherapy appeared to be inadequate prophylaxis and was rapidly replaced by a combination of HBIg and lamivudine. The first studies used intravenous HBIG at very high doses in combination with lamivudine monotherapy. They clearly demonstrated almost total eradication of hepatitis B recurrence and rapidly became the standard of care in most liver transplant centres. Mean infection rates were approximately 5%.[17] More recently, similar efficacy has been shown in several studies involving low-dose HBIG protocols in combination with lamivudine monotherapy.[18] HBIg is used as low as 400 IU/ml given intramuscularly with anti-HBs titres between 50–100 IU/L. It seems that these levels are sufficient in combination with direct antiviral agents to result in very low HBV recurrence. Of course for patients who were on lamivudine and adefovir therapy before liver transplantation for lamivudine resistance, HBIG was added. This combination therapy of lamivudine/adefovir and HBIG also resulted in very similar low levels of viral recurrence. After 1 year of therapy, the survival rate was 93% in the post liver transplant group.

The importance of withdrawing HBIG at some point post transplantation has been the subject of several studies. There is consistent emerging data now that long-term use of HBIG in this setting is unnecessary provided that the antiviral is not lamivudine monotherapy. HBIG can be discontinued and replaced with adefovir (i.e. lamivudine and adefovir therapy) with virtually no re-emergence of HBV infection.[19] As mentioned earlier, the role of continuing HBIG on patients who are on tenofovir and HBIG or entecavir and HBIG remains to be defined. With the use of more potent antiviral agents such approaches as attempting vaccination after or during HBIG are more likely to become redundant. A series of papers in the literature show that in a select group of liver transplantations, HBIG can be safely discontinued if anti-HBs seroconversion is induced with HBV vaccination.[16] The latter may occur in up to 50–80% of patients depending on the vaccine used. In one such study a novel adjuvant vaccine was used with quite high response rates.

With an increasing frequency of patients coming to liver transplantation on lamivudine and adefovir, entecavir or tenofovir alone (usually in the presence of HCC) the question of whether HBIG should be part of the protocol at all or whether these agents can be used as monotherapy is under regular discussion. Results from Australia and New Zealand indicate that use of lamivudine and adefovir (irrespective of previous lamivudine resistance) do not require HBIG to prevent recurrence 0/44 DNA and HBsAg negative (E. Gane, personal communication). Furthermore, initial results from Hong Kong indicate that entecavir monotherapy in this setting is effective in virtually eliminating HBV DNA recurrence although about 20% of patients are HBsAg positive (C.M. Lo, personal communication). It should be noted that this is occurring in the situation where many of the donors are anti-HBs positive and thus short-term HBIG therapy may still have a place. This may apply particularly to groups who are HBV DNA positive at the time of transplantation. This is a moot question. Recent results from Minnesota using tenofovir monotherapy and no HBIG also have excellent results with a recurrence rate of <10% (J. Lake, personal communication).

It seems we have moved to a post-HBIG era, where HBIG is only indicated in a few patients (those who are HBV DNA serum positive at transplant). Even in these patients, short-term low-dose intramuscular injection (IMI) therapy is likely to be enough.

Post-transplant de novo hepatitis B infection

This has mainly been described in liver transplant recipients from anti-HBcore antibody-positive donors. The risk of transmission is highest for anti-HcAb-negative and anti-HBs-negative recipients in the absence of any prophylaxis. Recent reviews of cohort studies indicate that lamivudine monotherapy used in HBsAg-negative recipients is sufficient in this setting to prevent HBV infection. It remains unclear whether this needs to be life-long treatment.[20]

Natural history of HCV post-transplant

Before discussing antiviral therapy, a review of the natural history of HCV recurrence post liver transplantation is required (Box 8.2). Unlike chronic HBV infection, currently there are no successful strategies to prevent HCV re-infection of the allograft. Recent studies show that HCV re-infection of the allograft can occur within 24 hours after liver transplantation, resulting in levels of viremia similar to pre-transplant levels within days.[21] Viral recurrence is then associated with peak viremia at about 3 months, which is usually at least one log higher than in the pre-transplant setting[22] and is associated with the onset invariably of acute hepatitis that may settle but always results in chronic hepatitis C in the allograft. A usual variant at this stage is the development of cholestatic HCV in approximately <10% of patients, which results in high levels of allograft failure.

Box 8.2 Chronic HCV: Factors definitely associated with worse outcomes[22]

Donor age
Severe hepatitis at 3 months
High viral load at 3 months
Evidence of SMA positivity on a biopsy at 3 months
F1 fibrosis at 12 months
High-dose pulse corticosteroids
OKT3 therapy

Once chronic hepatitis C is present in the allograft, then there may be progression to cirrhosis over a 5–10-year period. This is accelerated in many patients and can result in inferior outcomes for liver transplantation. Progression is variable, however, and the natural history of HCV recurrence at this stage has been studied at many levels. A major key variable in the prediction of progressive disease and increased fibrosis in the allograft are the features of the early hepatitis C recurrence episode at 3–4 months. Studies indicate that increased levels of hepatic inflammation in the allograft at that point predict later allograft fibrosis.[21] Levels of viral replication and detection of early markers of fibrosis such as smooth muscle actin (SMA) (in the absence of fibrosis in liver biopsy at this point) lead to increased levels of allograft loss or fibrosis at later time points.[23] After the 3-month point the 1-year liver biopsy is a key to prognosis. Evidence of even F1 fibrosis at this time point predicts advanced fibrosis at 5 years.[24]

There is much debate about whether different forms of immunosuppression alter outcomes. It is recommended that mild to moderate acute rejection episodes are not treated with pulse corticosteroid therapy but with an increase in background immunosuppression, as pulse steroids are detrimental. Only patients who have evidence of severe allograft rejection on liver biopsy (always in association with chronic hepatitis C) should be treated with pulse corticosteroids, however whether to completely withdraw corticosteroid (CS) is unclear. At least one study suggests that there is more rapid progression of disease when corticosteroids are withdrawn quickly.[25]

It is clear that OKT3 therapy (now not currently used at all) was associated with worse outcomes. The most controversial and highly debated issue is whether cyclosporin-based therapies or tacrolimus-based therapies affect HCV outcomes. Although isolated reports have supported worse outcomes of tacrolimus-based therapy, meta-analyses have not really supported this. More recently a multicenter randomized, controlled trial to study the effect of different immunosuppressive therapies has been carried out in the HCV-3 study, where three arms of immunosuppression were studied:[26]

1. Tacrolimus and corticosteroids
2. Tacrolimus, corticosteroids and mycophenolate
3. Mycophenolate, tacrolimus, and an IL-2 receptor antibody.

The results of disease progression in these three arms and clinical outcomes were identical in the first year, although there is some suggestion in the prednisone-free arm of mycophenolate and tacrolimus use that early IL-2 receptor induction has lessened disease progression in the second year. A full analysis of that result is to be awaited.

It is generally thought that hepatitis C patients should not be overimmunosuppressed and certainly quadruple immunosuppressive therapy is contraindicated. Other studies have indicated that genetic factors in the donor liver may affect outcomes of hepatitis C recurrence and one particular polymorphism of tumour necrosis factor has been associated with increased hepatic activity index in subsequent liver biopsies of the allograft.

The recommendations to prevent worse progressive allograft injury in the absence of antiviral therapy are to:

1. Monitor the viral load and minimize immunosuppression, not allowing the viral load to increase dramatically
2. Minimize cold ischemia in the graft
3. Avoid significant donor steatosis and significantly older donors
4. Taper immunosuppression slowly
5. Prevent CMV infection
6. Not treat acute rejection episodes blindly with pulse corticosteroid therapy.

Any one of these in isolation may not significantly affect the allograft outcome but combinations of these factors should be avoided. It is also important to recommend that control of body weight and alcohol intake (probably less than 5 drinks per week), known co-factors of disease progression in the pre-transplant state, be undertaken.

Despite these recommendations, allograft injury may be progressive and the ideal would be to control hepatitis C viral replication and obtain sustained virologic response with antiviral therapy.

Post-transplant antiviral therapy

Hepatitis C infection

There is now considerable data for this situation.[27] First, early use of interferon-based therapies in an attempt to minimize viral replication during the early months post transplant has been studied (so-called

Table 8.2 Chronic HCV: SVR following pegylated interferon and ribavirin[27]

Timepoint	Stage	Survival outcome
Non-transplant setting	G1	40–50%
	G2/3	70–80%
Pre-transplant (cirrhosis, portal hypertension, MELD <18)	G1	10–20%
Pre-transplant (cirrhosis, portal hypertension, MELD <18)	G2/3	40–50%
Post transplant	G1	20–30%
Post transplant	G2/3	30–50%

"pre-emptive" therapy) (Table 8.2). Such an approach has been compared to treating patients at later time points. Generally pre-emptive therapy is not recommended as there is no evidence that intervention at this stage has any greater benefit than treating the patient when required at later stages. It is also affected by poor tolerability of therapy. By far the greatest evidence for the use of antiviral therapy in the post-transplant setting occurs once there is established chronic infection and inflammation in the allograft. There are few randomized, controlled studies of this situation but data indicate the SVR rate is considerably lower than in the nontransplant setting. SVR rates are only obtained in 15–20% of genotype 1 patients and 30–40% of genotype 2/3 patients. There is, however, general agreement that if SVR is obtained then long-term outcomes in such patients are much improved compared to untreated patients or treated patients without an SVR. A major question revolves around when to start therapy. It has been previously recommended this should be undertaken at stage 2 fibrosis, however emerging data suggests that grade 1 fibrosis in the allograft at 12 months' post transplant is associated with worse outcomes. Increasingly antiviral therapy is being recommended once this level of fibrosis has been reached on a 12-month protocol biopsy.

One of the other controversial issues is whether ribavirin is well-tolerated in this situation as it would be expected to result in increasing complications. A recent Australian/New Zealand randomized, controlled trial compared pegylated interferon vs pegylated interferon and ribavirin in hepatitis C post liver transplantation.[28] Despite the increased complications of ribavirin, the SVR rates were considerably higher in the pegylated interferon and ribavirin arm vs pegylated interferon alone. Combination therapy is therefore indicated.

Outcomes of liver transplantation

Hepatitis B

There is no doubt that liver transplantation for hepatitis B has been one of the successful changing paradigms in liver transplantation medicine and surgery over the last 20 years. Before the introduction of direct antiviral agents, liver transplantation was often contraindicated in many western countries and outcomes were poor, however now, outcomes for liver transplantation for hepatitis B are probably one of the most successful in all patient subgroups, with 5-year survival rates of over 80%.[29]

Hepatitis C

Unlike hepatitis B infection, outcomes for liver transplant for hepatitis C seem worse in many centres over the past 10–15 years and outcomes are worse than in nonhepatitis C patients over long periods of time. More recently an Australia/New Zealand study indicated no improvement in HCV-related outcomes over a 20-year period despite significant improvement in nonhepatitis C patients.[30] It is thus expected that patients with hepatitis C have 5-year survival rates of approximately 70% compared to 80% for nonhepatitis C patients and at the 10-year mark 50% vs 70%, respectively. It is likely that some of these worsening outcomes of hepatitis C over this period of time have been associated with the use of older grafts and also certainly in some situations that lack of clear definition of hepatitis C recurrence alone in the allograft vs acute rejection and hepatitis C resulting in overimmunosuppression. It is also likely that improved outcomes in this situation will only arrive when new antiviral agents, such as the new HCV protease and polymerase inhibitors are introduced into practice in the pre- and post transplant setting. This will surely occur within the next 5 years and it is hoped that this will have revolutionized outcomes and approaches to hepatitis C in transplantation as have been seen in hepatitis B over the past 15 years.

Hepatitis delta

Of course some patients with HBV infection may be co-infected with the hepatitis delta virus (HDV). This occurs in the situation of simultaneous infection resulting in fulminant hepatitis and superinfection where HDV occurs in a patient with established chronic HBV. In the pretransplant setting therapies against HDV are not useful.[31] In the post-transplant setting the recurrence of HDV disease does not occur providing there is no HBV recurrence. HBV recurrence is minimal in this setting, even in the absence of the preventive approaches outlined previously,[32] however optimal prevention of HBV recurrence is required and should be used. The reason for this is that HDV itself may reinfect the allograft but will only become active if HBsAg returns as HBsAg is required for the production of HDV-replicating virions. If HBV reinfection does occur, however, there can be fulminant HDV disease. As mentioned earlier, this is now rare and patients with HDV probably have the best outcomes of all HBV-infected patients post transplant.

Hepatitis E

The hepatitis E virus (HEV) is well recognized to be a cause of fulminant hepatitis failure in endemic countries, however recent reports suggest that it can be associated with unexplained chronic hepatitis in the hepatic allograft. Such reports have come from at least two countries.[33] The prognosis and outcomes in this situation however remain to be defined.

References

1. Maddrey WC. Hepatitis B: an important public health issue. J Med Virol 2000;61:362–6.
2. El-Serag HB, Davila JA, Petersen NJ, et al. The continuing increase in the incidence of hepatocellular carcinoma in the United States: an update. Ann Intern Med 2003;139:817–23.
3. Lavanchy D. The global burden of hepatitis C. Liver Int 2009;29(Suppl 1):74–81.
4. Liaw YF. Natural history of chronic hepatitis B virus infection and long-term outcome under treatment. Liver Int 2009;29(Suppl 1):100–7.
5. Veldt BJ, Heathcote EJ, Wedemeyer H, et al. Sustained virologic response and clinical outcomes in patients with chronic hepatitis C and advanced fibrosis. Ann Intern Med 2007;147:677–84.
6. Merion RM, Schaubel DE, Dykstra DM, et al. The survival benefit of liver transplantation. Am J Transplant 2005;5:307–13.
7. Fontana RJ, Hann HW, Perrillo RP, et al. Determinants of early mortality in patients with decompensated chronic hepatitis B treated with antiviral therapy. Gastroenterology 2002;123:719–27.
8. Zoulim F, Radenne S, Ducerf C. Management of patients with decompensated hepatitis B virus associated [corrected] cirrhosis. Liver Transpl 2008;14(Suppl 2): S1–7.
9. Liaw YF, Sung JJ, Chow WC, et al. Lamivudine for patients with chronic hepatitis B and advanced liver disease. N Engl J Med 2004;351:1521–31.
10. Lok AS, Shetty K, Hussain M, et al. How to diagnose and treat hepatitis B virus antiviral drug resistance in the liver transplant setting. Liver Transpl 2008;14(Suppl 2):S8–14.
11. Ratziu V, Thibault V, Benhamou Y, et al. Successful rescue therapy with tenofovir in a patient with hepatic decompensation and adefovir resistant HBV mutant. Comp Hepatol 2006;5:1.
12. Lo CM, Fung JT, Lau GK, et al. Development of antibody to hepatitis B surface antigen after liver transplantation for chronic hepatitis B. Hepatology 2003;37:36–43.
13. Wong VW, Wong GL, Yiu KK, et al. Entecavir treatment in patients with severe acute exacerbation of chronic hepatitis B. J Hepatol 2011;54:236–42.
14. Everson GT, Trotter J, Forman L, et al. Treatment of advanced hepatitis C with a low accelerating dosage regimen of antiviral therapy. Hepatology 2005;42: 255–62.
15. Samuel D, Bismuth A, Mathieu D, et al. Passive immunoprophylaxis after liver transplantation in HBsAg-positive patients. Lancet 1991;337:813–5.
16. Angus PW, Patterson SJ. Liver transplantation for hepatitis B: what is the best hepatitis B immune globulin/antiviral regimen? Liver Transpl 2008;14(Suppl 2): S15–22.
17. Markowitz JS, Martin P, Conrad AJ, et al. Prophylaxis against hepatitis B recurrence following liver transplantation using combination lamivudine and hepatitis B immune globulin. Hepatology 1998;28:585–9.
18. Gane EJ, Angus PW, Strasser S, et al. Lamivudine plus low-dose hepatitis B immunoglobulin to prevent recurrent hepatitis B following liver transplantation. Gastroenterology 2007;132:931–7.
19. Angus PW, Patterson SJ, Strasser SI, et al. A randomized study of adefovir dipivoxil in place of HBIG in

combination with lamivudine as post-liver transplantation hepatitis B prophylaxis. Hepatology 2008;48: 1460–6.
20. Saab S, Waterman B, Chi AC, et al. Comparison of different immunoprophylaxis regimens after liver transplantation with hepatitis B core antibody-positive donors: a systematic review. Liver Transpl 2010;16: 300–7.
21. Ramirez S, Perez-Del-Pulgar S, Forns X. Virology and pathogenesis of hepatitis C virus recurrence. Liver Transpl 2008;14(Suppl 2):S27–35.
22. Gane EJ. The natural history of recurrent hepatitis C and what influences this. Liver Transpl 2008;14 (Suppl 2):S36–44.
23. Gawrieh S, Papouchado BG, Burgart LJ, et al. Early hepatic stellate cell activation predicts severe hepatitis C recurrence after liver transplantation. Liver Transpl 2005;11:1207–13.
24. Firpi RJ, Abdelmalek MF, Soldevila-Pico C, et al. One-year protocol liver biopsy can stratify fibrosis progression in liver transplant recipients with recurrent hepatitis C infection. Liver Transpl 2004;10:1240–7.
25. Brillanti S, Vivarelli M, De Ruvo N, et al. Slowly tapering off steroids protects the graft against hepatitis C recurrence after liver transplantation. Liver Transpl 2002;8:884–8.
26. Klintmalm GB, Washburn WK, Rudich SM, et al. Corticosteroid-free immunosuppression with daclizumab in HCV(+) liver transplant recipients: 1-year interim results of the HCV-3 study. Liver Transpl 2007;13:1521–31.
27. Terrault NA. Hepatitis C therapy before and after liver transplantation. Liver Transpl 2008;14(Suppl 2): S58–66.
28. Gane EJ, Strasser SI, Crawford DH, et al. A multicenter, randomized trial of combination pegylated interferon-alpha 2a plus ribavirin vs. pegylated interferon-alpha 2a monotherapy in liver transplant recipients with recurrent hepatitis C. Hepatology 2009;4(Suppl):393A–4A.
29. Lake JR. Do we really need long-term hepatitis B hyperimmune globulin? What are the alternatives? Liver Transpl 2008;14(Suppl 2):S23–6.
30. McCaughan GW, Shackel NA, Strasser SI, et al. Minimal but significant improvement in survival for non-hepatitis C-related adult liver transplant patients beyond the one-year posttransplant mark. Liver Transpl 2010;16:130–7.
31. Pascarella S, Negro F. Hepatitis D virus: an update. Liver Int 2010;31:7–21.
32. Samuel D, Zignego AL, Reynes M, et al. Long-term clinical and virological outcome after liver transplantation for cirrhosis caused by chronic delta hepatitis. Hepatology 1995;21:333–9.
33. Haagsma EB, van den Berg AP, Porte RJ, et al. Chronic hepatitis E virus infection in liver transplant recipients. Liver Transpl 2008;14:547–53.

9 Metabolic liver diseases

Maureen M.J. Guichelaar and Michael R. Charlton
Mayo Clinic, Mayo Clinic Transplant Center, Rochester MN, USA

Key learning points

- NASH will become the leading indication for OLT in the near future.
- After OLT, there is an increase in obesity and metabolic syndrome which has been related to a high prevalence of NAFLD recurrence and NAFLD-de-novo.
- With early diagnosis of hereditary hemochromatosis and its treatment (phlebotomies) the progression towards end-stage liver disease and OLT can be prevented
- Kayser Fleischer rings in Wilson's disease are often present (in adults) with neuropsychiatric disease, but are often absent (in children) if the presenting symptom is liver disease.
- Augmentation therapy in α1-antitrypsin deficiency will not contribute to improvement of liver disease.

Introduction

Metabolic liver disease comprises a broad array of liver diseases that includes hepatic manifestations of systemic disease (e.g. NASH, cystic fibrosis), diseases primarily affecting the liver (i.e. Wilson's disease, hemochromatosis, glycogen storage disease) and diseases that are based on metabolic defects in the liver but which are manifest extrahepatically (e.g. familial amyloidotic polyneuropathy, primary hyperoxaluria type 1)[1,2] (Table 9.1).

Orthotopic liver transplantation (OLT) for metabolic diseases of the liver is more common for pediatric patients than for adult patients, comprising about 20% of pediatric liver transplantation.[3] This chapter reviews metabolic indications for adult liver transplantation. Only a small proportion of adult liver transplantation is related to decompensated cirrhosis secondary to hemochromatosis, Wilson's disease and α1-antitrypsin deficiency. In contrast, cirrhosis due to NASH is increasing rapidly as an indication.[4] This increase is related to the increasing prevalence of obesity in the general population, of which a portion will eventually develop cirrhosis. It is projected that NASH will become the leading indication for liver transplantation in the next 10–20 years (Figure 9.1).

Non-alcoholic steatohepatitis

Non-alcoholic fatty liver disease (NAFLD) is a term that encompasses a spectrum of hepatic histologic manifestations for conditions ranging from simple steatosis to NASH with or without progressive fibrosis. NAFLD is closely related to the prevalence of obesity and the metabolic syndrome. Although only

Medical Care of the Liver Transplant Patient, Fourth Edition. Edited by Pierre-Alain Clavien, James F. Trotter and.

Table 9.1 Most common metabolic diseases in adults

Disease	Acquired/inherited	Pathophysiology	Clinical characteristics	Diagnostic testing	Liver pathology
NASH	Acquired, related to: –Insulin resistance –Hyperinsulinemia –Unbalanced adipokines	FFAs ↑ (uptake liver) Triglycerides ↑ (steatosis) Oxidation ↑ Inflammation ↑ Apoptosis ↑	Associated with obesity and metabolic syndrome	–US/CT: steatosis –Exclusion of other liver diseases –No history of alcohol abuse	NAFLD activity score: steatosis, lobular inflammation, hepatocyte ballooning, mallory bodies, fibrosis
Hereditary hemochromatosis	Autosomal recessive, mutations HFE gene: –80% C282Y/C282Y –6% C282Y/H63D –Other mutations also known	–Decreased hepcidin activity in liver → Macrophages and enterocytes release more iron in serum → Iron deposits in organs	–Often middle-aged patient –May present as HCC –Earlier onset in juvenile form, then also with more extrahepatic complications	–Transferrin saturation >45% –Ferritin ↑ Often >1000 ng/ml with liver disease	–Hepatic iron concentration (HIC) = mmol iron/g dry weight liver tissue –Hepatic iron index = HIC/age of patient >1.9 HH
Wilson's disease	Autosomal recessive Mutations WD gene (ATP7B) encoding for a copper-transporting P-type ATPase	–Less activity AT Pase → Less copper excreted in bile and binded to ceruloplasmin → Copper deposits in organs	–Children often have LD, sometimes acute liver failure –Adults also have LD, sometimes with neuropsychiatric symptoms	–Serum ceruloplasmin ↓ –Urinary copper excretion/24 hours ↑ –Kaiser–Fleischer rings –Serum copper ↑ with acute liver failure	–Measurements of hepatic copper content >250 ng/g dry weight –Chronic liver disease in WD may mimic other liver diseases, including autoimmune, NASH
α1AT deficiency	Autosomal recessive Mutated A1AT with ZZ, ZS alleles (MM alleles = normal production of A1AT)	–Mutated A1AT accumulates in liver –Less circulating A1AT: proteolytic destruction of pulmonary connective tissue matrix	–Children more often have LD, adults more often have pulmonary complications in addition to LD	–Serum A1AT ↓ –Protein phenotype evaluation (M = normal, Z en S with A1AT deficiency) –Genotyping for Z en S alleles	–di-PAS-positive globules, especially in periportal areas Other atypical findings may include steatosis in periportal areas

A1AT: α1-antitrypsin, ATPase: Adenosine triphosphate, CT: Computed tomogram, di-PAS: Periodic acid–Schiff-positive after diastase digestion, FFA: Free fatty acids, HCC: Hepatocellular carcinoma, HFE: Human hemochromatosis protein, HH: Hereditary hemochromatosis, HIC: Hepatic iron concentration, LD: Liver disease, NAFLD: Nonalcoholic fatty liver disease, NASH: Nonalcoholic steatohepatitis, US: Ultrasound, WD: Wilson's disease.

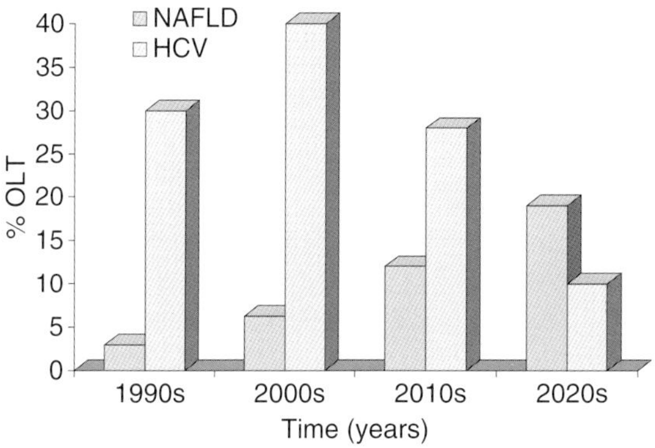

Figure 9.1 Predicted increase in NAFLD/NASH as indication for OLT over time

a small minority of obese patients develops NASH with progressive fibrosis, the high prevalence of obesity will result in parallel increases in the number of patients with NASH who develop end-stage liver disease and/or hepatocellular carcinoma (HCC).

Epidemiology and natural history

According to the most recent National Health and Nutrition Examination Survey 2007–2008 (NHANES), two-thirds of adults in the USA are overweight (BMI >25 kg/m^2) or obese (BMI >30 kg/m^2). The World Health Organization (WHO) estimated in 2005 that worldwide more than 1.6 billion adults are overweight and at least 400 million are obese.

The great majority of NAFLD is undiagnosed. A large study[5] assessed the prevalence of steatosis in 2287 adults with different ethnic backgrounds. Hepatic steatosis measured by proton H1 nuclear magnetic resonance spectroscopy was seen in one out of three patients. In most of these patients (79%) the serum aminotransferases were normal. From this study it is depicted that one out of every three people in the USA has NAFLD. What the actual impact of this high prevalence is on the number of patients with NASH was not clear from these findings. The natural history of NAFLD was studied in a large population-based cohort study[6] of 420 patients with a diagnosis of NAFLD. At the time of presentation it was found that 2% of this population had cirrhosis. Their findings showed that one out of 30 NAFLD patients may develop liver cirrhosis or another liver-related complication. Although NAFLD has been considered to be a relatively benign entity, between 1% and 5% of affected patients will develop cirrhosis. Patients with NASH-related cirrhosis have an estimated mean survival of 7 years, with mortality most commonly based on complications of end-stage liver disease and hepatocellular carcinoma.[7] The physiological basis for severity of disease among the minority of patients who develop NASH with progressive fibrosis is poorly understood.

The increase in end-stage liver disease related to NASH is further reflected by the increasing numbers of end-stage liver disease patients requiring OLT. A large proportion of cryptogenic cirrhotic patients requiring OLT have burnt-out NASH in which the histologic characteristics of NASH have faded away. The United Network for Organ Sharing (UNOS) registry showed that the combination of these primary diagnoses (NASH and cryptogenic cirrhosis) has increased from 3.6% to 6.9% in the 5 years between 2001 and 2005, while OLT for other indications did not change or decreased (i.e. hepatitis C) (Figure 9.1). These numbers may underestimate the actual figures, since patients with hepatocellular carcinoma on a background of cryptogenic cirrhosis or NASH are not included in these UNOS numbers. With increasing rates of NAFLD it is likely that more HCC will be seen in the future.

Pathogenesis

The pathogenesis of NASH involves multiple pathologic pathways related to insulin resistance, hyperinsulinemia, oxidative stress, and activated inflammatory cytokines. In order to outline two essential pathologic steps in NASH, a concept of a two-hit theory has been proposed. The first step is the accumulation of lipids in the liver. The second hit is related to the hepatic adaptive mechanisms for lipotoxicity resulting into oxidative and metabolic stress on the hepatocytes and abnormal cytokine production.[7]

Normal free fatty acid metabolism is characterized by hepatic uptake and de novo free fatty acid (FFA) synthesis. Within hepatocytes FFAs are oxidized to form triglycerides, which are then exported from the liver as very-low-density lipoprotein (VLDL) particles. Insulin resistance in peripheral adipose tissue causes enhanced oxidization of lipids, resulting in hepatic fatty acid oxidation to form triglycerides. Steatosis occurs when the rate of triglycerides overwhelms the capacity of VLDL synthesis and export. Owing to the increased oxidation of FFAs there is also an increased synthesis of by-products, including reactive oxygen species with initiation of inflammation and apoptosis pathways.

Insulin resistance is also associated with compensatory responses in pancreatic beta-cells leading to hyperinsulinemia. In the liver there are many cells expressing insulin receptors resulting in a variety of complex metabolic changes, such as increased lipogenesis and stimulation of stellate cell transformation into myofibroblasts.

Another important factor in NAFLD patients is the unbalanced adipocytokine production in adipose tissue, with increased TNF-alpha, resistin, angiotensinogen, plasminogen activator inhibitor, and decreased adiponectin. These changes have been related to a further release of FFAs from adipose tissue, promotion of insulin resistance, activation of inflammatory cascades in the liver, and antagonizing the effects of adiponectin. Adiponectin is produced in adipose tissue and has been associated with increased insulin sensitization and reduced lipid accumulation in the liver.

Diagnosis

Most patients with NAFLD are asymptomatic or have aspecific symptoms, including fatigue or right upper quadrant abdominal discomfort. Ultrasonography is often performed in the evaluation of patients who are eventually diagnosed with NAFLD/NASH. The use of ultrasonography in detecting steatosis has sensitivity and specificity rates of 90% and 97%, respectively, if hepatic steatosis is 30% or more.[7] Transaminases are typically mildly elevated, with little or no elevation in alkaline phosphatase or bilirubin. The diagnosis of NASH necessitates the exclusion of other diseases, i.e. alcoholic liver disease, viral hepatitis, α1-antitrypsin deficiency, autoimmune hepatitis, and Wilson's disease.

In the absence of portal hypertension, biochemical and radiologic assessment cannot distinguish simple steatosis from NASH. Currently the most accurate way to differentiate between the stages of NAFLD is by liver biopsy. There is no consensus about when to perform a liver biopsy in NAFLD patients. Liver biopsies are accompanied by risk of complications, cost, and the possibility of sampling error. Histologically significant disease (NASH with more than minimal fibrosis) is highly unusual in patients who have a BMI <28 kg/m^2 and/or are not insulin resistant. Ideally either a combination of clinical and biochemical markers or specific markers of fibrosis could be used for non-invasive staging of NAFLD patients. However, to date, although several of such panels have been proposed, none have been independently validated. Magnetic resonance elastography is emerging as a relatively sensitive and specific tool for non-invasive assessment of NAFLD.

Owing to the high prevalence of the metabolic syndrome in obese patients in general and specifically among patients with NASH (NASH has been referred to as a hepatic manifestation of the metabolic syndrome), consideration should be given to screening patients with NASH for other features of the metabolic syndrome. Young age at time of presentation of NASH-related complications should raise suspicion of hypopituitarism.

Management of NASH

Treatment of NASH remains a challenge, with the most important interventions being weight loss and increased physical activity. Weight loss has been shown to improve the aminotransferases, radiologic appearance and even to a certain extent the histologic appearance. Rapid weight loss, however, may exacerbate steatohepatitis and hepatic decompensation and should be avoided.[8] Most studies of pharmacotherapy of NASH have been small with short-term follow up, including only a few randomized, placebo-controlled trials. The most promising studies are related to insulin-sensitizing agents (thiazolidinediones), which act as agonists of the peroxisome proliferator-activated receptor gamma on ameliorating insulin resistance and improving glucose and lipid metabolism.[9] Thiazolidinediones have been shown to improve liver chemistry in NASH patients in addition to improving some histologic features, including steatosis, necroinflammation and fibrosis. Thiazolidinediones have also been associated with an increased BMI, and carry a risk for idiosyncratic cardiotoxicity. Other less well established treatment modalities in NASH include metformin, metronidazole, and ursodeoxycholic acid. Very limited data is available for clofibrate, gemfibrozil, vitamin E, n-acetyl cysteine and betaine in NASH. In a recent study[10] sponsored by the National Institutes of Health (the PIVENS study) pioglitazone was not effective in improving the histologic features of NASH, whereas vitamin E did improve histologic features, suggesting that vitamin E should be considered in NASH patients.

Owing to the known beneficial effects of weight loss in patients with NASH, bariatric surgery has become of increased interest to achieve clinical and histologic improvements.[11] Profound weight loss after surgery, however, has been related to increased risk of hepatic decompensation and the operation itself leads to significant adhesions in the upper abdomen, complicating a future OLT. Gastric bypass surgery can probably be safely used in the setting of obesity with simple steatosis alone. Sleeve gastrectomy has the advantage of preserving the gastric fundus (for management of variceal bleeding) and preserving access to the biliary tree. In addition the absorptive capacity is not much changed, which is essential in the setting of immunosuppressive treatment after OLT. Currently the timing of bariatric surgery in the setting of OLT has not been well established, but will likely evolve in the future.

NASH and liver transplantation

Patients with end-stage liver disease related to NASH are often morbidly obese, which has led to a significant debate about the concomitant risks of OLT.[12] Initial studies showed increased mortality rates in patients with increased BMIs, but after adjusting for ascites this risk appears to fade with good post-transplant survival rates, comparable to other indications.[13] These rates, however, apply to a selected group of patients, in which cardiovascular diseases have been excluded before activation for OLT. In addition, patients with an increased BMI have been shown to require longer hospital stays and have more post-transplant complications such as prolonged mechanical ventilation and reduced wound healing.

Approximately one-third of patients with normal weight at the time of transplant will become obese post-transplant, accompanied by an increased prevalence in metabolic syndrome.[14] There are multiple reasons for the increase in obesity and metabolic syndrome after OLT, including recovery of metabolic processes, as well as post-transplant immunosuppression. Immunosuppression has been shown to increase truncal fat (corticosteroids), hypertension (corticosteroids, calcineurin inhibitors), dyslipidemia (sirolimus, calcineurin inhibitors) and diabetes mellitus (DM) (corticosteroids and calcineurin inhibitors). Regarding these important effects of post-transplant immunosuppression, efforts should be made to taper corticosteroids early after OLT and stopping their admission during the first post-transplant year. In addition, calcineurin levels should be minimized.

Given the high prevalence of NASH-related risk factors after OLT, it is not surprising that NASH recurs after OLT or develops de novo in patients transplanted for other diseases.[15] Prospective histologic analysis showed that the probability of steatosis at 5 years post transplant was 100% in NASH patients, compared to 25% in patients transplanted for primary biliary cirrhosis (PBC) or alcoholic liver disease. Approximately 5–10% of patients transplanted for NASH will progress to cirrhosis after OLT, resulting in graft loss in 50% of these patients. NASH recurrence after OLT is often not well reflected by biochemical testing. The best way of assessing NASH recurrence or the novo NASH is by liver biopsy.

Hereditary hemochromatosis

Hereditary hemochromatosis (HH) is an autosomal recessive disorder characterized by deposits of iron in tissue and organs, including the liver. Most cases of hemochromatosis have been related to homozygous C282Y mutation of the HFE gene (located on chromosome 6). Mutations in other genes have also been related to hemochromatosis, e.g. hemojuvelin (HJV), ferroportin, transferring receptor 2 (Trf2). Probably most, if not all, of these mutations are associated with changes in hepcidin, which is thought to be the key regulator of iron homeostasis.[16] The recent discovery of hepcidin has also led to the assumption that hereditary hemochromatosis originates mainly in the liver and not the intestine. Recognition and treatment of the disease in an early stage is of key importance to prevent progression to end-stage liver disease requiring OLT.

Natural history

About 80% of patients with HH are homozygous for C282Y and 6% are compound heterozygotes (C282Y/H63D). These mutations are highly prevalent in northern Europe and its descendents in North America, with a prevalence variation of 1:200 to 1:250 homozygosity and 1:8 to 1:12 heterozygosity. The phenotypical expression of the disease is thought to be low; 30–60% of C282Y homozygotes develop increased ferritin and transferrin saturation with about 2–4% developing progressive tissue iron overload and clinical complications[2,17,18] but the phenotypical expression is higher in men.[18] In general, iron overloading related to C282Y homozygosity is a slow process, with clinical symptoms appearing in midlife. The major causes of death in patients with hereditary hemochromatosis have been related to decompensated cirrhosis, hepatocellular carcinoma, diabetes mellitus and cardiomyopathy. HCC is generally seen in HH patients with cirrhotic liver disease.

The compound heterozygotes C282Y/H63D have a lower expression of the disease, with only 0.5–1% of patients developing the clinical signs of iron overload. The H63D/H63D homozygotes may show increases in serum transferrin-saturation, but are in general not at risk to develop significant iron overload. Another mutation associated with HH is S65C but its contribution to clinical disease is thought to be low.[17]

A higher rate of iron overloading has been seen in the juvenile form of hemochromatosis, leading to clinical manifestations of iron overload by the second and third decades, including cardiomyopathy, diabetes, and hypogonadotropic hypogonadism. Most juvenile cases have been related to mutations in the HJV gene, encoding for hemojuvelin, which is a major transcriptional regulator of hepcidin.[2,16]

Pathogenesis

Patients with hereditary hemochromatosis absorb much more iron from the intestines than is physiologically necessary to compensate for daily losses. In normal patients, iron is stored as ferritin in enterocytes and released when serum ferritin levels fall, but in patients with HH the duodenal transfer of ferritin into plasma is inappropriately high. In addition, the macrophages in HH patients release more iron and retain less transferrin-bound iron.[16]

These disturbances have been associated with multiple mutations in genes, but they probably all relate to abnormalities of hepcidin levels. Hepcidin has been shown to downregulate ferritin release from enterocytes and macrophages. Its production originates in the hepatocytes, and is stimulated by serum iron, inflammatory stimuli, circulating regulators (i.e. bone morphogenetic protein, soluble HJV), and hepatocyte membrane-associated regulators (e.g. HJV, HFE, and TfR2).[16] Its actual function and relation with HH mutations has not been fully discovered although several observations support its important role.[19]

Diagnosis

Clinical manifestations in HH are related to iron overloading and include liver cirrhosis, diabetes mellitus, cardiomyopathy, hypogonadotrophic hypogonadism, hypothyroidism, and destructive arthritis. Other atypical symptoms such as fatigue and arthropathy may be less typical for HH since it also occurs in high prevalences in the general population.

A transferrin-saturation (serum iron divided by the serum total iron-binding capacity) of >45% raises the possibility of hereditary hemochromatosis. Liver disease is almost only seen in patients with ferritin levels >1000 ng/ml. Ferritin is an acute phase reactant that can lead to false-positive findings in the cases of inflammation and malignancy.

Genetic testing of mutations in the HFE gene (i.e. C282Y and H63D) is mainly used in the setting of suspected hemochromatosis (transferrin saturation >45%), and testing at-risk relatives. In the case of negative findings on standard genetic testing (C282Y and H63D) and high suspicion of hereditary hemochromatosis, it is possible to continue with second-line genetic testing (TfR2, HAP, HJV, etc).

Further evidence of iron overload can be derived from liver biopsy by measuring the hepatic iron concentration (HIC, expressed as micrograms/micromoles of iron per gram dry weight of liver). The hepatic iron index can then be calculated by dividing HIC by the age of the patient, to adjust for increasing liver iron stores with increasing age in HH. Normal values are

<1.0; homozygous C282Y patients have been associated with values >1.9.

Another diagnostic test for hemochromatosis is measuring iron excretion during phlebotomy, which can be helpful if liver biopsy cannot be performed. In normal patients with normal levels of hemoglobin, 500 cc of blood with phlebotomy will amount to 250 mg of iron. In HH patients this amount can easily exceed 4 g. Hepatic magnetic resonance imaging may be helpful in estimating the amount of iron in the liver by using the paramagnetic properties of iron. The advantage of using MRI is that it allows an estimation of the total iron content in the liver, taking into account the regional differences, but its role in the diagnosis of HH is not well established.

Management and liver transplantation

Patients who start iron-depleting therapy (phlebotomies) before the onset of cirrhosis and diabetes have a comparable survival to that of the general population. It is therefore of importance to make an early diagnosis. It has been recommended to start phlebotomies in patients with serum ferritin >1000 ng/ml. It may be delayed in patients with lower levels of ferritin (<1000 ng/ml) and no symptoms or liver function abnormalities. Treatment for hemachromatosis should include: phlebotomies (often started with phlebotomy (=500 ml/week) to continue until reaching normalization of iron stores (serum ferritin <50 ng/ml) with concomitant follow up of hematocrit (<20% change between phlebotomies). Levels <25 ng/ml indicate iron deficiency and require a temporary hold on phlebotomies. After the initiation phase, phlebotomies are less frequently planned, with maintaining ferritin of approximately 50 ng/ml.

Owing to effective treatment with phlebotomies, OLT is less common for end-stage liver disease but it is still seen for HCC complicating HH. Patients with significant iron staining before OLT (with or without HH) have been shown to have reduced outcomes after OLT.[20] The 1-, 3- and 5-year post-transplant survival rates have been reported to be 64%, 48% and 34%, respectively. Survival rates may have improved in the most recently transplanted patients due to reduction of cardiovascular complications following OLT.

Wilson's disease

Wilson's disease (WD), also known as hepatolenticular degeneration, is an autosomal recessive disease, caused by mutations of the WD gene (on the long arm of chromosome 13). The mutation results in abnormal hepatocyte copper transport with copper deposition in multiple organs, including the liver and brain. The prevalence of the disease is estimated to be one per 30 000 people, occurring worldwide. The diagnosis and therapy in these patients can be a challenge. With adequate copper-chelating therapy, the progression to end-stage liver disease can often be halted. OLT in WD patients has mainly been seen in the setting of acute liver failure.

Pathogenesis

Copper is absorbed from the gastrointestinal (GI) tract, bound to albumin and then transported to the liver. Patients with WD have mutations of gene ATP7B, which encodes for a copper-transporting P-type adenosine triphosphate (ATPase) expressed in hepatocytes. Genetic mutation in ATP7B can lead to diminished copper excretion into bile and a failure to incorporate copper into ceruloplasmin. Copper accumulates in the liver, and its overspill results in extrahepatic copper deposition (in the brain, kidney and cornea). This copper deposition stimulates cascades of processes resulting in increased production of reactive oxygen species, and cytokines.[21,22]

So far, more than 200 mutations have been detected in WD patients, most being missense mutations. Almost 35–50% of the WD cases in Europe or in populations of European descent have a mutation involving histidine to glutamine at position 1069 (H1069Q), whereas R778L is most often (50–60%) encountered in WD patients of Asian origin. Phenotypical expression of the disease, however, varies, even within families with similar genetic abnormalities.

Natural history

Most WD patients present with symptoms between the ages of 5 and 40, although younger and older patients (up to the eighth decade) have been reported. In general, younger patients (<20 years) tend to have more severe liver-related complications than adults, and may present with acute liver failure. Acute liver failure in the setting of WD is frequently accompanied with Coombs-negative hemolytic anemia and renal failure as a result of copper toxicity. The increased serum copper levels are the result of necrotizing hepatocytes shedding copper into the circulation.[22]

Neuropsychiatric symptoms tend to occur more in adults with more advanced stages of the disease, after accumulation of copper in the liver has occurred. Symptoms may include changes in behavior, lack of motor coordination, tremor, dysarthria, dystonia, and spasticity, as well as psychiatric manifestations (i.e. depression, anxiety, and psychosis). Chronic liver disease in the setting of WD often mimics findings of other liver diseases (biochemically and histologically) including autoimmune hepatitis, steatosis, and NASH.

Other symptoms related to copper deposition include renal disease, osteoporosis, cardiomyopathies, pancreatitis, and infertility. In some patients, low-grade hemolysis may exist for years without clinical evidence of liver disease. With adequate copper-chelating treatment, many presenting symptoms can be reversed, including liver disease. Liver transplantation for chronic liver disease with WD is therefore not often seen. Studies have reported low risk of HCC development in patients with WD. All patients with cirrhotic liver disease are at increased risk of developing HCC and some level of suspicion is warranted.

Diagnosis

The diagnosis of WD can be a challenge when typical findings are absent, such as reduced serum ceruloplasmin, increased urinary copper excretion, Kaiser–Fleischer (KF) rings, and increased quantitative levels of copper in liver tissue.[21]

KF-rings are present in the vast majority of WD patients with neuropsychiatric symptoms, but are often absent in patients with WD-related liver injury. KF rings can also occur with longstanding cholestasis. Ceruloplasmin is the major copper carrier in blood and is often reduced in WD patients (<20 mg/dl) due to the reduced half-life of apo-ceruloplasmin (ceruloplasmin without copper binding) when compared to ceruloplasmin. Ceruloplasmin increases with inflammation and increased estrogen levels (pregnancy and estrogen supplements), whereas reductions can be seen with renal or enteric protein loss and end-stage liver disease.

The 24-hour measurement of urinary copper reflects nonceruloplasmin-bound copper in the circulation and is often increased in symptomatic WD patients (>100 µg/24 hours or >1.6 µmol/24 hours). High levels of urinary copper (>1500 µg/24 hours) are seen with untreated WD. The American Association for the Study of Liver Diseases (AASLD)[21] recommends that lower levels of urinary copper, but exceeding the upper limit of normal (>40 µg/24 hours or >0.6 µmol/24 hours) also require further evaluation, since they may be seen with asymptomatic WD.

Owing to high variation in testing, serum copper is not often used in the process of diagnosing WD, although it can be useful in diagnosing acute liver failure associated with WD (then increased levels).

The diagnosis of WD in the setting of acute liver failure is especially a challenge. Ceruloplasmin is relatively increased with acute liver failure as an acute phase reactant, and measurements of 24-hour copper excretion are often inadequate due to the concomitant renal failure. In addition, KF rings are often absent in patients presenting with WD-related liver injury. Features that may lead to a suspicion of WD in acute liver failure are biochemical findings of high bilirubin with low or normal alkaline phosphatase and relatively modest elevations of transaminases, in addition to high serum levels of copper.

The measurement of hepatic copper in liver biopsies is probably the best and most adequate test for the diagnosis of WD. Hepatic copper content of ≥250 µg/g dry weight is diagnostic for WD. Although some patients may present with lower levels, it rarely is <50 µg/g dry weight of liver. Increases in hepatic copper content can also been seen in patients with chronic cholestasis. Sampling error may occur with increased stages of WD, due to large variations in hepatic copper distribution. Histological findings in WD may also mimic other liver diseases, such as autoimmune hepatitis, NASH, or drug-related hepatitis.

Siblings of a known WD patient can undergo detection of disease-specific ATP7B mutations, if the mutation is known in the patient. Owing to this high variability in phenotypic expression and amount of genetic mutations, genetic screening is mainly performed in patients with a high degree of suspicion for the disease or with a sibling known to have the disease.

Management and liver transplantation

Treatment of WD includes copper-chelating agents (D-penicillamine and trientine) and zinc salts (for reducing enteral copper absorption).[21] Owing to the rarity of the disease, large randomized studies in the treatment of WD are lacking.

Adequate treatment with D-penicillamine can reverse hepatic as well as other (neurologic, psychiatric, and ocular manifestations) of WD disease. D-penicillamine can still be used with advancing liver disease, with the exception of patients with acute liver failure, but its use has been limited due to side effects and complications, including lupus-like syndrome, nephritis, arthritis, leucopenia, thrombocytopenia, and skin fragility. Tolerability of D-penicillamine may be enhanced by slowly increasing doses until reaching maintenance dosing of 750–1000 mg/d administered in two doses with concomitant supplements of pyridoxine. After initiating treatment, 10–50% of patients may experience neurologic deterioration. The cessation of D-penicillamine treatment has been associated with a deterioration of liver disease in some cases. Patients with intolerance of D-penicillamine may benefit from trientine treatment (500–750 mg by mouth two times daily). The usual maintenance dose is 750–1000 mg/d in divided doses. In children the usual dose for trientine is 20 mg/kg rounded to the nearest 250 mg. Trientine should be taken 1–3 hours before meals. The actual effects of trientine for chelating copper is not known, but it has been shown to be effective in WD patients with a low risk for adverse effects. It is becoming more popular as a first-line treatment, although it is less well established. Zinc therapy (150 mg of elemental zinc by mouth per day in three divided doses) has also been shown to have hardly any side effect, and reduces intestinal uptake of copper. So far it has shown good efficacy in adults with less side effects, with the gluconate form being better tolerated than the acetate form. Its use in combination therapy (with trientine or penicillamine) is not well established, but may become of importance in the future. A newer treatment entity is ammonium tetrathiomolybdate, which interferes with intestinal uptake of copper as well as binding copper in plasma. Currently experience with this treatment is limited. In addition to medication, the restriction of food high in copper, such as liver, brain, chocolate, shellfish, nuts, and mushrooms may contribute to copper chelating, especially in the beginning of the treatment.

With adequate treatment, the progression of liver disease can be halted or reversed. Because of this, OLT for chronic liver disease is not common and the main indication for OLT in WD is acute liver failure. However, OLT for selected WD patients remains a good option with good post-transplant patient survival rates of 80–90%.[4,23] After OLT, neuropsychiatric improvements have been seen in many but not all WD patients. Longstanding neurological disease before OLT despite adequate medical therapy is unlikely to improve after OLT and is a contraindication for OLT.

α1-antitrypsin deficiency

α1-antitrypsin (A1AT) deficiency is an autosomal recessive disease that is relatively common in populations of European ancestry, in approximately one case per 3000 persons. The incidence of A1AT in white newborns is similar to that of cystic fibrosis. The inheritance of two deficiency alleles at the locus encoding for A1AT is related to abnormal action of the protein, which has been associated with the development of pulmonary emphysema and liver injury.

Pathophysiology

Normal synthesis of A1AT occurs within the endoplasmic reticulum of hepatocytes in the presence of 2 M-alleles. A1AT is essential to protect the lungs from inflammation. Although multiple mutations have been shown with phenotypical expression of A1AT deficiency, it is mainly related to homozygosity for Z-alleles (in some cases heterozygosity) also known as the Z-protein phenotype. This mutation results into aberrantly folding of the (mutated) A1AT protein, causing its accumulation in the cytoplasmic globules and later in endoplasmic reticulum of hepatocytes. The exact mechanisms that lead to A1AT-related liver injury have not been fully explored, but are thought to relate to increased apoptosis, mitochondrial injury and disruption of glycogen metabolism in the hepatocytes. Owing to entrapment of A1AT in the liver, less circulating A1AT is available, which may lead to uninhibited proteolytic destruction of the pulmonary connective tissue matrix.

The combination of alleles Z and M has been associated with a slightly increased risk of lung and liver disease, although this is not well established. The S allele is slightly more common than the Z allele and is associated with mildly reduced A1AT levels. The combination of alleles S and Z has been associated with increased risk for COPD, but at lower rates than that seen with the Z protein phenotype.[1,4,24]

Natural history

So far it has not been well established why only a portion (10–15%) of individuals with the ZZ allele develops clinical disease. In addition, the natural history of A1AT deficiency is not well known. An estimation of 1% of patients with COPD has A1AT deficiency, and it has been recommended by the American Thoracic Society and the European Respiratory Society to test for A1AT deficiency in all patients with chronic obstructive pulmonary disease (COPD), or asthma.

Of all newborns with ZZ or ZS alleles, approximately 25% have elevated liver enzymes and 5% will develop some form of liver disease. A1AT deficiency in children may present as a prolonged period of neonatal jaundice, hepatomegaly, failure to thrive, or as acute liver failure. Children present more often with liver-related complications than adults, whereas adults more often present with COPD or other pulmonary complications. Less common manifestations of A1AT deficiency include necrotizing panniculitis (painful localized necrosis of subcutaneous fat) and anti-proteinase-3-positive vasculitis.[1,4,24]

Diagnosis

A diagnosis is most often suspected in patients with early onset of COPD, with or without elevated liver enzymes. Diagnostic testing includes measurement of A1AT in serum, which is often decreased; serum levels of A1AT may, however, increase with inflammation (as part of an acute phase reaction). The finding of decreased A1AT levels requires further testing, including assessment of protein phenotyping or genotyping. With protein phenotyping the test identifies the type of A1AT protein produced by the liver (i.e. M, Z, or S protein). Most genotyping kits test for the most common A1AT allele variants (Z and S), which can lead to false-negative testing if missing one of the less common malfunctioning alleles. The combination of phenotypical and genotypical testing may provide further information. A liver biopsy is often not necessary to diagnose A1AT deficiency although it can be helpful to exclude other liver diseases and to assess the severity of the liver disease. Typical findings of A1AT deficiency in liver biopsies are the detection of periodic acid-Schiff positive after diastase digestion (di-PAS) intracytoplasmic eosinophilic globules, mainly seen in the periportal regions.

Baseline assessment of A1AT phenotype includes patient history of lung- or liver-related problems, as well as assessment of liver and pulmonary function (i.e. spirometry, lung volumes, diffusing capacity for carbon monoxide), which can then be followed annually. After identifying a patient with A1AT deficiency it has been recommended to test siblings for the presence of A1AT deficiency.

Management and liver transplantation

Patients should be advised to stop smoking, get vaccinated against pneumococcal infection and influenza, and to start early antibiotics in case of symptoms to decrease the neutrophil burden.

Patients with A1AT-related emphysema may benefit from parenteral augmentation therapy, using a plasma preparation of A1AT. This therapy has been proved by the Food and Drug Administration (FDA) for patients with A1AT <11 μmol/L and COPD). The therapy (i.v. administration once a week) has been shown to be safe with minor adverse reactions, but it is very costly and requires lifelong therapy.[25] With severe emphysema, patients may require bilateral lung transplantation.

A1AT augmentation therapy will not lead to prevention or treatment of liver disease. Currently there is no specific therapy for A1AT-related liver disease. General recommendations include the avoidance of obesity, alcohol or other toxic entities in order to prevent the development of end-stage liver disease. In addition, patients should be recommended to get hepatitic A and B vaccinations. End-stage liver disease related to A1AT deficiency is the most common inherited metabolic indication leading to liver transplantation in children and adults. Survival after liver transplantation has been shown to be good, with 1-year, 3-year and 5-year graft survival rates around 87%, 79% and 77% in adult patients.[1,4] After liver transplantation, the A1AT genotype converts to that of the donor with normalization of serum A1AT levels within weeks. In the future patients may benefit from gene therapy for A1AT deficiency.

Other liver diseases

Familial amyloidotic polyneuropathy

Familial amyloidotic polyneuropathy (FAP) is of autosomal dominant inheritance, resulting into multisystemic disease. Its prevalence is highest in Sweden, Portugal, and Japan, with symptoms presenting often around the third and fourth decades of life. The pathologic feature is a mutation of transthyretin (TTR), one of the prealbumins, which is most commonly caused by a single amino acid substitution of valine to methionine at position 30 (Val30Met). More than 80 other mutations have been reported as being associated with FAP. The disease penetration is probably low, with <10% of mutant carriers becoming symptomatic. The mutant TTR protein is mainly produced by the liver, but the aggregation of amyloid fibrils in connective tissues of organs results in many extrahepatic complications. The major symptoms of FAP are related to progressive peripheral and autonomic neuropathy, as well as insufficiency of visceral organs such as the heart, GI tract and kidneys. The diagnosis can be confirmed by identifying amyloid deposits in nerve tissue, by identifying TTR in the CSF by ELISA testing, or by identifying the genetic mutation of the TTR protein.[2,4,26]

The Familial Amyloidotic Polyneuropathy World Transplant Registry (FAPWTR) indicate that between 1990 and December 2009 more than 1000 liver transplantations for FAP have been performed, of which more than 700 in were carried out in Portugal (www.fapwtr.org). FAPWTR reported in 2004 the outcome of OLT in 539 FAP patients, transplanted in 54 centers in 16 countries. The 5-year patient survival rate was 77%, with an increased 5-year survival rate of 90% in the more recently transplanted patients (period 1995–2000).[27] The main cause of death was cardiac events in 39% of the patients studied. OLT has led to improvement of neuropathy and GI symptoms in almost half of the patients, whereas cardiovascular symptoms have been shown to improve in only 20% of patients.

Owing to the hepatic location of the abnormality, but without liver injury, liver transplantation is often done as domino-transplantation. This implies that the explanted liver of the FAP patient will then be transplanted into another patient with end-stage liver disease. With this new FAP liver the patient also receives the production of the mutant TTR protein, but the process of amyloid deposition has been thought to be slow. Domino liver transplantation has mainly been used in patients with a shorter life expectancy or higher chance of recurrence of disease. So far three cases have been reported in the literature with polyneuropathy de novo after domino liver transplantation with proven amyloid deposits. The three patients presented with symptoms 7–9 years after OLT.[28] Because of increasing follow up in patients after domino liver transplantation, new cases may become evident in the following years.

Glycogen storage disease type 1A

Glycogen storage diseases (GSDs) are inherited abnormalities of enzyme activity resulting in defects of glycogen synthesis or breakdown. The disease group comprises 11 disease variations of which glycogen Type 1A (or "Von Gierke disease") is the most common. It is an autosomal recessive disease, seen in one of 100 000 live births. GSD Type 1A is caused by an enzyme deficiency of glucose-6-phosphatase (G6PT), causing loss of glycogen degradation and accumulation of glycogen and fat in the liver, kidney and intestinal mucosa. Patients often present early in life (within the first year after birth) with a variety of symptoms, including hepatomegaly, hypoglycemia, lactic acidosis, seizures, hyperuricemia, hyperlipidemia, growth retardation, anemia, or leucopenia.[1,2,4]

The diagnosis can be made by elevated serum biotinidase, DNA testing for mutations, or liver biopsy (increased storage of glycogen, steatosis with or without fibrosis). Many metabolic changes can be reversed by maintaining an adequate level of glucose through the administration of uncooked cornstarch (glucose polymer) and avoiding food entities that require glucose-6-phosphatase activity (such as fructose and sucrose). Despite metabolic correction, glomerulosclerosis as a result of hyperfiltration has been shown to remain and sometimes deteriorate. Symptoms related to renal injury include arterial hypertension and proteinuria.

Patients with glycogen storage disease Type 1A have increased risk for developing liver adenomas typically developing in the second or third decades of life. The European Study of Glycogen Storage Disease (ESGSD) reported that the prevalence of adenomas increases with age, showing that the majority of patients older than 25 years had at least 1 lesion of which 50% were progressive in size and numbers.[29] OLT may be required in patients with large unresectable adenomas in order to prevent complications such as HCC. The outcome after OLT for type 1 GSD has been shown to be excellent. Not only does OLT result into the removal of the risk for HCC or other adenoma-complications, it also removes the underlying metabolic abnormality.

Primary hyperoxaluria type 1

Primary hyperoxaluria type 1 (PH1) is an autosomal recessive disease that has been associated with enzymatic defects resulting in enhanced conversion of glyoxalate into oxalate. The disease is related to an enzymatic defect of alanine-glyoxalate aminotransferase (AGT), resulting in less conversion of glyoxalate into glycine. The increased glyoxalate on its turn is converted into oxalate. Oxalate binds with calcium to form insoluble calcium oxalate in renal tubuli, causing complications.

Some patients present in the first year after birth with symptoms of chronic renal failure due to parenchymal accumulation of oxalate. The majority of patients present later in childhood (1–7 years) or early adulthood with symptoms related to urolithiasis or renal injury. In patients with a low glomerular filtration rate (GFR), the reduced rate of oxalate secretion results into deposition of calcium oxalate in a variety of tissues, including cardiovascular, osteoarticular and retinal. Diagnostic tests include findings of increased excretion of oxalate in urine, increased glycolate urinary excretion, increased plasma oxalate concentration and molecular genetic testing. In case of doubtful diagnosis a liver biopsy can be performed to evaluate AGT catalytic activity.[1–4]

Early diagnosis of PH1 and initiation of therapy may prevent renal failure. Pyridoxine (vitamin B6) stimulates the conversion pathway of glyoxalate to glycine, reducing the conversion to oxalate. The administration of orthophosphate, magnesium oxide, or potassium citrate reduces the capability to form calcium oxalate. Other measures include obtaining a high urinary output and avoidance of food with high oxalate content (chocolate, tea, spinach, and rhubarb). OLT accompanies kidney transplantation in the setting of renal failure for future protection of the transplanted renal graft. The European PH1 transplant registry reported the outcome of OLT in 126 patients with 1- and 5-year survival rates of 86% and 80%, respectively.[30] Pre-emptive liver transplantation (without renal transplantation) in stages with chronic renal insufficiency, not yet requiring renal transplantation, has been associated with improved growth and renal function.[31] Its role and timing in the treatment of PH1 has not been well established.

References

1. Zhang KY, Tung BY, Kowdley KV. Liver transplantation for metabolic liver diseases. Clin Liver Dis 2007; 11:265–81.
2. Pietrangelo A. Inherited metabolic disease of the liver. Curr Opin Gastroenterol 2009;25:209–14.
3. Kayler LK, Merion RM, Lee S, et al. Long-term survival after liver transplantation in children with metabolic disorders. Pediatr Transplant 2002;6: 295–300.
4. Weiss HK, Gotthardt D, Schmidt J, et al. Liver transplantation for metabolic liver diseases in adults: indications and outcome. Nephrol Dial Transplant 2007;22(Suppl 8):viii9–12.
5. Browning JD, Szczepaniak LS, Dobbins R, et al. Prevalence of hepatic steatosis in an urban population in the United States: impact of ethnicity. Hepatology 2004;40:1387–95.
6. Adams LA, Lymp JF, Sauver JST, et al. The natural history of non-alcoholic fatty liver disease: a population-based cohort study. Gastroenterology 2005;129: 113–21.
7. Lewis JR, Mohanty SR. Nonalcoholic fatty liver disease: a review and update. Dig Dis Sci 2010;55:560–78.
8. Neuschwander-Tetri BA. Lifestyle modification as the primary treatment of NASH. Clin Liver Dis 2009;12: 649–95.

9. Belfort R, Harrison SA, Brown K, et al. A placebo-controlled trial pioglitazone in subjects with non-alcoholic steatohepatitis. N Engl J Med 2006;355: 2297–307.
10. Sanyal AJ, Chalasani N, Kowdley KV, et al. Pioglitazone, vitamin E or placebo for non-alcoholic steatohepatitis. New Engl J Med 2010;362:1675–85.
11. Klein S, Mittendorfer B, Eagon JC, et al. Gastric bypass surgery improves metabolic and hepatic abnormalities associated with nonalcoholic fatty liver disease. Gastroenterology 2006;130:1564–72.
12. Nair S, Cohen DM, Cohen MP, et al. Postoperative morbidity, mortality, costs and long-term survival in severely obese patients undergoing orthotopic liver transplantation. Am J Gastroenterol 2001;96:842–5.
13. Leonard J, Heimbach JH, Malinchoc M, et al. The impact of obesity on long-term outcomes in liver transplant recipients – results of the NIDDK liver transplant database. Am J Transplant 2008;8:667–72.
14. Pagadala M, Dasarathy S, Eghtesad B, McCullough AJ. Posttransplant metabolic syndrome: an epidemic waiting to happen. Liver Transplant 2009;15: 1662–70.
15. Maor-Kendler Y, Batts KP, Burgart LJ, et al. Comparative allograft histology after liver transplantation for cryptogenic cirrhosis, alcohol, hepatitis C, and cholestatic liver diseases. Transplantation 2000;70:292–97.
16. Pietrangelo A. Hereditary hemochromatosis – A new look at an old disease. N Engl J Med 2004;350: 2383–97.
17. Pedersen P, Milman N. Genetic screening for HFE hemochromatosis in 6,020 Danish men: penetrance of C282Y, H63D, and S65C variants. Ann Hematol 2009;88:775–84.
18. Allen KJ, Gurrin LC, Constantine CC, et al. Iron-overload-related disease in HFE hereditary hemochromatosis. N Engl J Med 2008;358:221–30.
19. Gao J, Chen J, De Domenico I, et al. Hepatocyte-targeted HFE and TFR2 control hepcidin expression in mice. Blood 2010;115:3374–81.
20. Kowdley KV, Brandhagen DJ, Gish RG, et al. Survival after liver transplantation in patients with hepatic iron overload; the national hemochromatosis transplant registry. Gastroenterology 2005;129:494–503.
21. Robert EA, Schilsky ML. Diagnosis and treatment of Wilson disease; an update. AASLD practice guidelines. Hepatology 2008;47:2089–111.
22. El-Youssef M. Wilson disease. Mayo Clin Proc 2003;78:1126–36.
23. Medici V, Mirante VG, Fassati LE, et al. Liver transplantation for Wilson's disease: the burden of neurological and psychiatric disorders. Liver Transpl 2005;11:1056–63.
24. Silverman EK, Sandhaus RA. Alpha1-antitrypsin deficiency. N Engl J Med 2009;360:2749–57.
25. Chapman KR, Stockley RA, Dawkins C, et al. Augmentation therapy for alpha1 antitrypsin deficiency: a meta-analysis. COPD 2009;6:177–84.
26. Hou X, Aguilar MI, Small DH. Transthyretin and familial amyloidotic polyneuropathy. FEBS J 2007;274: 1637–50.
27. Herlenius G, Wilczek HE, Larsson M, et al. Ten years of international experience with liver transplantation for familial amyloidotic polyneuropathy: results from the familial amyloidotic polyneuropathy world transplant registry. Transplantation 2004;66:64–71.
28. Barreriros AP, Geber C, Birklein F, et al. Clinical symptomatic de novo systemic transthyretin amyloidosis 9 years after domino liver transplantation. Liver Transplant 2010;16:311–12.
29. Rake JP, Visser G, Labrune P, et al. Glycogen storage disease type 1: diagnosis, management, clinical course and outcome. Results of the European Study on Glycogen Storage Disease Type 1. Eur J Pediatr 2002; 161(Suppl 1):S20–34.
30. Jamieson NV. A 20-year experience of combined liver/kidney transplantation for primary hyperoxaluria (PH1): the European PH1 Transplant Registry Experience 1984–2004. Am J Nephrol 2005;25: 282–6.
31. Brinkert F, Ganschow R, Helmke K, et al. Transplantation procedures in children with primary hyperoxaluria type 1; outcome and longitudinal growth. Transplantation 2009;87:1415–21.

10 Cholestatic and autoimmune liver disease

Ulrich Beuers

Department of Gastroenterology and Hepatology, Academic Medical Center, University of Amsterdam, Amsterdam, The Netherlands

Key learning points

- Primary biliary cirrhosis (PBC) is an immune-mediated inflammatory disorder of small intrahepatic bile ductules in mostly middle-aged women that progresses to biliary cirrhosis. Its diagnostic hallmarks are elevated serum markers of cholestasis (γGT, alkaline phosphatase) and antimitochondrial antibodies in serum. Ursodeoxycholic acid (UDCA, 13–15 mg/kg/d) is the standard medical treatment for PBC today. Liver transplantation (LT) should be considered in decompensated cirrhosis.
- Primary sclerosing cholangitis (PSC) is characterized by chronic inflammation and fibrosis of both intra- and extrahepatic bile ducts in mainly younger men who often suffer from inflammatory bowel disease. The diagnostic hallmarks are irregular bile duct obliterations and strictures leading to liver cirrhosis and liver failure. UDCA (15–20 mg/kg/d) improves serum liver tests, but has not been shown so far to improve survival. LT should be considered in late-stage disease.
- Autoimmune hepatitis (AIH) is an inflammatory disease of the liver with a female preponderance (≤80%). Its diagnostic hallmarks are elevated serum transaminases, elevated serum IgG, the presence of serum autoantibodies (Type 1: ANA, ASMA, anti-SLA/LP; Type 2: LKM), and histopathologic findings of an interface hepatitis. The standard treatment of AIH with corticosteroids and azathioprine is successful in up to 80% of patients. Lack of adequate treatment response may lead to end-stage liver disease requiring LT.
- Features of ill-defined overlap syndromes of PBC/AIH and PSC/AIH are observed in up to 10% of patients with PBC and PSC.

Primary biliary cirrhosis

Summary

PBC is an immune-mediated inflammatory disorder of small intrahepatic bile ductules that progresses to biliary cirrhosis in late-stage disease and can affect about one in 1000 women at the age of 50 years. The diagnosis of PBC is based on elevated serum markers of cholestasis (γGT, alkaline phosphatase (AP)) and antimitochondrial antibodies (AMA) in serum. Liver biopsy is not mandatory, but delivers information on histologic stage and inflammatory activity of the disease.

At the time of diagnosis, about half of the patients are asymptomatic. Typical symptoms are fatigue and pruritus. Screening for other extrahepatic manifestations including sicca syndrome, osteopenia and osteoporosis, or deficiency of fat-soluble vitamins in late-stage disease or for associated diseases such as hypothyroidism due to thyroiditis Hashimoto is recommended to initiate prophylactic treatment for prevention of complications.

UDCA (13–15 mg/kg/d) is the standard medical treatment for PBC today. Up to two out of three patients adequately respond to UDCA treatment after 1 year (AP <3× normal (N), AST <2 × N, bilirubin

Medical Care of the Liver Transplant Patient, Fourth Edition. Edited by Pierre-Alain Clavien, James F. Trotter.

<1 mg/dl (17 μmol/L)) with a long-term prognosis over 15–20 years equal to an age- and gender-matched healthy population. Additional therapeutic approaches, particularly for patients not adequately responding to UDCA, are under evaluation.

LT should be considered in decompensated cirrhosis with an unacceptable quality of life or anticipated death within 1 year due to treatment-resistant ascites and spontaneous bacterial peritonitis, recurrent variceal bleeding, encephalopathy or hepatocellular carcinoma. Severe, treatment-resistant pruritus may merit consideration for transplantation. Patients should be referred to a liver transplant center for assessment when their bilirubin level approaches 6 mg/dl or 100 μmol/L, and the Mayo risk score is 7,8.[1]

Introduction

PBC is regarded as an organ-specific autoimmune disease characterized by immune-mediated destruction of small intrahepatic bile ducts and subsequent development of liver fibrosis and cirrhosis that occurs mainly in middle-aged women.[1–3] Major progress has been made in understanding key pathophysiologic mechanisms in PBC.[4,5] The formation of specific antibodies directed against the mitochondrial 2-oxo-acid dehydrogenase complexes (AMA-M2) had previously been regarded as an epiphenomenon in PBC, but has more recently been suspected as a potential step in its pathogenesis.[4] The induction of AMA-M2 formation (and simultaneously of PBC?) may be multifactorial: Modification of mitochondrial or bacterial proteins after exposure to reactant xenobiotics such as the cosmetic component, 2-nonynoic acid or hazardous aromatic hydrocarbons such as benzene or exposure to modified bacterial proteins with a high degree of sequence homology with the human mitochondrial 2-oxo-acid dehydrogenase complexes like those of *Novosphingobium aromaticivorans* or *Lactobacillus species* might induce loss of tolerance to human mitochondrial proteins in genetically susceptible individuals.

Aberrant expression of these modified proteins on cholangiocyte membranes by yet undefined mechanisms as observed in PBC may contribute to activation of an immune response leading to florid cholangitis and bile duct destruction in PBC.[4]

Clinical presentation and natural course

The most frequent symptoms of patients with PBC are fatigue and pruritus, which may affect up to 80% of patients during the course of disease. Other symptoms include dry eyes and dry mouth ("sicca syndrome"), and in advanced stages consequences of fat-soluble vitamin deficiencies (A, D, E, and K) and of liver cirrhosis like osteoporosis, variceal bleeding, ascites, and hepatic encephalopathy.

Fatigue is reported by the majority of patients with PBC in all stages of the disease and may be debilitating. Fatigue has recently been shown to be associated with sleep disturbance and excessive daytime somnolence. It is important to exclude other frequent causes of fatigue like hypothyroidism or anemia. Modafinil is the first agent shown in a small pilot study to be of potential benefit in severe fatigue in PBC[6] and deserves further evaluation in placebo-controlled trials.

Pruritus in cholestasis remains poorly understood and the pruritogens in PBC remain undefined although a striking correlation of serum levels of autotaxin and its product, lysophosphatidic acid (LPA), with cholestatic pruritus and pruritus intensity has recently been observed.[7] Clinical and experimental observations suggest that the pruritogens accumulate in the circulation, are biotransformed in the liver, are secreted into bile and undergo an enterohepatic circulation. Treatment of pruritus with anion exchangers like cholestyramine, the pregnane X receptor (PXR) ligand rifampicin, the opiate antagonist naltrexone, or the serotonin reuptake inhibitor sertraline are being recommended.[1] A meta-analysis underlined the effectiveness and safety of rifampicin and naltrexone in PBC-associated pruritus. While rifampicin is safe during short-term treatment for up to 2 weeks,[8] hepatotoxicity has been observed in up to 13% of patients after 3 months. Naltrexone is known to cause opioid withdrawal-like symptoms during the first days of treatment and should be started at very low doses in well-informed patients.

Without adequate treatment, PBC slowly progresses within 1–2 decades from early-stage to end-stage liver disease.

Standard treatment

UDCA is today widely regarded as the medical treatment of choice for PBC.[1–3] The beneficial effects of

UDCA on serum liver tests were reported in the late 1980s and early 1990s in randomized, controlled trials. Evidence for a beneficial effect of UDCA in halting histologic progression in PBC was first reported in 2000. Early meta-analyses questioned the long-term benefit of UDCA treatment in PBC, but were criticized for including trials of too short duration and insufficient dosage. A recent meta-analysis included only trials of acceptable duration for the evaluation of long-term prognosis and acceptable UDCA dosage ("mid-dose") and revealed a significant transplant-free survival benefit for patients with PBC under UDCA treatment in comparison to placebo-treated patients.[9]

Most recently, three large cohort studies with a duration of up to 20 years suggested that PBC patients in whom UDCA treatment at adequate doses (13–15 mg/kg/d) is started at an early histologic stage 1 or 2, have similar survival rates to a normal population matched for age, gender and duration of observation. In particular, patients who respond well to UDCA by normalization or at least a 40% decrease of AP serum activity after 1 year ("Barcelona criteria"),[10] or by reaching serum levels of AP <3 × ULN, AST <2 × ULN, and bilirubin <1 mg/dl (17 µmol/L) ("Paris criteria")[11,12] appear to have a good prognosis. The "Paris criteria" are regarded as a valuable endpoint for future therapeutic trials in PBC.[13]

Major mechanisms and sites of action of UDCA in PBC may include: 1) improvement of impaired hepatocellular and cholangiocellular secretion by mainly post-transcriptional mechanisms, 2) detoxification of bile, and 3) antiapoptotic effects.[14]

Patients not responding to standard treatment

Various immunosuppressive agents as well as nuclear receptor ligands have been recently discussed as potential candidates for combined treatment with UDCA, particularly of PBC patients who inadequately respond to UDCA treatment only.[3] The orally available glucocorticosteroid budesonide is characterized by a high first-pass effect of about 90%, leading to only low systemic serum levels of budesonide in PBC patients with early-stage disease.[15] Budesonide in combination with UDCA has shown beneficial effects on biochemical and histologic features in early-stage PBC[1] superior to those of UDCA alone. Large-scale trials over a sufficient long period of time are warranted to prove a potential long-term benefit of combined treatment with UDCA and budesonide in comparison to UDCA monotherapy in those patients who do not adequately respond to UDCA only. It is important to note that budesonide should be strictly avoided in cirrhotic PBC patients because it may cause severe side effects in patients with advanced disease due to altered pharmacokinetics.[15]

Results of pilot studies with drugs acting as agonists of nuclear receptors like the farnesoid X receptor (FXR), pregnane X receptor (PXR), or the vitamin D_3 receptor (VDR), which may induce expression of key transport proteins and biotransformation enzymes defective in cholestasis, are being awaited in the near future.

Patients with accompanying features of autoimmune hepatitis

Overlap syndromes of PBC and AIH have been reported in up to 10% of patients with PBC.[1] Overlap syndromes are ill-defined and still a matter of controversial discussion. Combined treatment of these disorders with UDCA and an immunosuppressive regimen is proposed in actual guidelines.[1,2]

Patients with end-stage PBC not responding to medical therapy

The majority of PBC patients improve after the start of UDCA treatment and show stabilization of liver function during long-term treatment. One-third of patients, however, slowly progress and may reach the final stage of PBC with decompensated liver cirrhosis, ascites, bleeding esophageal varices, hepatorenal failure or hepatic encephalopathy due to late diagnosis, inadequate treatment, or lack of treatment response. In these patients, LT is the only therapeutic option. The outcome after LT is excellent in PBC with survival rates of 78–92% after 5 years, but the recurrence rate of PBC was calculated to be 18% in patients during long-term follow up.[16] It should be kept in mind, however, that chronic graft rejection may mimic histologic features of recurrent PBC. PBC recurrence after LT does not usually have major clinical implications, probably due in part to the immunosuppressive treatment after LT.

Primary sclerosing cholangitis

Summary

Primary sclerosing cholangitis (PSC) is a chronic, cholestatic liver disease that is characterized by an inflammatory and fibrotic process affecting both intra- and extrahepatic bile ducts and leading to irregular bile duct obliteration with multifocal bile duct strictures and finally liver cirrhosis and liver failure. The typical patient is a young- to middle-aged man (male to female ratio 2:1) with concomitant inflammatory bowel disease (IBD in up to 80%), mostly ulcerative colitis (UC to Crohn's disease ratio 4–5:1).

A diagnosis of PSC is made in patients with biochemical markers of cholestasis not otherwise explained in whom cholangiography (by MRCP or ERCP, exceptionally pereutaneous transhepatic cholangiography (PTC)) shows typical findings and secondary causes are excluded. A liver biopsy is not mandatory for the diagnosis of PSC.

Patients with PSC have an enhanced risk to develop malignancies of the bile ducts and colon (in the presence of IBD), but also the gallbladder, liver, and pancreas, and should therefore be screened on a regular basis by annual abdominal ultrasound and by (bi-) annual colonoscopy in the presence of IBD.

There is no medical treatment with proven benefit on long-term survival. UDCA (15–20 mg/d) improves serum liver tests and surrogate markers of prognosis and might exert a chemopreventive effect on colorectal cancer in PSC, although more data from prospective trials are needed. Dominant bile duct strictures with significant cholestasis should be treated with biliary dilatation or short-term stenting under antibiotic prophylaxis.[1]

LT is recommended in patients with late-stage PSC and may be considered in patients with evidence of cholangiocyte dysplasia or severe recurrent bacterial cholangitis.[1,17]

Introduction

PSC is a chronic, inflammatory disease affecting both intra- and extrahepatic bile ducts and leading to irregular bile duct obliterations, cholestasis (AP and γGT elevated in the early stage), liver fibrosis, cirrhosis, and liver failure. The etiology of PSC is unknown. Genetic susceptibility is involved; the male to female ratio is 2:1. PSC can be diagnosed in children as well as in the elderly, but the mean age at diagnosis is 35 to 40 years. The vast majority (≤80%) of PSC patients have concomitant IBD, mainly ulcerative colitis (UC). The diagnosis of PSC is made in the presence of elevated biochemical markers of cholestasis (AP, γGT) when cholangiography (a high-quality MRCP recommended, otherwise ERCP; only exceptionally PTC) shows typical strictures and dilatations of intra- and/or extrahepatic bile ducts not otherwise explained. A liver biopsy is not mandatory, but allows: 1) assessment of the stage of the disease, 2) diagnosis of small-duct PSC if a high-quality MRCP is normal, and 3) diagnosis of additional/alternative diseases when serum transaminases and/or serum IgG levels or angiotensin-I-converting enzyme (ACE) levels are disproportionally elevated.

Clinical presentation and natural course

About 50% of PSC patients report symptoms at first presentation including fatigue, pruritus, pain in the right upper abdominal quadrant, episodes of fever and chills, and weight loss. Symptoms of decompensated liver cirrhosis like ascites and variceal hemorrhage are highly exceptional at diagnosis.[1] Jaundice, hepatomegaly, and splenomegaly are the most frequent clinical findings at diagnosis. Osteopenic bone disease and symptoms of fat malabsorption are observed in advanced, prolonged cholestasis. When untreated, patients with PSC had a median transplant-free survival of 10–12 years as reported in different studies.[1,17]

PSC is associated with an increased risk of hepatobiliary, pancreatic and colon malignancies. In a large cohort of 604 Swedish PSC patients followed for a median of 5.7 years, hepatobiliary malignancies (cholangiocarcinoma (CCA), gallbladder carcinoma, and hepatocellular carcinoma) were observed in 13.3%, corresponding to a risk 161 times that of the general population.[18] CCA is by far the most common hepatobiliary malignancy in PSC, with a cumulative life-time incidence of 10–15%, whereas gallbladder carcinoma and HCC are observed in up to 2–3% of PSC patients. Up to 50% of cases of CCA are diagnosed within the first year of diagnosis of PSC. After the first year, the yearly incidence rate is 0.5–1.5%.[19] The symptoms of CCA complicating PSC may be very difficult to differentiate from those of PSC without concomitant malignancy, but awareness of CCA must in particular be raised in cases of rapid clinical deterioration. The risk of colon carcinoma in patients with PSC and UC is higher than that of patients with UC only (odds ratio >4!).[20] Thus, (bi-)annual screening colonoscopy in patients with PSC and UC is recommended in actual guidelines.[1]

Standard treatment

Medical treatment

No proven benefit on long-term survival in PSC has been shown for any drug tested so far.[1,17] The requirements for a trial showing a survival benefit in PSC would include all of the following: 1) an adequate size of the study cohort, 2) an adequate disease stage of the study population for the drug and drug dosage to be tested, 3) an adequate period of treatment and follow-up, and 4) an adequate control of compliance. Up to 2010, no single clinical trial in PSC fulfilled all the criteria mentioned earlier, thus a true survival benefit in PSC by medical treatment has so far not been shown. This is mainly due to the fact that PSC is a rare and slowly progressive orphan disease.

UDCA UDCA has been demonstrated in the 1990s to induce biochemical and in some series histologic improvement in PSC patients using doses of 10–15 mg/kg/d.[1] Studies using 20–25 mg/kg/d demonstrated significant improvements in the histologic grade of liver fibrosis and the cholangiographic appearances of PSC, as well as the expected biochemical improvement.

A 2-year dose-ranging pilot study of 30 patients confirmed these findings by showing that the low dose (10 mg/kg/d) and the standard dose (20 mg/kg/d) tended to improve and the high dose (30 mg/kg/d) significantly improved projected survival.[21]

The Scandinavian UDCA trial recruited the largest group of PSC patients (n=219) for the longest treatment period (5 years) ever studied using a dose of 17–23 mg/kg/d.[22] It demonstrated a trend towards increased survival in the UDCA-treated group when compared with placebo, but it was still seriously underpowered (198 patients analyzed, 346 patients a priori calculated) to reach a statistically significant result. In comparison to other studies, the biochemical response was unexpectedly poor in this trial, which prompted questions about adequate compliance in a part of the study population.

An American multicentre study using high doses of 28–30 mg/kg/d of UDCA in 150 PSC patients over 5 years has been aborted recently because of an enhanced risk in the UDCA treatment group to reach a composite endpoint of death, LT, minimal listing criteria of transplantation, or development of varices, particularly in patients included with advanced disease while biochemical features improved in the whole UDCA group.[23] Thus, the role for UDCA in slowing the progression of PSC-related liver disease is as yet unclear and high-dose UDCA may be harmful in late-stage disease.[1]

Currently there is suggestive but limited evidence for the use of UDCA for chemoprevention of colorectal cancer in PSC. UDCA may be particularly considered in those patients with a strong family history of colorectal cancer, previous colorectal neoplasia or longstanding extensive colitis.[1]

Immunosuppressants Corticosteroids and other immunosuppressants are not indicated for treatment of PSC in adults unless there is evidence of an overlap syndrome.[1]

Endoscopic treatment

Dominant bile duct strictures with significant cholestasis should be treated with biliary dilatation.[1] Biliary stent insertion should be reserved for cases where stricture dilatation and biliary drainage are unsatisfactory. Prophylactic antibiotic coverage is recommended in this setting.[1]

Surgical treatment

LT is recommended in patients with late-stage PSC and may be considered in patients with evidence of cholangiocyte dysplasia or severe recurrent bacterial cholangitis.[1]

Differential diagnosis of PSC vs other forms of sclerosing cholangitis

Sclerosing cholangitis imitating PSC has been observed in patients: 1) with intraductal stone disease, 2) after surgical trauma from cholecystectomy or bile duct surgery, 3) after abdominal injury, 4) after intra-arterial chemotherapy, 5) after recurrent pancreatitis, and 5) in IgG4-associated cholangitis/autoimmune pancreatitis, eosinophilic cholangitis, mast cell cholangiopathy, portal hypertensive biliopathy, AIDS cholangiopathy, recurrent pyogenic cholangitis, ischemic cholangitis, and others. These conditions may need therapeutic approaches different from PSC and are not discussed here in detail as patients with these disorders usually are not candidates for LT.

Patients with accompanying features of autoimmune hepatitis

Overlap syndromes of AIH with PSC have been reported in children, adolescents, and young adults in about 8% of patients with these immune-mediated disorders.[1] Overlap syndromes are ill-defined and still a matter of controversial discussion. Combined treatment of these disorders with UDCA and an immunosuppressive regimen is proposed in actual guidelines.[1] LT is the only curative treatment in late-stage disease.

Patients with late/end-stage PSC

Patients with advanced cirrhosis, with symptoms and signs of decompensation as well as those with evidence of cholangiocyte dysplasia or severe recurrent bacterial cholangitis should be considered for LT, which represents the only potentially curative treatment for PSC. Outcome after LT is excellent in PSC, with survival rates around 90% after 5 years in most recent reports of experienced centers, but recurrence of PSC was calculated to be 11% in PSC patients after LT during long-term follow up.[16] Recurrence of PSC, however, is difficult to define due to similarities in bile duct damage with ischemic-type biliary lesions, infections, medication-induced injury, preservation injury, or chronic rejection.[1] Screening for colon carcinoma should be pursued after LT.

Autoimmune hepatitis

Summary

AIH is an inflammatory disease of the liver of yet unknown etiology that occurs worldwide in adults and children, and has a female preponderance (≤80%).

The diagnostic hallmarks of AIH are elevated serum transaminases, elevated serum IgG, the presence of serum autoantibodies (Type 1: ANA, ASMA, anti-SLA/LP; Type 2: LKM), and histopathologic findings of an interface hepatitis with lymphoplasmacytic infiltration of portal areas and periportal lymphoplasmacytic parenchymal invasion and piecemeal necrosis.

Standard treatment of AIH is successful in up to 80% of these patients. About 20% of patients present with "difficult-to-treat AIH" for different reasons and are at risk of developing end-stage liver disease requiring LT.

Patients not tolerating standard treatment form one subgroup of patients with "difficult-to-treat AIH". The elderly patient with diabetes mellitus and osteoporosis as well as the patient with severe side effects of corticosteroid or azathioprine treatment may need alternative treatment strategies. New generation corticosteroids in noncirrhotic patients such as budesonide with less systemic side effects at therapeutic doses and mycophenolate mofetil (MMF) represent therapeutic alternatives.

The pregnant patient with AIH apparently does not experience a maintenance treatment-related enhanced risk of complications for mother and fetus. Close monitoring of disease activity during and particularly shortly after pregnancy is mandatory to adequately treat flairs of AIH.

Patients not responding to standard treatment and at risk of developing cirrhosis and liver failure form the most challenging subgroup of patients with "difficult-to-treat AIH". The calcineurin inhibitors cyclosporine A and tacrolimus, have been successfully applied as potent alternative immunosuppressive strategies to induce remission and hinder disease progression in this patient group. Patients not responding to standard treatment or alternative medical approaches may have to undergo LT. These patients have a considerable risk of developing recurrence of AIH after LT, often not responding to standard treatment.

Introduction

AIH is an inflammatory disease of the liver that occurs worldwide in adults and children with a female preponderance (≤80%). Its pathogenesis is unresolved, but genetic as well as environmental factors play key roles in its development.[24,25] AIH is characterized biochemically and serologically by elevated serum transaminases, elevated serum IgG and the presence of autoantibodies (Type 1: ANA, ASMA, anti-SLA/LP; Type 2: LKM). The characteristic histopathologic finding is an interface hepatitis with lymphoplasmacytic infiltration of portal areas, periportal lymphoplasmacytic parenchymal invasion and piecemeal necrosis. Various toxic (drugs!), infectious (HBV, HCV), and metabolic (non-alcoholic steatohepatitis, (NASH); Wilson's disease) liver diseases may show features similar to AIH and have to be excluded before a firm diagnosis of AIH can be made. Simplified criteria for the diagnosis of AIH have recently been proposed and validated:[26–28] (**A**: ANA or SMA ≥1:40:1 point; ANA or SMA ≥1:80, LKM ≥1:40 or SLA/LP positive: 2 points; **B**: IgG >1 × ULN: 1 point; IgG >1.1 × ULN: 2 points; **C**: liver histology compatible with AIH: 1 point; liver histology typical of AIH: 2 points; **D**: absence of viral hepatitis: 2 points. **A + B + C + D = 6**: probable AIH; ≥7: definite AIH). About 40% of patients with AIH suffer from other autoimmune disorders such as autoimmune thyroiditis, rheumatoid arthritis, ulcerative colitis, diabetes mellitus, glomerulonephritis, vitiligo, alopecia, or nail dystrophies. Early diagnosis and treatment of AIH is crucial to hinder progression to cirrhosis and decompensation of liver disease.

Clinical presentation and natural course

AIH may start with an acute, sometimes severe hepatitis in almost 50% of patients, but may also take a smouldering course remaining undetected for years before the diagnosis is made. This explains why about 30% of patients present with cirrhosis at the time of diagnosis. The 10-year survival rate without treatment has been roughly estimated to be 10–30%[29] based on mainly retrospective data of heterogeneous patient cohorts from the past. These observations clearly show the need for adequate treatment from the time of clinical, serologic, and histologic diagnosis of AIH when serum transaminases and IgG are elevated.

Standard treatment

The standard treatment of AIH is an immunosuppressive regimen including corticosteroids alone or corticosteroids in combination with azathioprine for a period of 2 years to lifelong.[24] The therapeutic aim is complete remission with normalization of serum transaminases, serum IgG and histologic features of inflammation. Complete remission can be reached in up to 75% of patients after 2 years.

Corticosteroid monotherapy is started with predniso(lo)ne, 60 mg/d for 1 week followed by a dose reduction by 10 mg/week to 20 mg/d. Further tapering by 5 mg/week to 10 mg/d is possible as long as serum transaminases and IgG do not increase again under dose reduction. Maintenance therapy with 10 mg/d can be further tapered down during follow up by steps of 2.5 mg when serum transaminases and IgG remain normal.

Combination therapy with predniso(lo)ne 30–60 mg/d and azathioprine 50 mg/d can be initiated from the beginning or – as preferred by the author – after a 2–4-week period of predniso(lo)ne monotherapy in order to follow the initial pure corticosteroid response and to differentiate between potential corticosteroid- and azathioprine-induced gastrointestinal complaints. Corticosteroid tapering follows a course similar to the one mentioned for corticosteroid monotherapy. Long-term maintenance therapy can be performed with low doses of predniso(lo)ne and azathioprine[30] or with azathioprine only (1.5–2 mg/kg/d).[24,31]

Difficult-to-treat AIH

Elderly patient

AIH is a disease occurring at all ages. Patients aged 65 and older may present with relative contraindications against standard treatment more often than their younger fellow sufferers. Particularly osteoporosis and diabetes mellitus may put the patient under corticosteroid therapy at considerable risk for serious treatment-related complications.

The elderly patient with AIH more often presents with cirrhosis than younger patients, possibly due a smouldering course and failure to make an early diagnosis due to lack of symptoms.[32] However, the outcome of AIH in the elderly patient apparently does not differ from that in the younger patient, in part possibly due to a better response to standard treatment than in younger patients.[32]

AIH should be treated at all ages. The elderly may require alternative therapeutic strategies (see later) more often than the younger patient due to side effects of standard treatment, but not due to lack of treatment response.

Pregnant patient
The female predominance in AIH often leads to the question of whether a pregnancy poses an enhanced risk to both the mother with AIH and her child. A recent retrospective study analysed the course of 44 pregnancies in 22 patients with AIH and found: 1) adverse outcomes in 26% of pregnancies, in part associated with the presence of SLA/LP and Ro/SSA antibodies, 2) a postpartum flare in 52% of pregnancies, and 3) no difference in outcome between patients treated with or without azathioprine during pregnancy.[33] These retropective data may enable close monitoring of AIH patients during and particularly shortly after pregnancy, to continue azathioprine treatment during pregnancy when clinically needed, and to prospectively study the role of autoantibody profiles for the outcome of pregnancy in AIH.

Patient not tolerating standard treatment

Budesonide
Budesonide is a corticosteroid with an about 15- to 20-fold higher receptor binding affinity than predniso(lo)ne, but a 90% hepatic first-pass effect leading to significantly reduced systemic serum levels and reduced rates of corticosteroid-related side effects. Budesonide is contraindicated in cirrhosis with portal hypertension due to an enhanced risk for the development of portal vein thrombosis.[15] The so far largest randomized, placebo-controlled trial for the treatment of AIH in 207 noncirrhotic patients with AIH compared standard treatment with prednisone (initial dose 40 mg/d) + azathioprine with budesonide (initial dose 3×3 mg/d) + azathioprine and clearly showed more efficient induction of remission and a more favorable side-effect profile of budesonide in comparison to prednisone.[34] Budesonide may become an alternative first-line treatment for noncirrhotic AIH in the near future and may be particularly attractive for patients at high risk for corticosteroid-related side effects.

Mycophenolate mofetil
Mycophenolate mofetil (MMF), an inhibitor of inosine monophosphate dehydrogenases, impairs purine synthesis mainly of rapidly proliferating cells such as T- and B-lymphocytes and, thereby, exerts immunosuppressive effects. Small case series during the last decade have reported successful treatment of AIH with MMF, however the largest study so far, a recent retrospective analysis of 36 patients with AIH treated with MMF, revealed disappointing results in that only 39% of patients under MMF treatment showed a complete response.[35] Interestingly, a subclass analysis revealed that those patients who had not responded to azathioprine also did not adequately respond to MMF, thus MMF may be a therapeutic option for those AIH patients not tolerating standard treatment rather than for those not responding to standard treatment.

Patients not responding to standard treatment

Standard treatment with corticosteroids and azathioprine induces complete clinical, biochemical and histologic long-term remission in up to 80% of patients during long-term treatment. Alternative medications in nonresponders include the calcineurin inhibitors cyclosporine A and tacrolimus, the antimetabolites MMF and cyclophosphamide, and the mTor inhibitor rapamycin.

Cyclosporine A
The cyclic peptide cyclosporine A (CyA) derived from the fungus *Trichoderma polysporum* inhibits transcription of the interleukin 2 (IL2) gene by binding to cyclophilin and inhibiting calcineurin phosphatase activity. Its wide use in transplantation medicine has stimulated its use in open-label trials for adults and children with AIH in part not responding to standard treatment. CyA (at doses of 4–5 mg/kg/d or with target trough levels of 200–250 ng/ml) was shown to effectively induce remission in a majority of patients. Maintenance treatment with CyA, however, is hampered by the well-known risks of long-term CyA therapy including: arterial hypertension, renal insufficiency, hyperlipidemia, hirsutism, infection, and malignancy. Thus, a two-step strategy in AIH patients not responding to standard treatment with: 1) induction of remission with CyA, and 2) a careful switch to standard treatment under close monitoring of disease activity has been proposed and in single cases successfully reported.

Tacrolimus
The macrolide antibiotic tacrolimus (FK506) produced by *Streptomyces tsukubaensis* is a more potent immunosuppressive agent than CyA. Like CyA, tacrolimus inhibits calcineurin and, thereby, IL2 transcription in T-cells after forming a complex with an immunophilin, here FK binding protein. Low-dose tacrolimus is effective in AIH. In patients not responding to standard treatment, tacrolimus improved disease activity and degree of fibrosis (initial dose 1 mg twice daily; trough levels <6 ng/ml) and was reported to be effective alone or in combination with MMF in another cohort of patients not responding to or not tolerating standard treatment.[36] Tacrolimus may therefore be a valuable alternative to CyA in the treatment of AIH in patients not responding to standard treatment.

Cyclophosphamide
Cyclophosphamide (1–1.5 mg/kg/d) was successfully used in combination with prednisolone in three patients not responding to standard treatment.[37] The risk of severe hematologic side effects during long-term treatment argue against this experimental treatment option.

Methotrexate
The antimetabolite methotrexate (7.5 mg/week) had a steroid-sparing effect in a patient not responding to standard treatment.[38]

Patients with accompanying immune-mediated cholangitis

Overlap syndromes of AIH with PBC and AIH with PSC have been reported in 6–10% of patients with these immune-mediated disorders.[1] Overlap syndromes are ill-defined and still a matter of controversial discussion. Combined treatment of these disorders with UDCA and an immunosuppressive regimen is proposed in actual guidelines.[1]

UDCA
The hydrophilic bile acid UDCA is regarded as the standard therapy of PBC. UDCA does not act as an immunosuppressive agent, but has potent anticholestatic, anti-apoptotic and antifibrotic activity in PBC[1] and exerts anticholestatic effects in numerous other cholestatic disorders including PSC.[14] UDCA has been tested in "problematic" AIH in addition to corticosteroids with disappointing results.[39,40]

In contrast to patients with definite AIH, patients with an overlap syndrome of AIH and PBC and children and adolescents with an overlap syndrome of AIH and PSC may benefit from combined treatment with UDCA and a standard immunosuppressive regimen,[1] however randomized, controlled studies on this are lacking.

Patients with end-stage AIH not responding to medical therapy

Most AIH patients improve after starting immunosuppressive treatment and show stabilization of liver function during maintenance therapy. About 10% of patients, however, reach the final stage of AIH with decompensated liver cirrhosis, ascites, bleeding esophageal varices, or hepatic encephalopathy due to late diagnosis, inadequate treatment or lack of treatment response. In these patients, LT is the only therapeutic option. Outcome after LT is very good in AIH with survival rates around 80–90% after 5 years, but recurrence of AIH was calculated to be 22% in patients during long-term follow-up study.[16] AIH recurrence after LT carries the risk of not adequately responding to standard immunosuppressive therapy and represents a therapeutic challenge for the hepatologist as recurrent "difficult-to-treat AIH" (for experimental therapeutic approaches, see earlier.)

Abbreviations

AIH: autoimmune hepatitis, ANA: antinuclear antibodies, AP: alkaline phosphatase, ASMA: anti-smooth muscle antibodies, CyA: cyclosporine A, ERCP: endoscopic retrograde cholangiopancreatography, γGT: gamma-glutamyltransferase, HBV: hepatitis B virus, HCV: hepatitis C virus, IBD: inflammatory bowel disease, LC1: anti-liver cytosol Type 1 antibodies, LKM: anti-liver–kidney microsomal antibodies, LT: liver transplantation, MRCP: magnetic resonance cholangiopancreatography, pANCA: perinuclear antineutrophilic cytoplasmic antibodies, PBC: primary biliary cirrhosis, PSC: primary sclerosing cholangitis, PTC: percutaneous transhepatic cholangiography, SLA: anti-soluble liver antigen antibodies. UC: ulcerative colitis, UDCA: ursodeoxycholic acid, ULN: upper limit of normal.

References

1. EASL Clinical Practice Guidelines: Management of cholestatic liver diseases. J Hepatol 2009;51: 237–67.
2. Lindor KD, Gershwin ME, Poupon R, Kaplan M, Bergasa NV, Heathcote EJ. Primary biliary cirrhosis. Hepatology 2009;50:291–308.
3. Kaplan MM, Gershwin ME. Primary biliary cirrhosis. N Engl J Med 2005;353:1261–73.
4. Gershwin ME, Mackay IR. The causes of primary biliary cirrhosis: Convenient and inconvenient truths. Hepatology 2008;47:737–45.
5. Hohenester S, Oude-Elferink RP, Beuers U. Primary biliary cirrhosis. Semin Immunopathol 2009;31:283–307.
6. Jones DE, Newton JL. An open study of modafinil for the treatment of daytime somnolence and fatigue in primary biliary cirrhosis. Alim Pharm Ther 2007;25: 471–6.
7. Kremer AE, Martens JJ, Kulik W, et al. Lysophosphatidic acid is a potential mediator of cholestatic pruritus. Gastroenterology 2010;139:1008–18.
8. Khurana S, Singh P. Rifampin is safe for treatment of pruritus due to chronic cholestasis: a meta-analysis of prospective randomized-controlled trials. Liver Int 2006;26:943–8.
9. Shi J, Wu C, Lin Y, Chen YX, Zhu L, Xie WF. Long-term effects of mid-dose ursodeoxycholic acid in primary biliary cirrhosis: a meta-analysis of randomized controlled trials. Am J Gastroenterol 2006;101: 1529–38.
10. Pares A, Caballeria L, Rodes J. Excellent long-term survival in patients with primary biliary cirrhosis and biochemical response to ursodeoxycholic acid. Gastroenterology 2006;130:715–20.
11. Corpechot C, Abenavoli L, Rabahi N, et al. Biochemical response to ursodeoxycholic acid and long-term prognosis in primary biliary cirrhosis. Hepatology 2008;48: 871–7.
12. Kuiper EM, Hansen BE, de Vries RA, et al. Improved prognosis of patients with primary biliary cirrhosis that have a biochemical response to ursodeoxycholic acid. Gastroenterology 2009;136:1281–7.
13. Silveira MG, Brunt EM, Heathcote J, Gores GJ, Lindor KD, Mayo MJ. American Association for the Study of Liver Diseases endpoints conference: design and endpoints for clinical trials in primary biliary cirrhosis. Hepatology;52:349–59.
14. Beuers U. Drug insight: Mechanisms and sites of action of ursodeoxycholic acid in cholestasis. Nat Clin Pract Gastroenterol Hepatol 2006;3:318–28.
15. Hempfling W, Grunhage F, Dilger K, Reichel C, Beuers U, Sauerbruch T. Pharmacokinetics and pharmacodynamic action of budesonide in early- and late-stage primary biliary cirrhosis. Hepatology 2003;38: 196–202.
16. Gautam M, Cheruvattath R, Balan V. Recurrence of autoimmune liver disease after liver transplantation: a systematic review. Liver Transpl 2006;12:1813–24.
17. Chapman R, Fevery J, Kalloo A, et al. Diagnosis and management of primary sclerosing cholangitis. Hepatology;51:660–78.
18. Bergquist A, Ekbom A, Olsson R, et al. Hepatic and extrahepatic malignancies in primary sclerosing cholangitis. J Hepatol 2002;36:321–7.
19. Lazaridis KN, Gores GJ. Primary sclerosing cholangitis and cholangiocarcinoma. Semin Liver Dis 2006;26: 42–51.
20. Soetikno RM, Lin OS, Heidenreich PA, Young HS, Blackstone MO. Increased risk of colorectal neoplasia in patients with primary sclerosing cholangitis and ulcerative colitis: a meta-analysis. Gastrointest Endosc 2002;56:48–54.
21. Cullen SN, Rust C, Fleming K, Edwards C, Beuers U, Chapman R. High dose ursodeoxycholic acid for the treatment of primary sclerosing cholangitis is safe and effective. J Hepatol 2008;48:792–800.
22. Olsson R, Boberg KM, de Muckadell OS, et al. High-dose ursodeoxycholic acid in primary sclerosing cholangitis: a 5-year multicenter, randomized, controlled study. Gastroenterology 2005;129:1464–72.
23. Lindor KD, Kowdley KV, Luketic VA, et al. High-dose ursodeoxycholic acid for the treatment of primary sclerosing cholangitis. Hepatology 2009;50: 808–14.
24. Manns MP, Czaja AJ, Gorham JD, et al. Diagnosis and management of autoimmune hepatitis. Hepatology 2010;51:2193–213.
25. Vergani D, Longhi MS, Bogdanos DP, Ma Y, Mieli-Vergani G. Autoimmune hepatitis. Semin Immunopathol 2009;31:421–35.
26. Hennes EM, Zeniya M, Czaja AJ, et al. Simplified criteria for the diagnosis of autoimmune hepatitis. Hepatology 2008;48:169–76.
27. Czaja AJ. Performance parameters of the diagnostic scoring systems for autoimmune hepatitis. Hepatology 2008;48:1540–8.
28. Yeoman AD, Westbrook RH, Al-Chalabi T, et al. Diagnostic value and utility of the simplified International Autoimmune Hepatitis Group (IAIHG) criteria in acute and chronic liver disease. Hepatology 2009;50: 538–45.
29. Krawitt EL. Autoimmune hepatitis. N Engl J Med 2006;354:54–66.
30. Strassburg CP, Manns MP. Treatment of autoimmune hepatitis. Semin Liver Dis 2009;29:273–85.

31. Johnson PJ, McFarlane IG, Williams R. Azathioprine for long-term maintenance of remission in autoimmune hepatitis. N Engl J Med 1995;333:958–63.
32. Czaja AJ, Carpenter HA. Distinctive clinical phenotype and treatment outcome of type 1 autoimmune hepatitis in the elderly. Hepatology 2006;43:532–8.
33. Schramm C, Herkel J, Beuers U, Kanzler S, Galle PR, Lohse AW. Pregnancy in autoimmune hepatitis: outcome and risk factors. Am J Gastroenterol 2006;101: 556–60.
34. Manns MP, Bahr MJ, Woynarowski M, et al. Budesonide 3 mg tid is superior to prednisone in combination with azathioprine in the treatment of autoimmune hepatitis. J Hepatol 2008;49:S369.
35. Hennes EM, Oo YH, Schramm C, et al. Mycophenolate mofetil as second line therapy in autoimmune hepatitis? Am J Gastroenterol 2008;103:3063–70.
36. Chatur N, Ramji A, Bain VG, et al. Transplant immunosuppressive agents in non-transplant chronic autoimmune hepatitis: the Canadian association for the study of liver (CASL) experience with mycophenolate mofetil and tacrolimus. Liver Int 2005;25:723–7.
37. Kanzler S, Gerken G, Dienes HP, Meyer zum Buschenfelde KH, Lohse AW. Cyclophosphamide as alternative immunosuppressive therapy for autoimmune hepatitis – report of three cases. Z Gastroenterol 1997; 35:571–8.
38. Burak KW, Urbanski SJ, Swain MG. Successful treatment of refractory type 1 autoimmune hepatitis with methotrexate. J Hepatol 1998;29:990–3.
39. Czaja AJ, Carpenter HA, Lindor KD. Ursodeoxycholic acid as adjunctive therapy for problematic type 1 autoimmune hepatitis: a randomized placebo-controlled treatment trial. Hepatology 1999;30:1381–6.
40. Nakamura K, Yoneda M, Yokohama S, et al. Efficacy of ursodeoxycholic acid in Japanese patients with type 1 autoimmune hepatitis. J Gastroenterol Hepatol 1998; 13:490–5.

11 Hepatocellular carcinoma

Maria Reig[1], *Alejandro Forner*[2] *and Jordi Bruix*[3]
[1,2]BCLC Group, Liver Unit, Hospital Clinic, 1CIBERehd, IDIBAPS, University of Barcelona, Barcelona, Spain and [3]Head, BCLC Group, Liver Unit, Hospital Clinic, University of Barcelona, Barcelona, Spain

Key learning points

- Hepatocellular carcinoma (HCC) in cirrhosis may be diagnosed by non-invasive criteria.
- Liver transplantation is an effective treatment option for patients with early HCC.
- The shortage of organs forces the need to apply strict rules to the selection of patients in order to offer the best results.
- Live donation is an effective alternative to cadaver donation University of Barcelona,.

Introduction

The incidence of HCC has increased worldwide in the last decades. Chronic liver disease is the risk factor for HCC development and current data show that it is the main cause of death in patients with cirrhosis.[1] The incidence at 5 years of follow up in cirrhosis ranges between 10 and 20%.[1] The optimal strategy to decrease HCC-related mortality is to reduce excessive alcohol intake and avoid infection with hepatitis B or C viruses. Early treatment of viral infection with sustained response may also be effective, but if extensive liver damage (cirrhosis) is already present, cancer risk may be established and hence the only approach to reduce cancer-related death is early detection allowing effective treatment.[1] This is the rationale for involving the population at risk, namely cirrhotic patients, in surveillance programs based on ultrasound (US) every 6 months. The aim is to detect tumors at an early stage (Figure 11.1) when the patient may benefit from curative therapy.

It is well known that the prognosis for the patient with HCC does not depend only on the size and extent of the tumor (number of foci, vascular invasion, extrahepatic spread).[2] Hepatic function is an important parameter to select therapy for HCC. The clinical relevance of HCC symptoms in patients with HCC is also well established. Patients with weight loss, pain, fatigue or anorexia at initial diagnosis have a worse prognosis and those with impaired performance status have a poorer outcome.[2] Several scoring and staging systems have been proposed to predict the outcome of the patients diagnosed with HCC,[2] but up to now, the sole system that takes into account all these dimensions is the Barcelona Clinic Liver Cancer (BCLC) classification.[2] It has been extensively validated and has been endorsed by several associations and scientific groups (Figure 11.1).

Diagnosis of HCC can be established by biopsy or by imaging criteria (Figure 11.2). Tumor markers have very limited clinical usefulness.[1] Which tests should be used depends on the context. In a patient with cirrhosis, the diagnosis is established if magnetic resonance imaging (MRI) or computed tomography (CT) displays the specific pattern of intense arterial uptake of contrast followed by its washout in the

Medical Care of the Liver Transplant Patient, Fourth Edition. Edited by Pierre-Alain Clavien, James F. Trotter.

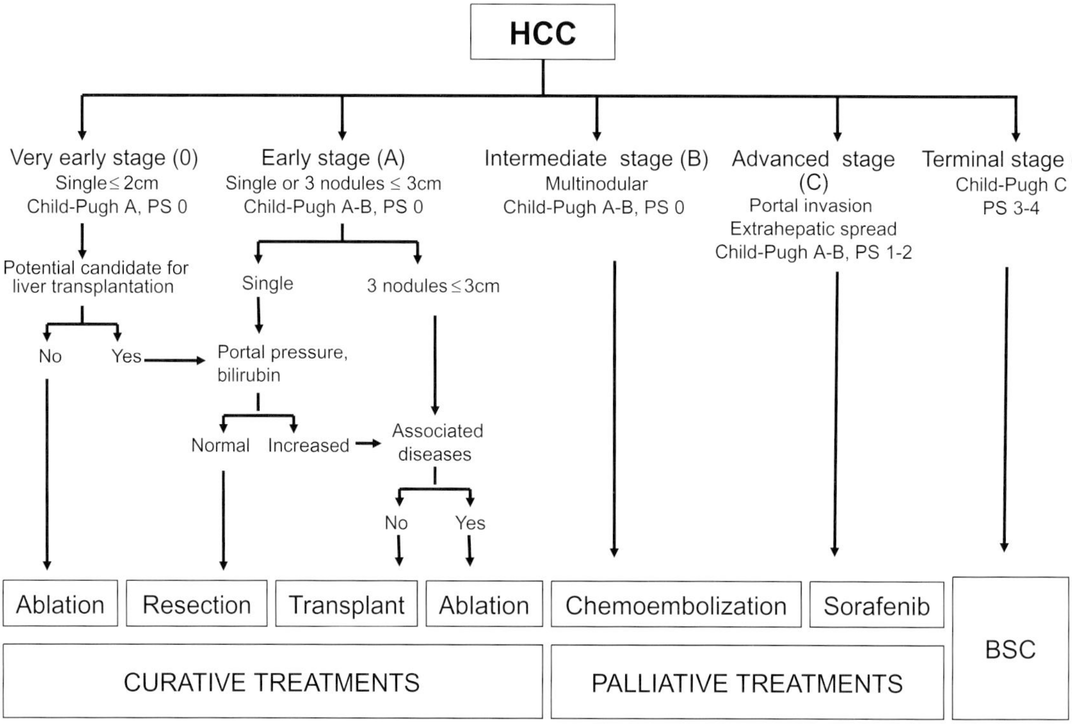

Figure 11.1 BCLC staging and treatment strategy for HCC patients. Patients diagnosed at an early stage (stage A) are considered for options that may provide long-term cure. Patients at intermediate stage (stage B) are considered for transarterial chemoembolization. If patients belong to an advanced stage (stage C), they are considered for sorafenib and if they fall into stage D, they just receive symptomatic therapy with avoidance of unnecessary suffering. Stage 0 includes those patients with very early HCC belonging to the so-called carcinoma in situ. This type of tumor is currently very difficult to diagnose prior to surgical resection as it lacks the characteristic radiologic pattern and biopsy is unable to reach confident diagnosis because of very well a preserved differentiation degree and architecture. (Reproduced from Forner A, Llovet JM, Bruix J. Hepatocellular Carcinoma. Lancet. 2011 In press.) HCC: hepatocellular carcinoma, PS: performance status, RFA: radiofrequency, TACE: transcatheter arterial chemoembolization

venous delayed phases.[2] If this is not observed, a biopsy should be required. In any case, either CT or MRI should be performed to determine the extent of the disease and provide the information to select the optimal therapy.

The number of patients diagnosed at early or very early BCLC stage and who are potential candidates for curative treatment is still limited. Curative options with potential disease-free survival at 5 years include surgery (resection and transplantation) and ablation (usually done percutaneously under US guidance). Liver transplantation will be extensively discussed in this chapter while the other options will be briefly summarized.

Liver resection is the first option for the noncirrhotic patient. If cirrhosis is present, the optimal candidates for resection are those patients with solitary tumors without evidence of vascular invasion or spread outside the liver.[2] The best results are obtained in Child–Pugh A individuals without significant portal hypertension and normal bilirubin concentration.[3] The validity of this criterion for outcome prediction has been confirmed in the East and West.[4] Optimal candidates should have almost no postoperative liver failure and associated mortality, and the expected 5-year survival rate may exceed 70%.[2] Unfortunately, even in carefully selected patients, the rate of tumor recurrence is high (>50% at 3 years).

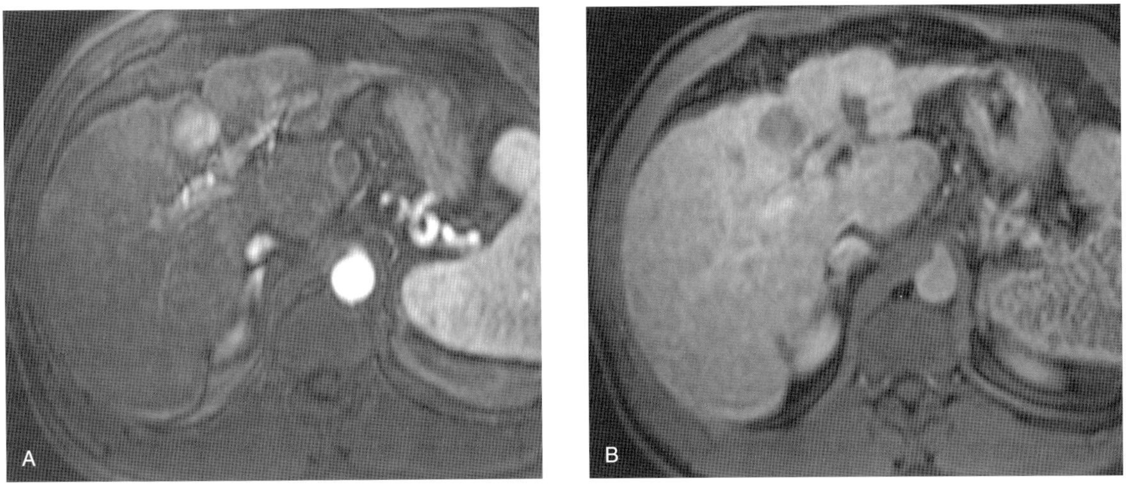

Figure 11.2 This patient was enlisted for liver transplantation for HCC. Diagnosis was carried out by non-invasive criteria. Dynamic magnetic resonance (MR) shows a nodule measuring 2.5 cm in segment IV. (**A**) This shows contrast uptake during the arterial phase indicated as hyperenhancement. (**B**) This shows the washout on delayed phase. (Courtesy of Dr J. R. Ayuso)

The most frequent cause of HCC is cell dissemination prior to treatment (metastatic nests) and the major predictors of recurrence are the presence of vascular invasion and/or satellite lesions.[5] The second mechanism is related to the oncogenic capacity of the underling liver, which can lead to metachronous tumor. Several options acting against these potential mechanisms have been proposed, including retinoid administration, selective localized radiotherapy and adoptive immunotherapy. The role of interferon to prevent recurrence has been evaluated in three meta-analyses,[6–8] and all suggest a benefit from its use. The limited quality of available trials, however, keep use of interferon controversial and, currently, there is no option that is established for conventional clinical practice. The positive data obtained on the use of sorafenib in patients with advanced HCC[9] have raised the potential of molecular-targeted therapies in this setting and several adjuvant trials are currently ongoing.

Patients treated by resection who develop recurrence could be considered for salvage transplantation, however this option has low applicability as most patients will present with multifocal disease exceeding enlistment criteria.[10] For this reason, the current authors offer transplantation to those patients who have received a resection and in whom pathology evidences a high risk of recurrence (with microvascular invasion or satellite lesions).[11] This is the sole prospective investigation assessing this strategy and validation is eagerly awaited.

Finally, tumor ablation is the best treatment option for patients with early-stage HCC who are not suitable for resection or transplantation. The two most widely used techniques are radiofrequency and ethanol injection. Radiofrequency has a more predictable necrotic capacity and requires fewer treatment sessions. While in tumors <2 cm both techniques are equally effective, radiofrequency has more efficacy in larger tumors. Other techniques such as laser, microwave, high-intensity ultrasound, cryotherapy or acetic acid injection are less common or less validated in terms of efficacy and safety.

Unfortunately, the majority of patients are diagnosed at intermediate or advanced stage and are only considered for palliative approaches.[2] The only two palliative treatments that have been proven to increase survival are chemoembolization[9,12] for intermediate stage (BCLC B) and sorafenib for advanced HCC (BCLC C). As mentioned earlier, this chapter discusses the issues regarding the selection, enlistment, and follow up of patients considered for liver transplantation (LT).

Selection of HCC patients for liver transplantation

Selection is the key to proper use of the limited number of livers that are available. Selection has to take into account age, co-morbidities, tumor burden and liver function. Diagnosis of HCC has to be unequivocal and staging has to be accurate to avoid understaging as much as possible. Non-invasive diagnosis based on imaging findings has a limited sensitivity (60%) in patients with early HCC.[2] Since cholangiocarcinoma may also appear in the setting of cirrhosis and be recognised as a hypervascular mass,[13] the need to obtain a positive diagnosis by biopsy should be taken into account. This is frequently challenged because of the potential risk of seeding due to tumor puncture. A critical review of the data confirms that the risk exists, but is less than 2%.[14] Ultimately, the risk of seeding should be balanced against the risk of misdiagnosis and wrong transplant indication with misuse of scarce resources. Clearly, as in all medical interventions, the decision-making process should be based on optimal technology and state-of-the-art expertise. This is what primed the recent consensus document by the National Conference on Liver Allocation in patients with HCC in the USA,[15] where a series of recommendations were exposed to perform and register the imaging findings.

There is now wide agreement in accepting the Milano criteria (single tumor ≤5 cm or up to the nodules ≤3 cm[16]) as the best selection criteria to enlist patients for LT if aiming to obtain long-term results similar to those of patients without malignancy. Experience from several other groups confirmed their validity and it is established that patients fitting into these definitions will achieve survival figures exceeding 70% at 5 years, while the recurrence rate will be less than 25%.[2]

Adherence to Milan criteria provides the best results in terms of survival, but several programs do not exclude patients from the list when follow-up staging while waiting exceeds entry criteria. If the tumor extent is not massive and there is no vascular invasion and/or extrahepatic spread, the results are progressively impaired and the outcome decreases to around 50% survival at 5 years, but with a higher recurrence rate. These figures could endorse the potential for an expansion[17–32] but the critical issue is how to define the new limits.[33] Table 11.1 shows the results from series reporting outcomes for applying expanded criteria to select HCC patients for liver transplantation.

Indeed the scarcity of livers has limited the application of less stringent criteria and currently there is no widely accepted definition for expansion of the tumor burden. In fact, in most proposals to expand the limits the findings are based on an analysis of explanted livers, and the information prior to surgery is not available. This is best exemplified by the recent "Metroticket" study,[17] which evaluated 1112 patients with HCC exceeding Milan criteria and 444 patients within Milan criteria at post-transplant pathology. It again evidenced that microvascular invasion is the major predictor of recurrence and survival as in its absence the tumor burden limits could be expanded to the "up-to-seven criteria" (HCC with seven as the sum of the largest tumor and the number of tumor). The 5-year survival rate could still be in the region of 72.2% if vascular invasion would be absent, but since this parameter is not available prior to treatment indication, no change in selection criteria could be established. Tumor differentiation has been proposed to be a predictor for microscopic vascular invasion,[22,34] but its assessment would require biopsy. Since large tumors are known to be heterogeneous, the accuracy of this strategy for use in clinical decision making would be suboptimal.

A second flaw of the encouraging suggestions of some studies is related to the fact that the small number of patients with expanded criteria are analysed together with the larger number of patients within Milan criteria (Box 11.1). This joint assessment dilutes the potentially poor outcome cohort within the cohort with good prognosis. This is evidenced in the analysis by Pelleter et al.[35] of the Organ Procurement Transplant Network Data in 2009, where only 11% of the patients exceeded the Milan criteria. Finally, the critical decision is not to what extent the enlistment criteria can be expanded, but by how much can the post-transplant life expectancy of the whole transplant cohort be lowered and still be acceptable, and what effect expanding the donor pool will have on mortality for non-HCC patients. These are ethical issues that have not been definitively resolved, thus, expanding the listing criteria is a very controversial issue, particularly when considering the shortage of donors. Because of all these considerations, the National Conference on Liver Allocation

Table 11.1 Results from series reporting outcomes for applying expanded criteria to select HCC patients for liver transplantation

Author, year	Selection criteria/method	Patients		5-year survival	
		All	Beyond Milan	All	Beyond Milan
Yao et al, 2001[19]	One tumor ≤6.5 cm or 3 tumors ≤4.5 cm Post-LT, pathology	70	N/A	75%	N/A
Roayaie et al, 2002[20]	Any HCC No extrahepatic spread No main portal invasion Pre-LT, radiology	80	80	25%	ITT: 25%* All LT 44%
Marsh and Dvorchik, 2003[21]	Any HCC Post-LT, pathology	393	145	N/A	67%
Molmenti and Klintmalm, 2002[23]	HCC >5 cm Post LT, pathology	790	181	50%	35%
Cillo et al, 2004[22]	Any Wel21mod differentiated HCC Pre-LT	33	13	75%	N/A
Decaens et al, 2006[24]	Any HCC No extrahepatic spread No main portal invasion Post-LT, radiology	479	199	60%	30%
Cillo et al, 2007[25]	No extrahepatic spread No main portal invasion No poor differentiate Pret-LT, radiology, pathology	100	40	ITT 73 %	ITT 79%
Duffy et al, 2007[26]	One tumor ≤6.5 cm or 3 tumors ≤4.5 cm Post-LT, pathology	467	294	52%	UCSF in: 64% UCSF out: 41%
Onaca et al, 2007[27]	One tumor ≤6 cm or 4 tumors ≤5 cm Post-LT, pathology	1206	575	55.1%	N/A
Ito et al, 2007[28]	≥10 nodules, ≤5 cm ≤11 nodules, >5 cm Pre-LT, radiology	125	55	68.3% MC: 78.3%	64
Lee et al, 2008[29]	Largest tumor ≤6 cm Less than 5 nodules Pre-LT, radiology	221	81	68%	44.5%
Toso et al, 2008[30]	Total tumor volume <115 cm^3 Post-LT, pathology	52 Alberta 154 Toronto 82 Colorado	30 69 32	75% 72% 80%	69% 68% 59%
Herrero et al, 2008[18]	One tumor ≤6 cm or 3 tumors ≤5 cm Pre-LT, radiology	85	26	70%	66%

(Continued)

Table 11.1 *Continued*

Author, year	Selection criteria/method	Patients		5-year survival	
		All	Beyond Milan	All	Beyond Milan
Silva et al, 2008[31]	Criteria not defined Pre-LT	257	26	63% ITT: 57%* MC: 68% MC ITT:62%*	69% ITT:66%*
Toso et al, 2009[32]	Total tumor volume <115 cm^3 and AFP ≤400 ng/ml Pre- LT	6437	169	MC: 71%	65%**
Mazzaferro et al, 2009[17]	Number of nodules ≤7 and Maximum diameter ≤7 Post-LT, pathology	1556	1112	MC: 73.3%	53.6

Includes only trials that indicated a 5 year survival rate.
*5-year survival according to intention to treat (ITT). AFP (alphafetoprotein), LT: liver transplantation, MC: Milan criteria, N/A: Not available
**3 year survival

Box 11.1 Barcelona expanded criteria for LDLT in HCC patients

Single HCC ≤7 cm

Multinodular HCC: 3 nodules ≤5 cm, 5 nodules ≤3 cm

Downstaging: parial response to any treatment lasting more than 6 months achieves the conventional criteria of cadaveric liver transplantation

Note: staging is based on imaging techniques

for patients with HCC suggested no change in the current policy regarding HCC criteria.[15]

The lack of sufficient liver donation is the major limitation for liver transplantation. There is always a waiting period between listing and transplantation; this varies among programs but if left long enough, the tumor will grow and develop major contraindications (vascular invasion, extrahepatic spread). The rate of exclusion on the waiting list may be as high as 25% if the time on the waiting list is longer than 12 months.[36,37] Obviously, if patients with more advanced tumors are included as a result of expanded listing criteria, the dropout rate will be higher and this will translate into poor survival figures on an intention-to-treat analysis.

Studies from Barcelona and San Francisco have shown that if the dropout rate due to advancing disease is 25% at 1 year, this will translate into a 60% survival rate for transplantation based on an intention-to-treat analysis of patients listed for transplant (rather than those who actually undergo transplantation).[36,38] Data from Mount Sinai describe a 50% dropout rate with an even worse survival if the criteria for transplant are expanded.[20] Furthermore, one of the most important issues is the lack of clearly defined criteria for removing patients from the waiting list because of excessive tumor growth while waiting.

If only major events (macroscopic vascular invasion and extrahepatic spread) are used to de-list patients, this will mean that some patients whose disease is too advanced to treat will undergo transplantation. This will ultimately impair the survival figures for transplantation for HCC and put the whole program at risk. The listing of patients using expanded criteria will further worsen this scenario and thus, prior to any change in listing policy, it is essential to define the exclusion criteria. Otherwise, the system will be completely saturated, mimicking a pharmacokinetic reaction with limited clearance capacity.[39]

Some groups have proposed to transplant patients who are initially beyond the Milan criteria, but are then successfully treated as tumor burden is reduced to fit into the enlistment limits. This policy is known as "downstaging" and despite enocouraging reports, it has not become a standard practice and the current recommendation is to develop prospective investigations with clear-cut inclusion and exclusion criteria. Until results from such investigations are available, it is not feasible to raise any robust recommendation.[15]

Waiting list management

As one of the major unsolved issues in LT is the shortage of donors, in order to make the best use of the few organs available it is fully justified to apply restrictive criteria to select the optimal candidates who will achieve the best possible long-term outcome. Nevertheless, even in countries with a high donation rate such as Spain, there is a continuously growing number of transplant candidates and this creates an expanding waiting time. During this period, the liver disease may progress and impede transplantation. There are no homogeneously accepted criteria to prompt exclusion. In most groups, exclusion is based on uncontrolled tumor progression leading to vascular invasion and/or extrahepatic spread. In contrast, in the USA the priority given to patients with HCC is cancelled when the patients exceed the restrictive limits accepted for enlisting.[15] There are several strategies to prevent exclusion while waiting. Health campaigns may increase the number of donations, and active policies within transplant teams may wisely use the so-called marginal livers (advanced age, statatosis) and those with metabolic disorders (amyloidosis, primary hyperoxaluria or with viral infection without significant liver injury). In addition, highly skilled surgeons may develop the split-liver technique.

The major impact is expected to come from live donation as commented on later in this chapter. A simultaneous strategy to impede progression is the application of adjuvant treatment with any of the available options known to be effective: resection, percutaneous ablation, and transarterial chemoembolization.

Treatment upon enlisting

There are no randomized, controlled trials (RCTs) comparing interventions with the best supportive care and thus, any suggestion of a therapeutic benefit is derived from cohort studies.[40] Unfortunately, most of these investigations merely describe the outcome of those patients who have been finally transplanted and do not offer information about those lost while waiting. The options that are most frequently applied are percutaneous ablation and intra-arterial locoregional treatment. Surgical resection might also be used as a bridge in those patients with moderate surgical risk. Clearly the decision to treat while waiting has to balance the risk of exclusion with the risk of side effects related to treatment, therefore the usual strategy is to avoid therapy if the expected waiting time is less than 6 months. Systemic chemotherapy has no efficacy and is hampered by severe side effects[1] and so should not be recommended.

Intra-arterial locoregional treatments include transcatheter arterial chemoembolization (TACE) and radioembolization. TACE using gelfoam and chemotherapy emulsified in lipiodol has been shown to delay progression and improve survival in patients with intermediate HCC.[41] Such data are not available for Ytrium-90 (Y-90).[42] The development of polyvinyl chloride spheres that release chemotherapy after being injected have improved the tolerance to TACE as they prompt a reduction of the side effects of the passage of chemotherapy into the systemic circulation.[43] In addition, since the spheres are calibrated, the arterial obstruction is predictable and the procedure is homogenised, while the antitumoral efficacy and safety are maintained, if not improved.

Chemoembolization results in extensive tumor necrosis that is associated with a reduced tumor growth rate. The portal vein should be patent and the liver function should be preserved. Child–Pugh C patients should not receive chemoembolization because of risk of death and Child–Pugh B patients may develop severe decompensation that ultimately may contraindicate transplantation.

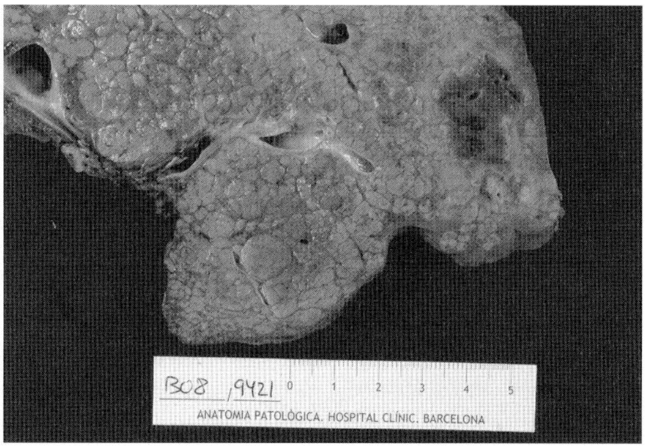

Figure 11.3 Percutaneous ablation of a small hepatocellular carcinoma (HCC) located in the right lobe of a cirrhotic liver. The patient was enlisted for liver transplantation and due to the long expected waiting time (more than 1 year) it was recommended to treat the HCC by radiofrequency. (Courtesy of Dr Sole)

Percutaneous ablation has been introduced more recently but it has rapidly shown its advantages and risks. The most common techniques to ablate tumors are ethanol injection and radiofrequency (RFA), with recent meta-analysis suggesting a higher efficacy by RFA[44] (Figure 11.3). Side effects are more frequent and severe with radiofrequency, but its efficacy is higher and more predictable.[45] For any ablation technique the major limitations for efficacy are tumor size and even for RF, the long-term local disease control is significantly impaired when tumor size exceeds 3 cm. Thereby, while complete tumor necrosis exceeds 95% in nodules measuring <2 cm, the success rate decreases to around 80% in HCC between 2 and 3 cm and to 50% long term in larger tumors. Long-term studies indicate that Child–Pugh A patients with successful tumor necrosis may achieve a 50% survival at 5 years; this compares well with the outcome of resection in those candidates who do not fit the optimal surgical profile.[2,4]

Analysis of explanted livers of patients who have received treatment upon enlistment indicate that the rate of complete responses is not as high as reported by radiologic examinations based on dynamic CT or MRI.[46] Treatment while waiting, however, does not aim to achieve complete eradication with long-term cure, but rather tumor mass shrinkage with avoidance of progression. It is clear that this might be achieved at least for a given period of time, but it is certain that the efficacy in preventing progression and exclusion will be reduced along with waiting time. Treatment, therefore, might be effective when the waiting time is kept below 12 months, while in waiting times beyond 24 months, almost any treatment will ultimately fail and not prevent the exclusion of the majority of the patients.

Priority policies

A second approach to diminish the risk of exclusion while waiting relies on the establishment of priority systems. This is a very controversial issue in patients with HCC as compared to patients with end-stage liver disease, in whom the Model for End-stage Liver Disease (MELD) system allows an accurate prediction of the risk of short time to death.[47] Such a predictive system is not available for HCC. There is very limited information from which to identify the parameters that may predict a higher likelihood of progression and thus of exclusion. Smaller tumors are less likely to present progressive growth, leading to exclusion and tumors that present progression while the patient is on the waiting list and exhibit an increased alphafetoprotein (AFP) concentration are higher risk tumors.

A legal mandate forced transplant centers in the USA to develop a priority policy in order to transplant the sickest patients and avoid time on the waiting list as the major determinant of transplantation. The MELD score[47] was used to establish priority in patients with end-stage disease, but initially it did not allocate points due to HCC development and thus was useless for HCC patients. To correct this unfair situation, HCC patients were given a fixed number of MELD points according to tumor size and number. The points given initially were excessive as HCC patients had a <90% probability of being transplanted in the first 3 months after enlisting, while the contrary was the case for patients without HCC. The reduction of points partially corrected that lack of equity and in the last modification that was implemented later on. Ultimately, it was decided that patients with solitary tumors <2 cm (Stage 1) would not get priority because of the low risk of exclusion. Only patients with Stage 2 tumors (solitary between 2 and 5 cm, or with up to three nodules measuring <3 cm each) would receive priority points. This new proposal was also expected to reduce the number of patients transplanted because of an HCC that ultimately is not confirmed in the explanted liver. In 2010 the policy was again modified.[15] Patients with HCC within MELD criteria and with MELD scores <15 are enlisted with 15 MELD points and patients with >15 MELD points because of liver failure receive their calculated MELD during the first 3 months. A MELD/HCC priority score is recalculated every 3 months and can increase or decrease according to change in tumor characteristics, however only candidates with at least Stage T2 tumors will receive additional HCC points. Candidates with T1 tumors or tumors outside MELD criteria are designated as having HCC at registration but do not get priority points. No additional points or priority is given because of increased AFP. The continuous analysis of the priority policy results will surely prompt new modifications aiming to obtain optimal results in HCC patients and also ensure that the access to transplant and long-term outcome is homogeneous in all categories of enlisted patients. In this regard, one of the concerns of priority policies upgrading patients with more advanced disease is the potential selection of patients with less favorable profiles and thus with lower probability of long-term survival.

Clearly, there is an urgent need to identify the strongest predictors of progression while waiting and it is expected that these will not come from rough assessment of size and number. Better knowledge of the genetic changes and molecular pathways that regulate tumor growth and dissemination[48] should provide the most accurate tools to predict biology and hence allow establishment of a more sensitive selection and priority policy.

Living-donor liver transplantation

Living-donor liver transplantation (LDLT) is considered an alternative to cadaver liver transplantation (CLT). In addition to the absence of a relevant waiting time between enlistment and transplantation, it offers the use of an optimal liver with less time between extraction and grafting. In adults, the most common approach is to use the right lobe of the donor. This will have undergone an extensive evaluation to diminish the risk related to major abdominal surgery as much as possible. Extensive informed consent from the donor and the recipient is of crucial importance because this is a complex intervention that should only be undertaken by expert surgeons to ensure the lowest morbidity and best outcome, not only to the recipient, but also to the donor. Complications may develop in 20–40% of the donors and the mortality risk for the donor is still 0.3–0.5%. Statistical modeling indicates that LDLT for early HCC offers substantial gains in life expectancy with acceptable cost-effectiveness ratios as compared with conventional CLT when waiting times for transplantation exceed at least 7 months and the outcome after transplant exceeds 70% at 5 years.

The outcome after LDLT in patients with HCC does not differ from that of patients receiving a cadaveric liver. All data validate the use of the Milan criteria, thereby if patients fit into the Milan criteria the survival rate at 3 years is around 80%, while if these are exceeded the long-term outcome is reduced as well known in cadaveric transplantation.[28,49–52] Years ago, there was major controversy about a higher severity of HCV graft infection after live donation. This was likely due to the confounding effect of biliary complications and when the learning curve for the surgical procedure is over, the outcome appears to be similar between cadaver and live donation.[53]

One of the major controversies raised by live donation is to which extent its indication should be restricted to the criteria used for cadaver livers or, if on the contrary, the criteria could be expanded. This would allow patients with cancer stage beyond the Milan criteria to benefit from transplantation and thus achieve long-term survival that otherwise would be unlikely. Following this reasoning, some groups have established a very liberal policy and proceed to live donation if there is no extrahepatic dissemination or invasion of a major blood vessel. Others have proposed a moderate expansion in terms of size and number of tumors, in part paralleling the proposals for expansion commented on before for cadaveric donation. Probably, the 50% survival at 5 years frequently proposed as the bottom figure in cadaveric donation should be implemented also in live donation. In keeping with this aim, in Barcelona the current authors have launched a pilot program of live donation with expanded definitions that are reflected in Box 11.1. The program runs under strict ethical controls and its application is expected to achieve a 5-year survival rate of 50%. Less than 10% of HCC patients fit into this indication and the final applicability only involves one-quarter of the potential candidates. In any case, staging of candidates for live donation should be as detailed as for cadaveric, in order to avoid the indication in too advanced patients in whom staging has been less strict. This is the basis for some suggestions of higher HCC recurrence after live donation, which has been later shown to be related to a more advanced stage at explant analysis.

Conclusion

In summary, LT is an effective therapy for patients diagnosed with HCC at an early stage. Its application is curtailed by the shortage of donors, which prompts a growing waiting time during which the tumor may progress. Adjuvant treatment upon enlistment may prevent this adverse event, but the best approach would be to increase the number of available livers either through increased cadaver donation or through live donation.

References

1. Bruix J, Sherman M. Management of hepatocellular carcinoma. Hepatology 2005;42:1208–36.
2. Forner A, LLovet JM, Bruix J. Hepatocellular Carcinoma. Lancet. 2011 In press.
3. Bruix J, Castells A, Bosch J, et al. Surgical resection of hepatocellular carcinoma in cirrhotic patients: prognostic value of preoperative portal pressure. Gastroenterology 1996;111:1018–22.
4. Ishizawa T, Hasegawa K, Aoki T, et al. Neither multiple tumors nor portal hypertension are surgical contraindications for hepatocellular carcinoma. Gastroenterology 2008;134:1908–16.
5. Imamura H, Matsuyama Y, Tanaka E, et al. Risk factors contributing to early and late phase intrahepatic recurrence of hepatocellular carcinoma after hepatectomy. J Hepatol 2003;38:200–7.
6. Miyake Y, Kobashi H, Yamamoto K. Meta-analysis: the effect of interferon on development of hepatocellular carcinoma in patients with chronic hepatitis B virus infection. J Gastroenterol 2009;44:470–5.
7. Breitenstein S, Dimitroulis D, Petrowsky H, Puhan MA, Mullhaupt B, Clavien PA. Systematic review and meta-analysis of interferon after curative treatment of hepatocellular carcinoma in patients with viral hepatitis. Br J Surg 2009;96:975–81.
8. Shen YC, Hsu C, Chen LT, Cheng CC, Hu FC, Cheng AL. Adjuvant interferon therapy after curative therapy for hepatocellular carcinoma (HCC): a meta-regression approach. J Hepatol 2010;52:889–94.
9. Llovet JM, Ricci S, Mazzaferro V, et al. Sorafenib in advanced hepatocellular carcinoma. N Engl J Med 2008;359:378–90.
10. Minagawa M, Makuuchi M, Takayama T, Kokudo N. Selection criteria for repeat hepatectomy in patients with recurrent hepatocellular carcinoma. Ann Surg 2003;238:703–10.
11. Sala M, Fuster J, Llovet JM, et al. High pathological risk of recurrence after surgical resection for hepatocellular carcinoma: an indication for salvage liver transplantation. Liver Transpl 2004;10:1294–1300.
12. Llovet JM, Real MI, Montana X, et al. Arterial embolisation or chemoembolisation versus symptomatic treatment in patients with unresectable hepatocellular carcinoma: a randomised controlled trial. Lancet 2002;359:1734–9.
13. Vilana R, Forner A, Bianchi L, et al. Intrahepatic peripheral cholangiocarcinoma in cirrhosis patients may display a vascular pattern similar to hepatocellular carcinoma on contrast-enhanced ultrasound. Hepatology 2010;51:2020–9.
14. Silva MA, Hegab B, Hyde C, Guo B, Buckels JA, Mirza DF. Needle track seeding following biopsy of liver lesions in the diagnosis of hepatocellular cancer: a systematic review and meta-analysis. Gut 2008;57:1592–6.
15. Pomfret E, Washburn K, Wald C, et al. Report of a national conference on liver allocation in patients with hepatocellular carcinoma in the United States. Liver Transpl 2010;16:262–78.
16. Mazzaferro V, Regalia E, Doci R, Andreola S, Pulvirenti A, Bozzetti F, Montalto F, et al. Liver transplantation for the treatment of small hepatocellular carcinomas in patients with cirrhosis. N Engl J Med 1996;334:693–9.
17. Mazzaferro V, Llovet JM, Miceli R, et al. Predicting survival after liver transplantation in patients with hepatocellular carcinoma beyond the Milan criteria: a retrospective, exploratory analysis. Lancet Oncol 2009;10:35–43.
18. Herrero JI, Sangro B, Pardo F, et al. Liver transplantation in patients with hepatocellular carcinoma across Milan criteria. Liver Transpl 2008;14:272–8.
19. Yao FY, Ferrell L, Bass NM, et al. Liver transplantation for hepatocellular carcinoma: expansion of the tumor size limits does not adversely impact survival. Hepatology 2001;33:1394–1403.

20. Roayaie S, Frischer JS, Emre SH, et al. Long-term results with multimodal adjuvant therapy and liver transplantation for the treatment of hepatocellular carcinomas larger than 5 centimeters. Ann Surg 2002;235:533–9.
21. Marsh JW, Dvorchik I. Liver organ allocation for hepatocellular carcinoma: are we sure? Liver Transpl 2003;9:693–6.
22. Cillo U, Vitale A, Bassanello M, et al. Liver transplantation for the treatment of moderately or well-differentiated hepatocellular carcinoma. Ann Surg 2004;239:150–9.
23. Molmenti EP, Klintmalm GB. Liver transplantation in association with hepatocellular carcinoma: an update of the International Tumor Registry. Liver Transpl 2002;8:736–48.
24. Decaens T, Roudot-Thoraval F, Hadni-Bresson S, et al. Impact of UCSF criteria according to pre- and post-OLT tumor features: analysis of 479 patients listed for HCC with a short waiting time. Liver Transpl 2006; 12:1761–9.
25. Cillo U, Vitale A, Grigoletto F, et al. Intention-to-treat analysis of liver transplantation in selected, aggressively treated HCC patients exceeding the Milan criteria. Am J Transplant 2007;7:972–81.
26. Duffy JP, Vardanian A, Benjamin E, et al. Liver transplantation criteria for hepatocellular carcinoma should be expanded: a 22-year experience with 467 patients at UCLA. Ann Surg 2007;246:502–9; discussion 509–11.
27. Onaca N, Davis GL, Goldstein RM, Jennings LW, Klintmalm GB. Expanded criteria for liver transplantation in patients with hepatocellular carcinoma: a report from the International Registry of Hepatic Tumors in Liver Transplantation. Liver Transpl 2007;13:391–9.
28. Ito T, Takada Y, Ueda M, et al. Expansion of selection criteria for patients with hepatocellular carcinoma in living donor liver transplantation. Liver Transpl 2007; 13:1637–44.
29. Lee SG, Hwang S, Moon DB, et al. Expanded indication criteria of living donor liver transplantation for hepatocellular carcinoma at one large-volume center. Liver Transpl 2008;14:935–45.
30. Toso C, Trotter J, Wei A, et al. Total tumor volume predicts risk of recurrence following liver transplantation in patients with hepatocellular carcinoma. Liver Transpl 2008;14:1107–15.
31. Silva M, Moya A, Berenguer M, et al. Expanded criteria for liver transplantation in patients with cirrhosis and hepatocellular carcinoma. Liver Transpl 2008;14: 1449–60.
32. Toso C, Asthana S, Bigam DL, Shapiro AM, Kneteman NM. Reassessing selection criteria prior to liver transplantation for hepatocellular carcinoma utilizing the Scientific Registry of Transplant Recipients database. Hepatology 2009;49:832–8.
33. Bruix J, Fuster J, Llovet JM. Liver transplantation for hepatocellular carcinoma: Foucault pendulum versus evidence-based decision. Liver Transpl 2003;9: 700–2.
34. Wayne JD, Lauwers GY, Ikai I, et al. Preoperative predictors of survival after resection of small hepatocellular carcinomas. Ann Surg 2002;235:722–30; discussion 730–1.
35. Pelletier SJ, Fu S, Thyagarajan V, et al. An intention-to-treat analysis of liver transplantation for hepatocellular carcinoma using organ procurement transplant network data. Liver Transpl 2009;15:859–68.
36. Yao FY, Bass NM, Nikolai B, et al. Liver transplantation for hepatocellular carcinoma: analysis of survival according to the intention-to-treat principle and dropout from the waiting list. Liver Transpl 2002;8:873–83.
37. Freeman RB, Mithoefer A, Ruthazer R, et al. Optimizing staging for hepatocellular carcinoma before liver transplantation: A retrospective analysis of the UNOS/OPTN database. Liver Transpl 2006;12:1504–11.
38. Llovet JM, Fuster J, Bruix J. Intention-to-treat analysis of surgical treatment for early hepatocellular carcinoma: resection versus transplantation. Hepatology 1999;30:1434–40.
39. Navasa M, Bruix J. Multifaceted perspective of the waiting list for liver transplantation: the value of pharmacokinetic models. Hepatology;51:12–15.
40. Schwartz M, Roayaie S, Uva P. Treatment of HCC in patients awaiting liver transplantation. Am J Transplant 2007;7:1875–81.
41. Bruix J, Sala M, Llovet JM. Chemoembolization for hepatocellular carcinoma. Gastroenterology 2004;127: S179–88.
42. Kulik LM, Carr BI, Mulcahy MF, et al. Safety and efficacy of 90Y radiotherapy for hepatocellular carcinoma with and without portal vein thrombosis. Hepatology 2008;47:71–81.
43. Varela M, Real MI, Burrel M, et al. Chemoembolization of hepatocellular carcinoma with drug eluting beads: efficacy and doxorubicin pharmacokinetics. J Hepatol 2007;46:474–81.
44. Cho YK, Kim JK, Kim MY, Rhim H, Han JK. Systematic review of randomized trials for hepatocellular carcinoma treated with percutaneous ablation therapies. Hepatology 2009;49:453–9.
45. Shiina S, Teratani T, Obi S, et al. A randomized controlled trial of radiofrequency ablation with ethanol injection for small hepatocellular carcinoma. Gastroenterology 2005;129:122–30.
46. Lu DS, Yu NC, Raman SS, et al. Radiofrequency ablation of hepatocellular carcinoma: treatment success as defined by histologic examination of the explanted liver. Radiology 2005;234:954–60.

47. Kamath PS, Wiesner RH, Malinchoc M, et al. A model to predict survival in patients with end-stage liver disease. Hepatology 2001;33:464–70.
48. Hoshida Y, Nijman SM, Kobayashi M, et al. Integrative transcriptome analysis reveals common molecular subclasses of human hepatocellular carcinoma. Cancer Res 2009;69:7385–92.
49. Gondolesi GE, Roayaie S, Munoz L, et al. Adult living donor liver transplantation for patients with hepatocellular carcinoma: extending UNOS priority criteria. Ann Surg 2004;239:142–9.
50. Todo S, Furukawa H. Living donor liver transplantation for adult patients with hepatocellular carcinoma: experience in Japan. Ann Surg 2004;240:451–9; discussion 459–61.
51. Jonas S, Mittler J, Pascher A, et al. Living donor liver transplantation of the right lobe for hepatocellular carcinoma in cirrhosis in a European center. Liver Transpl 2007;13:896–903.
52. Sugawara Y, Tamura S, Makuuchi M. Living donor liver transplantation for hepatocellular carcinoma: Tokyo University series. Dig Dis 2007;25:310–12.
53. Terrault NA, Shiffman ML, Lok AS, et al. Outcomes in hepatitis C virus-infected recipients of living donor vs. deceased donor liver transplantation. Liver Transpl 2007;13:122–9.

12 Cholangiocarcinoma

Howard C. Masuoka,[1] *Gregory J. Gores*[1] *and Charles B. Rosen*[2]
[1]Division of Gastroenterology and Hepatology, and [2]Division of Transplantation Surgery and Mayo Clinic William J. von Liebig Transplant Center, Mayo Clinic College of Medicine, Rochester, MN USA

Key learning points

- Cholangiocarcinoma (CCA) is a rare cancer that arises from the malignant transformation of biliary epithelial cells.
- Liver transplantation with neoadjuvant chemoradiotherapy has emerged as effective treatment for highly selected patients with early-stage unresectable hilar CCA and hilar CCA arising in PSC.
- Liver transplantation alone (without neoadjuvant therapy) is not an effective treatment for patients with CCA.
- Surgical resection and liver transplantation are the only potentially curative treatments.
- Percutaneous and endoscopic ultrasound-guided biopsy of the tumor should be avoided in liver transplant candidates.
- Antibiotics and adequate biliary drainage through endoscopic placement of plastic biliary stents are the mainstays of treatment of acute cholangitis in these patients.

Introduction

CCA is a primary neoplasm of the biliary system that arises from malignant transformation of cholangiocytes, the epithelial cells that line the biliary tree. CCA is the second most common primary hepatic cancer, and its incidence is increasing globally.[1] Nonetheless, CCA is a rare malignancy with an incidence of approximately 8 per million in the USA with 3500–5000 new CCA cases diagnosed annually.[2] The incidence varies across the world with the highest reported rate in northeast Thailand (96/100 000 in men and 38/100 000 in women) likely due to the high prevalence of infection by the liver flukes *Opisthorchis viverrini* and *Clonorchis sinensis*.

While most cases of CCA arise in the absence of an identifiable cause, chronic biliary inflammation and cholestasis are risk factors for CCA. Primary sclerosing cholangitis (PSC) carries a particularly high risk for the development of CCA with an incidence of 1.5% per year and a prevalence between 5% and 15%.[3] Interestingly, the risk of developing CCA is not associated with the duration or severity of PSC or inflammatory bowel disease.[4] Cystic diseases of the biliary tree, such as choledochal cysts and Caroli's disease also predispose to CCA. In Southeast Asia, a risk factor for CCA is infection with the liver flukes *Opisthorchis viverrini* and *Clonorchis sinensis*. The lifecycle of these organisms includes human consumption of raw fish bearing these organisms, which migrate into the biliary tree and produce eggs. Chronic inflammation from these eggs is thought to predispose to CCA. Another risk factor for CCA is exposure to the radiocontrast agent Thorotrast (a radioactive suspension of thorium dioxide particles) that was used from the 1930s through the 1960s. The risk for CCA and other hepatobiliary cancers is approximately 200 times that of non-exposed patients and the latency period for these cancers averages 35 years.

Medical Care of the Liver Transplant Patient, Fourth Edition. Edited by Pierre-Alain Clavien, James F. Trotter.

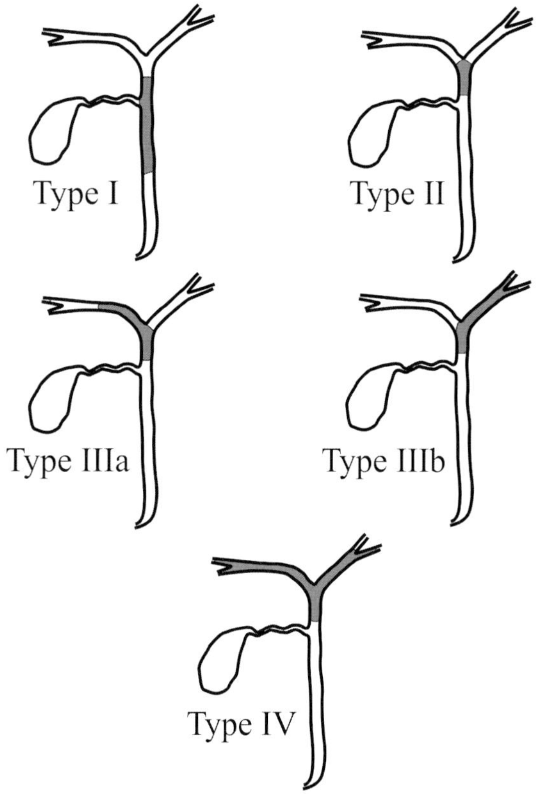

Figure 12.1 The Bismuth–Corlette Classification of Hilar Cholangiocarcinoma. (**Type I**) Involvement of the common hepatic duct. (**Type II**) Involvement of the bifurcation without involvement of the secondary intrahepatic ducts. (**Type IIIa**) Extends into the right hepatic duct. (**Type IIIb**) Extends into the left hepatic duct. (**Type IV**) Involvement of both right and left hepatic ducts

Pathologic classification

CCA is classified as either intrahepatic or extrahepatic based on its location in the biliary system. Extrahepatic CCA accounts for approximately two-thirds of all CCAs. Hilar CCAs, also known as Klatskin tumors, are the most common type of CCA and comprise roughly 60% of extrahepatic CCA. Hilar CCA is further classified based on the Bismuth–Corlette system (Figure 12.1), which classifies the tumor based on involvement of the biliary confluence and the right and left hepatic ducts.[5] Extrahepatic CCA usually has a sclerosing phenotype resulting in annular thickening of the bile ducts due to infiltration and fibrosis of the periductal tissues. Less commonly, extrahepatic CCA has a nodular or papillary phenotype. Intrahepatic CCA presents as a mass-forming hepatic neoplasm and is often confused with metastatic adenocarcinoma of unknown primary. More than 90% of CCAs are adenocarcinomas.[6] Microscopically CCA is usually a well- to moderately differentiated tubular adenocarcinoma within a prominent, dense, desmoplastic stroma. This fibrous stroma greatly increases the challenge of confirming CCA by fine-needle aspiration (FNA) or biopsy. Other histologic variants include papillary adenocarcinoma, signet-ring carcinoma, squamous cell or mucoepidermoid carcinoma, and lymphoepithelioma-like forms.

Clinical presentation and diagnosis

The clinical presentation of CCA depends on the tumor location. Extrahepatic CCA typically presents with obstructive symptoms such as jaundice, dark urine, pale stools, pruritus, malaise, abdominal pain, and weight loss. It is uncommon for patients to have cholangitis due to the insidious nature of the obstruction unless they have had previous episodes of cholangitis due to underlying PSC or have undergone instrumentation of the biliary tree. Laboratory tests frequently demonstrate a cholestatic picture with increased total and direct bilirubin, alkaline phosphatase and gamma-glutamyltransferase. Intrahepatic CCA most commonly presents with mild abdominal pain, weight loss, and gastrointestinal disturbances.

Ultrasonography is usually the best initial test for patients presenting with obstructive jaundice. Typically, ultrasonography will show dilation of the intrahepatic bile ducts. Ultrasonography can also determine the presence of intrahepatic metastases, occlusion of the hepatic arteries and the portal vein, or enlargement of lymph nodes, which are concerning for metastatic disease. The next test is usually computerized tomography (CT) of the chest, abdomen and pelvis. CT provides more detail needed for surgical consultation. Local invasion, relationship of the tumor to the hilar vessels, atrophy of the liver, regional and distant lymph node metastases, and distant metastases can all be readily appreciated with CT.

Imaging of the biliary system is critical in defining the location and extent of tumor. Endoscopic retrograde cholangiopancreatography (ERCP) provides the best definition of biliary strictures and permits brush cytology and biopsies of the bile ducts. Dilation and stenting of strictures may be done to alleviate obstruction or treat cholangitis. If neither of these is present the placement of a prophylactic stent is not recommended. For patients who may be transplant or resection candidates the current authors recommend placement of plastic rather than metallic biliary stents. Drainage of ducts involving the dominant hepatic lobe is usually sufficient. Drainage of both ductal systems is usually not necessary. Percutaneous transhepatic cholangiography (PTC) can also be employed, but the current authors recommend this approach only if ERCP is unsuccessful since PTC may cause seeding of tumor along the percutaneous tract. Magnetic resonance imaging (MRI) with concurrent magnetic resonance cholangiopancreatography (MRCP) may be obtained instead or in addition to CT. The advantages of MRI are that: 1) it is less invasive than ERCP, 2) it defines the anatomy beyond strictures too narrow to pass via ERCP, and 3) it defines involvement of surrounding structures (Figure 12.2). Indeed, MRI is able to provide information on cross-sectional imaging (i.e. segmental bile duct dilatation, atrophy, and intrahepatic metastasis), vascular encasement and cholangiographic images. MRI, therefore, has become the imaging modality of choice for this neoplasm.

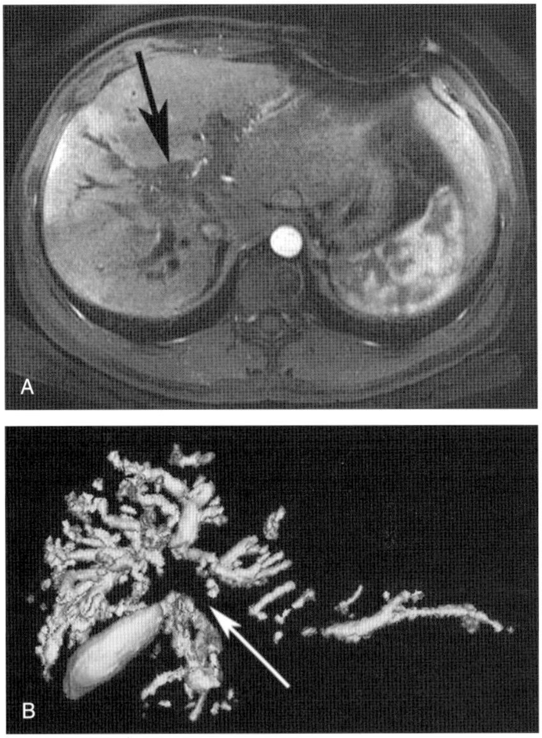

Figure 12.2 MRI appearance of cholangiocarcinoma. (**A**) A mass is visible at the junction of the right and left main hepatic ducts (black arrow). (**B**) An MRCP on the same patient demonstrating a stricture at the hilum seen as a filling defect (white arrow) with associated intrahepatic ductal dilatation

Imaging by CT or MRI can aid in the diagnosis of CCA and are a critical component in the evaluation of resectability. Studies, however, often fail to demonstrate a mass, especially in the setting of PSC. On abdominal CT, CCA occasionally appears as a hypodense lesion with delayed venous phase enhancement after IV contrast administration. On MRI, CCA appears hypointense on T_1-weighted images, hyperintense on T_2-weighted images, and enhances with MRI contrast. Visualization of CCA is improved with infusion of superparamagnetic iron (e.g. ferumoxides such as Feridex), which results in darkening of the surrounding hepatic parenchyma and with delayed gadolinium images. Unilobular bile duct obstruction often leads to atrophy of the affected hepatic lobe with hypertrophy of the unaffected lobe, a phenomenon known as the atrophy–hypertrophy complex. The presence of atrophy alone suggests vascular encasement of the affected lobe by CCA.

Endoscopic ultrasound (EUS)-guided aspiration of local, regional and distant lymph nodes is useful in determining the resectability of CCA or candidacy for neoadjuvant therapy and liver transplantation. In a small series of patients with CCA, EUS with nodal aspiration demonstrated nodal metastases in 17% that had not been previously visualized.[7] It cannot be overemphasized that endoscopic or percutaneous aspiration of hilar masses is not recommended due to the potential for tumor seeding, which has been observed in transplant candidates. Transperitoneal biopsy or aspiration via either a percutaneous or EUS route precludes transplantation as per the Mayo Clinic protocol.

Suspicious biliary lesions should be sampled for histologic and cytologic analyses. The sensitivity of routine cytology ranges from almost 20% to 60% and the specificity varies from 61% to 100% depending on the series.[8] Fluorescent in situ hybridization (FISH) is an advanced cytologic test for aneuploidy that aids early diagnosis of CCA, especially in high-risk patients.[9] FISH employs fluorescent probes to detect chromosomal amplification or loss. Using FISH in routine cytology increases the sensitivity without compromising the specificity for diagnosis of CCA. In the current authors' experience, the addition of FISH permits detection of an additional 14% of CCA in patients with PSC who had normal cytology.

Tumor markers, although nonspecific, can aid in the diagnosis of CCA. CA 19-9 has proven the most useful. CA 19-9 detects circulating high-molecular-weight mucin glycoproteins coated with sialylated blood group epitopes (i.e. sialyl Lewis). Importantly, other malignancies and bacterial cholangitis can result in an increase in CA 19-9. Also, approximately 7% of the population are Lewis negative and will always have an undetectable CA 19-9 level, even in the presence of malignancy.[10] A serum CA 19-9 of >100 U/ml is 89% sensitive and 86% specific for CCA in patients with PSC who do not have cholangitis, but it has a sensitivity of only 53% in patients without PSC.[11]

Treatment

Treatment of CCA remains a formidable challenge. To date, there are no nonsurgical therapies that have been shown to achieve a clear, substantial increase in patient survival. Surgical resection and neoadjuvant therapy with orthotropic liver transplantation in carefully selected patients offer the only potential for cure.

None of the currently available chemotherapeutic or radiation therapy regimens have been clearly shown to improve survival in CCA patients. The literature is difficult to interpret due to the small numbers of patients in each series, paucity of randomized, controlled trials, and inclusion of other tumors in locations such as the gallbladder, pancreas, or liver, which likely have a different response. A number of regimens have employed infusional 5-fluorouracil (5-FU) or gemcitabine alone or in combination with other agents such as cisplatin as well as radiation therapy. Targeted therapies such as antibodies to vascular endothelial growth factor and epidermal growth factor receptors are currently in trials and are exciting potential therapies.

Since biliary obstruction is a major cause of morbidity and mortality in these patients, biliary stenting is commonly required in patients with extrahepatic CCA. Palliative biliary stenting reduces this morbidity and results in modestly improved survival in patients with unresectable CCA from 3 months to 6 months.[12] The choice of biliary stent depends on what therapeutic interventions the patient may be a candidate for and their life expectancy.

Photodynamic therapy (PDT) is another palliative therapy that has shown some promise in the treatment of CCA. PDT involves the systemic infusion of a photosensitizing agent followed by endoscopic biliary application of laser light of the appropriate wavelength resulting in selective tumor toxicity. PDT can typically be repeated every 3 months. If patients require biliary stenting, the current authors recommend placement of plastic rather than metal stents, especially for patients intended to receive PDT. PDT has been demonstrated to increase median survival in unresectable extrahepatic CCA from 16–21 months compared to 3–7 months with biliary stenting alone.[13] PDT, however, is only available at a limited number of centers, and the improvement in survival is likely due to decreased biliary obstruction.

Surgical resection

Surgical treatment provides the only potential for curative therapy. Unfortunately, CCA usually presents late in the disease course, and most patients have unresectable disease at presentation. Criteria for unresectability include distant lymph node metastases, intra- and extrahepatic metastases, bilobar liver involvement including: 1) bilateral hepatic duct involvement up to the secondary radicals, 2) atrophy of one lobe of the liver with encasement of the contralateral vasculature, and 3) inadequate volume for the predicted residual liver. Ipsilateral portal vein embolization can occasionally be employed to induce contralateral lobe hypertrophy, thereby helping to provide sufficient liver mass for survival in the immediate postoperative setting. Resection is rarely possible in the setting of underlying liver disease, and PSC is a contraindication to surgical resection due to a survival rate of <5% at 3 years.[3,14]

Reported survival rates following resection vary widely. Differences are primarily due to patient selection and surgical technique. There has been a trend towards improved survival during the last 2 decades attributable to more aggressive surgical resection; in particular, the use of segmental hepatectomy with removal of the caudate for resection of hilar CCA has improved long-term survival and accounts for a minimal increase in postoperative mortality. Depending on the series, survival following resection of CCA is approximately 53–83% at 1 year, 30–63% at 2 years, 16–48% at 3 years, and 16–44% at 5 years.[15,16,17] The median survival is 12–44 months compared to 5 months for patients not treated with resection.[18] A positive resection margin, lymph node metastasis, multiple tumors, larger tumor size, vascular invasion, and lymphatic invasion have been identified as risk factors for recurrence.[19] Patients with positive surgical margins have survival rates comparable to those receiving only palliative therapy.[20,21] Sites of recurrence are typically biliary, hepatic, retroperitoneal or hilar lymph nodes, and peritoneal sites.

Adjuvant treatments with chemotherapy, radiation therapy, or both have not been shown to improve survival following resection.[22] Adjuvant external beam radiation therapy may even lead to hepatic decompensation.[23] Biliary drainage should be done only when necessary. Excessive stenting of poorly drained segments promotes cholangitis and is associated with more postoperative infectious complications. Conversely, the residual liver lobe needs to be adequately drained to ensure liver regeneration.

CCA liver transplantation protocol

Orthotropic liver transplantation (OLT) offers promise for treatment of CCA since it accomplishes a radical resection of the tumor, is not limited by bilateral ductal or vascular involvement, and treats underlying liver disease. Initial experiences with OLT for unresectable CCA were, however, disappointing due to frequent recurrence of CCA. The 5-year survival rate was only 5–15% in these early studies.[24,25] There were some long-term survivors; these patients had absence of extrahepatic disease and regional lymph node involvement.[26] These findings along with observations of patients treated with aggressive radiation therapy and chemotherapy prompted development of a protocol at the Mayo Clinic in 1993. The Mayo Clinic strategy was to combine neoadjuvant radiotherapy with chemotherapy, carefully select patients, and avoid transplantation for patients with regional lymph node metastases in order to achieve success with liver transplantation (Figure 12.3). The rationale was that neoadjuvant therapy prior to operative staging and liver transplantation would avoid tumor dissemination during the operative procedures and that operative staging would avoid transplantation for patients destined to develop metastases after transplantation. Hepatic complications of high-dose radiotherapy would be obviated by liver transplantation.

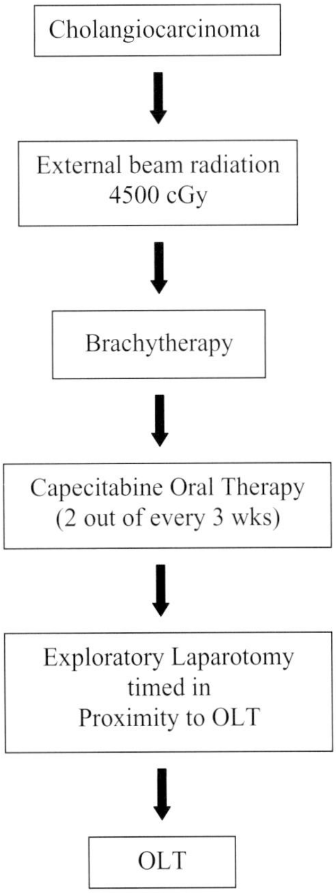

Figure 12.3 The Mayo Clinic CCA liver transplantation protocol

Results achieved with neoadjuvant therapy and liver transplantation have been very impressive. In a preliminary report of the first 11 patients transplanted for CCA, tumor-free survival was 45% with a median follow up of 7.5 years.[27] In a subsequent series at the Mayo Clinic, the survival rate following liver transplantation was 82% at 5 years.[28,29] From 1993 to April 2010, 196 patients have been enrolled in the CCA protocol at the Mayo Clinic. Following neoadjuvant chemoirradiation, 22% of these patients had findings at staging operation precluding transplantation and did not undergo OLT. A total of 126 patients have undergone OLT. The 5-year survival rate following transplant is 72%. This patient survival rate is higher than for those reported for resection, despite the fact that the patients either had unresectable disease or PSC precluding resection. A direct comparison with resection is not possible since intention to treat would need to be considered for both groups, which would include all patients started on neoadjuvant therapy for the transplant group and all patients explored for resection in the resection group. Importantly, survival for patients after transplantation is comparable to results achieved with liver transplantation for patients with other liver diseases and malignancies. Deceased- and living-donor transplantation have similar results in the Mayo Clinic experience. The success of this protocol is attributable to careful patient selection, neoadjuvant therapy with high-dose external beam radiation and intrabiliary radiation, and operative staging of all patients prior to liver transplantation to exclude those with intrahepatic, extrahepatic, and lymph node metastases.

Box 12.1 Diagnostic criteria for CCA

Definitive diagnostic criteria
- Biopsy (transluminal) positive for cancer
- Positive or suspicious cytology on brush cytology
- Mass lesion on cross-sectional imaging
- Malignant-appearing stricture combined with CA 19-9 >100 U/ml and/or FISH polysomy

Indeterminate diagnostic criteria
- FISH trisomy (chromosomes 7 or 3)
- Dysplasia
- FISH polysomy in absence of malignant-appearing stricture
- Malignant-appearing stricture in absence of mass lesion, positive cytology, biopsy, elevated CA 19-9 or FISH polysomy

Inclusion and exclusion criteria

Criteria for neoadjuvant therapy and liver transplantation are very selective. Patients must meet one of the definitive diagnostic criteria for CCA (Box 12.1). These criteria include either brush cytology or transluminal biopsy positive for adenocarcinoma, a malignant-appearing stricture on ERCP along with a serum CA 19-9 of >100 U/ml in the absence of cholangitis or polysomy on FISH analysis on brushings of the stricture, or a stricture with associated mass lesion on cross-sectional imaging. Patients are not eligible for the protocol if they have only dysplasia, trisomy on FISH, polysomy on FISH in the absence of a malignant-appearing stricture, or a malignant-appearing stricture with normal brushings and no mass. These patients are suspected of having cancer and are followed closely with repeat ERCP with brushings, cross-sectional imaging, and laboratory testing.

Patients must have extrahepatic CCA that is unresectable or arising in the setting of PSC. Criteria for anatomical unresectability include bilateral ductal involvement of second-degree biliary radicals, encasement of the main portal vein, unilateral segmental ductal extension with contralateral vascular encasement, or unilateral atrophy with either contralateral vascular or segmental ductal involvement. The presence of vascular encasement of the hilar vessels is not a contraindication to transplantation. It should be noted that liver transplantation is contraindicated in patients with intrahepatic CCA due to extremely high recurrence rates and lack of effective neoadjuvant or adjuvant therapy.

The criteria for protocol enrollment are designed to exclude patients with metastatic disease or with a low likelihood of responding to neoadjuvant therapy. Patients are excluded if there is a mass visible on cross-sectional imaging that is >3 cm in diameter. Patients are also excluded if there is metastatic disease including intrahepatic, extrahepatic, or regional lymph node metastases. Prior attempts at resection, percutaneous biopsy or FNA, or EUS-guided biopsy or FNA of the primary tumor are contraindications to enrollment in the protocol due to high rates of peritoneal and needle tract seeding. Patients with prior treatment with chemotherapy or radiation are also excluded. Candidates must have no active infections or medical conditions that would preclude neoadjuvant therapy or OLT.

Prior to initiation of neoadjuvant therapy, patients undergo evaluation to exclude metastatic disease. This evaluation includes a CT scan of the chest and abdomen, bone scan, and endoscopic ultrasound with fine-needle aspiration (EUS–FNA) of enlarged or suspicious regional lymph nodes. It should be emphasized that percutaneous or EUS-guided biopsy of the stricture or associated mass should not be carried out due to the significant risk of seeding tumor, and these procedures will exclude the patient from transplantation under the Mayo Clinic protocol. Since EUS–FNA was implemented in 2003, the percentage of patients with findings at the staging operation precluding transplantation decreased from 30–40% down to 15–20%. A positive EUS–FNA avoids the morbidity and mortality of high-dose neoadjuvant therapy and an unnecessary operation in patients destined to fall out of the protocol at operative staging.

Neoadjuvant therapy

All patients in the protocol receive neoadjuvant therapy consisting of continuous infusion 5-FU combined with external beam radiation therapy (40–45 Gy) administered over a 4-week period. This chemotherapeutic regimen is chosen due to its radiosensitization effects. At 2 weeks following external beam therapy, patients receive brachytherapy administered over 1 d via transcatheter radiation (20–30 Gy) to the tumor with iridium wires. Patients are then maintained on a protracted course of oral chemotherapy with capecitabine (Xeloda) given in 3-week cycles with 2 weeks on and 1 week off therapy until transplantation. All patients are begun on a proton pump inhibitor prior to initiation of external beam radiation due to the increased incidence of peptic ulcer disease, and these medications are continued through the completion of external beam radiation therapy.

Staging operation

All patients undergo pre-transplant staging exploratory laparotomy to evaluate for disease outside the bile ducts and liver.[28] Operative staging includes a thorough abdominal exploration, careful palpation of the liver to identify small previously undetected intrahepatic metastases, biopsy of any suspicious omental nodules, excision of a proximal proper hepatic artery lymph node (at the take-off of the gastroduodenal artery) and a pericholedochal lymph node posterior to the common bile duct just superior to the pancreas. The caudate process and retrohepatic vena cava are assessed for suitability of a caval-sparing hepatectomy (which is necessary for recipients of living-donor grafts). Presence of intrahepatic metastases, extrahepatic metastases including lymph node involvement, or locally extensive disease that precludes obtaining a negative surgical margin are all contraindications to transplantation. The staging operation was initially performed through a right subcostal incision with extension along the future liver transplant incision as necessary. During the past few years, the procedure is usually accomplished by hand-assisted laparoscopy utilizing a smaller right subcostal incision.

The timing of the staging operation is dependent on whether the patient will receive a deceased- or a living-donor transplant. For deceased-donor transplantation, the staging procedure is performed close to the expected time of transplantation based on anticipated waiting time. For living-donor transplantation the staging procedure is performed 2 d prior to transplantation. The staging procedure is performed as close to transplantation as practical in order to maximize the chance of detecting metastatic disease and to minimize extensive scar formation, which may develop afterward and increase the difficulty of the liver transplant procedure. There is always the potential for postoperative decompensation, especially for the patient with underlying PSC. If decompensation occurs, it may result in a rise in a patient's calculated MELD score. If the patient staged positive and is no longer a candidate for transplantation, however, the result is often fatal.

Unique issues in pre-transplant management

There are several issues in the pre-transplant management of CCA patients that are relatively unique to this condition.

Biliary obstruction is the major cause of morbidity in this patient population. Endoscopic biliary stenting is the preferred modality for biliary drainage given its negligible morbidity and mortality. Adequate drainage of a single functional hepatic lobe (30% of total liver volume) is sufficient to relieve cholestasis,[30] therefore, drainage of only one lobe is usually sufficient to relieve jaundice. More aggressive stenting is associated with an increased incidence of bacterial cholangitis and does not improve outcome. Metal stents are generally recommended only in patients who are not candidates for resection or liver transplantation. Percutaneous drainage can be performed when endoscopic intervention fails, but it has the disadvantage of external drains and the risk of bile leakage. Surgical biliary bypass is associated with high perioperative morbidity and mortality and is infrequently done – in fact it has been abandoned by most surgeons.

Acute cholangitis is a significant problem for CCA patients and is usually due to intubation to relieve jaundice or underlying biliary disease (PSC). Cholangitis is the most common cause for morbidity and mortality, especially if it is not appropriately treated in a timely fashion. Typically acute cholangitis does not become a significant issue until the patient has undergone instrumentation of the biliary system with placement of a biliary stent. Adequate biliary drainage of the infected biliary segment and prompt initiation of antibiotics are the cornerstones of treatment. It is important to emphasize that treatment with antibiotics in a patient without adequate biliary stenting can result in the development of highly resistant bacteria and formation of intrahepatic abscesses. There may also be no elevation of bilirubin when there is obstruction of up to half of the biliary system, so a normal bilirubin reading should not be taken as an indication of adequate biliary drainage. The current authors have found treatment with a course of fluoroquinolone to generally provide adequate coverage. The addition of metronidazole or other coverage targeted at anaerobic organisms is very rarely needed. It is their practice to administer prophylactic antibiotics immediately before ERCP and for 3–5 d following the procedure. They also provide patients with a prescription for antibiotics to be taken at the onset of symptoms of acute cholangitis.

Cholecystitis can develop in patients either due to tumor involvement of the cystic duct origin or due to compression by biliary stents. Diagnosis is made by history, examination and abdominal ultrasound. As with acute cholangitis, the initiation of antibiotics and adequate drainage are critical. Endoscopic drainage with placement of a cystic duct stent is preferred to operative therapy or percutaneous drainage. Endoscopic drainage can be technically difficult and requires an experienced endoscopist. A cholecystomy tube would be the next choice if the ERCP cannot be accomplished. If this cannot be accomplished then a cholecystectomy with care not to violate the tumor bed may be required. The current authors have only resorted to cholecystectomy in the setting of perforation. Awareness of the potential development of cholecystitis is important since delay in medical treatment may result in gall bladder necrosis and perforation, which requires an emergency operation.

Side effects of neoadjuvant therapy are very common. The current authors administer 5-fluorouracil as a continuous infusion rather than as bolus administrations due to improved tolerability. Capecitabine (Xeloda) is enzymatically converted to 5-fluorouracil and thus has a similar side-effect profile. Chemotherapy results in side effects in a significant portion of patients although side effects usually do not become significant until near the end of the chemotherapeutic course, i.e. during the last week of continuous infusion therapy with 5-FU and during the last few days of each 2-week course of capecitabine. Lethargy and malaise are common. Fortunately, these symptoms typically resolve within 2 weeks of completion of neoadjuvant therapy. Nausea, vomiting, anorexia, and diarrhea are common gastrointestinal side effects and are usually well controlled with medication and dietary changes. In addition, the current authors have observed that chemotherapy occasionally induces a flare of previously quiescent inflammatory bowel disease. If symptoms during neoadjuvant therapy are suggestive of a flare, they recommend performing a colonoscopy to exclude an infectious etiology. Flares of inflammatory bowel disease in this setting typically respond well to routine treatment.

Significant leucopenia, anemia, and thrombocytopenia can occur and the current authors recommend checking a complete blood count on a weekly basis to monitor for these changes since they can require a dose reduction. A painful rash most commonly involving the palms and soles (hand–foot syndrome), and stomatitis can develop and warrant dose reduction to prevent progression.

Radiation therapy results in a number of side effects. Patients receiving neoadjuvant therapy are at significant risk for duodenal ulcer formation likely secondary to radiation-induced injury. Several patients have required operative intervention for duodenal perforation or life-threatening hemorrhage from duodenitis and peptic ulceration. Therefore, ulcer prophylaxis is important in these patients. The current authors routinely administer a proton pump inhibitor daily throughout neoadjuvant therapy and extend this treatment for 1 month after completion of brachytherapy. Radiation therapy can result in significant impairment of gastric and duodenal motility. Symptoms include post-prandial nausea and vomiting. Onset can be delayed for weeks after radiation therapy and can extend well into the post-transplant period. Symptoms are particularly common when other exacerbating factors are present such as narcotics. Symptoms are typically managed by moving to a low-residue diet with frequent meals. Occasionally patients require a liquid diet or even jejunal feeding tubes for a limited period of time.

As with other cancers, weight loss is very frequently seen in CCA patients. Weight loss is likely mediated through immune system antitumor activity with production of factors such as tumor necrosis factor. Chemotherapy, antibiotics, and elevated bilirubin from impaired biliary drainage can all result in anorexia and dysgeusia that impair adequate oral intake. The current authors work to treat any correctable causes and to help patients maintain their weight through nutritional counseling, dietary changes, and nutritional supplements.

As with other adenocarcinomas, patients with CCA are hypercoagulable and are at increased risk for deep venous thrombosis and pulmonary embolism. These patients should therefore receive deep venous thrombosis prophylaxis whenever hospitalized for nonbleeding complications and especially during the perioperative staging period.

Liver transplantation

Liver transplantation for CCA is far more technically challenging than standard OLT. The operation is performed via a standard bilateral subcostal incision with vertical extension in the midline. Dissection can be difficult due to extensive scar tissue in the hepatoduodenal ligament as a result of both neoadjuvant radiation therapy and the previous staging procedure. Hilar dissection is avoided to minimize the risk of intraoperative dissemination of the tumor. The Mayo Clinic transplant group noted higher rates of arterial problems after transplantation for CCA than is usually seen with other indications, thus they prefer arterial reconstruction with a donor iliac artery interposition graft to the infrarenal aorta.

When an interposition graft is employed the deceased-donor arterial complication rate in patients transplanted for CCA is similar to patients undergoing OLT for other indications.[32] The bile duct is transected as close as possible to the pancreas and a short segment of the common bile duct can be enucleated from the head of the pancreas if necessary. The bile duct margin is submitted for frozen-section examination for microscopic tumor involvement. Bilioenteric continuity is restored with a choledochojejunostomy. The portal vein is divided as low as possible and is not dissected up into the hilus. Despite this low division of the recipient portal vein, the deceased-donor portal vein is almost always long enough for an end-to-end anastomosis. A caval sparing hepatectomy is performed in most cases and the donor suprahepatic vena cava is sewn to the left/middle hepatic vein trunk. If there is concern for tumor extension into the caudate lobe, the retrohepatic vena cava is excised, and the donor retrohepatic vena cava is sewn to the supra- and infrahepatic cavae as an interposition graft, usually with the use of porto- and veno-venous bypass.

The living-donor liver transplant (LDLT) is even more technically challenging but has been employed successfully in transplantation for CCA. Living-donor transplantation offers the potential for a shorter wait time for transplant with comparable survival to deceased-donor OLT. There are, however, higher rates of vascular and biliary complications. Radiation-induced injury to the hilar vessels and the location of the tumor result in a significant technical challenge given the short vessels of a living-donor allograft. There are several important differences in surgical technique in living-donor compared with deceased-donor OLT for CCA. The native artery is sewn directly to the living-donor artery during living-donor transplant since this technique results in a much lower rate of hepatic artery thrombosis compared with the use of a segment of the donor iliac artery as is employed in deceased-donor transplantation. A standard Roux-en-Y hepaticojejunostomy is employed to establish bilioenteric continuity. Since the living-donor graft has a very short portal vein, implantation requires use of a segment of deceased-donor iliac vein as an interposition graft between the donor right or left portal vein and the recipient portal vein.

If the distal bile duct is found to have microscopic carcinoma at the margin, a pancreaticoduodenectomy is performed when technically feasible. The addition of a pancreaticoduodenectomy greatly increases the technical complexity of transplantation and has a significant impact on postoperative morbidity and mortality. Of eleven patients who underwent OLT with concomitant pancreaticoduodenectomy at the Mayo Clinic, the 5-year survival was 56 ± 17% compared to 75 ± 5% overall.

Post-transplant management

There are a number of issues that deserve special attention in the management of patients after transplantation for CCA. The Mayo Clinic protocol does not include adjuvant therapy after transplantation, and immunosuppression management is similar to that for patients who undergo liver transplantation for benign disease. Since patients who undergo transplantation for CCA have received high-dose neoadjuvant radiation therapy, particular attention needs to be paid to late effects of radiation injury.

There is an increased incidence of late vascular complications in this patient population compared to patients who undergo OLT for other indications.[31] The rate of late portal vein stenosis (with or without thrombosis) is 20% in both living- and deceased-donor transplantation. The irradiated native common hepatic artery is employed in living-donor transplantation since it results in a lower rate of acute hepatic artery thrombosis compared with the use of a deceased-donor iliac artery graft as employed in deceased-donor transplantation, however, use of this vessel is associated with a 20% rate of late stenosis/thrombosis in these patients.[32] This arterial complication rate is higher than that observed after living-donor liver transplantation for other indications. All living-donor liver recipients are monitored closely with Doppler ultrasound to enable early detection of arterial stenosis. Intervention can often prevent sequelae of hepatic artery thrombosis such as cholangiopathy, intrahepatic abscesses, and graft loss.

LDLT is usually performed with a deceased-donor iliac vein interposition graft between the donor right or left portal vein and the recipient portal vein. When stenosis occurs it is located at the anastomosis of the native portal vein and the interposition graft, and this complication is seen in both living- and deceased-donor recipients with equal frequency. Late portal vein stenosis is usually apparent by 4 months post-transplant and can be detected by CT at that time. Even when asymptomatic, portal vein stenoses are treated by transhepatic angioplasty and stent insertion. Success with intervention is high, and the Mayo group has not experienced a graft loss due to this complication.

Impaired gastric motility is common following neoadjuvant therapy and can persist for some time during the post-transplant period. The postoperative state and narcotic pain medications tend to exacerbate this complication. These patients can develop postprandial nausea and vomiting without evidence of mechanical obstruction. Small, frequent meals that are primarily liquid are usually best. Symptoms tend to gradually but steadily improve, but an occasional jejunal tube feeding is required for a period to maintain nutrition. If symptoms are severe, gastrojejunostomy may be necessary.

Conclusion

CCA is a rare malignancy that arises in the biliary tree. The incidence of CCA is increasing globally. Primary sclerosing cholangitis and other conditions with chronic inflammation of the biliary tree are risk factors for the development of CCA. Hilar CCA usually presents with obstructive jaundice. Diagnostic techniques have significantly improved in the past 2 decades, enabling more accurate and less invasive evaluation. Surgical resection and liver transplantation in carefully selected patients are the only potentially curative treatments currently available. Liver transplantation following neoadjuvant therapy is effective therapy for patients with unresectable hilar CCA or hilar CCA arising in PSC. Preoperative issues include acute cholangitis, weight loss, and side effects of neoadjuvant chemotherapy and radiation therapy. Liver transplantation for CCA is technically challenging and associated with unique challenges and complications. Post-transplant management requires vigilance for late vascular complications. Standard immunosuppression is appropriate for these patients.

References

1. Khan SA, Taylor-Robinson SD, Toledano MB, Beck A, Elliott P, Thomas HC. Changing international trends in mortality rates for liver, biliary and pancreatic tumours. J Hepatol 2002;3:806–13.
2. Shaib Y, El-Serag HB. The epidemiology of cholangiocarcinoma. Semin Liver Dis. 2004 May;24(2): 115–25.
3. Rosen CB, Nagorney DM, Wiesner RH, Coffey RJ, Jr., LaRusso NF. Cholangiocarcinoma complicating primary sclerosing cholangitis. Ann Surg. 1991 Jan;213(1): 21–5.
4. Chalasani N, Baluyut A, Ismail A, Zaman A, Sood G, Ghalib R, et al. Cholangiocarcinoma in patients with primary sclerosing cholangitis: a multicenter case-control study. Hepatology. 2000 Jan;31(1):7–11.
5. Bismuth H, Corlette MB. Intrahepatic cholangioenteric anastomosis in carcinoma of the hilus of the liver. Surg Gynecol Obstet. 1975 Feb;140(2):170–8.
6. Nakajima T, Kondo Y, Miyazaki M, Okui K. A histopathologic study of 102 cases of intrahepatic cholangiocarcinoma: histologic classification and modes of spreading. Hum Pathol. 1988 Oct;19(10):1228–34.
7. Clary B, Jarnigan W, Pitt H, Gores G, Busuttil R, Pappas T. Hilar cholangiocarcinoma. Journal of Gastrointestinal Surgery. 2004 2004/0;8(3):298–302.
8. De Bellis M, Sherman S, Fogel EL, Cramer H, Chappo J, McHenry L, Jr., et al. Tissue sampling at ERCP in suspected malignant biliary strictures (Part 1). Gastrointest Endosc. 2002 Oct;56(4):552–61.
9. Baron TH, Harewood GC, Rumalla A, Pochron NL, Stadheim LM, Gores GJ, et al. A prospective comparison of digital image analysis and routine cytology for the identification of malignancy in biliary tract strictures. Clin Gastroenterol Hepatol. 2004;2(3):214–9.
10. Steinberg W. The clinical utility of the CA 19-9 tumor-associated antigen. Am J Gastroenterol. 1990;85(4): 350–5.
11. Nichols JC, Gores GJ, LaRusso NF, Wiesner RH, Nagorney DM, Ritts RE, Jr. Diagnostic role of serum CA 19-9 for cholangiocarcinoma in patients with primary sclerosing cholangitis. Mayo Clin Proc. 1993 Sep;68(9):874–9.
12. Prat F, Chapat O, Ducot B, Ponchon T, Fritsch J, Choury AD, et al. Predictive factors for survival of patients with inoperable malignant distal biliary strictures: a practical management guideline. Gut. 1998 Jan;42(1):76–80.
13. Zoepf T, Jakobs R, Arnold JC, Apel D, Riemann JF. Palliation of nonresectable bile duct cancer: improved survival after photodynamic therapy. Am J Gastroenterol. 2005 Nov;100(11):2426–30.
14. Stieber AC, Marino IR, Iwatsuki S, Starzl TE. Cholangiocarcinoma in sclerosing cholangitis. The role of liver transplantation. Int Surg. 1989 Jan-Mar;74(1): 1–3.
15. Okabayashi T, Yamamoto J, Kosuge T, Shimada K, Yamasaki S, Takayama T, et al. A new staging system for mass-forming intrahepatic cholangiocarcinoma: analysis of preoperative and postoperative variables. Cancer. 2001 Nov 1;92(9):2374–83.
16. Lai ECH, Lau WY. Aggressive surgical resection for hilar cholangiocarcinoma. ANZ Journal of Surgery. 2005 Nov;75(11):981–5.
17. Nagorney DM, Donohue JH, Farnell MB, Schleck CD, Ilstrup DM. Outcomes after curative resections of cholangiocarcinoma. Arch Surg. 1993 Aug;128(8): 871–7; discussion 7–9.
18. Nakeeb A, Tran KQ, Black MJ, Erickson BA, Ritch PS, Quebbeman EJ, et al. Improved survival in resected biliary malignancies. Surgery. 2002 Oct;132(4):555–63; discission 63–4.
19. Uenishi T, Hirohashi K, Kubo S, Yamamoto T, Yamazaki O, Kinoshita H. Clinicopathological factors predicting outcome after resection of mass-forming intrahepatic cholangiocarcinoma. Br J Surg. 2001 Jul;88(7): 969–74.
20. Jarnagin WR, Fong Y, DeMatteo RP, Gonen M, Burke EC, Bodniewicz BJ, et al. Staging, resectability, and outcome in 225 patients with hilar cholangiocarcinoma. Ann Surg. 2001 Oct;234(4):507–17; discussion 17–9.
21. Rea DJ, Munoz-Juarez M, Farnell MB, Donohue JH, Que FG, Crownhart B, et al. Major hepatic resection for hilar cholangiocarcinoma. Arch Surg. 2004;139(5): 514–25.

22. Kelley ST, Bloomston M, Serafini F, Carey LC, Karl RC, Zervos E, et al. Cholangiocarcinoma: advocate an aggressive operative approach with adjuvant chemotherapy. Am Surg. 2004 Sep;70(9):743–8; discussion 8–9.
23. Pitt HA, Nakeeb A, Abrams RA, Coleman J, Piantadosi S, Yeo CJ, et al. Perihilar cholangiocarcinoma. Postoperative radiotherapy does not improve survival. Ann Surg. 1995 Jun;221(6):788–97; discussion 97–8.
24. Iwatsuki S, Todo S, Marsh JW, Madariaga JR, Lee RG, Dvorchik I, et al. Treatment of hilar cholangiocarcinoma (Klatskin tumors) with hepatic resection or transplantation. J Am Coll Surg. 1998;187(4):358–64.
25. Jonas S, Kling N, Guckelberger O, Keck H, Bechstein WO, Neuhaus P. Orthotopic liver transplantation after extended bile duct resection as treatment of hilar cholangiocarcinoma. First long-terms results. Transplamt Int. 1998;11(Suppl 1):S206–8.
26. Shimoda M, Farmer DG, Colquhoun SD, Rosove M, Ghobrial RM, Yersiz H, et al. Liver transplantation for cholangiocellular carcinoma: Analysis of a single-center experience and review of the literature. Liver Transpl. 2001 Dec;7(12):1023–33.
27. Sudan D, DeRoover A, Chinnakotla S, Fox I, Shaw B, Jr., McCashland T, et al. Radiochemotherapy and transplantation allow long-term survival for nonresectable hilar cholangiocarcinoma. Am J Transplant. 2002 Sep;2(8):774–9.
28. Heimbach JK, Gores GJ, Haddock MG, Alberts SR, Nyberg SL, Ishitani MB, et al. Liver transplantation for unresectable perihilar cholangiocarcinoma. Seminars in Liver Disease. 2004;24(2):201–729.
29. Rea DJ, Heimbach JK, Rosen CB, Haddock MG, Alberts SR, Kremers WK, et al. Liver transplantation with neoadjuvant chemoradiation is more effective than resection for hilar cholangiocarcinoma. Ann Surg. 2005 Sep;242(3):451–8; discussion 8–61.
30. De Palma GD, Galloro G, Siciliano S, Iovino P, Catanzano C. Unilateral versus bilateral endoscopic hepatic duct drainage in patients with malignant hilar biliary obstruction: results of a prospective, randomized, and controlled study. Gastrointest Endosc. 2001 May;53(6):547–53.
31. Mantel HT, Rosen CB, Heimbach JK, Nyberg SL, Ishitani MB, Andrews JC, et al. Vascular complications after orthotopic liver transplantation after neoadjuvant therapy for hilar cholangiocarcinoma. Liver Transpl. 2007 Oct;13(10):1372–81.
32. Heimbach JK. Successful liver transplantation for hilar cholangiocarcinoma. Curr Opin Gastroenterol. 2008 May;24(3):384–8.

13 Rare indications for liver transplantation

Stevan A. Gonzalez

Annette C. and Harold C. Simmons Transplant Institute, Baylor All Saints Medical Center, Fort Worth and Baylor University Medical Center, Dallas, TX, USA

Key learning points

- Rare indications for liver transplantation (LT) include vascular disorders such as Budd–Chiari syndrome (BCS), sarcoidosis, nonhepatocellular malignancies, and congenital hepatobiliary disorders.
- Patients with extrahepatic diseases that occur as a result of metabolic defects originating within the liver such as primary hyperoxaluria and familial amyloid polyneuropathy may benefit from LT.
- Mortality risk associated with rare malignancies, congenital disorders, or metabolic defects may not be reflected in conventional organ prioritization measures such as the Model for End-stage Liver Disease (MELD) score.
- Selection of liver transplant candidates with favorable clinical features and low risk of recurrent disease is essential to ensuring optimal post-transplant outcomes, particularly in the setting of nonhepatocellular malignancies.

Introduction

Rare indications for LT include vascular disorders, nonhepatocellular malignancy, congenital liver disorders, and progressive extrahepatic diseases resulting from primary metabolic defects originating within the liver. Although some disorders are not associated with hepatic synthetic dysfunction or portal hypertension, LT may offer the most definitive form of therapy with a significant long-term survival benefit. Consequently, mortality risk associated with rare malignancies, congenital disorders, or metabolic defects may not be reflected in conventional organ prioritization measures such as the MELD score. In some cases, exception must be granted by regional review boards in order to advance prioritization. Selection of appropriate candidates with favorable clinical features who would benefit most from LT in this setting is essential to ensuring optimal post-transplant outcomes.

Budd–Chiari syndrome

Primary BCS is defined by hepatic outflow obstruction secondary to thrombosis at the level of the hepatic veins or suprahepatic inferior vena cava (IVC) in the absence of cardiac disease.[1] A key factor in the pathogenesis of BCS is the presence of an underlying prothrombotic condition, which can be identified in the majority of cases. Some data suggest that at the time of presentation, a significant proportion of patients with BCS have multiple risk factors occurring simultaneously.[2,3] Secondary BCS can result from extrinsic compression or vascular invasion of the hepatic outflow tract by tumor and must be distinguished from primary BCS.

Clinical evaluation of patients presenting with BCS includes an assessment for the presence of an underlying prothrombotic condition. Myeloproliferative disorders (MPD) account for up to one-half of all BCS

Medical Care of the Liver Transplant Patient, Fourth Edition. Edited by Pierre-Alain Clavien, James F. Trotter.

Box 13.1 Risk factors associated with primary BCS

Myeloproliferative disorders
Factor V Leiden mutation
Factor II mutation
G20210A prothrombin mutation
Protein C or S deficiency
Antithrombin deficiency
Plasminogen deficiency
MTHFR mutation
Hyperhomocysteinemia
Antiphospholipid syndrome
Paroxysmal nocturnal hemoglobinuria
Use of oral contraceptives
Pregnancy
Behçet's disease
Inflammatory bowel disease

MTHFR: methylenetetrahydrofolate reductase

cases.[2] In particular, the V617F Janus tyrosine kinase-2 (JAK2) mutation associated with MPD is a major risk factor, as the majority of BCS cases secondary to MPD are positive for this mutation. Other risk factors include use of oral contraceptives, antiphospholipid syndrome, and factor V Leiden mutation (Box 13.1).[1,2,4] Disorders such as protein C, protein S, or antithrombin deficiency may be difficult to assess in the setting of compromised hepatic synthetic function.

The clinical presentation of BCS varies greatly, ranging from asymptomatic disease to fulminant hepatic failure. In chronic BCS, long-term hepatic venous outflow obstruction can result in progressive centrilobular hepatic fibrosis and severe portal hypertension. Presenting features associated with BCS may include abdominal pain, fever, hepatomegaly, splenomegaly, lower extremity edema, and ascites. The diagnosis of BCS can be made through imaging studies such as ultrasound with Doppler or cross-sectional contrast-enhanced imaging including computed tomography (CT) scan or magnetic resonance imaging (MRI). Imaging studies may reveal compensatory caudate lobe hypertrophy, as venous outflow from the caudate lobe directly to the IVC may be unobstructed.[2]

All patients presenting with BCS should be considered for immediate anticoagulation therapy.[5] Hepatic vein thrombus may coincide with vascular stenosis; thus, hepatic vein angioplasty and stent placement may be effective in some cases. Transjugular intrahepatic portosystemic shunt (TIPS) placement should also be considered, as over half of patients with BCS may benefit from this form of treatment.[6] The use of systemic thrombolytics has been described, although data demonstrating any significant benefit is limited. Ultimately LT should be considered in those who fail anticoagulation, hepatic vein angioplasty, and TIPS placement. According to data derived from large cohorts in Europe and the USA, survival following LT in patients with BCS has been reported to be 72–75% at 3 years, and as high as 71% at 5 years.[6,7]

Sarcoidosis

Sarcoidosis is a multisystemic disease of unknown etiology characterized by the presence of noncaseating granulomas in affected organs. The global epidemiology of sarcoidosis is difficult to assess as it varies greatly based on geography and ethnicity. The highest incidence of sarcoidosis has been reported in Scandinavian and Northern European populations in which the disease occurs in up to 40 cases per 100 000 individuals.[8] Among American populations, the incidence varies by ethnicity and occurs more frequently in African Americans compared with Caucasians.[8,9] Sarcoidosis is most commonly associated with pulmonary disease, however other organ systems can be affected, including the skin, lymph nodes, eyes, and liver.[9]

Sarcoidosis is the most common identifiable cause of hepatic granulomatous disease. Granulomas may be present on liver biopsy in up to 75% of patients with systemic sarcoidosis.[10] Although advanced liver disease is rare, significant involvement of the liver has been reported to occur in 11.5% of patients according to one large multicenter case–control study, in which African Americans were more than twice as likely to have liver disease compared with Caucasians.[9] Clinical features associated with hepatic sarcoidosis may include fever, arthralgias, pruritis, abdominal pain, hepatomegaly, and jaundice, although many patients are asymptomatic. Liver enzymes are frequently characterized by elevations in serum alkaline phosphatase. The diagnosis of sarcoidosis requires the presence of clinical features, radiographic evidence, and tissue histopathology demonstrating noncaseating granulomas in one or more organ systems.[8] Over one-half of patients with sarcoidosis may have an elevated angiotensin-converting enzyme (ACE) level, which is produced by sarcoidal granulomas; however the diagnostic utility of this test is not well established. An important component of the diagnostic evaluation of hepatic sarcoidosis is the exclusion of alternative diseases associated with hepatic granulomas including infection, primary biliary cirrhosis, lymphoma, and drug-induced liver injury.

Histopathologic features of hepatic sarcoidosis may reveal cholestatic, necroinflammatory, or vascular patterns of liver injury.[11] As a defining characteristic of sarcoidosis, granulomas are present in all cases and are typically identified in periportal areas. Features associated with cholestasis include bile duct injury with inflammation, periductal fibrosis in the absence of inflammation, or ductopenia. In patients with a necroinflammatory pattern, chronic portal inflammatory changes can be seen in addition to foci of necrosis. Vascular changes occur less frequently and may be associated with sinusoidal dilation or nodular regenerative hyperplasia. A key aspect in the histologic diagnosis of sarcoidosis is confirming the absence of mycobacterial, fungal, or parasitic infections through special staining and laboratory studies.

Treatment of sarcoidosis most commonly involves corticosteroid therapy. Use of corticosteroids in hepatic sarcoidosis has been associated with biochemical and symptomatic improvement; although no clear long-term histologic benefit has been demonstrated.[12] When indicated, recommended medical therapy includes prednisone 20–40 mg/d and ursodiol 15 mg/kg/d.[8] Small studies have suggested a potential benefit from alternative agents including tumor necrosis factor (TNF)-α inhibitors and methotrexate, yet the role of these agents in the treatment of sarcoidosis involving the liver is unclear.

Although only a minority of patients with systemic sarcoidosis develop significant liver disease, it can result in progressive hepatic fibrosis, portal hypertension, and end-stage liver disease (ESLD).[12] Some patients may develop portal hypertension in the absence of nodular cirrhosis on liver biopsy, representing a subgroup of patients in whom TIPS placement may be beneficial. Data describing outcomes in patients undergoing LT for hepatic sarcoidosis are limited; however post-transplant survival appears to be comparable to other chronic liver diseases, with 5-year patient survival reported to be as high as 80%.[13,14] Recurrent sarcoidosis in the liver allograft has been described, but does not result in allograft dysfunction in most cases.

Primary and metastatic tumors

Epithelioid hemangioendothelioma

Epithelioid hemangioendothelioma (EHE) is a rare mesenchymal soft tissue vascular tumor that frequently affects the liver and is characterized histologically by epithelioid morphology. EHE is considered to be of intermediate malignancy in the spectrum of epithelioid vascular tumors including benign lesions such as hemangioma and more aggressive tumors such as angiosarcoma.[15] EHE is more common in women, typically presents in the second to third decades of life, and can occur as a primary tumor in various tissues including lung, bone, and liver. Although the potential exists, the incidence of metastatic disease in primary hepatic EHE is relatively low and has been described in up to 27% of cases after a median follow up of longer than 4 years.[15]

The clinical presentation and disease course associated with hepatic EHE varies widely. Many patients with hepatic EHE are asymptomatic; although some cases may present with portal hypertension, BCS, or progressive hepatic failure. Symptoms and clinical features noted on presentation include abdominal pain, weight loss, fatigue, jaundice, and hepatomegaly.[15] Laboratory studies typically reveal elevated liver enzymes, most commonly with elevations in alkaline phosphatase. Multifocal disease is seen in the majority of cases with multiple tumors in both the right and left hepatic lobes.[16] Imaging studies including ultrasound, CT, or MRI may reveal patterns described as multinodular disease or diffuse tumor infiltration, the latter of which typically represents more advanced disease. A central region of sclerosis with surrounding cellular proliferation may give a target appearance to some tumors on MRI imaging, while others are characterized by a central area of hemorrhage or necrosis.[16]

The diagnosis of EHE is made histologically. Typical features on biopsy include the presence of infiltrating clusters of eosinophilic epithelioid or dendritic cells in a myxohyaline stroma. The infiltration of tumor cells occurs within vascular spaces such as hepatic sinusoids, portal veins, and terminal hepatic venules.[15] An additional feature of tumor cells includes the presence of intracytoplasmic lumina. Immunohistochemistry is important in confirming the diagnosis, as all EHE tumors express the endothelial markers factor VIII-related antigen, CD31, and CD34. Histopathologic features such as increased mitotic activity, atypia, and necrosis do not appear to correspond with poor outcome in EHE,[17] however the degree of tumor cellularity may predict more aggressive disease.[15]

As systemic chemotherapy is not effective, curative surgical resection or LT are the treatments of choice for hepatic EHE. In rare cases with tumor confined to the right or left hepatic lobes, partial resection may be considered. As the majority of patients present with multinodular disease involving both hepatic lobes, LT is the most common form of treatment. Patients who undergo LT for EHE appear to have a low rate of recurrence, even in the presence of extrahepatic metastases, although data are limited. In the three largest series to date, overall survival at 5 years following LT ranged from 54% to as high as 83%.[16,18,19] In a study utilizing data from the European Liver Transplant Registry, 10 patients with hepatic EHE and evidence of extrahepatic disease had no difference in survival compared to those with disease localized to the liver; however the presence of vascular invasion may be associated with decreased post-transplant survival at 5 and 10 years.[18] In the setting of tumor recurrence following transplantation, aggressive treatment with chemotherapy and ablative techniques should be considered.

Neuroendocrine tumors

Gastroenteropancreatic neuroendocrine tumors (NETs) are a rare group of neoplasms derived from hormone-producing cells found throughout the digestive tract. Neuroendocrine cells originate from multipotent gastrointestinal stem cells and undergo a process of differentiation into distinct cell types that produce specific peptides or neuroamines that regulate digestive and endocrine functions within the gut.[20] Although many subtypes of NET are generally thought to be associated with a benign clinical course, tumors may vary greatly with regard to clinical presentation, disease severity, and malignant potential. Most cases of NET are sporadic, however they may occur in association with familial endocrine cancer syndromes.[21]

The liver is the most common site of NET metastasis, which may occur in up to 85% of cases, depending on the primary site of origin.[20]A significant proportion of patients with NET are asymptomatic with nonfunctioning tumors and tend to present late in the course of disease. In contrast, some NETs present with abnormal secretory function resulting in distinct clinical syndromes based on their cell type (Table 13.1). Carcinoid syndrome most frequently occurs in the presence of liver metastases.[21] Carcinoid

Table 13.1 Most common gastroenteropancreatic NETs based on cell type, secretory product, and clinical syndrome

Tumor	Cell type	Product	Clinical syndrome
Carcinoid	Enterochromaffin	Serotonin (5-HIAA)	Flushing, diarrhea, abdominal pain, bronchospasm
Insulinoma	β	Insulin	Hypoglycemia
Gastrinoma	G	Gastrin	Peptic ulcer disease (Zollinger–Ellison)
VIPoma	VIP	VIP	Watery diarrhea, hypokalemia, achlorhydria (Verner–Morrison)
Glucagonoma	α	Glucagon	Necrolytic migratory erythema, diabetes, weight loss, weakness, venous thrombosis, depression
Somatostatinoma	D	Somatostatin	Steatorrhea, diabetes, cholelithiasis

5-HIAA: 5-hydroxyindoleacetic acid, VIP: vasoactive intestinal peptide crisis is a severe life-threatening variation of the syndrome characterized by tachycardia, arrhythmias, and rapid fluctuations in blood pressure that may occur at the time of manipulation, resection, or ablation of tumors. A key step in the diagnostic evaluation of NET is the use of imaging studies to assess the extent of disease and potentially identify the primary tumor site.[21]Imaging modalities commonly include CT, MRI, endoscopic ultrasound (EUS), and somatostatin receptor scintigraphy (SSRS). SSRS may be particularly useful, as the majority of NETs express somatostatin receptors, and this technique is the most sensitive in the assessment of liver metastases or extrahepatic disease.[20,21] Measurement of plasma chromogranin A may also be useful as both a diagnostic and surveillance tool, as it is produced by all NETs including nonfunctioning tumors.

Surgical management of NET is the principal means of definitive treatment, although many patients present with extensive metastatic disease and surgical options may be limited.[21]Surgical resection of the primary and metastatic lesions, if possible, is essentially curative and is associated with excellent long-term survival. Other forms of therapy include somatostatin analogues, ablative therapies, debulking or palliative surgery, and chemotherapy. Somatostatin analogues are particularly effective in controlling symptoms associated with hypersecretory syndromes and should be given prior to surgical procedures involving carcinoid tumors in order to minimize the risk of carcinoid crisis.[20,21]

LT has become an important treatment option for NET in the setting of unresectable liver metastases or uncontrolled symptoms, although appropriate selection of candidates is essential. The largest studies describing LT for metastatic NET reported overall post-transplant patient survival to be approximately 50% at 5 years.[22,23] Other smaller studies have reported more favorable post-transplant outcomes with patient survival ranging from 80–90%; however this may reflect differences in patient selection. Factors associated with decreased post-transplant survival have included age >50, requirement for upper abdominal exenteration or pancreatoduodenectomy, increased proliferation index by immunohistochemistry, and duodenal or pancreatic site of the primary lesion. Although clear criteria have yet to be defined, LT is a viable treatment option in metastatic NET, particularly in younger patients with favorable clinical features and no evidence of extrahepatic metastases.

Hepatic cavernous hemangioma

Cavernous hemangiomas are the most common benign tumors encountered in the liver, with an incidence reported to be as high as 20%. Hemangiomas occur more frequently in women and the majority are solitary, <4 cm in size, asymptomatic, and are usually discovered incidentally with abdominal imaging studies.[24] Lesions >4 cm in size are referred to as "giant cavernous hemangiomas." Histopathologic assessment reveals a vascular lesion characterized by ectatic vascular channels lined with endothelial cells and separated by fibrous septa.[25]

The diagnosis of cavernous hemangioma is typically made with imaging studies. Characteristic features can be seen on ultrasound, CT, and MRI. MRI is generally regarded as the preferred imaging modality with the highest specificity.[25] Although the vast majority of patients are asymptomatic with normal laboratory studies, presenting features in symptomatic patients with giant cavernous hemangiomas may include abdominal pain, hepatomegaly, nausea, vomiting, and weight loss.[26] Complications such as intratumoral hemorrhage, rupture, or Kasabach–Merritt syndrome (KMS) are uncommon. KMS is a rare but life-threatening syndrome characterized by thrombocytopenia and coagulopathy resulting from entrapment of platelets by proliferating endothelium within the lesion, platelet activation, secondary consumption of clotting factors, and subsequent intratumoral hemorrhage leading to rapid enlargement of the hemangioma.

A definitive surgical approach is usually taken if treatment is indicated, with enucleation of the lesion as the preferred technique.[25,26] Lesions with persistent or worsening symptoms, progressive enlargement, acute complications, or inability to exclude malignancy should be considered for surgical management. LT is rarely performed in the treatment of giant cavernous hemangiomas, although it may be considered in unresectable cases or in the setting of KMS. The majority of reported transplants for giant cavernous hemangiomas have been performed in patients who presented with KMS, while severe symptomatic disease is a less common indication.[24]

Polycystic liver disease

Fibropolycystic liver diseases are inherited congenital disorders associated with abnormal portobiliary development. Defective remodeling of the ductal plate during embryologic development of the hepatobiliary system leads to a range of bile duct abnormalities with variable presentations and disease courses. Ductal plate malformations may occur within small, medium, or large bile ducts resulting in distinct manifestations of biliary disease known as congenital hepatic fibrosis, Caroli syndrome (CS), and Caroli disease (CD).[27] Autosomal dominant forms of polycystic liver disease that occur in association with autosomal dominant polycystic kidney disease (ADPKD) or in isolation result from autonomous proliferation of intrahepatic bile duct epithelial cells and subsequent intralumenal secretory function, remodeling, and neovascularization.[28] Although fibropolycystic liver diseases generally do not alter hepatocellular function, some cases may lead to progressive liver disease characterized by portal hypertension, infectious complications, and an increased risk of malignancy.

Congenital hepatic fibrosis and CD

Congenital hepatic fibrosis (CHF) is characterized by ductal plate malformations occurring at the microscopic interlobular bile ducts with associated portal vein abnormalities and periportal fibrosis. The diagnosis of CHF is made through histopathologic assessment. Liver biopsies in patients with CHF reveal increased numbers of embryonic bile ducts in portal areas arranged in a primitive ductal plate configuration.[27] Bridging fibrosis extending between portal tracts may be present without evidence of bridging to central veins or nodular cirrhosis. CHF is most commonly associated with autosomal recessive polycystic kidney disease (ARPKD). The clinical presentation of CHF is highly variable and may be associated with features including splenomegaly, ascites, and gastroesophageal varices resulting from portal hypertension. In addition, CHF may be associated with an increased risk of hepatocellular carcinoma (HCC). Although periportal fibrosis occurring in the setting of CHF can be progressive, hepatocellular function is well preserved.

CD occurs as a result of ductal plate malformations within medium to large bile ducts and can be seen with hepatic imaging studies.[27] Biliary cystic disease in CD leads to multifocal saccular or fusiform ectasias in continuity with the intrahepatic biliary ductal system. The diagnosis of CD is made through direct cholangiography or noninvasive methods such as magnetic resonance cholangiopancreatography (MRCP). CS refers to CD in the presence of concomitant CHF. In CS, cystic changes occur within large bile ducts in addition to interlobular duct abnormalities and perioportal fibrosis seen on liver biopsy. As in CHF, patients with CS may present with clinical manifestations of portal hypertension and renal fibrocystic disease associated with ARPKD. Major complications associated with CD include hepatolithiasis, cholangitis, and cholangiocarcinoma. Ursodiol therapy, therapeutic endoscopy, and surgical methods have been described in the treatment of complications associated with CD; however LT should be considered in those with diffuse progressive hepatobiliary disease. Data derived from large liver transplant registries in Europe and the USA have demonstrated favorable outcomes in patients with CD who undergo LT, with 5-year survival estimates ranging from 77–86%.[29,30] In patients with CHF or CS who have ARPKD-associated renal disease, combined kidney and LT may be considered.

Autosomal dominant polycystic liver disease

Polycystic liver disease (PLD) is a fibrocystic liver disorder defined by the presence of multiple hepatic cysts embedded within the liver parenchyma. In contrast to CD, cysts that occur in PLD are not in continuity with the intrahepatic biliary ductal system and occur as a result of autonomous proliferation of intrahepatic bile duct epithelial cells.[28] PLD is most frequently associated with ADPKD. A less common variant of PLD, autosomal dominant polycystic liver disease (ADPLD) occurs in the absence of fibrocystic renal disease. Most forms of PLD follow an autosomal dominant inheritance pattern.

The prevalence and number of liver cysts associated with ADPKD or ADPLD increases with age and female gender.[28] In the setting of ADPKD, the majority of affected patients develop concomitant PLD and the prevalence of liver involvement increases with severity of fibrocystic renal disease. Most patients with PLD are asymptomatic, although some may present with abdominal pain or symptoms related to mass effect. PLD can be distinguished from CD through the use of hepatic imaging studies including MRCP and molecular genetic testing can be used to confirm the presence of mutations associated with ADPKD or ADPLD. Although hepatocellular function remains normal in most cases, some patients with PLD may develop progressive disease and complications associated with portal hypertension, infection, intracystic hemorrhage, or rupture. As no effective medical therapy exists, patients with progressive disease associated with PLD may benefit from LT or combined kidney and LT, in which 5-year post-transplant survival has been reported to be as high as 69 and 76%, respectively.[28]

LT for extrahepatic disease

Primary hyperoxaluria Type 1

Primary hyperoxaluria Type 1 (PH1) is a rare autosomal recessive disorder defined by excessive hepatic oxalate synthesis. The metabolic defect associated with PH1 occurs as a result of deficient or absent peroxisomal alanine/glyoxylate aminotransferase (AGT) activity within the liver.[31] Oxalate is primarily excreted by the kidneys and excessive urinary concentrations can lead to progressive renal dysfunction, end-stage renal disease, and significant systemic disease.

As a result of elevated urinary oxalate excretion, patients with PH have a high propensity to form calcium oxalate crystals within the renal tubules and interstitium, leading to urolithiasis and medullary nephrocalcinosis, respectively. Renal interstitial fibrosis and recurrent urinary obstruction may in turn lead to progressive renal failure. Further reductions in glomerular filtration rate (GFR) lead to the inability to excrete oxalate. Systemic oxalosis may then occur as a consequence of elevated serum oxalate levels and deposition of calcium oxalate crystals in tissues apart from the kidneys including bone, skin, retina, and myocardium. The risk of oxalosis is highest in patients with reductions in GFR to <30–40 ml/min/1.73m^2.[31] The phenotypic expression of disease in PH is variable, with the age of presentation ranging from infancy to adulthood. PH1 is the most common form of PH, accounting for up to 80% of all cases, and it more frequently results in severe systemic disease.

PH1 results from mutations occurring at the *AGXT* gene that disrupt production of the AGT protein. Although the role of genetic sequencing may become increasingly important, a liver biopsy with assessment of tissue AGT enzymatic activity is the most effective means of establishing the diagnosis of PH1.[31] Undertaking 24-hour urine testing also contributes to the diagnosis of PH1, in which urinary oxalate is elevated as well as urine glycolate. PH1 must be distinguished from primary hyperoxaluria Type 2 (PH2), which occurs as a result of deficient glyoxylate reductase/hydroxypyruvate reductase (GRHPR) activity, and is characterized by elevated urine L-glyceric acid. PH2 is associated with a more favorable prognosis, in which LT may not be clinically indicated.[31] A less common form of primary hyperoxaluria known as non1, non2 primary hyperoxaluria has also been described; however data regarding the natural history of this subtype are limited. The differential diagnosis of PH1 includes various conditions that may lead to secondary hyperoxaluria, most commonly as a result of excessive absorption of dietary oxalate in the digestive tract. Causes of secondary hyperoxaluria are typically associated with fat malabsorption such as inflammatory bowel disease, short bowel syndrome, and cystic fibrosis.

Treatment of PH1 involves efforts to reduce hepatic oxalate production and urinary calcium oxalate crystal formation, as well as provide renal replacement therapy in the setting of progressive renal dysfunction. Administration of pyridoxine, which acts as a cofactor for AGT, may increase AGT activity in some individuals. Alkali citrate may also be given to reduce calcium oxalate formation within the kidneys. The use of probiotics has been described as a method of altering intestinal absorption and excretion of oxalate. Ultimately, some patients develop progressive renal disease and require initiation of renal replacement therapy in order to reduce the risk of systemic oxalosis.

As the primary metabolic defect associated with PH1 occurs within the liver, hyperoxaluria can persist following kidney transplantation. Thus, simultaneous liver and kidney transplantation is the definitive form of treatment of PH1 once renal failure occurs. In contrast with PH1, kidney transplant alone in patients with PH2 is associated with favorable long-term outcomes and LT is not required. Transplantation for PH1 is generally considered once renal replacement therapy is initiated for progressive renal dysfunction despite attempts at medical therapy. Post-transplant patient survival for mostly combined kidney and LT has been reported to be 80% at 5 years according to a large European series.[32] The use of pre-emptive LT in PH1 has been described, although this approach has been met with considerable controversy in light of the variable natural history of the disease, risk to the recipient, and concerns regarding organ availability.

Familial amyloid polyneuropathy

Familial amyloid polyneuropathy (FAP) is a severe autosomal dominant form of hereditary amyloidosis leading to excessive production of amyloid proteins, systemic amyloidosis, and progressive neurologic disease. The most common amyloid protein associated with FAP is amyloidogenic mutated transthyretin (ATTR), which is produced in the liver as a result of mutations in the transthyretin (TTR) gene. Many mutations associated with ATTR production have been identified, of which the point mutation ATTR Val30Met is the most common.[33] Progressive multisystemic disease can result from accumulation of amyloid protein in various tissues with a typical presentation occurring within the second to third decades of life. Although the incidence and severity of clinical disease varies greatly among individuals with FAP, a significant proportion of patients will develop progressive neurologic, cardiac, and renal dysfunction.

Most patients with FAP present with progressive neuropathic symptoms characterized by a lower-extremity sensorimotor peripheral neuropathy and autonomic neuropathy. Symptomatic disease associated with autonomic neuropathy may include gastrointestinal dysmotility, orthostatic hypotension, cardiac arrhythmias, urinary retention, and erectile dysfunction. In addition, cardiac diastolic dysfunction, conduction defects, and renal insufficiency with proteinuria may occur as a result of amyloid deposition within myocardial and renal interstitial tissues.[33] Diagnosis of FAP generally requires molecular genetic analysis.

LT is accepted as the most effective treatment of FAP. Over 90% of ATTR is produced within the liver and transplantation results in clearance of the protein as well as improvement of FAP-associated disease in many cases. Up to half of FAP patients who receive liver transplants experience significant improvements in symptoms including motor disability, sensory loss, and gastrointestinal symptoms related to autonomic neuropathy.[33] Based on data from a large cohort of patients enrolled in the FAP World Transplant Registry, post-transplant survival was reported to be 77% at 5 years.[34]

An important consideration in LT related to FAP is the risk of coexisting cardiovascular disease in affected individuals. Timing of transplantation early during the course of FAP-related disease is associated with improved post-transplant outcomes, while some data suggest longer duration of disease prior to transplantation is associated with a decline in post-transplant survival.[33] This trend may occur as a result of cardiovascular complications, which are the leading cause of death following LT in patients with FAP.[34] An extensive cardiovascular evaluation, therefore, is warranted in patients with FAP prior to undergoing transplantation in order to accurately determine cardiovascular risk. In cases of progressive cardiomyopathy resulting from FAP, combined heart transplantation and LT has been described.[35]

As patients with FAP have otherwise anatomically and functionally normal livers apart from the aberrant production of the ATTR protein, FAP livers have been used as donor organs. This practice, known as sequential or "domino" LT, is based on the natural history of FAP in which 20–30 years are required to develop clinical disease related to amyloidosis. Domino transplantation may be an acceptable alternative for some patients awaiting transplant, particularly in candidates with a hepatocellular or metastatic malignancy who would otherwise require longer waiting times.

References

1. Valla DC. Primary Budd–Chiari syndrome. J Hepatol 2009;50:195–203.
2. Darwish Murad S, Plessier A, Hernandez-Guerra M, et al. Etiology, management, and outcome of the

Budd–Chiari syndrome. Ann Intern Med 2009;151: 167–75.
3. Denninger MH, Chait Y, Casadevall N, et al. Cause of portal or hepatic venous thrombosis in adults: the role of multiple concurrent factors. Hepatology 2000;31: 587–91.
4. DeLeve LD, Valla DC, Garcia-Tsao G. Vascular disorders of the liver. Hepatology 2009;49:1729–64.
5. Janssen HL, Garcia-Pagan JC, Elias E, et al. Budd–Chiari syndrome: a review by an expert panel. J Hepatol 2003;38:364–71.
6. Segev DL, Nguyen GC, Locke JE, et al. Twenty years of liver transplantation for Budd–Chiari syndrome: a national registry analysis. Liver Transpl 2007;13: 1285–94.
7. Mentha G, Giostra E, Majno PE, et al. Liver transplantation for Budd–Chiari syndrome: A European study on 248 patients from 51 centres. J Hepatol 2006;44: 520–8.
8. Iannuzzi MC, Rybicki BA, Teirstein AS. Sarcoidosis. N Engl J Med 2007;357:2153–65.
9. Baughman RP, Teirstein AS, Judson MA, et al. Clinical characteristics of patients in a case control study of sarcoidosis. Am J Respir Crit Care Med 2001;164: 1885–9.
10. Rose AS, Tielker MA, Knox KS. Hepatic, ocular, and cutaneous sarcoidosis. Clin Chest Med 2008;29: 509–24, ix.
11. Devaney K, Goodman ZD, Epstein MS, et al. Hepatic sarcoidosis. Clinicopathologic features in 100 patients. Am J Surg Pathol 1993;17:1272–80.
12. Kennedy PT, Zakaria N, Modawi SB, et al. Natural history of hepatic sarcoidosis and its response to treatment. Eur J Gastroenterol Hepatol 2006;18: 721–6.
13. Casavilla FA, Gordon R, Wright HI, et al. Clinical course after liver transplantation in patients with sarcoidosis. Ann Intern Med 1993;118:865–6.
14. Lipson EJ, Fiel MI, Florman SS, et al. Patient and graft outcomes following liver transplantation for sarcoidosis. Clin Transplant 2005;19:487–91.
15. Makhlouf HR, Ishak KG, Goodman ZD. Epithelioid hemangioendothelioma of the liver: a clinicopathologic study of 137 cases. Cancer 1999;85:562–82.
16. Mehrabi A, Kashfi A, Fonouni H, et al. Primary malignant hepatic epithelioid hemangioendothelioma: a comprehensive review of the literature with emphasis on the surgical therapy. Cancer 2006;107: 2108–21.
17. Mentzel T, Beham A, Calonje E, et al. Epithelioid hemangioendothelioma of skin and soft tissues: clinicopathologic and immunohistochemical study of 30 cases. Am J Surg Pathol 1997;21:363–74.
18. Lerut JP, Orlando G, Adam R, et al. The place of liver transplantation in the treatment of hepatic epitheloid hemangioendothelioma: report of the European liver transplant registry. Ann Surg 2007;246: 949–57.
19. Rodriguez JA, Becker NS, O'Mahony CA, et al. Long-term outcomes following liver transplantation for hepatic hemangioendothelioma: the UNOS experience from 1987 to 2005. J Gastrointest Surg 2008;12: 110–6.
20. Modlin IM, Oberg K, Chung DC, et al. Gastroenteropancreatic neuroendocrine tumours. Lancet Oncol 2008;9:61–72.
21. Ramage JK, Davies AH, Ardill J, et al. Guidelines for the management of gastroenteropancreatic neuroendocrine (including carcinoid) tumours. Gut 2005;54 (Suppl 4):iv1–16.
22. Lehnert T. Liver transplantation for metastatic neuroendocrine carcinoma: an analysis of 103 patients. Transplantation 1998;66:1307–12.
23. Le Treut YP, Gregoire E, Belghiti J, et al. Predictors of long-term survival after liver transplantation for metastatic endocrine tumors: an 85-case French multicentric report. Am J Transplant 2008;8: 1205–13.
24. Lerut JP, Weber M, Orlando G, et al. Vascular and rare liver tumors: a good indication for liver transplantation? J Hepatol 2007;47:466–75.
25. Bioulac-Sage P, Laumonier H, Laurent C, et al. Benign and malignant vascular tumors of the liver in adults. Semin Liver Dis 2008;28:302–14.
26. Yoon SS, Charny CK, Fong Y, et al. Diagnosis, management, and outcomes of 115 patients with hepatic hemangioma. J Am Coll Surg 2003;197: 392–402.
27. Gunay-Aygun M. Liver and kidney disease in ciliopathies. Am J Med Genet C Semin Med Genet 2009;151C:296–306.
28. Everson GT, Taylor MR, Doctor RB. Polycystic disease of the liver. Hepatology 2004;40:774–82.
29. De Kerckhove L, De Meyer M, Verbaandert C, et al. The place of liver transplantation in Caroli's disease and syndrome. Transpl Int 2006;19: 381–8.
30. Millwala F, Segev DL, Thuluvath PJ. Caroli's disease and outcomes after liver transplantation. Liver Transpl 2008;14:11–7.
31. Hoppe B, Beck BB, Milliner DS. The primary hyperoxalurias. Kidney Int 2009;75:1264–71.
32. Jamieson NV. A 20-year experience of combined liver/kidney transplantation for primary hyperoxaluria (PH1): the European PH1 transplant registry experience 1984–2004. Am J Nephrol 2005;25:282–9.

33. Monteiro E, Freire A, Barroso E. Familial amyloid polyneuropathy and liver transplantation. J Hepatol 2004;41:188–94.
34. Herlenius G, Wilczek HE, Larsson M, et al. Ten years of international experience with liver transplantation for familial amyloidotic polyneuropathy: results from the Familial Amyloidotic Polyneuropathy World Transplant Registry. Transplantation 2004;77: 64–71.
35. Grazi GL, Cescon M, Salvi F, et al. Combined heart and liver transplantation for familial amyloidotic neuropathy: considerations from the hepatic point of view. Liver Transpl 2003;9:986–92.

14 Liver Transplantation in HIV patients

Marion G. Peters[1] *and Peter G. Stock*[2]

Departments of [1]Medicine and [2]Surgery, University of California at San Francisco, San Francisco, CA, USA

Key learning points

- Human immunodeficiency virus (HIV) patients with decompensated liver disease should be considered for liver transplantation (LT).
- Specific selection criteria exist for HIV patients with decompensated liver disease.
- There are multiple drug–drug interactions in HIV patients, especially post LT with calcineurin inhibitors.
- Coinfection with HCV represents a considerable challenge in the post-transplant management of HIV patients.

Introduction

Since the introduction and widespread use of highly active antiretroviral therapy (HAART), HIV-positive patients are now living longer. Unfortunately they are developing comorbidities related to co-infection with viral hepatitis and complications of HIV disease and HAART. In particular, viral hepatitis with cirrhosis and its complications has become a major health problem, with liver disease being the leading cause of non-AIDS-related death among viral hepatitis co-infected patients.[1] When patients develop decompensated liver disease with HIV, LT is now accepted as part of the management strategy. Much of the care of HIV patients, both pre and post transplantation, is similar to that of non-HIV patients. However there are special issues that pertain to the care of the HIV patient and this chapter will address these issues.

End-stage liver disease in individuals with HIV

Scope of the problem

Worldwide there are approximately 40 million individuals living with HIV. As noted earlier, liver disease is the second most common cause of death in HIV patients from North America, Western Europe and Australia.[1] The deaths are mainly due to viral hepatitis B (HBV) and C (HCV). Co-infection with HBV occurs in about 10% of HIV-infected individuals but is higher in areas of high endemicity of HBV, such as sub-Saharan Africa and Asia.[2] Co-infection with HCV occurs in about 20% of HIV-infected individuals. Rates of co-infection vary depending upon the population studied; they are much higher in certain transmission groups, such as hemophiliacs and intravenous drug users.

Cirrhosis in HIV patients

Progression of liver fibrosis is more rapid in HIV-infected individuals with viral hepatitis.[3] It is important to note the alanine aminotransferase (ALT) is not a good marker of liver disease in HIV patients and significant liver fibrosis has been reported in up to 25–40% of co-infected patients with normal ALT. "Silent" cirrhosis has been reported in nearly 15% of HIV patients infected with viral hepatitis.[4] The time to decompensated cirrhosis and survival after development of decompensated liver disease is shorter in co-infected patients than in non-HIV patients with

Medical Care of the Liver Transplant Patient, Fourth Edition. Edited by Pierre-Alain Clavien, James F. Trotter.

viral hepatitis, with a mean of 13 months in one study.[5] Management of variceal hemorrhage, ascites and hepatic encephalopathy are similar to the HIV-negative individual.[6]

All cirrhotic patients should have imaging performed at least yearly to rule out hepatocellular carcinoma (HCC). HCC occurs more frequently in HIV patients than in HIV-negative patients. If HIV patients acquire HCC, they should be offered all conventional therapies, including transplant. Upper endoscopy should be routine in all cirrhotic patients to evaluate for esophageal varices and treat as appropriate with nonselective beta-blockers. HIV patients with ascites should have prophylaxis for spontaneous bacterial peritonitis with weekly ciprofloxacin 750 mg or daily co-trimoxazole. The choice of prophylaxis depends upon what other drugs the patient is taking and if any sulfa allergies exist. Many HIV patients experience diarrhea due to HAART and may not tolerate lactulose therapy for hepatic encephalopathy. These patients would benefit from zinc and rifaximin therapy.

Hepatotoxicity

Co-infected patients are more likely to develop drug toxicity than HIV patients without viral hepatitis.[2] Studies of hepatotoxicity in HIV patients have shown higher rates in patients with viral hepatitis B and C.[7] When HCV is successfully treated, there is clearance of HCV, regression of liver fibrosis,[8] and a reduced risk of antiretroviral-related hepatotoxicity.[9] It is often difficult to determine which drug is involved in HIV patients on multiple medications. HAART itself consists of many medications and HIV patients are usually on other drugs for HIV-related illnesses or HAART-related complications. Currently, drug-induced liver injury is largely a diagnosis of exclusion, thus there may be multiple drug candidates to consider in evaluating hepatotoxicity in HIV patients. It may be due to HAART, therapy for other infections (anti-TB, antifungal and antibiotics), neuropsychiatric medications, nonsteroidal anti-inflammatory drugs (NSAIDs) or over-the-counter medications. It is critical that physicians probe the patient to determine all prescribed medications as well as over-the-counter medications, alternative therapies, and herbal remedies.

All classes of antiretrovirals have been associated with some hepatotoxicity and overall 6.2% of patients have grade 3 or 4 toxicity.[10] Nucleoside reverse transcriptase inhibitors (NRTIs) are associated with mitochondrial toxicity, steatosis, hyperlactatemia, and lactic acidosis. The triad of mitochondrial toxicity, steatosis, and lactic acidosis can present as an acute, severe syndrome. The relative risk is increased by 3.7 if the patient has either HCV or HBV co-infection. More commonly, a chronic low-grade hyperlactatemia is observed. This is manifest by normal lactate (<5 mmol/L), lack of acidosis, and an asymptomatic state. The degree of inhibition of DNA polymerase γ correlates with the hepatotoxicity most commonly associated with the use of stavudine, didanosine, and zalcitabine. This toxicity is less commonly associated with abacavir, zidovudine, and lamivudine.

Non-nucleoside reverse transcriptase inhibitors (NNRTIs) are associated with hepatotoxicity. Nevirapine has been associated with immune-mediated hepatotoxicity with severe allergic reactions such as Stevens–Johnson syndrome or toxic epidermal necrolysis and death.[5] At particularly high risk are pregnant patients and patients with high CD4 counts. There appears to be no agreement on the value of drug levels in predicting nevirapine toxicity, but toxicity is increased in patients co-infected with viral hepatitis.[10]

Protease inhibitors have been reported to cause hepatotoxicity.[11] Severe hepatotoxicity (ALT >5 times upper limit of normal) has been noted with tipranavir, indinavir and lopinavir (with or without ritonavir boosting). Indinavir and atazanavir are also associated with increased unconjugated bilirubin, which is not liver toxicity but inhibition of glucuronyl transferase: this is not a reason to stop HAART. It is important to remember that toxicity is higher in patients with elevated baseline ALT or with viral hepatitis. The Food and Drug Administration (FDA) states that the combination of ALT >3 times the upper limit of normal with total bilirubin >1.5 times the upper limit of normal is an indicator for clinical concern (see www.fda.gov/downloads/drugs/scienceresearch/researchareas/ucm091457.pdf).

Selection criteria for LT

As a result of the exacerbation of liver fibrosis in co-infected HIV patients, there are increasing numbers of patients who develop ESLD and present for evaluation for LT. The severity of liver disease should be assessed in the same manner as with HIV-negative patients and similar criteria are used for listing. The probability of survival of a patient with ESLD on the waiting list is predicted by the Model for End-stage Liver Disease (MELD) scoring system.[12] This score is used in the allocation process of all patients awaiting LT including HIV patients. Unfortunately, HIV-infected candidates may deteriorate at a lower MELD score than their HIV-uninfected counterparts,[5] thus HIV patients and their providers need to consider other options to increase the chance of transplantation with lower MELD scores. These include the use of "higher risk" donors or living donors. While all transplant centers encourage early referral to decrease the high death rate of HIV-infected liver transplant candidates while on the waiting list, alternative methods are still in development to obtain LT early in order to optimally benefit the HIV patient.

Pre-LT management of HIV patient with viral hepatitis

In patients with HBV co-infection, the use of two anti-HBV drugs is now the standard of care for HIV patients.[2] Most HIV patients are HBeAg positive and require life-long therapy, both pre and post LT. More than 80% have lamivudine-resistant HBV and are co-infected patients, but lamivudine is no longer first-line therapy. With the advent of high potency anti-HBV nucleotide analogs (tenofovir and entecavir) most patients will have undetectable HBV DNA prior to LT. The presence of viral hepatitis increases the chance of hepatotoxicity as noted earlier. If patients stop HBV therapy they may develop life-threatening flares of HBV. Patients treated with HAART that does not include anti-HBV drugs (rare nowadays) can develop severe immune reconstitution when CD4 counts improve. Because the majority of anti-HBV drugs also have anti-HIV activity, they must be taken as part of HAART and cannot be used in isolation.

For those co-infected with HCV pre LT, interferon and ribavirin therapy can be used in stable cirrhotics,[2] however the response rate is lower than seen in monoinfected HCV patients. When the patient develops decompensated liver disease, therapy is not an option, as patients with ESLD are less able to tolerate interferon and ribavirin. More investigation is required to improve outcomes of HIV/HCV co-infected patients pre and post LT. Large prospective studies are needed to assess this challenging group of transplant candidates. The large cooperative effort of 17 centers, sponsored by the University of California at San Francisco (UCSF) and supported by the National Institute of Allergy and Infectious Diseases (NIAID)/National Institutes of Health (NIH), has aimed to evaluate the safety and efficacy of solid-organ transplantation in people with HIV disease. This prospective, multi-center cohort study looks at HIV-infected patients who undergo kidney and LT (www.HIVtransplant.com). Data from this NIH multicenter trial of LT recipients show that patients with HCV have a poorer outcome if ESLD is associated with renal disease or low body mass index (www.HIVtransplant.com).

Candidacy for transplant in HIV-infected recipient

Careful interaction of hepatologists with HIV physicians is critical to ensure that the patient is a candidate from an HIV point of view.[5] Exclusion criteria include progressive multifocal leukoencephalopathy (PML), chronic cryptosporidiosis, drug-resistant fungal infections and visceral Kaposi sarcoma. CD4 counts are required to be at least 100/mm^3 for listing for LT. These CD4 counts are lower than required for renal transplantation as many cirrhotic patients have portal hypertension and hypersplenism. Poorer outcomes are noted in patients unable to tolerate post-transplant HIV medication. This may be difficult to ascertain if pre-transplant HAART is stopped pre transplantation, when ALT becomes more elevated because of concern for hepatotoxicity. If the patient is not taking HAART, the assessment of liver transplant candidacy may be more difficult. HIV resistance testing is particularly useful in this situation.

Postoperative management

Immunosuppression

Initially it was thought that patients with HIV would require less immunosuppression because of an already immunocompromised state. In fact liver transplant studies demonstrated similar acute rejection rates in HIV-infected and HIV-uninfected recipients.[5] Interestingly, in the HIV-infected kidney transplant recipients, a significantly higher incidence of rejection has been seen as compared to HIV-negative recipients, suggestive of a dysregulated immune system rather than immune deficiency.

The majority of centers utilize standard maintenance immunosuppression with steroids, mycophenylate (MMF), and a calcineurin inhibitor (CNI). MMF has virostatic as well as antiproliferative action. The anti-HIV action is thought to result from the depletion of guanoside nucleosides required for the completion of the virus lifecycle, and the inhibition of immune activation and cellular proliferation. Both calcineurin inhibitors, cyclosporine (CsA) and tacrolimus have well-documented anti-retroviral effects, thought to be due to selective inhibition of infected cell growth and interference with the function of HIV proteins, leading to reduction of HIV production. Both CNI and protease inhibitors (PIs), used in HAART regimens, are known to be diabetogenic, which may exacerbate post-transplant glucose control. Since many HIV-infected transplant patients experience some degree of renal insufficiency, sirolimus, a target of rapamycin (TOR) inhibitor and an anti-proliferative agent has been used instead of calcineurin inhibitors. Sirolimus also exerts some antiretroviral activity. This HIV effect occurs via suppression of T-cell activation and professional antigen presenting cell function, and disruption of infective HIV replication. In addition, sirolimus decreases the expression of CCR5 receptors on monocytes and lymphocytes, which may have additional benefit by inhibiting viral entry. Sirolimus has been shown to benefit patients with Kaposi's sarcoma (KS) post-transplant through inhibition of vascular endothelial growth factor (VEGF). Maintenance of adequate CNI levels can be difficult in patients on NNRTIs, because induction of the cytochrome P450 system by NNRTIs leads to lower CNI levels. In contrast, PIs lead to potent inhibition of the cytochrome P450 system, which leads to CNI toxicity without prompt dose adjustment. Thus, great care and attention are required in dosing and adjusting immunosuppression in HIV patients, as a change in immunosuppression or HAART may lead to under or over-immunosuppression with potential life-threatening consequences.

For the HIV-positive liver transplant recipients, induction therapy with lymphodepleting agents has not been necessary, based on the ability to control rejection with standard maintenance agents. Early experience with lymphocyte depletion following LT in HIV-infected recipients resulted in severe bacterial sepsis, and the use of these induction agents is strongly discouraged in the postoperative period. The use of anti-IL25 monoclonal induction agents has not been utilized in most liver transplant protocols, as adequate control of rejection can be achieved with calcineurin inhibitors and mycophenolate mofetil.

Strategies for HAART

HIV patients who are selected for transplantation are required to have stable HIV disease.[5] Post-transplant control is usually achieved by maintaining recipients on the pre-LT regimen if they had controlled, stable HIV disease pre LT. Post transplantation, HIV recipients do not show progression of their HIV to AIDS. Those patients who were not on HAART as a result of hepatotoxicity require HIV resistance testing and input from HIV physicians to determine the appropriate post-LT HAART regimen. After transplantation, HAART is usually not started until postoperative days 4–7, when immunosuppression doses are more stable. If any toxicity of HAART occurs, all HAART must be stopped at the same time to avoid emergence of HIV drug-resistant strains. When HAART is stopped, it is critical to adjust immunosuppression accordingly to avoid over- or underimmunosuppression as noted eariler. HAART may be stopped post LT for several weeks, without little increase in HIV viral load or change in CD4 T-cell count. If HAART must be stopped for a toxic event, HIV physician input is required to choose a new, different HAART regimen.

Pharmacokinetic interactions

This is a difficult and complicated issue in HIV patients post transplantation. It is clear that patients with HIV have complicated pharmacokinetic interactions that lead to substantial changes in most drug plasma levels. These changes can lead to toxic side effects, organ rejection or breakthrough of HIV disease. For this reason, intensive monitoring and titration of drug levels must be undertaken. CNIs inhibit both membrane efflux transporters and the cytochrome P450 system. Inhibition of P-glycoprotein (P-gp) and CYP3A4 activity leads to increased intestinal uptake, decreased hepatic metabolism and excretion of both CNIs and PIs. NNRTIs induce CYP3A4 activity and decrease CNI levels. CsA doses in HIV patients on protease inhibitors are 20% of the dose required for the HIV-negative post-transplant patient, and even less if the regimen is boosted with ritonavir. Similarly, the doses of tacrolimus and sirolimus that achieve adequate blood levels are decreased more than fivefold, and for those patients on tacrolimus (FK) or sirolimus, not only is the required CNI dose markedly decreased, but the dosing interval increased more than fivefold.[5] HIV patients may also require antifungals (e.g. fluconazole) or macrolide antibiotics (e.g. clarithromycin and azithromycin), which further inhibit the CYP3A4 system.

If proton pump inhibitors (PPIs) are taken in conjunction with steroids, the absorption and plasma concentration of atazanavir may be reduced. Indeed patients on PPIs may need ritonavir boosting with atazanavir, thus careful monitoring and knowledge of the effects of all HIV and liver transplant medications are required to find the best treatment of both HIV and immunosuppression of the liver graft. Assistance from and team interaction with hepatologists, HIV physicians, and pharmacologists are optimal in managing these challenging patients.

HBV management

Control of HBV post LT has been revolutionized by the use of hepatitis B immune globulin (HBIg) and potent nucleoside analogs. This has led to HBV having one of the best outcomes post LT in monoinfected patients.[13] Co-infected patients also have good outcomes post LT. As noted earlier, HIV- and HBV-infected patients require two anti-HBV medications as part of HAART.[2] Lamivudine resistance is almost universal and the majority of nucleoside analogs have anti-HIV activity. This represents a special challenge as all HAART must be started or stopped at the same time. For this reason HAART is usually initiated as soon as possible post transplant in these patients in order to have adequate anti-HBV activity. Appropriate dose adjustment for renal insufficiency is required for all nucleoside analogs. Currently approved medications for the treatment of chronic HBV are alpha interferons, adefovir, entecavir, lamivudine, telbivudine, and tenofovir. Emtricitabine is approved for HIV therapy with tenofovir and has anti-HBV activity similar to lamivudine. Successful prevention of HBV recurrence post transplantation can be achieved in HIV/HBV co-infected patients with prophylactic therapy consisting of HBIg, and dual therapy with lamivudine or emtricitabine and tenofovir. In these patients, HBIg therapy is administered indefinitely, at doses depending upon antibody titers.

HCV management

As noted earlier, liver disease is now the leading cause of death in HIV/HCV-infected patients and HCV remains the most common reason for LT in all patient studies.[5] Unfortunately, unlike the successful experience with HIV/HBV transplant patients, rapid recurrence of HCV post LT continues to be a major problem in HIV/HCV recipients for reasons that are not well defined. The timing and effectiveness of antiviral therapy for HCV in these patients is not yet clear. Some studies show successful control of HCV recurrence using post-transplantation administration of interferon and ribavirin therapy, while others do not.[5] Routine liver biopsies are often performed to monitor patients post transplantation. Interferon and ribavirin therapy should be administered when there is histologic evidence of progressive fibrosis in HCV/HIV patients.

Pharmacokinetics and hepatotoxicity in these patients are special challenges for their management post LT. CsA has both anti-HIV and anti-HCV activity. Many centers recommend CsA over tacrolimus for immunosuppression therapy for this reason. Steroid boluses can increase HCV RNA and perhaps exacerbate liver disease and should be avoided if possible in HIV/HCV co-infected recipients. In contrast to the deleterious effects of LT on HCV, there have been several reports on spontaneous clearance of HCV in HCV/HIV co-infected patients, both before and after transplantation. Further study of this fascinating outcome is critical to understanding the interaction of both viruses post LT and to aid in the management of HIV/HCV co-infected patients.

Immunizing HIV patients

Immunization of HIV patients is the same as for HIV-negative patients. All patients (HIV positive and negative) require immunization against pneumococcal, hepatitis A and B prior to transplantation and initiation of immunosuppression. Any adult patients who have not been exposed to chicken pox should not receive the varicella vaccine, but immunoglobulin G treatment after exposure. Household contacts of LT patients should be advised not to receive any live-attenuated vaccines such as oral polio or smallpox inoculations.

Prophylaxis for opportunistic infection

All LT patients require prophylaxis for cytomegalovirus, fungal infections and *Pneumocystitis carinii* pneumonia in the early post-LT period. HIV patients also require prophylaxis for *Mycobacterium avium* complex (MAC) when CD4 counts drop below 75 cells/μl.

HIV-associated malignancy risks in the transplant recipient

All LT patients have an increased risk of cancer associated with immunosuppression; this is increased in HIV recipients. All LT recipients remain at risk for skin cancers and monitoring is essential. Lung, liver, and stomach cancers are increased post LT but not further increased in HIV patients. There appear to be increased rates of brain and testicular cancer post LT in HIV-infected patients,[5] thus routine post-LT care of HIV-infected patients must include screening for cancers including malignancies particular to HIV, those common in the aging population, and those seen in all transplant recipients.

HIV-infected patients are at risk for specific cancers: AIDS-related cancers, Kaposi sarcoma (KS) and non-Hodgkin lymphoma (NHL) are associated with an immunodeficient state. Since the advent of HAART, the prevalence of these cancers has declined. Viral-mediated cancers such as cervical, anal, and liver cancer are noted to be higher in HIV patients pre LT. Whether this is increased post LT is unclear, nor is it clear whether immunosuppression leads to progression of human papillomavirus (HPV)-mediated anal and cervical lesions. HIV patients have a tenfold increased risk of these cancers and require routine screening both pre and post LT. The UCSF screening guidelines recommend that these patients should be screened with Papanicolaou (Pap) test smears of the cervix and/or anal canal annually. This is followed with repeat smears, and colposcopy and/or anoscopy depending on the stage of the lesion (www.analcancerinfo.ucsf.edu).

Summary

Progression of HIV disease following LT and immunosuppression has not been a significant issue. Patients undergoing LT for HIV/HBV co-infection have similar patient and graft survival rates as compared to the HBV mono-infected cohort as a result of the ability to control HBV post transplant.

Recurrence of hepatitis C has been problematic, with poorer overall survival as compared to HCV mono-infected patients. Nonetheless, there have been several HIV/HCV co-infected patients who have cleared HCV post transplant, and this may in part be related to the administration of anti-retroviral therapy. Pharmacokinetic interactions between the anti-retrovirals and the immunosuppressive agents need close attention to avoid life-threatening toxicities. Finally, the development of HPV-mediated cancers may be problematic in the HIV co-infected liver transplant recipient, and anal and cervical Paps should be performed annually. HIV co-infection should no longer be a contraindication for LT in recipients with well-controlled HIV disease.

Acknowledgments

Authors were supported in part by the Solid Organ Transplantation in HIV: Multi-Site Study (A1052748) and Women's Interagency HIV Study (U02 AI034 989), funded by the National Institute of Allergy and Infectious Diseases.

References

1. Weber R, Sabin CA, Friis-Moller N, et al. Liver-related deaths in persons infected with the human immunode-

ficiency virus: the D:A:D study. Arch Intern Med 2006;166:1632–41.

2. Koziel MJ, Peters MG. Viral hepatitis in HIV infection. N Engl J Med 2007;356:1445–54.
3. Martin-Carbonero L, Benhamou Y, Puoti M, et al. Incidence and predictors of severe liver fibrosis in human immunodeficiency virus-infected patients with chronic hepatitis C: a European collaborative study. Clin Infect Dis 2004;38:128–33.
4. Sterling RK, Contos MJ, Sanyal AJ, et al. The clinical spectrum of hepatitis C virus in HIV coinfection. J Acquir Immune Defic Syndr 2003;32:30–7.
5. Tan-Tam CC, Frassetto LA, Stock PG. Liver and kidney transplantation in HIV-infected patients. AIDS Rev 2009;11:190–204.
6. Peters MG. End-stage liver disease in HIV disease. Top HIV Med 2009;17:124–8.
7. Sulkowski MS, Thomas DL, Chaisson RE, Moore RD. Hepatotoxicity associated with antiretroviral therapy in adults infected with human immunodeficiency virus and the role of hepatitis C or B virus infection. JAMA 2000;283:74–80.
8. Soriano V, Labarga P, Ruiz-Sancho A, Garcia-Samaniego J, Barreiro P. Regression of liver fibrosis in hepatitis C virus/HIV-co-infected patients after treatment with pegylated interferon plus ribavirin. AIDS 2006;20: 2225–7.
9. Uberti-Foppa C, De Bona A, Morsica G, et al. Pretreatment of chronic active hepatitis C in patients coinfected with HIV and hepatitis C virus reduces the hepatotoxicity associated with subsequent antiretroviral therapy. J Acquir Immune Defic Syndr 2003;33: 146–52.
10. Sulkowski MS. Management of hepatic complications in HIV-infected persons. J Infect Dis 2008;197(Suppl 3):S279–93.
11. Sulkowski MS, Mehta SH, Chaisson RE, Thomas DL, Moore RD. Hepatotoxicity associated with protease inhibitor-based antiretroviral regimens with or without concurrent ritonavir. AIDS 2004;18:2277–84.
12. Kamath PS, Kim WR. The model for end-stage liver disease (MELD). Hepatology 2007;45:797–805.
13. Kim WR, Poterucha JJ, Kremers WK, Ishitani MB, Dickson ER. Outcome of liver transplantation for hepatitis B in the United States. Liver Transpl 2004;10: 968–74.

15 Living-donor liver transplantation

Robert S. Brown Jr
Center for Liver Diseases and Transplantation, Columbia University College of Physicians and Surgeons, New York, NY, USA

Key learning points

- Living-donor liver transplantation (LDLT) is frequently used in Asian countries, where deceased donors are scarce, but comprise <10% of transplant activity in most countries in the West.
- Though the risk of mortality for the living liver donor is <1%, it is higher than for kidney donors and there is significant morbidity, which may temper interest in LDLT.
- When it is performed in experienced centers, LDLT decreases the waiting list and overall mortality rate from the time of listing.
- Protection of donor safety and autonomy is of paramount importance and requires a dedicated donor team.
- Optimal application of LDLT in patients with HCV and HCC is evolving as the pre-transplant therapy for these diseases improves.

Introduction

The first adult-to-adult LDLT was performed in Hong Kong in 1993. The first LDLT was performed in the USA in 1998 and was followed by a rapid increase in utilization, which peaked in 2001. Currently, over 90 centers in the USA have performed at least one LDLT, though most procedures are done in a smaller number of larger volume centers. In other parts of the world where deceased-donor transplant is unavailable or severely limited, particularly Asia, virtually all transplant centers perform LDLT for the majority of transplant procedures. The majority of LDLTs are for adults using right-lobe grafts, though interest in using smaller left-lobe grafts has persisted due to improved donor safety and acceptance. Right hepatectomy almost always provides the recipient with sufficient hepatic mass to replace the cirrhotic liver while still leaving the donor with enough functioning hepatocytes. In 2000 there was great enthusiasm for adult LDLT, with 49 centers performing at least one LDLT. The enthusiasm was quickly tempered by the death of a donor in January 2002, the second reported death of an adult living transplant donor in the USA.

The current author and colleagues previously reported that 76% of liver transplant programs that had not performed LDLT planned on starting a program, but since then the climate for living donation had changed.[1] From 2001–2006, the number of centers performing LDLT and the number of procedures declined, though it appears to have stabilized at ~250/cases per year, about half of the peak in 2001[2] (Figure 15.1).

There are several possible reasons why the number of centers performing LDLT and the total number of LDLTs performed has declined beyond reticence following the donor deaths. The changes in organ allocation system to a Model for End-stage Liver Disease (MELD)-based allocation system with priority for HCC have decreased waiting list mortality, which was a major driver of need for LDLT. Second, recognized complication rates in donor and recipient may have created increased reticence among donors and recipients to proceed with LDLT, especially when there was no perceived survival benefit to LDLT.

Medical Care of the Liver Transplant Patient, Fourth Edition. Edited by Pierre-Alain Clavien, James F. Trotter.

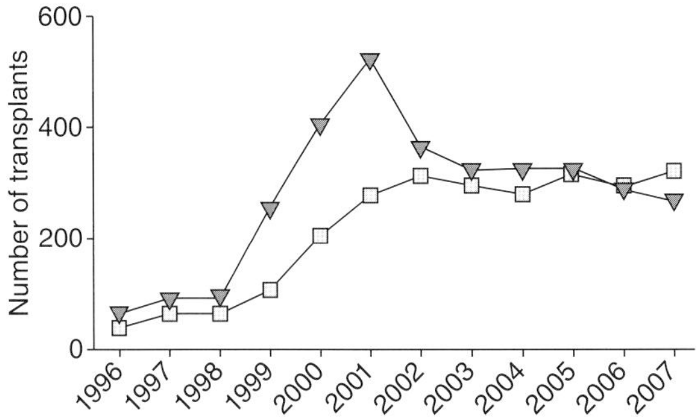

Figure 15.1 Evolution of living donor liver transplantation in Europe and the USA. ■ European data from the European Liver Transplant Registry. ▼ US data from the Organ Procurement and Transplantation Network[3]

Finally, the increased use of extended-criteria donor (ECD) livers, which includes those from older donors (over 60–70 years old), donation after cardiac death (DCD, formerly called nonheart-beating donors), and liver with steatosis or exposure to/infection with hepatitis B or C, has allowed an alternate to LDLT for those who wanted expedited transplantation. Worldwide the number and volume of centers performing LDLT has continued to grow, highlighting that demand for the procedure has not changed.

In the USA over 2000 LDLTs have been performed and four early deaths and two liver transplants have occurred in adult living liver donors. There have been several additional late deaths though these were not clearly related to donation. After the second donor death, a number of position papers, conferences, and review boards took place.[4–6] Similar rates of death have been reported worldwide[7–8] and questions have been raised about the quality of reporting of donor outcomes.[9–10] New York State created a review committee and document mandating guidelines for transplant centers and physicians who perform LDLT.[6]

The United Network for Organ Sharing (UNOS) now collects 2-year follow-up data on all donors and has developed standards for evaluating programs as well as resource documents to help standardize the donor consent and evaluation processes. Additionally, a more detailed study of LDLT, A2ALL, is an NIH-sponsored multicenter prospective study of LDLT at nine centers in the USA and Canada. The study has now been renewed and has followed LDLT candidates and controls for over 7 years. This group has published excellent recipient outcomes including a survival benefit for candidates on the waiting list who pursue LDLT[11] as well as quantifying donor risk and outcomes. A2ALL will continue for an additional 5 years to collect long-term data on donors and recipients that will further guide our decision-making process.

Selection of LDLT recipient candidates

Currently in the USA, most programs require that recipients considered for LDLT should fulfill the same criteria established for deceased-donor liver transplantation (DDLT). Some transplant physicians and surgeons believe that LDLT should be extended to patients not felt to be candidates for deceased-donor grafts, e.g. those with metastatic tumors and acute alcoholic hepatitis. This raises an ethical conundrum. The principle of autonomy states donors and recipients should be allowed to make an independent decision even if the risk is prohibitive or a deceased-donor transplant is felt to be contraindicated. In many of these situations, though the outcome for LDLT is worse than for other candidates for the procedure, it is still better than the potential recipient's survival without a transplant. LDLT may be pursued by families when the outcome with transplantation is far less than expected for a standard orthotopic liver transplantation (OLT) (e.g. 1-year survival <50%) or when traditional criteria for the transplant are not met (e.g. 6 months of abstinence from alcohol) but the chance of surviving to and/or obtaining a transplant is virtually nil. In these cases, LDLT clearly offers a survival benefit. The converse is the ethical question of whether it can be justified to expose a healthy donor to risk to perform a transplant that society or the transplant center do not feel is justified with a deceased-donor graft. This is a paternalistic standpoint based on an assumption that the donor cannot reach true informed understanding. When no other options exist, LDLT is perceived as overly coercive to the potential donor.

Most of the problems and concerns stated earlier relate to organ scarcity. If deceased-donor organs were unlimited, many transplants currently viewed as contraindicated might be performed. Emergency nontransplant surgery with expected outcomes of 20–50% in the long term is widely accepted. The current author would propose the following ethical construct: Does the expected outcome justify the procedure with a deceased-donor graft if organs were unlimited? If the answer is "yes", and the candidate would be suitable for a deceased-donor organ at this time, then the candidate is acceptable for LDLT.

The potential recipient who derives the maximal benefit from LDLT is someone who would have a good chance of surviving transplantation if it is carried out immediately but is unlikely to receive a deceased-donor graft prior to dying or becoming too ill due to waiting list priority, age, or other co-morbidities. On the other hand, since the major benefit of LDLT is to reduce waiting time mortality, it is possible that patients may receive LDLT too early in their disease course, negating that survival benefit. Prior to the implementation of MELD, a substantial proportion (43%) of patients undergoing LDLT were UNOS status 3 (i.e. Child Class B and at home) at the time of transplantation, unlike those undergoing DDLT, who were usually Status 2 (i.e. Child Class C or hospitalized with complications of liver disease).[12] During the proliferation of LDLT, the system for organ prioritization in the USA and some other countries has changed from a waiting time-based system to a severity-of-illness system based on the Model for End-stage Liver Disease (MELD) score. The optimal MELD score at which patients undergoing LDLT derive a sustained survival benefit by reducing waiting time mortality that is not offset by post-transplant mortality is yet to be determined. It was initially felt to be >15 in most clinical situations,[13] but now further data suggests that patients with MELD scores above 11 or 12 also derive a benefit from LDLT.[14]

Selection of LDLT donor candidate

The goal of the donor evaluation is to determine if the donor is medically and psychologically suitable for living donation. Equally important, is to ensure that the donor is well informed of the risks and benefits of the procedure and is making an autonomous and noncoerced decision. Most living donors are in excellent health. Although there is no definitive age cutoff, donors are typically between 21 and 55 years old. New York State mandates an upper age limit of 60 years. Donors under 18 are generally felt unacceptable except for an emancipated minor donating to their child.

Donors should not have liver disease or significant co-morbidities, such as coronary artery disease or cerebrovascular disease. The presence of mild systemic disease, such as well-controlled mild hypertension or diet-controlled diabetes, is not necessarily a contraindication to donation. Individuals who are significantly obese, with a body mass index over 35 likely are excluded as living donors in many programs due to fear of postoperative complications or the presence of hepatic steatosis. The current author and colleagues have shown, however, that selected obese donors with BMIs up to 40 can donate safely with good outcomes for both donor and recipient.[15] Because the presence of hepatic steatosis may compromise the function of the graft, some centers perform liver biopsies on all donor candidates, while other centers rely upon physical examination, risk factors for hepatic steatosis, and imaging studies.[16–17]

Potential donor candidates undergo a similar medical evaluation as the recipient with serologic testing for viral hepatitis, HIV antibody, as well as testing for other chronic liver diseases.[17] An independent transplant physician, usually a hepatologist who is not the primary hepatologist of the recipient, should evaluate the LDLT donor candidate. An independent donor advocate who is not part of the transplant team has been recommended by UNOS, the Advisory Council on Transplantation (ACOT) and the New York State Commission. We have an independent donor advocate team (IDAT) that evaluates all donors and meets separately from our recipient selection committee. Evaluation of vascular and biliary anatomy can be achieved non-invasively with CT or MR angiography or invasively with conventional angiography and ECRP. The approach varies from to center to center although most centers use non-invasive methods.[1] All living-donor candidates should undergo a psycho–social evaluation to determine if coercion is present and if they truly understand the risks of the procedure. Between 15–45% of donors who present for evaluation may be suitable candidates who eventually proceed with LDLT.[1,17–19] In the multicenter A2ALL consortium the donor acceptance rate overall was 40% but varied markedly between centers and over time.[19]

Determining if the donor has adequate hepatic mass to provide both a functional graft and remnant is a key component to LDLT evaluation. A graft-to-body-weight ratio (GRBW) of 0.8% has been recommended as the minimum cut-off for the recipient.[16] A GRBW of <0.8% may be associated with impaired liver graft function in the recipient, or small-for-size syndrome characterized by ascites, jaundice, and hepatic congestion, but this is rare with right hepatectomy unless the donor is much smaller than the recipient. Other centers estimate the actual graft volume typically with CT or MRI. There are less clear rules for the minimum left lobe size that remains in the donor, who can also suffer from small-for-size syndrome if the left lobe remnant is inadequate for immediate postoperative metabolic needs. Small-for-size syndrome usually resolves spontaneously over 10–14 d.

Living-donor hepatectomy

The performance of LDLT relies upon an understanding of the vascular and biliary anatomy of the liver. The left lateral lobe consists of Couinaud segments 2 and 3, the median left lobe is Couinaud segment 4, and Couinaud segments 5, 6, 7 and 8 comprise the right hepatic lobe (Figure 15.2). Couinaud segment 1 is the caudate lobe. Most often segments 5–8 or the right hepatic lobe, comprising 50–60% of hepatic volume are resected from the living donor and transplanted into the recipient in adult-to-adult LDLT. In some circumstances, usually when the recipient is

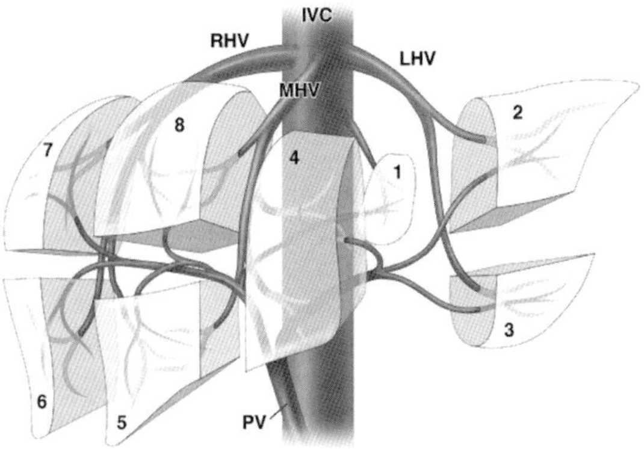

Figure 15.2 Segmental anatomy of the liver using the Couinaud segments

smaller than the donor, the left hepatic lobe (segments 2–4) can be used. For babies, the left lateral segment, comprising segments 2 and 3 or ~20% of hepatic mass are used. In most right-lobe liver donation, the liver is divided to the right of the middle hepatic vein with or without inflow occlusion. Some programs in Asia include the middle hepatic vein in the graft to provide improved outflow and hepatic mass to the recipient but the majority of programs in the USA dictate that the increased risk of small-for-size syndrome in the donor cannot be justified in a healthy person who did not need the operation. The benefit to the recipient of improved graft outflow is not clearly justified by increased risk to the donor. The recipient hepatectomy is usually begun concurrently with the donor operation to minimize cold ischemia time. The biliary anastomosis is established either through a choledochojejunostomy with a Roux-en-Y anastomosis, to the donor's right hepatic duct(s) or a duct-to-duct choledochocholedochostomy between the donor's right hepatic duct and recipient's common bile duct remnant. Because of variations in biliary anatomy, multiple bile duct anastomoses may need to be performed.

The most common complications with LDLT involve the biliary tree. Anomalous biliary anatomy is present in up to 40% of donors.[16] The most common complications reported in donors and recipients are early bile duct leaks and early and late biliary strictures. These complications are more frequent than with whole-graft DDLT. It is now recognized that a learning curve exists with a lower complication rate and improved graft survival over time. In the A2ALL consortium, the rate of biliary complications in the recipients was 30% in the first 20 cases and decreased to 11% thereafter.[20] Vascular complications in the recipient include hepatic artery thrombosis and hepatic venous congestion and are the most common cause of graft loss.[20] Vascular complications in the donor are rare.

Recipient outcomes for LDLT

Impact of severity of disease

It was initially believed that receiving a whole liver is preferable to receiving a partial liver graft, however in experienced living-donor centers, the outcomes for living- and deceased-donor transplantation from the

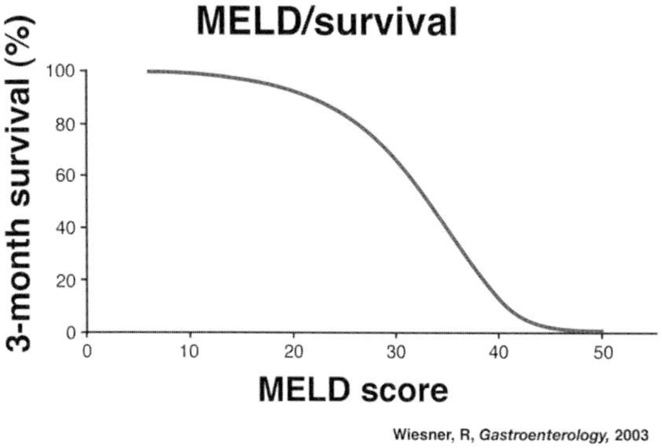

Figure 15.3 The relationship between MELD scores and likelihood of 3-month survival. From Wiesner R, Edwards E, Freeman R, et al. Model for end-stage liver disease (MELD) and allocation of donor livers. Gastroenterology 2003;124:91–6

time of transplant were shown to be equivalent for comparable patient populations at the time of listing.[11] Additionally, because of the organ shortage, most transplant centers do not have the luxury of transplanting all of their patients in need of transplantation with MELD-allocated deceased-donor organs before they die or become too ill. Overall mortality is also driven by pre-transplant deaths on the waiting list and the efficiency of transplant. These factors with post-OLT survival will determine the overall impact of any liver replacement therapy. The waiting list mortality increases in patients with advanced liver disease (Figure 15.3) and patients with a MELD score of 25 have a 20% 3-month mortality rate.[21] There is marked regional variability in MELD at transplant across the UNOS regions[22] and between different countries. Thus, depending on the region, the availability of deceased-donor organs and the average MELD score at the time of transplant, LDLT may offer patients a substantially higher likelihood of transplantation than waiting for a deceased-donor liver.

When assessing a liver transplant candidate for LDLT, the adequacy of a partial graft for transplantation depends on the candidate's severity of liver disease. A balance needs to be struck where the severity of the recipient's liver disease is sufficient to justify transplantation, but not be so advanced that a partial graft will not provide adequate hepatic mass. Although LDLT has been performed in patients with fulminant liver failure and patients with very advanced liver disease (ICU-bound patients or with MELD scores >30), historically, post-transplant survival rates are poor in this group of patients.[23–25] In one series, patient survival was 57% with an average stay of 23 days in the intensive care unit. In comparison, 1-year patient survival is 82% in deceased-donor transplant recipients who were ICU-bound as UNOS status 2A at the time of transplant.[25] This has led most centers in the USA to abandon LDLT in the most severely ill patients with high MELD scores, especially now that they are given high priority on the UNOS waiting list. Since short-term mortality without liver transplantation approaches 100% in these critically ill patients with high MELD scores in areas with low deceased-donor organ availability, the decreased post-transplant survival rates with LDLT may be superior to the alternative of the high mortality on the waiting list, especially as outcomes with LDLT improve. This has led to the use of LDLT in this situation in Asia with good outcomes in some studies.[26]

We do not have an absolute MELD cut-off for LDLT. Decisions on LDLT are made on a case-by-case basis, but in general it is uncommon to proceed with LDLT in patients with MELD scores above 30. A lower limit of MELD score with LDLT is more controversial and varies from center to center. Since for patients with MELD scores <15 and certainly <12, the likelihood of 1 year of survival is *less* with transplant than remaining on the waiting list,[13] some have advocated to not proceed with LDLT in candidates with MELD scores <15. However, in the A2ALL cohort the average MELD score at LDLT was 14, and a survival benefit was seen with longer follow up than 1 year,[11] therefore decisions need to be made on a case-by-case basis. Particular attention needs to be taken in patients with HCV for whom recurrent HCV could decrease life expectancy if a transplant is performed too early in the absence of pre-transplant viral eradication (see later). The current author tends to avoid LDLT at low MELD scores (<12) except in patients with hepatocellular carcinoma (HCC), a suspicious biliary stricture or dysplasia in the setting of primary sclerosing cholangitis, or significant impairment of quality of life (e.g. refractory pruritus or metabolic bone disease in PBC, or difficult-to-control ascites and encephalopathy) is present.

Complications in the living-donor recipient

Biliary and vascular complications are the major complications that occur in the recipient after LDLT, although wound infection, pneumonia and other typical postoperative complications can occur. Biliary complications, either bile leak or stricture at the anastomotic site or cut edge of the transected liver were reported in 15–60% of recipients in most reports.[27–30] The leak rate in the A2ALL study was 31%.[31] Stenting the biliary anastomosis has been used to attempt to reduce the rate of bile leaks and strictures, but it is of unproven benefit. Complications are probably underreported and a standardized reporting system has been recommended for LDLT. Many use the Clavien grading scheme but it may not capture all the necessary elements of LDLT.

Vascular complications include thrombosis of the right hepatic artery at the anastomosis between the recipient and donor artery. Because of the small size of the right hepatic artery, in comparison to the proper hepatic artery in deceased donor liver transplantation, the anastomosis between the recipient's right hepatic artery and donor's right hepatic artery may increase the risk of thrombosis. It has become increasingly recognized that small tributaries 3–5 mm in diameter of the middle hepatic vein that drain segments 5 and 8 should be included in the anastomosis to the recipient hepatic vein or inferior vena cava to prevent hepatic venous congestion of the transplanted right lobe in the recipient.

Postoperatively, regeneration occurs rapidly in the recipient. Initial reports suggested that >85% of hepatic volume was restored 1 week after transplantation.[32] Based on MRI imaging of the abdomen, the left lobe increases in mass by 100% in the donor and the right lobe increases by 87% in the recipient. Subsequent studies, however, suggest regeneration continues over 6 months.[33]

Outcomes for hepatitis C

Hepatitis C remains the most common indication for liver transplant. Early data suggested that patients with HCV who received an LDLT had worse outcomes than did recipients of DDLT.[34–35] These early studies in which LDLT has been associated with increased graft failure have attributed the difference to more rapid HCV progression in the regenerating LDLT graft. Several in vitro studies suggest that dividing hepatocytes are more vulnerable to HCV infection; this could lead to increased levels of viremia, which is seen in cholestatic HCV, in LDLT recipients. This may also have been due to an increased rate of biliary complications or other problems seen during the learning curve of early LDLT experience. It was thought that biliary complications were synergistic in their adverse impact on HCV outcomes, but this has not been supported by subsequent data.[36]

More recent data suggests that there is no difference in recurrent HCV between recipients of DDLT and LDLT. These studies were usually based on protocol biopsies and included a later experience with LDLT. In a study of 23 LDLT recipients and 53 of DDLT, protocol biopsies at 6 and 12 months were compared for inflammation and fibrosis and there was no difference in mean inflammation scores or fibrosis at any of the time points measured.[37] Of the recipients of DDLT, 21% suffered acute rejection compared to 14% of the LDLT recipients; this difference was not statistically significant. Graft and patient survival rates between the two groups were similar: at 48 months, 82 and 82% for DDLT patients and 76 and 79% for LDLT patients (P = NS). Results from this study, which looked at liver histology do not support the idea that recurrent HCV is more prevalent among recipients of LDLT. Additional studies have also concluded that rates of HCV recurrence are not different among recipients of LDLT.[12,37]

The A2ALL data on HCV comparing 181 HCV-positive LDLT recipients to 94 HCV-positive DDLT recipients[38]showed similar patient survival but a lower 3-year graft survival in LDLT recipients than in DDLT recipients (68% compared to 80%, $P = 0.04$).

Center experience was a confounder on the relationship between donor type and outcome. Once the center had performed 20 cases, graft survival was equivalent between DDLT and LDLT recipients. For centers performing <20 LDLTs, the 3-year graft survival was only 55% compared to 79% and 80% for centers performing >20 LDLTs and DDLTs, respectively. There was equivalent and excellent patient survival rate between centers performing >20 LDLTs and DDLTs as well: 91% and 87%, respectively. Unfortunately, the majority of patients studied in the retrospective arm of the A2ALL group did not have protocol liver biopsies. Of the 63 patients who were biopsied, there was no difference in total necroinflammatory or fibrosis scores between DDLT and LDLT at 1 year post transplant, thus the majority of recent data suggests that outcomes for HCV are similar for LDLT and DDLT at experienced centers and HCV is an acceptable indication for LDLT.

Outcomes for HCC

Prior to the implementation of MELD-based allocation in the USA, a large proportion of LDLTs were performed for HCC.[39] Long waiting times and high rates of drop-out on the list made LDLT the only viable option for many patients. Currently, the increased MELD priority (to 22 points with additional points every 3 months) given to patients who meet the Milan (T2) criteria, i.e. with a single lesion ≤5 cm or 2–3 lesions each measuring <3 cm, provides access to DDLT for many patients who meet these criteria. Patients just outside these criteria (e.g. those between the Milan and the more expanded, UCSF criteria) will typically have very long wait list times that make transplant unfeasible. In some regions and many places outside the USA, even patients within Milan criteria may have a 9–12-month wait for DDLT. LDLT therefore remains an important option for the treatment of HCC, particularly in situations where the risk of disease progression on the wait list is substantial.

Although it seems obvious that patients with HCC would benefit from earlier transplant and thus LDLT, data to date has not supported superior outcomes or lower recurrence with LDLT compared to DDLT. Much of this may have to do with differences between LDLT and DDLT recipients and study design. One retrospective study looked at outcomes of transplant in 43 living-donor recipients and compared them to the outcomes of 17 deceased-donor recipients.[40] All of these patients met Milan or UCSF (solitary tumor <6.5 cm or ≥3 tumor nodules, each measuring <4.5 cm with a total maximum size of <8 cm) criteria. The MELD scores, Child Pugh Turcotte (CPT) scores, and etiology of liver disease and tumor stage in the explant were comparable in both groups, but there were more patients with Child's A or MELD <10 in the LDLT group. Of the LDLT group, 10 out of 40 (25%) of recipients underwent a salvage transplant after resection or ablation compared to one out of 12 (8%) of the patients who received a DDLT. Tumor recurrence developed in 10 out of 43 (23%) LDLT patients and none of 17 DDLT patients.

Multivariate analysis revealed that salvage transplant (relative risk (RR) 5.2) and tumor outside of UCSF criteria (RR 4.1), but not LDLT, were the only independent predictors of disease recurrence. This study is limited by the small sample size and the fact that despite the similarities in gross staging, the patients differed in terms of prior therapy and microscopic disease, suggesting that more aggressive tumors were disproportionately undergoing LDLT. The authors conclude that the higher recurrence rate seen in LDLT is due to confounding by more advanced disease.

The A2ALL group has also studied LDLT in the setting of HCC. A total of 106 patients were studied retrospectively: 58 LDLT and 34 DDLT recipients. While LDLT recipients enjoyed shorter waiting times compared to DDLT recipients (mean 160 d vs 469 d, $P < 0.0001$), HCC recurrence was more common in LDLT recipients at 3 years (29% vs 0%, $P = 0.002$).[41] There was no difference in overall mortality between the two groups.

The most likely explanation for this observed difference is that the groups are not truly comparable. It is important to compare HCC recipients of DDLT and LDLT with caution; LDLT is often used as salvage transplant for patients who have failed to respond to resection or ablation or in patients who are progressing rapidly. This group of patients may represent a particularly aggressive type of tumor that has a high risk of recurrence with any type of transplant. The reason these patients do not recur post-DDLT is that they do not exist; if they do not receive a LDLT they likely progress rapidly while on the transplant list and drop out or die prior to receiving DDLT. The wait list serves as a Darwinian selection mechanism for patients who have favorable tumor biology and a lower recurrence risk. This results in a paradoxical situation in which longer waiting times translate into better outcomes, reflecting more favorable tumor biology rather than an impact of waiting time or type of transplant. The increased recurrence in LDLT recipients, therefore, may reflect selection of patients with more aggressive disease, not suboptimal therapy.

The A2ALL results support this theory. Additionally, "fast-tracked" transplants, which were defined as recipients who met the Milan criteria and received additional MELD points through exception or who underwent LDLT, had higher rates of tumor recurrence post transplant compared to recipients of nonfast-tracked transplants who received transplants on the waiting list prior to being able to receive MELD exception points.[42] These results underscore the concept that increased waiting times may provide a filter for patients whose tumor biology is amenable to cure with transplant, not that the operations fundamentally differ in outcomes.

In addition, these studies focus only on post-transplant outcomes. From the patient perspective, only overall (pre- and post-transplant) survival matters. Future studies need to analyze mortality from the time of listing, including drop-out due to tumor progression pre-transplant and post-transplant recurrence to adequately assess the impact of LDLT on outcome. If the drop-out rate pre transplant with DDLT significantly exceeds the tumor recurrence post transplant with LDLT, it may be that LDLT offers a substantial overall survival benefit. Additionally, improved methods to risk stratify patients with HCC, and better adjuvant and neoadjuvant treatment regimens are needed. As more is discovered about HCC biology, it will become easier to identify patients with more virulent cancers, who may not benefit from transplant or require more aggressive locoregional or systemic anticancer therapy. LDLT may allow optimization of these therapies and controlled timing of transplantation.

Other single-center data has been more supportive of LDLT for patients with HCC. In a study comparing 36 cases of HCC, 53% outside the Milan criteria, who were treated with LDLT to a cohort of 165 recipients of deceased-donor organs, no significant difference was found regarding survival or recurrence rates.[43] Furthermore, data suggest that LDLT for patients with HCC not only results in similar disease-free survival rates as DDLT, but that for patients with advanced HCC, outside of Milan criteria, LDLT was shown to provide a 3-year survival rate of 60%.[44]

Future studies need to address the role of LDLT in patients with HCC. A true comparison of LDLT and DDLT for HCC should encompass both post-OLT recurrence as well as progression to death or delisting pre-transplant on the waiting list for both groups. For high-risk tumors and those not eligible for MELD exceptions, it is likely that tumor progression on the waiting list has a higher risk of mortality than recurrence rates post LDLT.

Donor outcomes

Donor safety is paramount in LDLT. To date, five donor deaths after right-lobe donation have been reported in the USA, four of which occurred within the first postoperative month and were clearly related to the procedure for an overall mortality rate of 0.15%. One donor died from complications of aspiration pneumonia and one donor died of complications partly related to sepsis.[45] One donor died of recreational drug use or suicide 23 months after donation.[1,27] There have also been three liver transplants in living donors for postoperative liver failure. Worldwide other donor deaths have been reported in Europe and Asia, with an overall worldwide estimate of 19 and a donor mortality rate of 0.15%, but the exact number is not known.[46]

A wide range of complication rates has been reported in the literature in donors after LDLT. Overall complication rates ranged from 0–67%, with an overall crude complication rate of 31%.[47] Biliary complications have been reported in 0–7% of donors, including bile leaks and strictures. Complications related to major abdominal surgery occur in 9–19% of donors, including wound infections, small bowel obstruction, pneumonia, and incisional hernia. There are reports of aborted donor hepatectomy at the time of surgery as a result of unexpected findings, including the presence of significant hepatic steatosis, but these figures have not been collected rigorously so the exact number is unknown. Comprehensive data on donor outcomes has been limited due to the lack of a national registry and the majority of data available is generated from single centers with small numbers of patients or self-reported data in national surveys. Additionally it has not been clear whether complication rates reported have included only problems that require substantial intervention or all deviations from standard of care.

Earlier studies reported complication rates of 15–32%, likely reflecting differences in the rigor of the donor selection process, the experience of the center, and differences in reporting.[48] National data was obtained via voluntary survey of all centers performing LDLT after an early NIH meeting on the topic.

Based on this data from 84 different centers, the national overall donor complication rate was estimated to be 14.5%, with a re-hospitalization rate of 8.5%, and a donor mortality rate of 0.2%.[1] Currently, overall donor complication rates are estimated at 10%, with mortality rates between 0.2–0.4%, based on a survey of 30 different transplant centers in the country.[49] This study also revealed higher complication rates in centers that performed fewer transplants.

The A2ALL donor complication data was 38% when all deviations from standard of care were included.[50] Of these, 27% were Clavien Grade 1 and only 0.8% of these were life threatening. UNOS now requires follow-up reporting on all living donors for a minimum of 2 years. The combination of detailed data from a smaller number of large-volume centers and registry data on all donors will allow a more accurate assessment of donor risk and outcomes.

Because of variation in complication rates and lack of uniform criteria used by centers for defining complications, a standardized system for reporting complications is necessary.[51–52] The Clavien system has been modified to include complications that may occur after liver transplantation. This system can be applied to both the living donor and recipient after LDLT and has been adopted by the A2ALL consortium among others.[52]

Long-term complications are not well characterized after right donor hepatectomy because the procedure was not performed on a substantial number of patients until 1999. Therefore, 10 years of data are available on very few patients and 5-year data are just becoming available. The major issue that will evolve is obtaining long-term data from donors because practice patterns for centers following donors after living donation are quite variable as far as the frequency and duration of visits after living donation.[53] Furthermore, years after LDLT healthy donors may be lost to follow up or difficult to contact due to a real or perceived lack of need for medical care, insurance barriers, or access to care.

Donor quality of life

Studies assessing donor quality of life after LDLT demonstrate that virtually all donors state that they would donate again, irrespective of recipient outcomes.[54–55] Most (96%) of donors were able to return to work after a mean of 10 weeks after surgery. A substantial proporation (71%) of donors reported abdominal symptoms several months after surgery that they attributed to surgery.[55] A report on 30 donors at varying time points post donation reported quality of life at or above US norms on a general quality of life survey.[56] In a larger study of 68 Japanese donors at a mean of longer than 4 years post donation, there were two donors who indicated that they would not donate again; in both of these cases the recipients had died. This correlation between recipient outcome and donor satisfaction is not seen in pediatric living donation, where few parents express regret regardless of the outcome in the child. There was no difference in score between donors who sustained complications themselves and those who had no complications.[57]

Although overall quality-of-life data is important, there are specific areas that may be a source of stress and concern to donors, including finances and return to work, and expected recipient outcomes should be addressed both before and after donation.[58] Severe psychiatric disturbances have been reported in some living donors.[59] A notable limitation to all of these studies is the disproportionately high lack of response from donors whose recipients had serious complications and that the instruments used in these quality-of-life studies have been general quality-of-life instruments, e.g. Short Form (SF)-36, which may not capture symptoms or complaints specific to right donor hepatectomy.

Ethical issues

LDLT and performing a right hepatectomy in a healthy individual on the surface challenges the basic Medicine tenet of "first do no harm". The premise of living donation has to be based on a psychological benefit to the donor from donation. That benefit can be either due to providing a direct benefit to the recipient or satisfaction with the attempt to provide life-saving therapy. In order to properly weigh the ethical issues, a precise understanding of the risks and benefits to the donor and recipient are needed.

Living-donor kidney transplantation has been performed for over 4 decades with an estimated mortality risk to the donor of 0.03%.[60] The mortality rate for the donor is fivefold greater in LDLT compared to living kidney donation. This may be an unfair comparison because there has been over 40 years of experience with living-donor kidney transplantation and only 10 years of experience with adult-to-adult LDLT. There is reason to believe that with experience and improved selection criteria the mortality rate will decrease. Right donor hepatectomy, however, will always be a more morbid procedure compared to living kidney donation and a real risk of mortality to the donor is unavoidable.[60–61]

The main ethical dilemma is in assessing the level of acceptable risk of mortality to the donor and determining whether this is an absolute measure or one that is subject to the clinical situation and the donor preferences. The absolute risk is small and very small compared to the ~20% risk of mortality on the waiting list for the recipient. The principle of autonomy places the perspective of the donor as the most important. The donor must be informed of the risks associated with the procedure. Coercion of the donor needs to be excluded during an independent, confidential evaluation. What mortality rate is acceptable when the donor understands the risks and coercion has been excluded? Donors may be willing to accept high rates of mortality if the life of a loved one is in jeopardy, higher than the level acceptable to the transplant physicians and surgeons. In a single study, laypeople indicated a willingness to donate with a ~20% mortality risk undergoing hepatectomy for a ~50% anticipated recipient survival.[62] There has to be a balance between the risk incurred by the donor and what is acceptable to society and the medical community.

Recipient outcomes are incorporated into decision making about LDLT. From a medical perspective if patient or graft survival rates are markedly lower compared to DDLT then LDLT may be perceived as a failure. However, from a patient and donor perspective, if survival after LDLT is better compared to survival on the waiting list without a liver transplant then LDLT may be acceptable. This issue arises for patients with hepatocellular carcinoma who do not meet the current UNOS criteria for additional MELD priority or those with acute alcoholic hepatitis. With a high risk of death on the list or a current contraindication to transplant and no likelihood of recovery, LDLT may be considered ethical as the potential benefits outweigh the potential risks to both donor and recipient. We currently limit consideration of LDLT to patients we would perform DDLT on if a liver was available. Dilemmas exist, however, if patients and donors are willing to accept lower post-transplant survival rates if survival to DDLT is negligible. Similar arguments can be made in the setting of HIV and advanced liver disease or retransplantation for hepatitis C-related cirrhosis. Thus far, we have elected to apply the same criteria to LDLT that is applied to DDLT, but these standards may be challenged by a society faced with organ shortages.

Costs

There are numerous studies on factors associated with the cost of DDLT, but there are few studies comparing the cost of LDLT to DDLT.[63–66] DDLT is accepted as a cost-effective therapy for end-stage liver disease (ESLD). The effectiveness of LDLT is established but its cost effectiveness relative to DDLT has not been well defined.

The first study of the costs of LDLT compared to DDLT reported costs in arbitrary units and not number of dollars and found that total costs in the deceased-donor group were 21% lower compared to the LDLT group, although this difference was not statistically significant.[64] On average the cost of LDLT was $25 000–30 000 higher in the LDLT group. Included in the analysis were costs of donor evaluation (and rejection) and cost of 1 year of donor follow-up care, including re-transplantation, if applicable. Notably, there were four retransplants in the LD group, which markedly increases cost, and all of which occurred in the first 10 cases. If the study was performed further along the program's learning curve, it is reasonable to assume that costs would be lower with LDLT. A recent modeling study using A2ALL data showed that LDLT added additional life-years when added to a DDLT program but at a greater cost.[67] The current author and colleagues showed that LDLT does not cost more than DDLT during the MELD era when only the later experience, after the learning curve is analyzed.[68]

Overall, it is likely that LDLT costs the same or marginally more and is cost effective relative to the alternative of potential DDLT alone. Future research should make an attempt to include all associated costs, including both donor costs and the costs associated with waiting list morbidity and mortality.

Additionally, donors should be informed that they might be responsible for costs in certain settings. For example, the living donor may be responsible for some costs that occur after initial hospital discharge, including complications that are a result of the procedure, such as incisional hernia. These costs may be substantial and require a financial counselor to review what the recipient and donor's health insurance will cover and any potential financial liabilities for the donor.

In one study the mean out-of-pocket expenses for the donor were $3660.[55] Complications occur in 15–30% of donors and donors should be aware that they may be responsible for costs that are not covered by the recipient's insurance, even if it is related to a complication. After right hepatectomy donors can anticipate not returning to work for at least 2–3 months and they should contemplate whether their household can support this period of time off and if their employer will allow it.

Benefits of LDLT

In order to balance the risks and costs outlined earlier, some quantification of benefit is needed. As indicated earlier the major benefit to the donor would be increased likelihood of transplant and potential survival and quality-of-life benefit to the recipient. One of the main reasons LDLT is offered is to reduce waiting time mortality due to the deceased-donor organ shortage.[69] Two initial studies of LDLT, conducted in Asia and the USA, reported higher rates of transplantation and lower waiting time mortality rates in the group of patients with living-donor volunteers compared to a group without living-donor volunteers.[70–71] The survival benefit to LDLT was more clearly quantified in the A2ALL consortium. We studied mortality rates in patients who had a donor evaluated for possible LDLT and compared two groups: 1) recipients of LDLT, and 2) patients who did not receive a LDLT (including those who received a DDLT, those who remained on the list at study completion, and those who died on the list).[11] LDLT recipients had an adjusted mortality hazard ratio of 0.56 (95% CI 0.42–0.74; $P < 0.001$) relative to patients who were evaluated for but did not receive a living-donor graft, controlling for clinical differences at the time of evaluation. This benefit was significantly increased at centers with experience (defined as case number >20), with a hazard ratio of 0.47 (95% CI 0.32–0.69, $P < 0.001$) associated with LDLT.[11] This study, which most closely approximates an "intention-to-treat" analysis, quantifies the reduction in waiting list mortality for LDLT patients compared to remaining on the waiting list as post-transplant survival was the same in DDLT and LDLT groups at experienced centers (i.e. >20 cases).

Studies from the time of evaluation have all demonstrated substantial benefits of pursuing LDLT on waiting time mortality. Patients are interested in their *overall* survival, not only if they survive to transplant. It appears that except for patients with high MELD scores, LDLT offers equivalent results to DDLT from the time of transplant at experienced centers, despite an initial belief that for any given severity of illness a whole organ should result in superior or equivalent outcomes compared to a partial organ. Moreover, most centers offer LDLT because transplant candidates die waiting for a whole organ or may become very ill prior to transplantation, complicating their post-transplant recovery.

Conclusion

Adult living-donor liver transplantation offers improved access to a life-saving transplant for patients with ESLD in areas where waiting time mortality is high and availability of deceased-donor organs falls short of the need of the population. There are significant risks to the living donor, including the risk of death and substantial morbidity that must be taken into account before patients, physicians, and transplant programs embark on LDLT. Significant improvements in outcomes have been seen over recent years that have now been reported in larger multicenter studies. Despite this, the rate of LDLTs performed remains relatively stagnant. Data support the use of LDLT in patients with ESLD due to HCV as well as HCC, although there remain questions about which patients with HCC are most suitable for LDLT.

It is clear that centers with more experience have better outcomes. Future research needs to address optimal donor evaluation, as well as identify the most suitable LDLT donors and recipients. Results of the

A2ALL and other multicenter studies in Europe and Asia will help quantify donor risk and recipient outcome, and hopefully allow growth and development of the procedure.

References

1. Brown RS Jr, Russo MW, Lai M, et al. A survey of liver transplantation from living adult donors in the United States. N Engl J Med 2003;348:818–25.
2. Gruttadauria S, Marsh JW, Cintorino D, et al. Adult to adult living-related liver transplant: report on an initial experience in Italy. Dig Dis Liver 2007;39:342–350. (http://www.unos.org/data/about/viewDataReports.asp. 2007) (accessed December 15 2007).
3. Dutkowski P, de Rougemont O, Müllhaupt B, and Clavien P-A. Current and future trends in liver transplantation in Europe. Gastroenterology 2010; 138:802–809.
4. American Society of Transplant Surgeons' position paper on adult-to-adult living donor liver transplantation. Liver Transpl 2000;6:815–7.
5. Cotler SJ, Cotler S, Gambera M, Benedetti E, Jensen DM, Testa G. Adult living donor liver transplantation: perspectives from 100 liver transplant surgeons. Liver Transpl 2003;9:637–44.
6. Report by New York State Committee on Quality Improvement in Living Liver Donation (http://www.health.state.ny.us/nysdoh/liver_donation/pdf/liver_donor_report_web.pdf. 2002) (accessed December 15 2007).
7. Akabayashi A, Slingsby BT, Fujita M. The first donor death after living-related liver transplantation in Japan. Transplantation 2004;77:634.
8. Coelho JC, de Freitas AC, Matias JE, et al. Donor complications including the report of one death in right-lobe living-donor liver transplantation. Dig Surg 2007;24: 191–6.
9. Ringe B, Strong RW. The dilemma of living liver donor death: to report or not to report? Transplantation 2008;85:790–3.
10. Bramstedt KA. Living liver donor mortality: where do we stand? Am J Gastroenterol 2006;101:755–9.
11. Berg CL, Gillespie BW, Merion RM, et al. Improvement in survival associated with adult-to-adult living donor liver transplantation. Gastroenterology 2007;133: 1806–13.
12. Russo MW, Galanko J, Beavers K, Fried MW, Shrestha R. Patient and graft survival in hepatitis C recipients after adult living donor liver transplantation in the United States. Liver Transpl 2004;10:340–6.
13. Merion RM, Schaubel DE, Dykstra DM, Freeman RB, Port FK, Wolfe RA. The survival benefit of liver transplantation. Am J Transplant 2005;5:307–13.
14. Schaubel DE, Guidinger MK, Biggins SW, et al. Survival benefit-based deceased-donor liver allocation. Am J Transplant 2009;9:970–81.
15. Moss J, Lapointe-Rudow D, Renz JF, et al. Select utilization of obese donors in living donor liver transplantation: implications for the donor pool. Am J Transplant 2005;5:2974–81.
16. Marcos A. Right lobe living donor liver transplantation: a review. Liver Transpl 2000;6:3–20.
17. Trotter JF, Wachs M, Trouillot T, et al. Evaluation of 100 patients for living donor liver transplantation. Liver Transpl 2000;6:290–5.
18. Trotter JF, Campsen J, Bak T, et al. Outcomes of donor evaluations for adult-to-adult right hepatic lobe living donor liver transplantation. Am J Transplant 2006;6: 1882–9.
19. Trotter JF, Wisniewski KA, Terrault NA, et al. Outcomes of donor evaluation in adult-to-adult living donor liver transplantation. Hepatology 2007;46:1476–84.
20. Olthoff KM, Merion RM, Ghobrial RM, et al. Outcomes of 385 adult-to-adult living donor liver transplant recipients: a report from the A2ALL Consortium. Ann Surg 2005;242:314–23, discussion 23–5.
21. Wiesner R, Edwards E, Freeman R, et al. Model for end-stage liver disease (MELD) and allocation of donor livers. Gastroenterology 2003;124:91–6.
22. Pomfret EA, Fryer JP, Sima CS, Lake JR, Merion RM. Liver and intestine transplantation in the United States, 1996–2005. Am J Transplant 2007;7:1376–89.
23. Kam I. Adult–adult right hepatic lobe living donor liver transplantation for status 2a patients: too little, too late. Liver Transpl 2002;8:347–9.
24. Marcos A, Ham JM, Fisher RA, et al. Emergency adult to adult living donor liver transplantation for fulminant hepatic failure. Transplantation 2000;69:2202–5.
25. Testa G, Malago M, Nadalin S, et al. Right-liver living donor transplantation for decompensated end-stage liver disease. Liver Transpl 2002;8:340–6.
26. Liu CL, Fan ST, Lo CM, Wong J. Living-donor liver transplantation for high-urgency situations. Transplantation 2003;75:S33–6.
27. Ghobrial RM, Saab S, Lassman C, et al. Donor and recipient outcomes in right lobe adult living donor liver transplantation. Liver Transpl 2002;8:901–9.
28. Marcos A, Ham JM, Fisher RA, Olzinski AT, Posner MP. Single-center analysis of the first 40 adult-to-adult living donor liver transplants using the right lobe. Liver Transpl 2000;6:296–301.
29. Miller CM, Gondolesi GE, Florman S, et al. One hundred nine living donor liver transplants in adults and

children: a single-center experience. Ann Surg 2001;234: 301–11; discussion 11–12.
30. Bak T, Wachs M, Trotter J, et al. Adult-to-adult living donor liver transplantation using right-lobe grafts: results and lessons learned from a single-center experience. Liver Transpl 2001;7:680–6.
31. Freise CE, Gillespie BW, Koffron AJ, et al. Recipient morbidity after living and deceased donor liver transplantation: findings from the A2ALL Retrospective Cohort Study. Am J Transplant 2008;8:2569–79.
32. Marcos A, Fisher RA, Ham JM, et al. Liver regeneration and function in donor and recipient after right lobe adult to adult living donor liver transplantation. Transplantation 2000;69:1375–9.
33. Akamatsu N, Sugawara Y, Kaneko J, et al. Effects of middle hepatic vein reconstruction on right liver graft regeneration. Transplantation 2003;76:832–7.
34. Garcia-Retortillo M, Forns X, Llovet JM, et al. Hepatitis C recurrence is more severe after living donor compared to cadaveric liver transplantation. Hepatology 2004;40: 699–707.
35. Gaglio PJ, Malireddy S, Levitt BS, et al. Increased risk of cholestatic hepatitis C in recipients of grafts from living versus cadaveric liver donors. Liver Transpl 2003;9:1028–35.
36. Verna EC, De Martin E, Burra P, et al. The impact of hepatitis C and biliary complications on patient and graft survival following liver transplantation. Am J Transplant 2009;9:1398–405.
37. Shiffman ML, Stravitz RT, Contos MJ, et al. Histologic recurrence of chronic hepatitis C virus in patients after living donor and deceased donor liver transplantation. Liver Transpl 2004;10:1248–55.
38. Terrault NA, Shiffman ML, Lok AS, et al. Outcomes in hepatitis C virus-infected recipients of living donor vs. deceased donor liver transplantation. Liver Transpl 2006;13:122–9.
39. Rudow DL, Russo MW, Hafliger S, Emond JC, Brown RS Jr. Clinical and ethnic differences in candidates listed for liver transplantation with and without potential living donors. Liver Transpl 2003;9:254–9.
40. Lo CM, Fan ST, Liu CL, Chan SC, Ng IO, Wong J. Living donor versus deceased donor liver transplantation for early irresectable hepatocellular carcinoma. Br J Surg 2007;94:78–86.
41. Fisher RA, Kulik LM, Freise CE, et al. Hepatocellular carcinoma recurrence and death following living and deceased donor liver transplantation. Am J Transplant 2007;7:1601–8.
42. Kulik L, Abecassis M. Living donor liver transplantation for hepatocellular carcinoma. Gastroenterology 2004;127:S277–82.
43. Gondolesi GE, Roayaie S, Munoz L, et al. Adult living donor liver transplantation for patients with hepatocellular carcinoma: extending UNOS priority criteria. Ann Surg 2004;239:142–9.
44. Todo S, Furukawa H. Living donor liver transplantation for adult patients with hepatocellular carcinoma: experience in Japan. Ann Surg 2004;240:451–9; discussion 9–61.
45. Miller C, Florman S, Kim-Schluger L, et al. Fulminant and fatal gas gangrene of the stomach in a healthy live liver donor. Liver Transpl 2004;10:1315–9.
46. Trotter JF, Adam R, Lo CM, Kenison J. Documented deaths of hepatic lobe donors for living donor liver transplantation. Liver Transpl 2006;12:1485–8.
47. Beavers KL, Sandler RS, Shrestha R. Donor morbidity associated with right lobectomy for living donor liver transplantation to adult recipients: a systematic review. Liver Transpl 2002;8:110–7.
48. Trotter JF, Wachs M, Everson GT, Kam I. Adult-to-adult transplantation of the right hepatic lobe from a living donor. N Engl J Med 2002;346:1074–82.
49. Renz JF, Roberts JP. Long-term complications of living donor liver transplantation. Liver Transpl 2000;6: S73–6.
50. Ghobrial RM, Freise CE, Trotter JF, et al. Donor morbidity after living donation for liver transplantation. Gastroenterology 2008;135:468–76.
51. Ghobrial RM, Busuttil RW. Future of adult living donor liver transplantation. Liver Transpl 2003;9:S73–9.
52. Clavien PA, Camargo CA Jr, Croxford R, Langer B, Levy GA, Greig PD. Definition and classification of negative outcomes in solid organ transplantation. Application in liver transplantation. Ann Surg 1994;220: 109–20.
53. Beavers KL, Cassara JE, Shrestha R. Practice patterns for long-term follow up of adult-to-adult right lobectomy donors at US transplantation centers. Liver Transpl 2003;9:645–8.
54. Pascher A, Sauer IM, Walter M, et al. Donor evaluation, donor risks, donor outcome, and donor quality of life in adult-to-adult living donor liver transplantation. Liver Transpl 2002;8:829–37.
55. Trotter JF, Talamantes M, McClure M, et al. Right hepatic lobe donation for living donor liver transplantation: impact on donor quality of life. Liver Transpl 2001;7:485–93.
56. Kim-Schluger L, Florman SS, Schiano T, et al. Quality of life after lobectomy for adult liver transplantation. Transplantation 2002;73:1593–7.
57. Miyagi S, Kawagishi N, Fujimori K, et al. Risks of donation and quality of donors' life after living donor liver transplantation. Transpl Int 2005;18:47–51.
58. Verbesey JE, Simpson MA, Pomposelli JJ, et al. Living donor adult liver transplantation: a longitudinal study of the donor's quality of life. Am J Transplant 2005; 5:2770–7.

59. Trotter JF, Hill-Callahan MM, Gillespie BW, et al. Severe psychiatric problems in right hepatic lobe donors for living donor liver transplantation. Transplantation 2007;83:1506–8.
60. Surman OS. The ethics of partial-liver donation. N Engl J Med 2002;346:1038.
61. Russo MW, Brown RS. Ethical issues in living donor liver transplantation. Curr Gastroenterol Rep 2003;5: l26–30.
62. Cotler SJ, McNutt R, Patil R, et al. Adult living donor liver transplantation: Preferences about donation outside the medical community. Liver Transpl 2001;7:335–40.
63. Sagmeister M, Mullhaupt B, Kadry Z, Kullak-Ublick GA, Clavien PA, Renner EL. Cost-effectiveness of cadaveric and living-donor liver transplantation. Transplantation 2002;73:616–22.
64. Trotter JF, Mackenzie S, Wachs M, et al. Comprehensive cost comparison of adult–adult right hepatic lobe living-donor liver transplantation with cadaveric transplantation. Transplantation 2003;75:473–6.
65. Russo MW, Brown RS Jr. Financial impact of adult living donation. Liver Transpl 2003;9:S12–5.
66. Russo MW, Brown RS Jr. Is the cost of adult living donor liver transplantation higher than deceased donor liver transplantation? Liver Transpl 2004;10:467–8.
67. Northup PG, Abecassis MM, Englesbe MJ, et al. Addition of adult-to-adult living donation to liver transplant programs improves survival but at an increased cost. Liver Transpl 2009;15:148–62.
68. Lai JC, Pichardo EM, Emond JC, Brown RS Jr. Resource utilization of living donor versus deceased donor liver transplantation is similar at an experienced transplant center. Am J Transplant 2009;9:586–91.
69. Everhart JE, Lombardero M, Detre KM, et al. Increased waiting time for liver transplantation results in higher mortality. Transplantation 1997;64:1300–6.
70. Liu CL, Lam B, Lo CM, Fan ST. Impact of right-lobe live donor liver transplantation on patients waiting for liver transplantation. Liver Transpl 2003;9:863–9.
71. Russo MW, LaPointe-Rudow D, Kinkhabwala M, Emond J, Brown RS Jr. Impact of adult living donor liver transplantation on waiting time survival in candidates listed for liver transplantation. Am J Transplant 2004;4:427–31.

16 Fulminant hepatic failure

Michael A. Heneghan and William Bernal
Institute of Liver Studies, King's College Hospital, London, UK

Key learning points

- The most common cause of fulminant hepatic failure (FHF) is acetaminophen toxicity.
- While acute hepatitis is common, the feature required for the diagnosis of FHF is hepatic encephalopathy.
- Cerebral edema is a common complication in FHF and a frequent cause of death.
- Liver transplantation, including auxiliary and living donor liver transplantation (LDLT), is an effective therapy for properly selected patients with FHF.

Introduction

FHF describes a pattern of clinical symptoms associated with abrupt arrest of normal hepatic function.[1,2] The defining state is the presence of hepatic encephalopathy with coagulopathy and jaundice. In many cases, the clinical picture is complicated by cerebral edema, renal impairment, sepsis, and multiorgan failure. Liver transplantation (LT) is an important treatment option in the management of severe liver failure and constitutes approximately 10% of liver allograft usage in both the USA and Europe. However, the process of selecting appropriate candidates for transplantation remains problematic. Prior to reaching a decision in favor of surgery, physicians must be able to identify patients whose prognosis is otherwise poor without operative intervention.

This chapter reviews the clinical and laboratory characteristics that are associated with a poor prognosis in acute liver failure (ALF) and that accordingly serve as a basis for selecting patients for transplantation. Etiological and management issues are also considered, including the steps to be taken by physicians prior to the transplant center referral. The paradigm should, however, be early discussion, referral and transfer of patients to the transplant center because the key to successful management and outcome of ALF is the maintenance of other organ function such that the option of transplantation is preserved.

Definitions

The first effort to define FHF was by Trey and Davidson[3] (as part of a surveillance study of liver damage after halothane anesthesia in the USA), who described it as "a potentially reversible condition, the consequence of severe liver injury, with the onset of hepatic encephalopathy within 8 weeks of the first symptoms and in the absence of pre-existing liver disease." Within this group of patients are those who present unwell without any symptom referable to the liver and accordingly it causes difficulty in defining the onset of illness. This definition primarily served to differentiate between patients with true acute deterioration in hepatic failure and those with decompensation or exacerbation of chronic liver disease.

Medical Care of the Liver Transplant Patient, Fourth Edition. Edited by Pierre-Alain Clavien, James F. Trotter.

Other definitions have categorized patients into two, and, more recently, into three groups of liver failure based on the timing between the development of jaundice and the onset of hepatic encephalopathy.[4] All definitions serve to subdivide patients into prognostic categories. Time considerations have become clear as important indicators of likely progress, and paradoxically groups of patients with the most rapid onset of encephalopathy are those with the best chance of spontaneous recovery. To account for this, an umbrella term of "acute liver failure" has been proposed within which three categories exist:[4] 1) **hyperacute liver failure** is used to describe those patients who develop encephalopathy within 7 d of the onset of jaundice, 2) **acute liver failure** (ALF) includes those with a jaundice-to-encephalopathy time of 8–28 d, and 3) **subacute liver failure** is suggested to describe patients with a jaundice-to-encephalopathy time of 5–12 weeks. The majority of patients in the hyperacute liver failure group have acetaminophen poisoning but other common causes include acute hepatitis A and B virus infections. The majority of patients within the ALF group have viral hepatitis, whereas the bulk of patients in the subacute liver failure group have nonA, nonB (seronegative) hepatitis. Table 16.1 summarizes the characteristics of patients presenting with each of the three categories of ALF. For the purpose of this discussion, all patients without pre-existing liver disease and who present with jaundice, encephalopathy, and coagulopathy will be termed an FHF.

Causes of FHF

The list of potential causes of FHF is long (Table 16.2). Although considerable differences existed in the past pertaining to the etiology of hepatic failure based on geographical location,[1–9] these differences have become less pronounced. In a report from a workshop in the mid-1990s, viral hepatitis accounted for 62% of all causes of ALF in the USA, with hepatitis B being the most common agent.[7] In contrast, a recent publication from the US Acute Liver Failure Study Group (US ALFSG) involving 17 centers identified acetaminophen toxicity as the most common cause of FHF (46% of cases), with idiosyncratic drug reactions accounting for a further 11%.[8] Viral hepatitis A and B combined were implicated in only 10% of cases, whereas 14% of cases of FHF were of indeterminate cause. Hepatitis A virus as a cause of fulminant or subfulminant hepatic failure varies from 13% in the UK to 50% in France and 90% in India.[9] Indeed, in the UK, acetaminophen hepatotoxicity accounted for approximately 70% of all FHF in the 1980s and 1990s.[2,4] Legislation restricting analgesic pack sizes introduced in September 1998, however, changed the pattern of deaths by suicidal

Table 16.1 Characteristics of subgroups and etiology of liver failure in patients with acute liver failure classified according to O'Grady et al. (1993)

Factor	Hyperacute liver failure	Acute liver failure	Subacute liver failure
Encephalopathy	Yes	Yes	Yes
Duration of jaundice (days)	0–7	8–28	29–84
Cerebral edema	Common	Common	Rare
Prothrombin time	Prolonged	Prolonged	Least prolonged
Bilirubin	Least raised	Raised as subacute	Raised as acute
Prognosis	Moderate	Poor	Poor
Acetaminophen	Common	Never	Never
Hepatitis A	Common	Common	Rare
Hepatitis B	Common	Common	Rare
NANB hepatitis	Rare	Common	Common
Idiosyncratic drug reaction	Common	Common	Rare

Table 16.2 Etiology of acute liver failure

Etiology	Frequency
Viral hepatitis	
A/B, B with D superinfection	Common in developed world
C	Rare
E	Common in endemic areas, especially in pregnant women
NANB	Common cause of acute and subacute liver failure
Herpesviruses 1, 2, and 6	Rare except in immunocompromise
Varicella-zoster	Rare except in immunocompromise
CMV/EBV/adenovirus	Rare except in immunocompromise
Hemorrhagic fever viruses	Rare
Drugs	
Acetaminophen	Common
Isoniazid, ketoconazole, tetracycline, cocaine, phenytoin, valproate, carbamazepine, halothane, nonsteroidal anti-inflammatory agents	Relatively common
Herbal remedies	
Germander/chaparal/Jin bu huan	Increasingly common
Others	
Veno-occlusive disease/Budd–Chiari	Common
Wilson's disease	Rare
Pregnancy-related liver disease/Acute fatty liver/HELLP/ liver rupture	Rare
Circulatory failure/ischemic hepatitis	Rare if less than 50 years old
Amanita phalloides	Rare
Malignancy/leukemia	Rare
Heatstroke	Rare

overdose with acetaminophen, salicylates, and ibuprofen.[10] Concurrently, the numbers of patients admitted to liver units, listed for LT, and undergoing transplantation for acetaminophen hepatotoxicity have all fallen.[10] Suicidal deaths from acetaminophen and salicylates were reduced by 22% in the year after the change in legislation, and this reduction persisted in the next 2 years. Liver unit admissions and liver transplants for acetaminophen hepatotoxicity were reduced by around 30% in the 4 years after the legislation. Numbers of acetaminophen and salicylate tablets consumed in nonfatal overdoses were reduced in the 3 years after the legislation. Large overdoses were reduced by 20% (9–29%) for acetaminophen and by 39% (14–57%) for salicylates in the second and third years after the legislation. Ibuprofen overdoses increased after the legislation, but with little or no effect on deaths.

Currently there are over 200 formulations containing acetaminophen in the USA. With increasing acetaminophen use, higher rates of morbidity and mortality have been seen in patients with accidental overdose than in patients who attempted suicide, even though the latter group had ingested more acetaminophen.[11] This may be accounted for by higher frequency of chronic alcohol abuse, starvation, or by concomitant ingestion of other enzyme-inducing drugs such as phenytoin, carbamazepine, primidone, phenobarbital, rifampicin, and isoniazid. Approximately two-thirds of the acetaminophen overdoses leading to FHF in the USA are due to formulations with a narcotic including oxycodone and hydrocodone.[12] In addition, recent publications indicate that as many as 18% of cryptogenic cases may be caused by acetaminophen, detected by the presence of a serum acetaminophen-cysteine adduct.[13] Hepatitis

E virus as a cause of FHF is common in subtropical areas, especially in pregnant women, where it is associated with high mortality.[14,15]

Management of FHF

Severe FHF, once established follows a predictable course. For this reason, it is appropriate to consider advance treatment options in such patients.[1,2,16] The principles of management of FHF include:

1. Recognition of the tempo of liver failure with attention to the rapidity of onset of encephalopathy from the appearance of jaundice
2. Establishment of likely etiology (history, physical examination, laboratory studies, radiology)
3. Institution of antidotes where appropriate
4. Early discussion with the transplant center
5. Anticipation and prevention of complications of FHF or aggressive treatment (acidosis, renal failure, sepsis, cerebral edema, circulatory failure) where established
6. Institution of organ support (ventilatory, renal replacement therapy (RRT), inotropes, bioartificial liver/extracorporeal liver assist device (ELAD))
7. Early consideration of transplantation (orthotopic, auxiliary, living donor).

Making the diagnosis

There is no substitute for a detailed clinical history from the patient, a close relative, or a friend. This should include history of recent surgery, prescribed drug intake, transfusions, extent of alcohol intake, recreational drug ingestions (e.g. amphetamines, cocaine), family history, travel history, and sexual practice. Issues such as the premorbid personality should be also discussed as some patients may not be appropriate transplant candidates based on a history of severe psychiatric disease or multiple previous suicidal attempts. Many patients with FHF are not transplant candidates because of psychiatric contraindications.

Treatment of FHF for the most part follows general supportive care guidelines, but notable exceptions occur, especially in patients whose disease results from specific hepatotoxic insults. In patients who have consumed the wild death cap mushroom *Amanita phalloides*, penicillin and silibinin may prevent death.[17] Such patients present with marked muscarinic symptoms followed by a period of wellness and subsequent FHF. Transplantation may be the only option if diagnosis and treatment is delayed beyond 12 h of ingestion. The use of N-acetylcysteine (NAC) is clearly beneficial in cases of acetaminophen toxicity. It may be potentially useful in other cases of fulminant hepatic liver failure, where its benefit arises not from donation of sulfur groups but rather from its antioxidant effects, which prevent the inflammatory response initiated by oxidative damage, and by improvement in microcirculatory blood flow through restoration of normal vascular responsiveness to endothelial-derived relaxing factor.[18] A recent publication from the US ALFSG reported a marginal benefit in transplant-free survival in patients receiving NAC (40%) compared to controls (27%), $P = 0.043$, however, the benefits were limited to patients with early-stage encephalopathy.[19]

Syndromes causing FHF that merit further attention include FHF occurring in the context of pregnancy. Liver dysfunction, especially prolongation of the prothrombin time (PT), should trigger expeditious delivery in all cases irrespective of etiology (hypertension-related liver disease, Hemolysis, Elevated Liver enzyme Levels and low Platelet count (HELLP) syndrome, acute fatty liver of pregnancy).[20] A trial of labor can be attempted in selected cases that have no evidence of encephalopathy. In general, the paradigm of management should be parenteral steroid administration to aid maturation of the fetal lung followed by early delivery. Severe unrecognized liver disease may be present and delay in delivery can result in catastrophic consequences including hepatic infarction, subcapsular hematoma, liver rupture, and death. Successful LT has been carried out for FHF occurring in this setting.

In any patient who presents with a marked transaminitis and coagulopathy, it is important to also consider whether or not patients might be presenting with FHF of unusual cause. In some situations such as an acute presentation of Wilson's disease, prognosis without LT is dismal and a high index of suspicion should be present among young adults with FHF of unknown cause with Coomb's negative hemolytic anemia. Although Kayser–Fleischer rings representing copper deposition in Descemet's membrane of the cornea are associated with the condition, they are not pathognomonic and absence thereof should not preclude diagnosis and transplantation. Other useful clues to the diagnosis may be the presence of an elevated serum bilirubin concentration that is out of proportion compared with other hepatic enzymes, a low normal alkaline phosphatase, moderate transaminitis, and a low uric acid level (resulting from a renal tubular defect from copper accumulation). In fact, the common liver function tests may be a more accurate means to confirm the dose rapidly compared to specific tests for Wilson's disease.[21] An alkaline phosphatase (AP) to total bilirubin (TB) ratio <4 has a sensitivity of 94% and specificity of 96% for the diagnosis of fulminant Wilson's.

In contrast to acute presentation of Wilson's disease, where LT is appropriate, patients who demonstrate an unusual presentation of other disease processes need to be carefully excluded from transplantation. This includes etiologies such as infiltrative liver disease from acute leukemia, lymphoma, breast carcinoma, melanoma, or small-cell lung carcinoma.[22,23] Other etiologies that preclude transplantation include ischemic/hypoxic hepatitis and liver failure occurring in the setting of severe sepsis.

Box 16.1 Criteria adapted for identifying patients who are considered for transplantation in King's College Hospital, London (King's criteria), see O'Grady et al. (1989)

Acetaminophen

pH <7.30 (irrespective of encephalopathy grade after volume resuscitation)

or

PT >100 s (INR >6.5) + serum creatinine >300 μmol/L if in Grade III or IV coma

Nonacetaminophen

PT >100 s (INR >6.5) (irrespective of encephalopathy grade)

or

Any three of the following (irrespective of encephalopathy grade):

- Etiology (NANB/indeterminate hepatitis/halothane/drug reaction)
- Age <10 or >40 years
- Jaundice-to-encephalopathy interval >7 d
- PT >50 s (INR >3.5)
- Serum bilirubin >300 μmol/L

Wilson's disease

Encephalopathy alone in patient with FHF

Budd–Chiari syndrome

Encephalopathy and renal failure in patient with FHF

Prognosis without LT

In considering further management of these patients, particularly those with Grade III or IV coma, specific factors need to be examined in relation to listing for transplantation. Several criteria have been defined, but the commonest in use (King's College Hospital (KCH)) is outlined in Box 16.1 and offers specificity of 90% in predicting mortality from FHF. Other authors have suggested that LT should be tentatively offered to all patients who have Grade III or IV encephalopathy, but the decision to proceed to transplant should be deferred until an organ is identified for that patient.[24] An alternative proposal suggests performing volumetric computed tomography (CT) among patients in whom doubt exists and transplanting all patients whose ratio of (calculated liver volume)/(standard liver volume) <0.80.[25] However, the latter two concepts have not been subjected to rigorous prospective evaluation.

The difficulty with most currently applied criteria is that they fail to predict those patients who do not need LT. In patients with FHF from acetaminophen toxicity, however, blood lactate levels may be helpful.[26] Blood lactate levels may reflect both hepatic dysfunction and the degree of tissue oxygenation in patients with FHF.[27] Threshold values that best identified individuals likely to die without transplantation were derived from a retrospective initial sample of 103 patients with acetaminophen-induced FHF and applied to a prospective validation sample of 107 patients. Predictive value and speed of identification were compared with those of KCH criteria. In the initial sample, median lactate concentration was significantly higher in nonsurviving patients than in survivors both in the early samples (8.5 vs 1.4 mmol/L, $P < 0.0001$) and after fluid resuscitation (5.5 vs 1.3 mmol/L, $P < 0.0001$). A threshold value of 3.5 mmol/L applied to the validation sample early after admission had sensitivity of 67%, specificity of 95%, positive likelihood ratio of 13, and negative likelihood ratio of 0.35. Combined early and post-resuscitation lactate concentrations had similar predictive ability to KCH criteria but identified nonsurviving patients earlier in the clinical course. Addition of post-resuscitation lactate concentration to KCH criteria increased sensitivity from 76 to 91% and lowered negative likelihood ratio from 0.25 to 0.10. Therefore, arterial blood lactate measurement rapidly and accurately identifies patients who will die from acetaminophen-induced FHF and its use could improve the speed and accuracy of selection of appropriate candidates for transplantation.

Management issues

Given the general lack of treatments of certain efficacy, except in those cases in which an antidote can be administered, the most fitting place for management of the patient with FHF is the intensive care unit (ICU). Although criteria for admission to intensive care facilities differ from center to center, any patient with altered mental status in conjunction with a prolongation in PT should be managed in this setting on the basis that further deterioration is likely and may occur precipitously, and that the development of complications may be pre-empted by early recognition of other organ system dysfunction. The issues of greatest importance in the management of patients with FHF are discussed further.

General considerations

All patients should have a urinary catheter inserted, cardiac monitoring instituted, and a triple-lumen central venous catheter inserted. The most appropriate routes of venous access are the internal jugular and femoral vein approaches. In patients with severe coagulopathy, the subclavian vein should be avoided. In most instances, an arterial line for hemodynamic monitoring and blood sampling should be inserted and Swan–Ganz pulmonary artery pressure monitoring should be undertaken in any patient in whom arterial hypotension exists and/or urine output is poor. Intubation and ventilation should be considered early in any patient with Grade III or IV encephalopathy. Despite profound coagulopathy, bleeding is rarely a problem in patients with FHF and fresh–frozen plasma should only be given if active bleeding occurs. The foremost difficulty in treating coagulopathy is that it disallows interpretation of the PT as a prognostic indicator, especially in patients with acetaminophen-induced FHF. In contrast, platelet infusions are appropriate in the setting of thrombocytopenia and severe coagulopathy for all procedures.

Intracranial hypertension

Cerebral edema leading to intracranial hypertension occurs in between 50 and 80% of patients with severe FHF (Grade III or IV coma) in whom it is a leading cause of death.[28] Customary measures include placement of the patient in a quiet area with the head elevated at 10–20° above the horizontal. In general, sedation of any kind should be avoided in the early stages of coma. Assisted ventilation should be undertaken in all patients with Grade III or IV coma. Gagging, fevers, seizures, arterial hypertension, agitation, head turning, and endotracheal suction are all associated with elevations in intracranial pressure (ICP) and should be avoided. Although paralysis may be needed if patients are particularly difficult to ventilate or if severe hypoxia exists, paralyzing agents should be avoided as seizure activity may be masked.

Invasive monitoring of cerebral pressure using the Camino® fiberoptic catheter tip system is used most commonly in patients with FHF, and if aggressive correction of coagulopathy and thrombocytopenia is carried out prior to insertion of the extradural monitor, its use is associated with few complications. In most centers, it is inserted in patients who have developed pupillary abnormalities or in patients with Grade III/IV coma who are to undergo transplantation. When used in conjunction with jugular venous bulb oxygen saturation measurement, it allows accurate assessment of cerebral perfusion and oxygenation.

The goals of management should be to maintain cerebral perfusion pressure (CPP) >40 mmHg and mean arterial pressure >60 mmHg. In many centers, a CPP of <40 mmHg for 2 successive hours is a contraindication to transplantation, although frequent successes have been reported in patients with CPP below this level for longer periods of time. Surges in ICP above 20 mmHg for longer than 5 min or pupillary changes should be treated with mannitol given as a bolus over 30 min (0.5–1.0 g/kg, 20% solution). However, the use of invasive monitoring of intracerebral pressure varies widely from center to center and it's utility has never been formally proven. A report from the US ALFSG found that only 28% of patients in their cohort were monitored. While the monitored patients were more likely to receive a transplant, there was no indication that cerebral monitoring affected outcome; there was no difference in 30-day post-transplant survival (85% in both groups).[29] A recent novel approach to the management of elevated ICP in FHF is the establishment of moderate hypothermia (in keeping with the principles of neurosurgical management of cerebral trauma victims); however, these promising observations need confirmation prospectively.[30]

Close attention should also be paid to serum electrolytes such as magnesium, calcium, and sodium. In a recent randomized, controlled trial, the effect of induced hypernatremia to maintain serum sodium concentrations of 145–155 mmol/L using 30% hypertonic saline was examined.[31] In patients randomized to hypertonic saline, the norepinephrine dose requirement was less and ICP decreased significantly relative to baseline over the first 24 h. Moreover, the incidence of intracranial hypertension, defined as a sustained increase in ICP to a level of >25 mmHg, was significantly higher in the control group. The objectives of therapy in all cases are to avoid cerebral herniation and the occurrence of fixed dilated pupils on examination.

Circulatory disturbance

Patients with FHF typically have poor oral intake prior to hospitalization and are dehydrated and hemoconcentrated. Paradoxically, vasodilatation and capillary leak may also be present as a result of Gram-negative sepsis and cytokine release from liver necrosis. Additionally, increased muscle tone and a stress response results in release of epinephrine. The clinical situation is usually one of volume depletion and hypotension in a patient with warm peripheries and tachycardia. The principles of management relate to volume resuscitation with colloid while avoiding high arterial pressure associated with the development of cerebral edema. A pulmonary capillary wedge pressure of 12–14 mmHg is desirable.

The hypotension observed in FHF is frequently seen in association with a reduction in systemic vascular resistance and a hyperdynamic circulation. If pulmonary artery pressures remain low, vascular filling is required and if it persists despite this, fungal or bacterial sepsis should be suspected and treated prophylactically. If arterial hypotension persists and urine output is low, norepinephrine may be required to restore arterial pressure. Prostacyclin, a microcirculatory vasodilator, causes a fall in systemic vascular resistance but mean arterial pressure is maintained by virtue of significant increases in cardiac output. Prostacyclin use also results in an increase in both oxygen delivery and oxygen consumption, suggesting a marked tissue oxygen debt exists in patients with FHF. As previously discussed, NAC also results in improving cardiac output and oxygen delivery in FHF.[18]

Metabolic and renal disturbance

Hypoglycemia occurs early in the clinical course of FHF and results from impaired gluconeogenesis, an inability to mobilize glycogen stores, and an increase in circulating insulin. Blood glucose levels should be monitored every 4–6 h in patients with FHF and the blood sugar concentration maintained using 10 and 20% dextrose solutions. Patients with FHF should also be fed via the enteral route if possible: nasogastric feeding is appropriate in ventilated patients. Hypophosphatemia and hypomagnesemia are seen in those who maintain urine output.

Metabolic acidosis is a frequent finding in FHF. Although originally attributed to liver dysfunction and impaired lactate metabolism, it has been established that much of the acidosis is related to the presence of tissue hypoxia and increased peripheral lactate production. RRT may be appropriate in this situation, even prior to the development of renal failure. Renal failure (urine output <300 ml/24 h) occurs in up to 70% of severe acetaminophen-induced FHF and 30% of FHF from other causes, with sepsis, hypovolemia, and reduced intravascular filling important contributory factors in its development.[32] Initial management should consist of aggressive volume loading and if oliguria persists "renal dose" dopamine can be instituted. If no effect occurs, intravenous furosemide infusion may be tried. However, it is unlikely that any of these approaches will be successful in the anuric patient, and this should prompt early consideration of RRT. RRT of some form should be instituted if acidosis, fluid overload, hyperkalemia, or a rising creatinine develops. Access should be achieved via a double-lumen catheter. Continuous venovenous hemodiafiltration (CVVHD) or high-volume hemofiltration are the most appropriate forms of RRT. Intermittent hemodialysis should be avoided, as significant hypotension frequently accompanies hemodialysis and critical falls in CPP are detrimental in these cases. An important concept in the management of FHF is the observation that ALF and septic shock share many clinical features, including hyperdynamic cardiovascular collapse. Adrenal insufficiency may result in a similar cardiovascular syndrome.[33] In septic shock, adrenal insufficiency, defined using the short synacthen test (SST), is associated with hemodynamic instability and poor outcome. Abnormal SSTs have been reported in 62% of patients with FHF.[34] Those who required norepinephrine for blood pressure support had a significantly lower cortisol increment following synacthen compared with patients who did not. Moreover, increment and peak cortisol concentrations following SST were lower in patients who required ventilation for the management of encephalopathy. In addition, the increment was significantly lower in those who fulfilled liver transplant criteria or who died compared with those who survived.

Sepsis

Severe immunocompromise typically accompanies FHF, and prevention of infection is a major goal in the management of such patients. Daily blood cultures should be drawn in all cases. Typical markers of infection such as fever and leukocytosis are frequently absent in these patients even in the presence of positive blood cultures. In a recent analysis of 206 ALF patients, 72 (35%) developed bacteremia.[35] Gram-negative organisms (52%) were the most common, followed by Gram-positive organisms (44%) and fungus (5%). Median time to first bacteraemia was 10 d (range 7–16 d) and a Systemic Inflammatory Response Syndrome (SIRS) score >1 was independently predictive of bacteremia. A change in clinical status should result in collection of culture materials from all body fluids and close attention to antimicrobial coverage. The use of prophylactic antibiotics is controversial and their institution should probably be deferred until clinically indicated.

A recent study of 227 consecutive patients with Stage I–II encephalopathy prospectively enrolled in the US ALFSG examined the role of infection as a factor in progression of encephalopathy.[36] On multivariate analysis, acquisition of infection during Stage I–II encephalopathy was a predictive factor for worsening encephalopathy in patients with acetaminophen-induced FHF. In patients who progressed to deep encephalopathy, the first confirmed infection preceded progression in 15 out of 19 acetaminophen patients and in 12 out of 23 non-acetaminophen patients. In patients who did not demonstrate positive microbiologic cultures, a higher number of components of the SIRS at admission was associated with more frequent worsening of encephalopathy. The use of prophylactic antibiotics in these patients and the mechanisms by which infection triggers hepatic encephalopathy clearly requires further investigation.

Orthotopic, auxiliary, and living donor transplantation in FHF

Liver transplantation is the best therapy for selected patients with FHF. The outcomes of liver transplant candidates and recipients have been reported from the US ALFSG.[37] Of the 308 patients evaluated, 73% of patients were women and the median age was 38 years. Only 29% of patients received a liver transplant while 43% survived without a transplant and the remaining 28% died. The long-term post-transplant survival rates for FHF are comparable to other indications. However, the 1-year mortality rates after FHF (18.1%) are slightly higher than noncholestatic disease (15.4%) related to their underlying critical illness.[38] There has been concern that psychiatric problems in liver recipients with acetaminophen-induced FHF, which are more common in these patients, would impact long-term survival. A recent analysis of 60 patients transplanted for acetaminophen-induced FHF, however, reported that of the 44 surviving to discharge, there was no difference in long-term survival rates compared to recipients with FHF from other etiologies.[39] The incidence of psychiatric illness was ten times more common in the acetaminophen patients (43%) and their long-term compliance was lower. These data provide support for liver transplantation in this difficult group of patients.

Apart from the conventional techniques of orthotopic liver transplant for treatment of FHF, some novel approaches to liver replacement therapy have occurred as a result of organ shortage. One of these novel approaches includes an auxiliary LT, whereby a lobe of liver from the patient with FHF is removed and replaced with a cadaveric lobe.[40–42] Following transplantation, immunosuppression is instituted in a similar fashion as for a conventional liver transplant recipient. Over subsequent months, the native liver regenerates and when normal liver function has recovered, immunosuppression is withdrawn to facilitate regeneration of the native liver and atrophy of the transplanted lobe. Up to 62.5% of patients undergoing auxiliary transplant for FHF for ALF have regeneration of the native liver to full recovery to the extent that immunosuppression can be reduced, and in the vast majority (80%), suspended.[42] Patients with FHF from acetaminophen toxicity in particular fared particularly well with full native liver recovery occurring in 100% of surviving patients.

Another alternative approach has been LDLT of either the complete right or the left hepatic lobes in adult patients, and left lateral segments (segments 2 and 3 of the left hepatic lobe) in children. Data from the Adult-to-adult living donor liver transplant (A2ALL) study group reported outcomes in 14 patients evaluated for LDLT that were comparable to deceased-donor recipients and acceptable rates of donor morbidity and mortality.[43] LDLT for FHF, however, is rarely performed outside of Asia, due to the difficulty in completing the donor evaluation and the severity of illness in this rapidly progressive disease.

Steps in referral prior to transfer

Criteria to define which patients with FHF should be transferred from nontransplant to transplant centers are unclear, but the keys to survival are early contact, frequent discussion with the transplant center, early initiation of intensive care management, and early transfer, if appropriate. With this in mind, all patients with encephalopathy of any grade, acidosis, prolonged PT, rising creatinine, and rising bilirubin levels should be discussed with the transplant center. Indeed, the absence of encephalopathy should not discourage contact. A further issue to clarify at an early point in discussions is the preferred transplant center of the patient's insurance carrier, as this will avoid reduplication of effort. Referral should not be delayed while a diagnosis is being sought, the label of FHF being sufficient to warrant discussion regarding transfer to the transplant center.

Although delay may exist on the part of the transplant center, it is usually in the context of arranging accommodation, and communication should continue by frequent phone contact. In the interval between referral and transfer, key pieces of data can be obtained such as blood group, HIV status, hepatitis serology, acetaminophen levels, ultrasound examination of the liver, and past medical and psychiatric history. In contrast to patients with chronic liver disease, the need for urgent clarification on these issues is vital. Box 16.2 summarizes the appropriate steps in referral. Contraindication to transplantation does not preclude transfer. Undeniably, greater resources can be made available to FHF patients in a transplant center than in smaller hospitals, where management of this complex metabolic disturbance is not commonplace.

Role of artificial liver support

In the same way that RRT is life-saving among patients with acute renal failure, it is certain that a proportion of patients could recover fully from the syndrome of FHF if supported through the period of extreme organ dysfunction and physiological stress. This could alter the role or need for LT for this disease, allowing regeneration of the damaged liver and recovery of hepatocyte function. With this goal in mind, several systems that show considerable promise including the bioartificial liver (BAL) and the ELAD exist. The HepatAssist™ liver support system is an extracorporeal porcine hepatocyte-based BAL.[44] In a prospective, randomized, controlled, multicenter trial in patients with severe ALF, a total of 171 patients were enrolled. Although there was no statistically significant difference in survival at 30 d between BAL-treated vs control patients for the complete patient cohort, subgroup analysis identified the group of patients with fulminant or sub-FHF as being more likely to benefit from therapy.[44] The molecular adsorbent recirculating system (MARS) is an emerging option for patients with liver failure, which encompasses a cell-free, albumin dialysis device that enables the removal of albumin-bound substances. The

Box 16.2 Steps in referral of patients to a liver transplant center

Step I Determine the following:
- Presence of fulminant to hepatic failure
- Detailed history
- Laboratory studies (HIV test, ABO blood group, syphilis, acetaminophen level, etc.)
- Radiographic investigation (chest films and liver ultrasound)
- Orders for daily blood cultures

Step II
- Discuss possibility of liver transplantation with patient and family
- Identify social support network

Step III
- Contact the patient's insurance carrier
- Identify the preferred transplant center

Step IV
- Contact the transplant team
- Inform transplant team of patient's clinical status

Step V
- Determine means of transportation with the transplant team (air/ground)
- Provide transplant team with contact names and numbers (medical/family)

Step VI
- Inform the patient and family of travel arrangements
- Assemble records (history/laboratory data/x-rays) for transfer
- Designate physician family member to travel with patient

Step VII
- Designate physician and nurse to travel with patient
- Assemble adequate resuscitation equipment, fluids, and drugs for transfer
- Anticipate potential complications during transfer
- Inform transplant center of departure and anticipated arrival time

proponents of albumin dialysis postulate that substances such as bilirubin and bile acids, metabolites of aromatic amino acids, fatty acids, and cytokines may be responsible for some of the systemic manifestations of FHF and might offer either a bridge to transplant or an alternative treatment choice. In fact, in patients with cirrhosis and encephalopathy, the MARS treatment may provide marginal improvement in hepatic encephalopathy without a survival benefit.[45] Despite positive results from nonrandomized trials and case reports, a recent meta-analysis suggests that MARS treatment does not appear to reduce mortality for patients either with FHF or in patients with acute-on-chronic liver failure compared with standard medical treatment.[46] The goal, however, will be to provide a device with longer term capabilities.

References

1. Polson J, Lee WM. AASLD position paper: the management of acute liver failure. Hepatology 2005;41: 1179–97.
2. Bernal W, Auzinger G, Dhawan A, Wendon J. Acute liver failure. Lancet 2010;376:190–201.
3. Trey C, Davidson LS. The management of fulminant hepatic failure. In: Popper H, Schaffner F, editors. Progress in liver failure. New York: Grune and Stratton; 1970:282–98.
4. O'Grady JG, Schalm S, Williams R. Acute liver failure: redefining the syndromes. Lancet 1993;342:373–5.
5. O'Grady JG, Alexander GJM, Hayllar KM, Williams R. Early indicators of prognosis in fulminant hepatic failure. Gastroenterology 1989;97:439–45.
6. Escorsell A, Mas A, de la Mata M. Spanish Group for the Study of Acute Liver Failure. Acute liver failure in Spain: analysis of 267 cases. Liver Transpl 2007;13: 1389–95.
7. Hoofnagle JH, Carithers RL Jr, Shapiro C, Ascher N. Fulminant hepatic failure: summary of a workshop. Hepatology 1995;21:240–52.
8. Lee WM, Squires RH Jr, Nyberg SL, Doo E, Hoofnagle JH. Acute liver failure: Summary of a workshop. Hepatology 2008;47:1401–15.
9. Acharya SK, Dasarathy S, Kumer TL, et al. Fulminant hepatitis in a tropical population: clinical course, cause and early predictors of outcome. Hepatology 1996;23: 1448–55.
10. Hawton K, Simkin S, Deeks J, et al. UK legislation on analgesic packs: before and after study of long term effect on poisonings. Br Med J 2004;329:1076–80.
11. Schiødt FV, Rochling FA, Casey DL, Lee WM. Acetaminophen toxicity in an urban county hospital. N Engl J Med 1997;337:1112–7.
12. Larson AM, Polson J, Fontana RJ, et al. Acetaminophen-induced acute liver failure: results of a United States multicenter, prospective study. Hepatology 2005;42: 1364–72.

13. Khandelwal N, James LP, Sanders C, Larson AM, Lee WM and the Acute Liver Failure Study Group. Unrecognized acetaminophen toxicity as a cause of indeterminate acute liver failure. Hepatology 2011;53: 567–76.
14. Jilani N, Das BC, Husain SA, et al. Hepatitis E virus infection and fulminant hepatic failure during pregnancy. J Gastroenterol Hepatol 2007;22:676–82.
15. Patra S, Kumar A, Trivedi SS, Puri M, Sarin SK. Maternal and fetal outcomes in pregnant women with acute hepatitis E virus infection. Ann Intern Med 2007;147:28–33.
16. Stravitz RT, Kramer AH, Davern T, et al. Intensive care of patients with acute liver failure: recommendations of the US Acute Liver Failure Study Group. Crit Care Med 2007;35:2498–508.
17. Mas A. Mushrooms, amatoxins and the liver. J Hepatol 2005;42:166–9.
18. Harrison PM, Wendon JA, Gimson AE, Alexander GJ, Williams R. Improvement by acetylcysteine of hemodynamics and oxygen transport in fulminant hepatic failure. N Engl J Med 1991;324: 1852–7.
19. Lee WM, Hynan LS, Rossaro L, et al. Intravenous N-acetylcysteine improves transplant-free survival in early stage non-acetaminophen acute liver failure. Gastroenterology 2009;137:856–64.
20. Westbrook RH, Yeoman AD, Joshi D, et al. Outcomes of severe pregnancy-related liver disease: refining the role of transplantation. Am J Transpl 2010;10: 2520–6.
21. Korman JD, Volenberg I, Balko J, et al. Screening for Wilson disease in acute liver failure: a comparison of currently available diagnostic tests. Hepatology 2008; 48:1167–74.
22. Nazario HE, Lepe R, Trotter JF. Metastatic breast cancer presenting as acute liver failure. Gastroenterol Hepatol (NY) 2011;7:65–6.
23. Rowbotham D, Wendon J, Williams R. Acute liver failure secondary to hepatic infiltration: a single centre experience of 18 cases. Gut 1998;42:576–80.
24. Van Thiel DH. When should a decision to proceed with transplantation actually be made in cases with fulminant or subfulminant hepatic failure: at admission to hospital or when a donor organ is made available? J Hepatol 1993;17:1–2.
25. Yamagishi Y, Saito H, Ebinuma H, et al. A new prognostic formula for adult acute liver failure using computer tomography-derived hepatic volumetric analysis. J Gastroenterol 2009;44:615–23.
26. Craig DG, Ford AC, Hayes PC, Simpson KJ. Systematic review: prognostic tests of paracetamol-induced acute liver failure. Aliment Pharmacol Ther 2010;31: 1064–76.
27. Bernal W, Donaldson N, Wyncoll D, Wendon J. Blood lactate as an early predictor of outcome in paracetamol-induced acute liver failure: a cohort study. Lancet 2002;359:558–63.
28. Larsen FS, Wendon J. Prevention and management of brain edema in patients with acute liver failure. Liver Transpl 2008;14:S90–6.
29. Vaquero J, Fontana RJ, Larson AM, et al. Complications and use of intracranial pressure monitoring in patients with acute liver failure and severe encephalopathy. Liver Transpl 2005;11:1581–9.
30. Stravitz RT, Larsen FS. Therapeutic hypothermia for acute liver failure. Crit Care Med 2009;37:S258–64.
31. Murphy N, Auzinger G, Bernel W, Wendon J. The effect of hypertonic sodium chloride on intracranial pressure in patients with acute liver failure. Hepatology 2004; 39:464–70.
32. Ellis A, Wendon J. Circulatory, respiratory, cerebral and renal derangements in acute liver failure: pathophysiology and management. Semin Liver Dis 1996;16: 379–88.
33. O'Beirne J, Holmes M, Agarwal B, et al. Adrenal insufficiency in liver disease – what is the evidence? J Hepatol 2007;47:418–23.
34. Harry R, Auzinger G, Wendon J. The clinical importance of adrenal insufficiency in acute hepatic dysfunction. Hepatology 2002;36:395–402.
35. Karvellas CJ, Pink F, McPhail M, et al. Predictors of bacteraemia and mortality in patients with acute liver failure. Intensive Care Med 2009;35:1390–6.
36. Vaquero J, Polson J, Chung C, et al. Infection and the progression of hepatic encephalopathy in acute liver failure. Gastroenterology 2003;125:755–64.
37. Ostapowicz G, Fontana RJ, Schiødt FV, et al. Results of a prospective study of acute liver failure at 17 tertiary care centers in the United States. Ann Intern Med 2002;137:947–54.
38. OPTN/SRTR Annual Report (http://optn.transplant.hrsa.gov/ar2009/908a_rec-dgn_li.htm) (accessed July 1 2010).
39. Cooper SC, Aldridge RC, Shah T, et al. Outcomes of liver transplantation for paracetamol (acetaminophen)-induced hepatic failure. Liver Transpl 2009;15:1351–7.
40. Faraj W, Dar F, Bartlett A, et al. Auxiliary liver transplantation for acute liver failure in children. Ann Surg 2010;251:351–6.
41. Jaeck D, Pessaux P, Wolf P. Which types of graft to use in patients with acute liver failure? (A) Auxiliary liver transplant (B) Living donor liver transplantation (C) The whole liver. (A) I prefer auxiliary liver transplant. J Hepatol 2007;46:570–3.
42. Quaglia A, Portmann BC, Knisely AS, et al. Auxiliary transplantation for acute liver failure: Histopathological study of native liver regeneration. Liver Transpl 2008;14:1437–48.

43. Campsen J, Blei AT, Emond JC, et al. Outcomes of living donor liver transplantation for acute liver failure: the adult-to-adult living donor liver transplantation cohort study. Liver Transpl 2008;14:1273–80.
44. Demetriou AA, Brown RS, Busuttil RW, et al. Prospective, randomized, multicenter, controlled trial of a bioartificial liver in treating acute liver failure. Ann Surg 2004;239:660–7.
45. Hassanein TI, Tofteng F, Brown RS, et al. Randomized controlled study of extracorporeal albumin dialysis for hepatic encephalopathy in advanced cirrhosis. Hepatology 2007;46:1853–62.
46. Khuroo MS, Farahat KL. Molecular adsorbent recirculating system for acute and acute-on-chronic liver failure: a meta-analysis. Liver Transpl 2004;10: 1099–10.

PART TWO

Donor Issues and Management in the Perioperative Period

17 Extended-criteria donor

Ashraf Mohammad El-Badry and Mickael Lesurtel
Swiss HPB (Hepato–Pancreato–Biliary) and Transplantation Centers, Department of Surgery, University Hospital Zurich, Zurich, Switzerland

Key learning points

- Extended-criteria donor allografts from deceased donors were previously thought to be associated with an unacceptably high risk of graft failure.
- The main recognized donor risk factors are age over 60, reduced height, nonwhite race, other causes of donor death than trauma, partial graft and long cold ischemic time (>10 h).
- In case of extended criteria donor, cold ischemic time must be shortened as much as possible.
- Donor risk index, including values for each of the underlying donor co-risk factors, is directly related to a corresponding predicted rate of graft survival and may help to match donor and recipient.

Introduction

A large and global imbalance between the supply of donor organs for orthotopic liver transplantation (OLT) and the pool of potential liver transplant recipients continues to fuel efforts to maximize utilization from existing donors, increase the overall number of donors, and identify new donor sources. According to the 2009 United Network for Organ Sharing (UNOS) data, 6300 OLTs were performed in 2009 in the USA while more than 11 000 patients were listed at the same period.[1] Until recently, deceased-donor OLT was largely confined to donors with ongoing cardiac activity, who were diagnosed with brain death. Currently, many transplant programs have begun to transplant extended-criteria allografts, which were previously thought to be associated with an unacceptably high risk of graft failure.[2] These include transplants using livers from, among others, older donors, and those whose hearts have stopped beating, termed "donation after cardiac death" (DCD, see Chapter 18). Efforts to expand the donor pool have included the development of novel surgical approaches to split a single liver to transplant two recipients.[3] In recent years, as each of these forays into previously uncharted donor territory has been undertaken, several reports suggested that liver transplant candidates could be served by these innovations. At the same time, experience has demonstrated that each option is associated with an incremental risk of graft failure when compared to whole-liver transplants from young deceased donors.

Beyond the issues mentioned earlier, which affect graft function, there is an entirely separate concept of donor risk factors that concerns the possibility of transmissible disease (e.g. hepatitis viruses, human immunodeficiency virus, or malignancy). These issues are discussed in Chapter 19.

This chapter will review the dramatic evolution of donor characteristics that emerged in the recent years and cover the impact of extended-criteria donors on OLT outcome. These criteria will be divided into graft (cold ischemia time (CIT), steatosis, split liver, hypernatremia and abnormal liver tests) and donor (age, race, gender, weight and height of donor, cause of death)-related factors.

Medical Care of the Liver Transplant Patient, Fourth Edition. Edited by Pierre-Alain Clavien, James F. Trotter.

Definitions

An accepted definition of extended-criteria donor livers has not yet been established by the liver transplant community. In 2007 the International Liver Transplantation Society organized a consensus conference in Paris, France to clarify issues related to expanded-criteria donors and propose guidelines.[2] An extended criteria donor implies higher risk in comparison with a reference donor. The risk may manifest as increased incidence of poor allograft function, allograft failure, or transmission of a donor-derived disease. In the past, a reference (or ideal) donor was defined according to the following criteria: age <40 years, trauma as the cause of death, donation after brain death, hemodynamic stability at the time of procurement, no steatosis or any other underlying chronic liver lesion. Additional factors such as transmissible disease, which do not directly affect the risk of graft failure, must also be considered in the definition of extended criteria.

There is still ongoing debate about the distinction between an ideal allograft and an ideal donor. The ideal allograft category may be influenced by variables that are introduced following procurement, such as the prolonged CIT, or technical variants, such as those occurring with allograft reduction (e.g. split-liver allograft). It was then suggested that these variables should not be included in the definition of an extended-criteria donor because the aim was to assess risk at procurement.

Graft factors

Cold ischemic time

Cold ischemia occurs purposely during organ retrieval when the liver is cooled, perfused and then stored in a cold preservation solution. Morphologic changes of the sinusoidal endothelial cells such as cell swelling and loss of cytoplasmic processes are observed during cold preservation as a result of pathologic processes involving the cytoskeleton and extracellular matrix.[4] Most of the sinusoidal endothelial cells tolerate cold ischemia; nonetheless they slough into the sinusoidal lumen on reperfusion. Endothelial cell detachment is directly related to the duration of CIT.[4] A long period of cold ischemia is an independent risk factor for the development of delayed function and primary nonfunction of the graft.[5] A complicated postoperative course manifested by increased hepatocellular injury and decreased graft survival is associated with prolonged CIT.[6] Two surveys from Europe and the USA demonstrated that recipient survival is negatively affected by CIT over 12 and 10 hours, respectively.[7,8] Analysis of data from 20 023 OLTs, in which liver grafts were obtained from deceased donors and implanted in adult recipients, showed that the risk of graft loss increases by 1% for each additional hour of cold ischemia.[9] In a retrospective study on 186 OLTs performed in Pittsburgh, PA, USA, significant impairment of graft function was observed when graft transport distance exceeded 600 miles due to prolongation of the cold ischemic time.[10] Therefore the results emphasize that further efforts must be exerted to shorten CIT as much as feasible, especially in the case of the extended-criteria donor.

Steatosis

The incidence of steatosis in liver grafts is expected to rise, due to the global increase in the prevalence of hepatic steatosis.[11] For instance, about one-third of the American population in Dallas, TX, USA exhibit some degree of liver steatosis.[12] Microscopic evaluation of fat content in hepatocytes represents the current gold standard to characterize hepatic steatosis.[13] Quantitative estimation is defined by the percent of hepatocytes containing lipid droplets (mild: <30%, moderate: 30–60%, and severe >60%). Alternatively, a qualitative assessment considering the size of lipid droplets and displacement of the hepatocyte nucleus separates fatty liver into micro- and macrosteatosis. During OLT procedures, the liver graft is inherently exposed to cold preservation and rewarming ischemia.[13] Fat accumulation in the cytoplasm of the hepatocytes is associated with an increase in the cell volume, which may result in partial or complete obstruction of the hepatic sinusoidal space and subsequently sinusoidal perfusion failure after portal and hepatic arterial reconstruction.[13] In animal models of steatosis, impairment of hepatic microcirculation has been demonstrated to be influenced also by the polyunsaturated fatty acid content of intrahepatic lipids.[14] Steatotic liver grafts show a defective regenerative power, which is fundamental for recovery of the liver functions, particularly after partial OLT.[13]

Table 17.1 Clinical studies on the effect of steatosis on graft and patient survival after liver transplantation

Author (year)	No. of patients	Graft survival	Patient survival
Marsman et al.[18] (1996)	116	Decreased with mild steatosis	Decreased with mild steatosis (83% at 4 months)
Hayashi et al.[23] (1999)*	338	nr	Decreased with severe steatosis (0% at 5 years)
Soejima et al.[24] (2003)*	52	No significant effect with macrosteatosis	nr
Afonso et al.[20] (2004)	48	nr	No significant effect
Perez-Daga et al.[17] (2006)	294	nr	Decreased with severe steatosis (59% at 3 months)
McCormack et al.[21] (2007)	60	No significant effect	No significant effect
Angele et al.[22] (2008)	225	No significant effect	nr
Noujaim et al.[19] (2009)	118	Decreased with severe steatosis	Decreased with severe steatosis (76% at 1 month)

*LDLT, nr: not reported

In a study on 860 OLTs that have been carried out in 784 patients, a group from Italy reported that macrosteatosis affecting more than 15% of the graft was the only independent variable associated with shorter patient and graft survival.[15] The prognosis was further deteriorated if more than 15% macrovesicular steatosis was associated with a total ischemia time more than 10 h, donor age >65 years or a hepatitis C virus (HCV)-positive recipient.[15] While severe grades of steatosis can be reasonably expected by the gross examination, detection of mild and moderate grades seems more tricky and in some cases liver biopsy is mandatory.[2]

In the UK, 38% of liver transplant surgeons proceed to biopsy when steatosis is suspected at inspection while 50% never integrate histopathologic assessment into making a decision. In the USA, the Organ Procurement and Transplantation Network data demonstrate that only 28% of all 7593 cadaveric livers considered for OLT in 2005 were actually biopsied.[6] In particular situations, the decision on implantation of an organ is entirely based on frozen-section biopsy, which allows rapid assessment of liver architecture, fibrosis, steatosis, inflammation, and extent of hepatocyte necrosis.[2] Of note, biopsy is the only reliable method for assessment of superimposed pathologies, such as fibrosis and inflammation, which may preclude transplantation.[2]

Despite being the current "gold standard" for evaluation of liver steatosis, assessment of liver sections by four expert pathologists from well-known European and North American centers demonstrated poor concordance as to the degree of total, macro- and microsteatosis. The inconsistency extended to the semiquantitative evaluation; for example a diagnosis of marked steatosis (≥30%) varied from 22 to 46%. Obvious disparity regarding the assessment of the parameters of steatohepatitis (lobular and portal inflammation, hepatocyte ballooning and Mallory's hyaline) as well as the overall diagnosis was also reported.[16] These data may explain the inconsistency among several published studies (Table 17.1) on the influence of liver steatosis on graft function and graft and patient survival after OLT.

There is a number of studies demonstrating negative effects of graft steatosis on the outcome of OLT. For instance, the rates of severe renal failure and early (90 d) mortality were reported to be significantly higher in recipients of severely steatotic organs.[17] In 57 recipients of donor livers with up to 30% steatosis who were matched to 59 patients who received grafts without fatty infiltration, the median transaminase value at the second postoperative day was significantly higher in the fatty liver group.[18] Moreover, steatosis was an independent risk factor for graft loss and correlated with significant decrease of the

4-month graft survival and in 2-year patient survival.[18] In another study, the clinical outcome of OLT in 115 patients who were categorized according to the grade of steatosis into four groups was prospectively analyzed. There were no significant differences among all groups with regard to the demographic data, etiology of liver disease, indication of OLT and Model for End Stage Liver Disease (MELD) score.[19] Graft survival at 1-year was significantly lower with severe compared with the absent and even mild and moderate steatosis groups. Severe graft steatosis exerted significant influence on 1-year patient survival compared with non- and mildly steatotic organs.[19]

Sharply contrasting the previous reports, some studies did not document any negative impact of steatosis on the morbidity and mortality after OLT. Liver grafts with more than 50% steatosis exhibited adequate initial graft function and no reduction in early (30 d) patient survival.[20] However, this positive outcome could be attributed to avoidance of prolonged ischemia and absence of other risk factors among recipients of fatty organs.[20] In Zurich, despite the higher rate of primary graft dysfunction, renal failure, prolonged intensive care unit, and hospital stay for patients with severe steatosis, 60-day mortality and 3-year patient survival were not negatively affected.[21] Conforming with the current authors' data, a study on the cumulative graft survival in recipients of mildly steatotic grafts compared patients who received grafts with moderate and severe grades of steatosis showed no significant difference despite impaired graft function postoperatively.[22]

In a large Japanese series of living-donor liver transplantation (LDLT), implantation of organs with mild and moderate steatosis resulted in comparable graft and patient survival with normal grafts while severe steatosis worsened the outcome.[23] In another study on LDLT,[24] graft biopsy showed no, mild (1–20%) or moderate (21–50%) degrees of steatosis. The peak transaminase levels were significantly higher with steatosis and both groups showed comparable 1-year graft survival.[24] These results highlight the urgent need to establish a reliable alternative approach for accurate assessment of liver steatosis.

Split-liver transplantation

Split-liver transplantation (SLT), a procedure in which one cadaver liver is divided to provide for two recipients, has existed for over a decade. Despite the potential for expanding the cadaver-donor pool and decreasing reliance upon living donation, SLT is seldom performed.[3] The main limitation is its technical challenges including: 1) the creation of sufficient liver volume to meet the metabolic demands of the recipient, 2) graft positioning to optimize vascular flow and biliary drainage, and 3) an appreciation of anatomic variations that necessitate complex biliary or vascular reconstruction. Frequent complications among partial-liver allograft recipients include: 1) parenchymal bile leak, 2) hepatic arterial thrombosis, 3) hepatic venous outflow obstruction, 4) infection from remnant necrotic tissue, and 4) poor graft function secondary to insufficient hepatic volume. Surveys in western populations indicate that SLT in adults is associated with significant increases (about 10%) in graft failure and recipient morbidity.[2] This is supported by the recent analysis of the large Scientific Registry of Transplant Recipients database, where split or partial grafts were associated with 52% higher risk of graft failure.[9]

Historically, the principal beneficiaries of SLT have been adult–pediatric recipient pairs; however, the current scarcity of cadaver organs has renewed interest in expanding these techniques to include two adult recipients for one adult cadaver donor.[25] SLT for two adults has been performed in select transplant centers with better results for right vs left allografts.[3] Adult transplantation with a left graft remains a challenging technical procedure with a high risk of primary nonfunction due to insufficient parenchymal volume and often complex biliary and vascular anastomosis.[26] A data request from the Organ Procurement and Transplant Network Liver and Intestinal Transplantation Committee was submitted to provide outcomes of SLT right lobe (right trisection) allografts in adults.[27] Assuming that SLT is restricted to optimal donors, partial right allograft outcomes were compared with two groups: 1) a comparable group of whole-organ cadaver donors between 18 and 40 years of age, and 2) a surrogate extended-criteria donor group consisting of cadaver whole-organ donors older than 60 years. Between 1994 and 2001, 215 SLT right allografts were identified; these included 33 partial, 42 *in situ*, and 140 *ex vivo* allografts that were compared with 2901 allografts procured from donors older than 60 years and 9802 allografts procured from donors 18–40 year old. Graft failure and death occurred in 32 and 26% of right SLT recipients, respectively. This outcome was comparable to that of whole-organ allografts from donors older than 60 years and inferior to cadaver whole-organ donors 18–40 years old. SLT allograft data were comparable to those of the extended-criteria donor group with overall graft failure and death not statistically different. Thus, SLT of optimal donors yielded adult allografts that functioned similarly to cadaver extended-criteria donor whole organs.

Recently Wilms et al.[28] reported a match pair analysis comparing 70 SLTs (right trisection liver) recipients with 70 recipients of whole-liver transplantation. Matching criteria were indication for transplantation, UNOS status, recipient age, donor age, CIT, and year of transplantation. The authors did not document any difference between the two groups regarding the 5-year patient survival rates (78% after SLT vs 75%, after whole liver) and the 5-year graft survival rates (77% after SLT vs 66% after whole liver). No significant difference between the two groups in terms of short- and long-term morbidity was observed. The authors concluded that these favorable results could be achieved by improvements in surgical technique and the allocation of the leftover liver by the splitting surgeon to a suitable second recipient in the same center, thus minimizing CIT. Splitting of a deceased-donor liver should always be considered if no contraindication is obvious.

Unless significant technical advances are achieved, the use of left allografts cannot be widely applied in adults. SLT using the right lobe slightly increases the rate of graft failure, however, this should not represent a disincentive for using SLT as this technique expands the donor pool, particularly for pediatric recipients.[2]

Hypernatremia

Hypernatremia is frequently encountered in donors who received aggressive treatment of cerebral edema and those who suffered from reduced antidiuretic hormone levels or inappropriate fluid administration.[5] Hepatocytes increase their osmolality to diminish cellular damage associated with the extracellular hypertonicity. During correction of hypernatremia, enhanced intracellular accumulation of water may result in cell swelling and injury. Therefore, lack of proper management of hypernatremia could result in detrimental effects on postoperative graft functions.[5] A Pittsburgh group studied the influence of correction of donor sodium levels on early graft dysfunction after 181 consecutive OLTs. According to the donor serum sodium levels before organ procurement, patients were divided into three groups: 1) with serum sodium level ≤155 mEq/L (group A), 2) peak >155 mEq/L and final level ≤155 mEq/L (group B), and 3) final level >155 mEq/L (group C). Compared with groups A and B, the rate of graft loss was significantly higher in group C,[29] therefore, a pre-cool perfusion with 1 L of 5% dextrose in water for donor serum sodium levels above 160 mEq/L prior to explantation for correction of hypernatremia was suggested to abrogate its negative effect.[30]

Abnormal liver tests

Perturbations of liver tests are very common at the time of donor evaluation. The interpretation of such abnormalities remains difficult since they may be the result of hemodynamic instability, underlying chronic hepatopathy, or sepsis; therefore no liver procurement should be excluded on the basis of abnormal liver tests. On the other hand, normal liver tests do not preclude liver disease. Abnormal liver tests have never been identified as a donor prognostic factor in several studies that targeted such factors.[8,9,31] A clear upper limit in serum transaminases that contraindicates use in transplantation does not clearly exist. In cases of markedly elevated serum transaminases, donor hemodynamics is an essential consideration. A rapid decrease in serum transaminases over time in potential donors indicates resolving hepatocellular injury, which should promote them as candidates for organ donation. Recently, the Paris consensus meeting on expanded-criteria donors stated that a marked increase in the GGT level (>200 UI/L) is a concern, utilization of their organs should be carefully weighed in light of other donor factors, and liver biopsy is warranted.[2] A low prothrombin index and increased international normalized ratio (INR) are not contraindications for transplantation. In deceased donors with major brain trauma, these changes are more likely to be due to disseminated intravascular coagulation than to altered liver function.

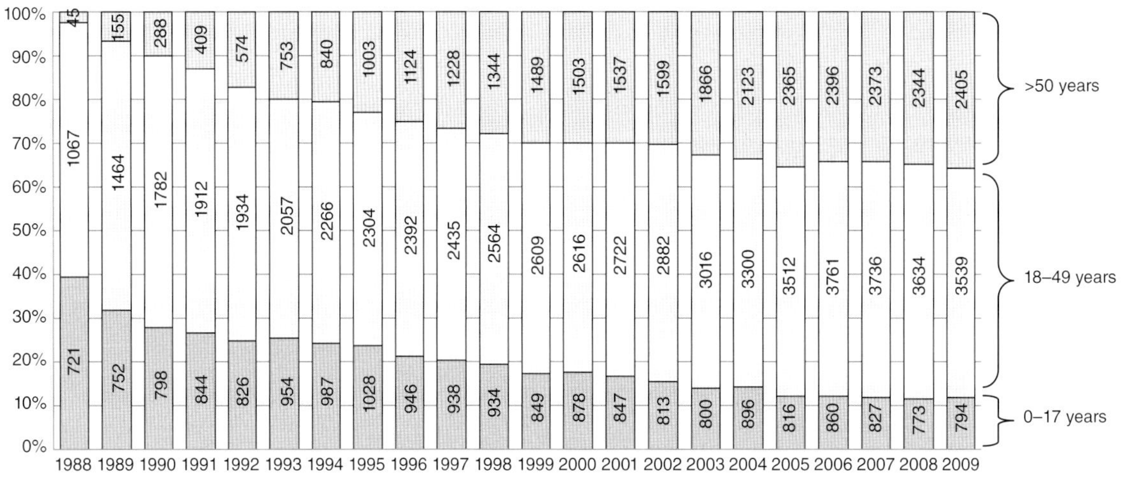

Figure 17.1 Distribution of deceased donor age for liver donors by year, 1988–2009[1]

Donor factors

Donor age, race, gender, weight, and height

Donor age has steadily increased over recent decades. In 1989, <10% of deceased donors in the USA were 50 years or older (Figure 17.1). Ten years later, this percentage increased to 30%, and in 2009, 35% of the donors were older than 50 years of age. Reports from various liver transplant registries have shown that donor age is a significant risk factor for graft failure and recipient patient mortality. Donor age over 60 years significantly increased 3-month patient mortality in the analysis of the European Liver Transplant Registry.[32] However, single-center comparative studies have generally failed to demonstrate significant differences in primary graft nonfunction or graft and patient survival after OLT using donors older than 60 or 70 years.[33,34] In 2002, Berenguer et al.[35] described a possible relationship between donor age and a worse outcome in hepatitis C virus (HCV)-positive recipients. A 5-year graft survival of <50% was described with donors older than 70 years among HCV-positive patients.[36] The reasons for the worse outcome after OLT in HCV-positive patients using elderly donors are not well known, however, it has been proposed that the progression of fibrosis and development of cirrhosis could be related to hepatocyte telomere shortening correlated with senescence.[37]

Recipient selection seems to be paramount with elderly grafts. An ideal recipient for donors older than 70 years has been described as a patient younger than 45 year old, with a body mass index <35, no HCV infection as an indication for OLT, and not undergoing emergency or re-transplant with a CIT <8 h.[38] With these ideal recipients, OLT using donors older than 70 years resulted in graft and patient 3-year survivals that were comparable with ideal (with a recipient younger than 40 years) donors: 75 and 81% vs 77 and 81%, respectively.

Even though the donor gender (female) has been identified as a risk factor for post-OLT outcome in some studies,[39] this could not be confirmed by others.[9] Race, however, consistently seems to affect recipient outcome with livers from black donors having a higher risk of graft failure compared to those from white donors.[9,39] Interestingly, of the two parameters reflecting donor size, only height but not weight was independently associated with recipient outcome.[9]

Causes of donor death

In the early years of liver transplantation the typical cause of death of an organ donor was related to cerebral trauma. In more recent years cerebral trauma as a cause of death of organ donors has gradually decreased, while cerebrovascular causes increased.[40] According to the study by Feng et al.[9] cause of death other than trauma was associated with a 16% (cerebrovascular accident) and 20% (other causes) increased risk of graft failure, respectively. The success of renal transplantation from nonheart beating donors also referred to as "donation after cardiac death" has led to a renewed interest in the liver transplant community as a potential way to increase the donor pool.[41] Chapter 18 of this book is dedicated to this topic.

Donor risk index

Several risk factors that are associated with an increase rate of liver allograft failure have been identified in the USA and UK[9,42] (Table 17.2). In the US series, seven characteristics were identified in a multivariable Cox regression model of time to graft failure or death.[9] These included three donor demographic characteristics (age, race, and height), two relating to cause of donor death (cerebrovascular accident or causes other than cerebrovascular accident, trauma, or anoxia), one related to type of donor death (DCD), and use of a split or partial graft.

Compared with a reference group of donors younger than 40 years of age, increasing age was associated with a significant and monotonic increase in the risk of graft failure. For example, donor age was an extremely important risk factor for graft failure (relative risk 1.53 and 1.65, for donors age 61–70 and >70, respectively; both $P < 0.0001$). Livers

Table 17.2 Significant donor risk factors

Significant donor risk factors	5 donor and 2 transplant risk factors identified in the US[9]		6 donor and 1 transplant risk factor identified in the UK[42]	
	Risk factor reference value	Increased risk of graft failure Relative risk	Risk factor Reference value	Increased risk of graft failure Relative risk
Donor risk factors				
Age	Age <40	61–70: 1.53 >70: 1.65	Age	Increase by 1.05 per decade
Race	White	African American: 1.19	White	Nonwhite: 2.17
Size	Height	Increase by 1.07 per 10 cm decrease in height	nr	
Cause of donor death	Cause of donor death: Trauma	CVA*: 1.16 Other†: 1.20 DCD‡: 1.51	nr	
Type of graft	Full graft	Partial/split: 1.52	Full graft	Reduced/split: 1.93
BMI	ns		BMI	Increase of 1.01 per unit increase
Graft appearance	No data		Normal	Suboptimal: 1.31
Diabetes	ns		No diabetes	Diabetes: 1.41
Transplant risk factors				
Cold ischemia time	Cold ischemia time	Increase of 1.01/h	Cold ischemia time	Increase of 1.02/h
Sharing outside local area	Local area	Same region: 1.11 National: 1.28	nr	

*cerebrovascular accident, †cause of death not trauma, cerebrovascular accident or anoxia, ‡donation after cardiac death, ns: not significant, nr: not reported

from black donors had a 19% higher risk of graft failure in comparison with those from white donors (relative risk 1.19; $P < 0.0001$). Although two parameters reflecting donor size were assessed, the association of height was stronger than, and independent of, the association of weight. Compared with trauma as a cause of death, cerebrovascular accident and other causes of death (not trauma, cerebrovascular accident, or anoxia) were associated with 16 and 20% higher risks of graft failure, respectively (both $P < 0.02$). DCD status and split/partial grafts were associated with a 51 and 52% higher risk of graft failure ($P < 0.001$). Two transplant-related factors, CIT and sharing outside of the local donor service area, were also found to be significantly associated with increased risk of graft loss.

Taken together, these factors can be incorporated into a single equation to generate the combinatorial overall donor risk index (DRI) for each donor, given the values for each of the underlying co-risk factors (Table 17.2). The DRI for each particular combination is directly related to a corresponding predicted rate of graft survival, which varies from 86% at 1 year for donors younger than 40 years of age with no other risk factors to 24% for DCDs or split grafts from donors over the age of 70 years. As an example, consider a brain-dead liver donor of white race, age 64 years, with a height of 170 cm who died of a traumatic brain injury, and whose liver was transplanted locally after a CIT of 8 h. The calculated DRI would be 1.53, meaning that there is a 53% higher risk of graft failure than a reference donor younger than 40 with the same characteristics. If that same donor had died of a stroke instead of a traumatic injury, the DRI would rise to 1.77 and further to 1.88 if the CIT were 14 h instead of 8 h. Table 17.3 gives some examples of specific combinations of donor risk factors and the corresponding DRI using the formula shown below the table.

At the time when a donor liver is offered for a candidate on the liver transplant waiting list, a choice must be made to either accept the risk of transplantation with that particular organ or to decline the offer in favor of waiting for a subsequent donor, which may or may not have a more favorable profile. This decision requires prognostic information about the donor graft being offered as well as knowledge of the risk of death from progressive liver disease if the offered graft is declined. The DRI provides substantial data regarding the first issue, and published reports show that the risk of death on the waiting list can be reasonably estimated using the MELD.[43] Recently, the same team estimated survival benefit according to cross-classifications of candidate MELD score and deceased DRI using sequential stratification based on US data from the Scientific Registry of

Table 17.3 Specific combinations of donor risk factors and the corresponding DRI (From Feng et al.[9])

Donor factor	Reference donor	Example 1	Example 2	Example 3	Example 4	Example 5
Age	Under 40	**64**	**64**	**64**	25	25
Cause of death	Trauma	Trauma	**Stroke**	**Stroke**	Trauma	Trauma
Race	White	White	White	White	White	White
DCD	No	No	No	No	No	**Yes**
Partial/split	No	No	No	No	No	No
Height (cm)	170	170	170	170	170	170
Location	Local	Local	Local	Local	Local	Local
Cold time (h)	8	8	8	**14**	**14**	**14**
Donor risk index*	1.00	1.53	1.77	1.88	1.06	1.60

*Calculation: donor risk index = exp[(0.154 if 40 ≤ age < 50) + (0.274 if 50 ≤ age < 60) + (0.424 if 60 ≤ age < 70) + (0.501 if 70 ≤ age) + (0.079 if COD = anoxia) + (0.145 if COD = CVA) + (0.184 if COD = other) + (0.176 if race = African American) + (0.126 if race = other) + (0.411 if DCD) + (0.422 if partial/split) + (0.066 ((170 − height)/10)) + (0.105 if regional share) + (0.244 if national share) + (0.010 × cold time)]

Transplant Recipients (SRTR) on 28 165 adult liver transplant candidates waitlisted between 2001 and 2005.[44] Covariate-adjusted hazard ratios were calculated for each liver transplant recipient at a given MELD with an organ of a given DRI, comparing post-transplant mortality to continued waitlisting with possible later transplantation using a lower-DRI organ. High-DRI organs were more often transplanted into lower-MELD recipients and vice versa. Compared with waiting for a lower-DRI organ, the lowest MELD category recipients (MELD 6–8) who received high-DRI organs experienced significantly higher mortality (HR = 3.70; $P < 0.0005$). All recipients with MELD of >20 had a significant survival benefit from transplantation, regardless of DRI. Transplantation of high-DRI organs is effective for high but not low-MELD candidates. Pairing of high-DRI livers with lower-MELD candidates fails to maximize survival benefit and may deny lifesaving organs to high-MELD candidates who are at high risk of death without transplantation.

Conclusion

With the increasing waiting time for OLT, donor organs remain in short supply. Because of this lack of organs, more centers are transplanting livers that were previously considered unacceptable. The deleterious effects of extended-criteria donors on graft function seem additive with the presence of multiple marginal characteristics. In an effort to maximize successful use of extended-criteria donors, donor risk factors have been established and extended-criteria donor grafts must be considered as part of an appropriately matched graft–recipient pair, rather than as isolated entities.

Until there are enough donors to meet the needs of the transplant waiting list, marginal donors may represent a viable option to expand the donor pool.

Abbreviations

CIT: cold ischemia time, DCD: donation after cardiac death, DRI: donor risk index, LDLT: living-donor liver transplantation, MELD: model for end-stage liver disease, OLT: orthotopic liver transplantation, SLT: split-liver transplantation.

References

1. United Network for Organ Sharing. (http://www.cebm.net/) 2010.
2. Durand F, Renz JF, Alkofer B, et al. Report of the Paris consensus meeting on expanded criteria donors in liver transplantation. Liver Transpl 2008;14:1694–707.
3. Renz JF, Yersiz H, Reichert PR, et al. Split-liver transplantation: a review. Am J Transplant 2003;3: 1323–35.
4. Selzner N, Rudiger H, Graf R, et al. Protective strategies against ischemic injury of the liver. Gastroenterology 2003;125:917–36.
5. Alkofer B, Samstein B, Guarrera JV, et al. Extended-donor criteria liver allografts. Semin Liver Dis 2006;26:221–33.
6. Mullhaupt B, Dimitroulis D, Gerlach JT, et al. Hot topics in liver transplantation: organ allocation – extended criteria donor – living donor liver transplantation. J Hepatol. 2008;48(Suppl 1):S58–67.
7. Adam R, Cailliez V, Majno P, et al. Normalised intrinsic mortality risk in liver transplantation: European Liver Transplant Registry study. Lancet 2000;356:621–7.
8. Cameron AM, Ghobrial RM, Yersiz H, et al. Optimal utilization of donor grafts with extended criteria: a single-center experience in over 1000 liver transplants. Ann Surg 2006;243:748–53; discussion 53–5.
9. Feng S, Goodrich NP, Bragg-Gresham JL, et al. Characteristics associated with liver graft failure: the concept of a donor risk index. Am J Transplant 2006;6:783–90.
10. Totsuka E, Fung JJ, Lee MC, et al. Influence of cold ischemia time and graft transport distance on postoperative outcome in human liver transplantation. Surg Today 2002;32:792–9.
11. Everhart JE, Bambha KM. Fatty liver: think globally. Hepatology 2010;51:1491–3.
12. Szczepaniak LS, Nurenberg P, Leonard D, et al. Magnetic resonance spectroscopy to measure hepatic triglyceride content: prevalence of hepatic steatosis in the general population. Am J Physiol Endocrinol Metab 2005;288: E462–8.
13. Selzner M, Clavien PA. Fatty liver in liver transplantation and surgery. Semin Liver Dis 2001;21:105–13.
14. El-Badry AM, Graf R, Clavien PA. Omega 3 – Omega 6: What is right for the liver? J Hepatol 2007;47: 718–25.
15. Salizzoni M, Franchello A, Zamboni F, et al. Marginal grafts: finding the correct treatment for fatty livers. Transpl Int 2003;16:486–93.
16. El-Badry AM, Breitenstein S, Jochum W, et al. Assessment of hepatic steatosis by expert pathologists: The end of a gold standard. Ann Surg 2009;250;720–8.

17. Perez-Daga JA, Santoyo J, Suarez MA, et al. Influence of degree of hepatic steatosis on graft function and postoperative complications of liver transplantation. Transplant Proc 2006;38:2468–70.
18. Marsman WA, Wiesner RH, Rodriguez L, et al. Use of fatty donor liver is associated with diminished early patient and graft survival. Transplantation 1996;62: 1246–51.
19. Noujaim HM, de Ville de Goyet J, Montero EF, et al. Expanding postmortem donor pool using steatotic liver grafts: a new look. Transplantation 2009;87:919–25.
20. Afonso RC, Saad WA, Parra OM, et al. Impact of steatotic grafts on initial function and prognosis after liver transplantation. Transplant Proc 2004;36:909–11.
21. McCormack L, Petrowsky H, Jochum W, et al. Use of severely steatotic grafts in liver transplantation: A matched case–control study. Ann Surg 2007;246: 940–8.
22. Angele MK, Rentsch M, Hartl WH, et al. Effect of graft steatosis on liver function and organ survival after liver transplantation. Am J Surg 2008;195:214–20.
23. Hayashi M, Fujii K, Kiuchi T, et al. Effects of fatty infiltration of the graft on the outcome of living-related liver transplantation. Transplant Proc 1999;31:403.
24. Soejima Y, Shimada M, Suehiro T, et al. Use of steatotic graft in living-donor liver transplantation. Transplantation 2003;76:344–8.
25. Burdelski MM, Rogiers X. What lessons have we learned in pediatric liver transplantation? J Hepatol 2005;42:28–3.
26. Azoulay D, Castaing D, Adam R, et al. Split-liver transplantation for two adult recipients: feasibility and long-term outcomes. Ann Surg 2001;233:565–74.
27. Renz J, Emond JC, Yersiz H, Ascher NL,Bussutil RW. Split-liver transplantation in the United States: outcomes of a national survey. Ann Surg 2004;239: 172–81.
28. Wilms C, Walter J, Kaptein M, et al. Long-term outcome of split liver transplantation using right extended grafts in adulthood: A matched pair analysis. Ann Surg 2006;244:865–72.
29. Totsuka E, Dodson F, Urakami A, et al. Influence of high donor serum sodium levels on early postoperative graft function in human liver transplantation: effect of correction of donor hypernatremia. Liver Transpl Surg 1999;5:421–8.
30. Busuttil RW, Tanaka K. The utility of marginal donors in liver transplantation. Liver Transpl 2003;9:651–63.
31. Moore DE, Feurer ID, Speroff T, et al. Impact of donor, technical, and recipient risk factors on survival and quality of life after liver transplantation. Arch Surg 2005;140:273–7.
32. Burroughs AK, Sabin CA, Rolles K, et al. 3-month and 12-month mortality after first liver transplant in adults in Europe: predictive models for outcome. Lancet 2006;367:225–32.
33. Grande L, Rull A, Rimola A, et al. Outcome of patients undergoing orthotopic liver transplantation with elderly donors (over 60 years). Transplant Proc 1997;29: 3289–90.
34. Grazi GL, Cescon M, Ravaioli M, et al. A revised consideration on the use of very aged donors for liver transplantation. Am J Transplant 2001;1:61–8.
35. Berenguer M, Prieto M, San Juan F, et al. Contribution of donor age to the recent decrease in patient survival among HCV-infected liver transplant recipients. Hepatology 2002;36:202–10.
36. Mutimer DJ, Gunson B, Chen J, et al. Impact of donor age and year of transplantation on graft and patient survival following liver transplantation for hepatitis C virus. Transplantation 2006;81:7–14.
37. Wiemann SU, Satyanarayana A, Tsahuridu M, et al. Hepatocyte telomere shortening and senescence are general markers of human liver cirrhosis. FASEB J 2002;16:935–42.
38. Segev DL, Maley WR, Simpkins CE, et al. Minimizing risk associated with elderly liver donors by matching to preferred recipients. Hepatology 2007;46:1907–18.
39. Ioannou GN. Development and validation of a model predicting graft survival after liver transplantation. Liver Transpl 2006;12:1594–606.
40. Markmann J, Markmann JW, Markmann DA, et al. Preoperative factors associated with outcome and their impact on resource use in 1148 consecutive primary liver transplants. Transplantation 2001;72:1113–22.
41. Weber M, Dindo D, Demartines N, Ambuhl PM, Clavien PA. Kidney transplantation from donors without a heartbeat. N Engl J Med 2002;347: 248–55.
42. Dawwas MF, David C, Barber KM, Watson CJ, Neuberger J, Gimson AE. Developing a liver transplantation donor risk index in a national registy. Hepatology 2007;46:235A.
43. Wiesner RH, McDiarmid SV, Kamath PS, et al. MELD and PELD: application of survival models to liver allocation. Liver Transpl 2001;7:567–80.
44. Schaubel DE, Sima CS, Goodrich NP, et al. The survival benefit of deceased donor liver transplantation as a function of candidate disease severity and donor quality. Am J Transplant 2008;8:419–25.

18 Liver transplantation using donors after cardiac death

Paolo Muiesan, Laura Tariciotti and Chiara Rocha
Liver Unit, Queen Elizabeth Hospital, Birmingham, UK

Key learning points

- History of liver transplantation with DCD grafts and classification of the donors according to Maastricht Criteria.
- Uncontrolled DCD liver allografts: first clinical experiences with Maastricht categories 1 and 2 donors and technical aspects including the use of ECMO
- Controlled DCD liver allografts: expanding the donor pool but vulnerable to primary non function and biliary complications
- Assessment and allocation of the graft: criteria to identify and select the ideal DCD liver donor
- Matching donor liver to recipient as a strategy to improve outcomes
- Open ethical issues and future developments towards extra corporeal machine perfusion devices

Introduction

The first human liver transplant was performed in 1963 by the surgical team led by Dr Thomas Starzl of Denver, CO, USA. The initial attempts at human liver transplantation produced short-term survival, and only in 1967 the same group reported the first series of liver transplants with improved outcomes, and one survival of almost 1 year. As the criteria for brain death had not yet been established, at that time organs were retrieved after the donors died of cardiopulmonary arrest after withdrawal from respiratory support.

The only source of cadaveric allografts remained donation after cardiac death (DCD) until 1968, when the Harvard neurological definition and criteria for brain death were published.[1] Once brain death criteria were introduced in clinical practice, interest in DCD declined because of the better outcomes obtained with heart-beating donor grafts. The organs remained perfused during retrieval, thus suffering minimal warm ischemia. Therefore DCDs were almost universally abandoned.

During the past decade, the rising discrepancy between the number of patients listed for transplantation and the shortage of organs from brain-dead donors, and the stagnating donation rates in many countries, have brought new interest in organ donation after death by cardio-pulmonary criteria. Requests by potential donor families have also contributed to the re-exploration of donation after cardiac death by transplant centers.

To increase graft supply, several strategies have been successfully implemented, including the use of marginal, split, living, and domino donor livers. Following the successful use of DCD kidney grafts for transplantation, where the long-term outcomes are equivalent to the ones of donors after brain death (DBD), interest has moved to the use of extra-renal organs, including liver, pancreas, lung and, more recently, the heart.

Since the 1970s a great deal of progress has been made in the areas of immunosuppression, organ preservation, and surgical technique, so that DCD in the modern era has true potential to provide better quality organs.

Medical Care of the Liver Transplant Patient, Fourth Edition. Edited by Pierre-Alain Clavien, James F. Trotter.

Yet there has been great caution in using DCD livers for transplantation and the selection process is of vital importance to avoid the main problems associated with the additional damage of donor warm ischemia time (DWIT), including primary nonfunction (PNF), delayed graft function, and ischemic-type biliary strictures (ITBS).

Classification

According to the setting in which cardiac death occurs, DCDs are divided into two categories: controlled or uncontrolled.[2]

Controlled donors are generally victims of a catastrophic brain damage of diverse etiology, deemed incompatible with meaningful recovery, but whose condition does not meet formal criteria for brain death and whose cardiopulmonary function ceases before organs are retrieved. The attending physician and the family of the injured patient agree to withdraw life support treatment. This decision is independent from, and precedes, the one to donate. The procedure of withdrawal of life-sustaining therapy is planned by the medical team attending the patient and cardiac arrest occurs within an intensive care unit (ICU) or in the operating room (Maastricht category 3). Occasionally the next of kin of a brain-dead donor will ask for the retrieval to take place only after cardiac arrest (Maastricht category 4).

On the other hand, uncontrolled donation refers to donation after death that occurred suddenly and was not anticipated. The typical patient has an unexpected cardiopulmonary arrest outside the hospital and is dead at arrival in hospital (Maastricht category 1) or dies within the emergency room or hospital wards (Maastricht category 2) and death is declared only after failure of resuscitation attempts. Cardiac arrest following the determination of brain death in the ICU (Maastricht category 4) may also be considered uncontrolled in case it happens under unexpected circumstances and required a rapid retrieval. The ethics, assessment, techniques of retrieval, and outcomes of transplant are very different with controlled- and uncontrolled-liver DCDs (Figure 18.1).

Uncontrolled liver donation

Worldwide the majority of uncontrolled DCDs are category 1 or 2 donors and constitute the best part of patients considered eligible for DCD in Spain and

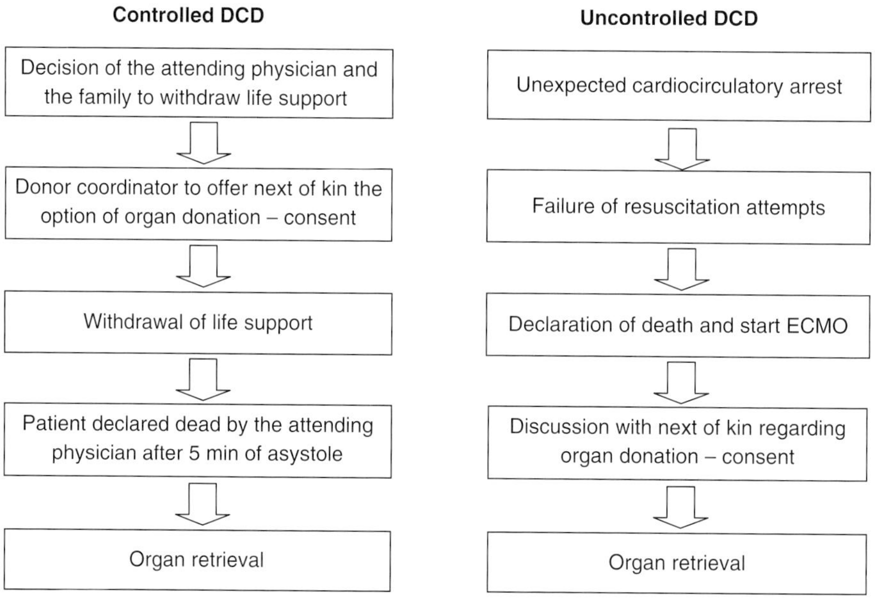

Figure 18.1 Different pathways of uncontrolled and controlled DCD

France. Uncontrolled DCDs are more likely to be trauma victims, younger and *healthier* individuals, yet the use of these grafts is still limited. Death often occurs after prolonged periods of resuscitation maneuvers, leading to substantial injury from warm ischemia. The real extent of DWIT is difficult to assess due to the unanticipated nature of cardio-circulatory arrest that may have not occurred within the medical setting. As donation interventions need to be initiated quickly, the surrogate decision makers are unlikely to be immediately available to provide consent.

The early results of transplantation with uncontrolled DCD were disappointing. In 1995 Casavilla et al. reported the Pittsburgh experience with poor post-transplant graft survival of DCD livers, particularly those from uncontrolled donors, mainly due to PNF and vascular complications.[3] Despite the poor results reported in the early studies at the beginning of the DCD experience, recent series showed improving outcomes (Table 18.1).

Procedure

When a potential category I or II donor suffers cardiac arrest and all resuscitation attempts fail, cardiopulmonary resuscitation (CPR) is suspended for a 5–10-minute interval, after which death is declared. CPR is resumed manually or by means of a mechanical compression device, either in the mobile ICU unit or in the Emergency room after death is certified. External thoracic compressions maintain some degree of circulation to keep organs viable. Once in the Emergency department, the femoral artery used to be cannulated with a double balloon triple lumen catheter to provide access for perfusion of the abdominal organs with copious cold preservation solution. As cold perfusion failed to provide viable uncontrolled DCD livers for transplantation, a change of strategy was put into practice.

The concept is that of artificial restoration of circulation of blood in the abdominal aorta using an extracorporeal membrane oxygenation (ECMO) circuit. Monitoring of blood parameters and bypass flow are maintained until cold preservation is established at retrieval.[4]

The procurement follows and is divided in three phases:

1. Phase 1: Dissection phase while on ECMO
2. Phase 2: Discontinuation of CPR/ECMO
3. Phase 3: Organ perfusion with cold preservation solution using standard retrieval technique.

Mechanical ventilation and external massage, extracorporeal perfusion, or in situ preservation are all means to maintain organ viability until permission can be obtained from the family to proceed to donation. ECMO, by providing prolonged organ

Table 18.1 Liver transplantation from uncontrolled DCD: main series

Author	OLT centre	Year	No. UDCDs	PNF (%)	HAT (%)	BC (%)	Re OLT (%)	Graft survival (%)	Patient survival (%)	Follow up (months)
Casavilla et al.	Pittsburgh	1995	6	33	17	–	50	17	67	12
Busutill and Tanaka	UCLA	2003	16	6.25	–	–	–	75	88	12
Otero et al.	La Coruna	2003	20	25	0	5	25	55	80	24
Quintela et al.	La Coruna	2005	10	10	0	0	10	90	90	57
Fondevila et al.	Barcelona	2007	10	10	10	10	25	50	70	23
Suarez et al.	La Coruna	2008	27	18	3.6	25	–	49	62	60
Jimenez-Galanes et al.	Madrid	2009	20	10	0	5	15	80	85.5	12

BC: biliary complication, HAT: hepatic artery thrombosis, OLT: orthotopic liver transplantation, PNF: primary nonfunction, UDCD: uncontrolled donor after cardiac death preservation, grants more time to locate the next of kin, allowing the family the opportunity to decide on organ donation.

The decision about the timing, initiation, and discontinuation of CPR, declaration of death, and consent of the recipient are all features of this procedure that raise various ethical issues. Interestingly, the rate of family refusals among potential DCDs is lower than among families of brain-dead individuals. Possible explanations include a greater understanding of death because the heart is not beating and less time of uncertainty about death.

The organization required to cope with an uncontrolled DCD program is unique and needs a dedicated on-call team 24 hours per day. In Madrid, for example, special ambulances, staffed with a physician and nurse trained in critical care are equipped to provide intensive medical care to seriously ill patients. A few Spanish transplant coordination teams have developed a policy for uncontrolled DCDs within the pre-hospital health care system.

Despite the longer DWIT, uncontrolled donation may have a theoretical advantage. It has been hypothesized that brain death may lead to an upregulation of pro-inflammatory mediators and cell-surface molecules in peripheral organs to be engrafted, thus making them more susceptible to inflammatory and immune responses in the host.[5] Owing to the rapidity of events, uncontrolled donors are expected to be spared by the negative effects of severe brain injury. On the contrary, controlled DCDs are likely to be affected to a degree by the "cytokine storm" given the longer duration of the central nervous system injury.

Maastricht DCD categories 1 and 2 have been revisited mostly in Spain, where withdrawal of life support and controlled donation are not supported for medico–legal reasons. The difference between categories is important for both the logistics of retrieval and expected outcome after transplantation.

Category 1: dead on arrival at hospital

This category includes the so-called deaths "in the streets" – all the patients who die of cardiac arrest outside a hospital setting. It is essential that the moment of cardiac arrest is witnessed and recorded by bystanders for individuals in this category to become potential donors. The timings of preadmission resuscitation must also be well documented. Alvarez and colleagues reported 111 potential DCDs, of which 53 became actual category 1 donors.[6] Out of 12 retrieved livers, eight were transplanted, all with good early function but the report lacks further details on the outcomes of the recipients. Category 1 donors, given the longer and indeterminate DWIT, are more likely to donate only kidneys and rarely provide liver grafts suitable for transplantation.

Category 2: unsuccessful resuscitation

Individuals in this category have experienced cardiac arrest in a hospital setting, usually within the Accident and Emergency department, where all CPR, timings, the interval and efficiency of resuscitation can be adequately documented. Therefore DWIT is better defined compared to category 1 donors. In the setting of uncontrolled DCD, liver grafts from category 2 donors appear to have better outcomes.

The results from a series of 20 liver transplants from Maastricht category 2 DCD was compared with 40 liver transplants from heart-beating donors in a report by Otero and colleagues.[7] They found that using a mechanical device to continue chest and abdominal compressions and establishing extracorporeal perfusion proved more effective in preserving the liver compared to swift cold perfusion, which was associated with a high rate of PNF. However, graft survival remained significantly lower (55%) compared to that of livers from DBD and a 2-year patient survival rate of 80% was maintained only by means of an aggressive re-transplantation policy. The overall incidence of PNF, liver dysfunction, and biliary complications remained greater among livers from DCD compared with those from DBD. The group from Juan Canalejo University Hospital described 10 DCDs maintained by means of the method of chest and abdominal compression–decompression.[8] There was only one PNF-related graft loss and all the other grafts showed good early and medium-term results. Very recently the same group reported a very high incidence of biliary complications (41.7%) of uncontrolled DCD liver transplants.[9]

A normothermic ECMO was successfully used in uncontrolled donors by the group in Barcelona.[4] Of 40 potential DCDs, 10 livers were transplanted. All but two transplants had good hepatic function: one

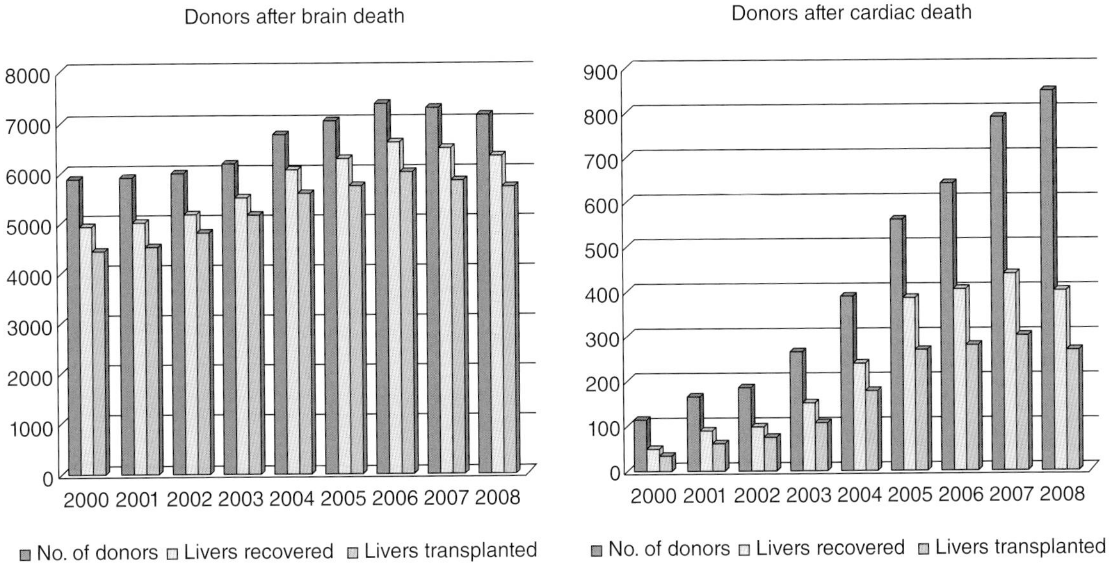

Figure 18.2 UNOS data on donors after brain death and cardiac death (2000–2008). Note the lower yield, in proportion, of livers from DCDs. http://optn.transplant.hrsa.gov/

graft was lost to PNF and the other to hepatic artery thrombosis (HAT). To assess graft suitability for transplantation the authors reviewed several parameters including CPR and ECMO times, transaminase serum levels during ECMO, and donor age. Good results were achieved at a cost of a strict selection of DCD liver grafts.

More recently, in a study from Madrid, where the authors used a similar normothermic ECMO protocol in 20 DCD liver recipients, the overall patient and graft survival with uncontrolled donors were similar to those of DBD.[10]

In the future, uncontrolled DCD liver donation may represent a valuable additional source of grafts. Yet, currently, there is a gap in liver graft survival comparing conventional cadaveric donors and uncontrolled DCDs largely due to higher PNF rates and a greater incidence of biliary complications, specifically of ITBS. It is crucial that techniques of extracorporeal liver machine perfusion are developed to successfully resuscitate organs and allow better graft selection. Research should also progress towards new strategies to minimize organ ischemia-reperfusion injury. These steps would be necessary to safely expand the organ pool for liver transplantation into Maastricht category 2, and possibly category 1.

Controlled liver donation

According to the UNOS database, the number of donors after cardiac death has been progressively growing in the USA, and currently represent 5% of the whole donor pool (Figure 18.2). The number of donors referred as controlled DCD has been expanding rapidly in the last 12 months in the UK (Figure 18.3). The procedure of withdrawal of treatment, when it is considered futile to continue, has been accepted and regulated in several countries including Canada, the USA, the UK, Belgium, the Netherlands, Switzerland and Australia. Without a legal framework of withdrawal of treatment, controlled (Maastricht category 3) donation after cardiac death cannot take place.

The decision to withdraw life support is taken by the attending physician (intensivist, neurosurgeon) in agreement with the family, as a result of the ascertained futility of further therapeutic efforts and in the best interest of the patient. Such decision precedes and must be independent of any consideration of donor suitability.

To minimize both real and perceived conflicts of interest for ICU staff between their therapeutic duty to the critically ill patient and their nontherapeutic

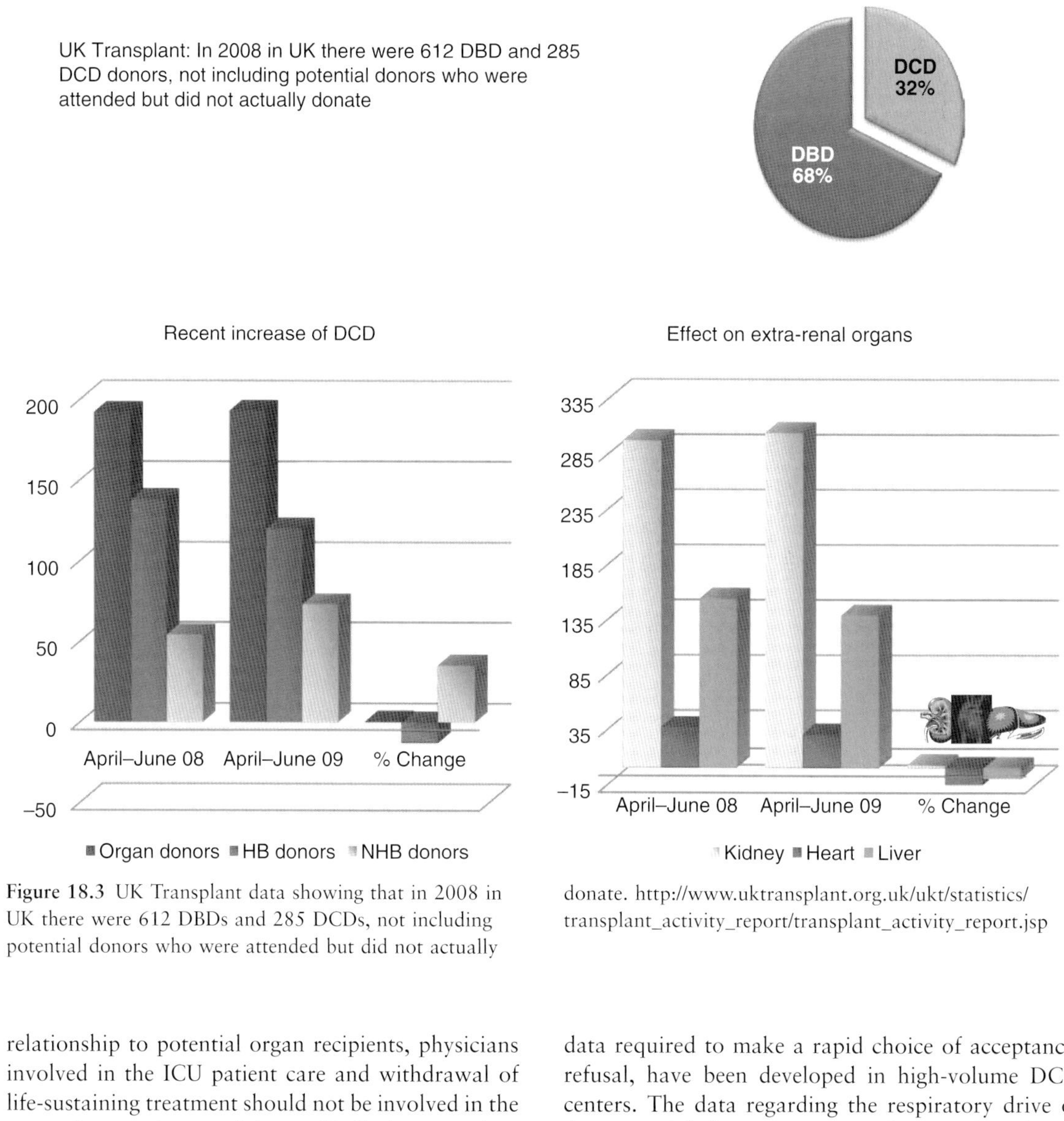

Figure 18.3 UK Transplant data showing that in 2008 in UK there were 612 DBDs and 285 DCDs, not including potential donors who were attended but did not actually donate. http://www.uktransplant.org.uk/ukt/statistics/transplant_activity_report/transplant_activity_report.jsp

relationship to potential organ recipients, physicians involved in the ICU patient care and withdrawal of life-sustaining treatment should not be involved in the care of transplant recipients. Similarly transplant physicians should not be involved in the decision to withdraw treatment or certify of death.

Efficient coordination is a critical step for a successful DCD liver donation given the greater sensitivity to DWIT of the liver compared to the kidney, pancreas, or lung.

The transplant coordinators offer the organs to the appropriate centers in a concise way, including only the essential information due to the constraints of time. Specific DCD referral forms, with the essential data required to make a rapid choice of acceptance/refusal, have been developed in high-volume DCD centers. The data regarding the respiratory drive of the potential donor are very relevant, though still difficult to interpret when deciding whether to send a team to the referring hospital. The group from Wisconsin described an algorithm based on respiratory and cardiocirculatory data for predicting whether cardiac arrest will or will not occur early in the potential donor, though it has not yet been validated in other centers.[11]

The majority of liver transplant units would not consider using a DCD liver unless cardiac arrest intervenes within 30 minutes after withdrawal.

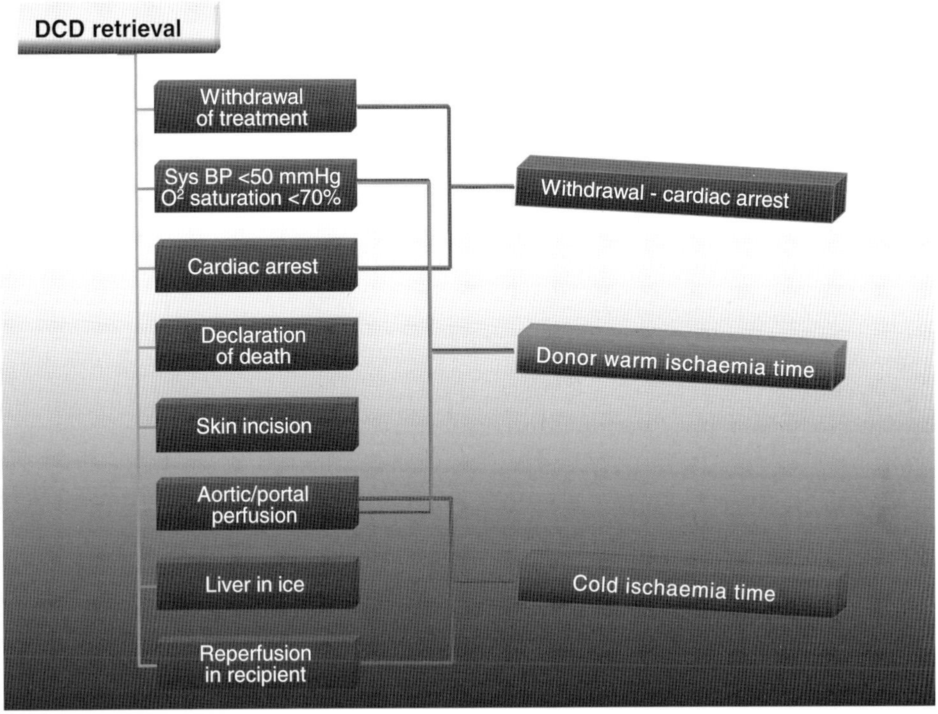

Figure 18.4 Steps of controlled donation after cardiac death

Approximately 40% of the potential DCDs do not suffer cardiac arrest within 60 min and liver donation is abandoned.

Treatment is withdrawn in accordance with local practice and policies and it is usually by extubation and interruption of drugs supporting the blood pressure. In the UK, withdrawal commonly takes place either in the ICU or in the anesthetic room. Withdrawal in the operating room is frequent practice in the USA. Such practice has the advantage of minimizing DWIT but it may limit the wishes of the family to assist their dying relative and may not allow a complete partition of the physician declaring death from the surgeon waiting to perform the procedure.

Documentation of regular observations at 5-minute intervals, including pulse, blood pressure and oxygen saturations, is completed by the transplant coordinator and provides additional information to help the transplant surgeon in the assessment of suitability of the retrieved organs for grafting.

Following asystole, death is certified by the attending physician. The time required to declare death following cardiac arrest varies in different centers and countries and it is still a subject of active debate. A controlled DCD pediatric heart transplant program in Denver accepts a 66-second time lag after circulatory cessation to certify death. The Pittsburgh protocol advocates an interval of 2 min between asystole and surgical retrieval.[12] The Institute of Medicine in the USA suggests a "no-touch period" of 5 min. Death is declared after at least 5 min from detection of cardiac arrest. Following certification of death the patient is rapidly transferred to the operating room to proceed with the surgical retrieval (Figure 18.4). In Italy DCD kidney transplants have been performed despite the legal requirement to observe a 20-minute interval from cardiac arrest to certification of death.

Definitions of warm ischemia time also vary among centers retrieving DCD organs. In the UK the start of DWIT is defined by the advent of hypotension (systolic blood pressure <50 mmHg) or hypoxia (saturation <70%) to better reflect effective hypoperfusion of the organs.[13] Given the great disparity in definitions of

DWIT in the USA, a consensus conference recently defined warm ischemia as the interval of time between withdrawal of treatment and initiation of cold perfusion.[14] The latest ASTS, recommended practice guidelines for DCD distinguish between **Total DWIT** (from withdrawal of treatment to initiation of cold perfusion) and **True DWIT** (defined as the interval between a drop in mean arterial pressure below 60 mmHg and initiation of perfusion).[15] True DWIT is similar to the DWIT definition in the UK and other European centers, and its upper acceptable limit, to safely utilize DCD livers, is set to 30 min.

Cold ischemia time (CIT) extends from the initiation of cold preservation of the liver to reperfusion after implantation in the recipient. For DCD, liver transplantation CIT should be shorter than 8 h. When the CIT exceeds 8 h or 12 h, the incidence of liver graft failure within 60 days of transplantation has been shown to increase to 30% and 58%, respectively.[16]

Surgical procedure

The standard retrieval procedure is the super-rapid technique, originally described by Casavilla et al.[3] The procedure begins with a midline laparotomy and rapid isolation and cannulation of the distal aorta followed by perfusion with a low viscosity preservation solution containing heparin (Figure 18.5). The inferior vena cava (IVC) is vented in the abdomen or in the chest. The thoracic aorta is clamped just above the diaphragm. In DCD liver retrievals dual perfusion is advisable as the abdominal aorta often contains clots that may embolize into the vasculature of the abdominal organs. Moreover perfusion of the aorta by gravity flow of University of Wisconsin (UW) solution or histidine–tryptophan–ketoglutarate (HTK) solutions achieves only suboptimal pressures in the hepatic artery of 19 mmHg and 16 mmHg, respectively.[17] Therefore pressure perfusion at 200 mmHg, applied at the solution bag, is desirable to improve perfusion pressure in the liver and other abdominal organs. The portal vein is then cannulated and perfused with UW solution also containing heparin. The abdominal cavity is topically cooled using copious saline ice slush.

In summary, the modifications of the retrieval procedure reduce liver congestion, improve organ perfusion, and facilitate surgical dissection thus further reducing DWIT. Minor changes to the Casavilla technique, aiming at speeding aortic cannulation have been described.

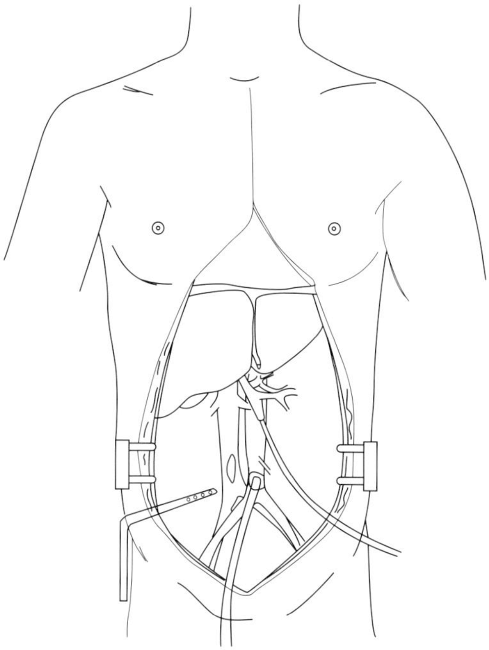

Figure 18.5 Super rapid procedure for controlled DCDs. Initial laparotomy and rapid cannulation and perfusion of the aorta

Choice of preservation solution

Effective washout of the DCD liver microvasculature during retrieval is essential for optimal preservation. If the blood remnants in the liver are not completely washed out of the microcirculation, perfusion of the biliary tree and graft viability may be compromised. Most DCD livers are transplanted with CIT just short of 8 h; therefore most of the current crystalloid-based low-viscosity preservation solutions should be suitable, including Euro-Collins, Marshall, HTK and Celsior solution. HTK has recently gained popularity as a wash-out and preservation solution for DCD livers. Advantages of HTK compared to UW include lower viscosity, faster cooling rates, and a low potassium content that avoids the need for the portal flush prior to reperfusion. An analysis of the UNOS database, comparing 575 liver grafts UW-preserved and 254 HTK-preserved, showed that HTK was independently associated with 44% increased risk of graft loss compared to UW.[18] As in situ aortic perfusion has been shown to be inadequate in delivering physiological pressures in hepatic artery, high pressure in situ and ex situ perfusion has been suggested as a technique to improve perfusion of the hepatic arterial tree, therefore more effectively flushing the microcirculation of the bile ducts, aiming at reducing biliary complications.

Although machine perfusion of the liver with cold preservation solutions may have theoretical advantages, it has not reached widespread clinical use as with kidney transplantation. Guarrera first demonstrated the safety and reliability of hypothermic machine perfusion (HMP) with a pilot case-controlled series of 20 adults transplanted with HMP-preserved livers at the Columbia University Medical Center.[19]

Clinical experience with controlled DCD and ischemic cholangiopathy

The first experience at Pittsburgh revisiting 24 potential liver donors after cardiac death between 1989 and 1994 showed a very high rate of early graft failure and a high rate of vascular complications.[3] This was followed in 1995 by a series of five recipients of DCD livers at the University of Wisconsin with one graft loss due to primary nonfunction. In 2005 the same group[20] reported up-to-date results on 36 recipients transplanted with DCD livers. Both 3-year graft and patient survival (68% and 56%) were inferior compared with recipients of DBD allografts (84% and 80%). There was no significant difference in the incidence of PNF between the two groups but hepatic artery stenosis occurred with greater frequency in DCD liver recipients. Interestingly this finding was confirmed by others and could be attributable to a greater possibility of traumatic arterial intimal injuries when using the super rapid retrieval technique.

Abt et al. first reported a high incidence of biliary complications in five out of 15 DCD liver recipients, the majority being intrahepatic strictures,[21] resulting in multiple interventional procedures, retransplantation, or death. ITBS were later universally recognized as a severe complication of transplantation of DCD liver grafts and were confirmed as one of the main causes of graft loss by the majority of reports. In animal DCD models it has been shown that irreversible biliary tract damage occurs after 40 min of DWIT.[22] The greatest impact of biliary damage and of ITBS in particular, is on patient re-listing, retransplantation and quality of life as several radiologic diagnostic and treatment procedures may be required.

The first insult contributing to biliary damage is certainly ischemic, though there is still poor understanding in the sequence of events leading to ITBS. Some studies point the finger at the liver microcirculatory dysfunction related to hypotension and cardiac standstill. The resulting ischemic injury to the microvascular endothelium leads, in the preservation phase, to cell disruption and may contribute to microvascular thrombosis, which prevents effective revascularization and exacerbates ischemic injury to the biliary epithelium.

Damage to the biliary epithelial cells seems to be central to the eventual formation of stenoses, and may occur before or after organ retrieval because of energy stores depletion. Hydrophobic bile salts cause further biliary epithelial damage, which could be reduced by copiously flushing the biliary tree free of bile during liver retrieval. In addition, the infusion of a cold perfusate into the biliary tree through a naso-biliary tube or directly with a syringe during the various phases of organ retrieval may further reduce ischemic injury by reducing the metabolic requirements of biliary epithelial cells. Moreover, the activation of neutrophils, promoting the release of free radicals causes oxidative stress, further damaging vulnerable epithelial cells. The end result is the loss of epithelium in the biliary tree leading to ulcer formation, which may serve as a foundation for formation of biliary sludge. The ulcerations in the epithelial lining are associated with growth of granulation tissue on the underlying stroma, and the progressive fibrosis, promotes the development of biliary strictures.

Skaro et al.[23] identified a significantly higher retransplant rate of DCD (22%) vs DBD transplant patients (7%), due to severe biliary complications (53% vs 22%) despite a strict selection and a low threshold to discard grafts that didn't perfuse completely with 2–3 liters of preservation solution. These results were not modified when analyzing separately the early and late experience of the center.

Chan et al.[24] also reported a higher incidence of ITBS among the DCD transplant patients compared to the DBD group (13.7% vs 1%), but the factors linked with the poorer outcome in their study included donor weight and age and a CIT >9 hours. Donor age and CIT also correlated well with the Donor Risk Index concept.[25] As to donor weight, a high BMI is likely to lengthen the time from skin incision to cannulation and perfusion. The livers are also expected to be steatotic, thus interfering with the flushing of the smaller arterioles feeding the biliary tree and triggering ischemic damage. A high BMI is also associated with diverse co-morbidity, including cardiovascular disease, dyslipidemia, metabolic syndrome, type 2 diabetes mellitus and high blood pressure, thus increasing the degree of risk associated with these donors.

Other single-center experiences from London and Philadelphia[14,26] reported excellent graft and patient survival in two respective series of 19 and 32 DCD liver recipients comparable to standard outcomes of DBD liver transplantation. The incidence of biliary complications in the King's College Hospital group was similar to the one of recipients of standard cadaveric donor livers. There were no graft losses due to ITBS. Though no significant differences were found by Fujita et al. in the incidence of biliary strictures between 24 DCD and 1209 DBD graft recipients, all cases affected by ITBS in the DCD group eventually lost the graft, and needed re-grafting.[27]

Two large single-center experiences were recently published, one from Jacksonville Florida, showing no difference in graft and patient survival between 108 DCD and 1328 DBD recipients and the other from Pittsburgh, Pennsylvania, which reported significantly worse long-term graft outcomes for 141 DCD recipients accurately matched with 282 DBD transplants. Longer DWIT, CIT and older donors were related with poorer graft survival and recipient factors (age, BMI and male graft into female recipient) to graft failures.

Large DCD studies on liver transplantation have utilized registry data United Network for Organ Sharing/Scientific Registry of Transplant Recipients (UNOS/SRTR). Abt et al. in 2004 analyzed the outcomes of 144 DCD and 26 856 DBD liver transplants from the UNOS database and identified the significance of cold ischemic time as a predictor of graft failure in DCD grafts.[16] Merion et al. compared the results of 472 DCD and 23 598 DBD liver grafts from the SRTR database, confirming the findings of Abt et al. of inferior DCD graft survival outcomes.[28]

Mateo et al. looked at UNOS data and defined a recipient cumulative relative risk (RCRR) using significant risk factors identified from a Cox regression analysis including age, medical condition at transplantation, regraft status, need for dialysis, and serum creatinine.[29] Graft survival from DCD was significantly inferior to DBD but low-risk recipients with low-risk DCD livers (DWIT <30 min and CIT <10 h) achieved similar graft survival rates to recipients with DBD allografts.

Lee et al. developed a DCD risk index to stratify the DCD transplants in four risk groups using data of the UNOS database. Graft survival of the most favorable DCD group (donor age <45 years, DWIT <15 min, and CIT <10 h) was comparable to that of DBD liver transplants irrespective of recipient condition. Increasing donor age was highly predictive of poor outcomes in DCD compared to DBD, especially in sick recipients. The data confirmed the exponential increase in the usage of DCD grafts in the USA, but also their lower survival rates at 3 and 5 years.[30]

Selck et al. highlighted the tendency of selecting recipients of DCD grafts in a study of 855 DCD and 21 089 DBD liver transplants from the SRTR data. DCD recipients were older than DBD patients but had lower Model for End-stage Liver Disease (MELD) scores and were less likely to be in the ICU or have a high-urgency status. DCD listing for retransplantation and graft failure progressed continuously over 6 months compared to 20 days in the DBD group.[31] This pattern of temporal distribution of graft failure proved disadvantageous for DCD patients needing regrafting as they waited longer and received higher risk grafts. A change of liver allocation policy has been advocated to address those disadvantaged by a failing DCD graft. The main reports on liver transplantation from controlled DCD are summarized in Table 18.2.

Pediatric liver transplantation and hepatocyte transplantation

Abt and colleagues reviewed the outcomes of 19 pediatric DCD liver recipients from the UNOS database over a 10-year period.[32] A total of 16 patients received livers from pediatric donors and three from adult donors. Graft survival was excellent and comparable to DBD grafts. Seven children transplanted with segmental liver grafts were reported to be all alive and with good graft function at the end of the study

Table 18.2 Liver transplantation from controlled DCD: main series

Author	OLT centre	Year	No. of DCDs/ DBD	PNF (%)	HAT (%)	BC (%)	Re-OLT (%)	Graft survival (%)	Patient survival (%)	Follow up (years)
Muiesan et al.	King's College, London	2005	32/–	3.1/–	6.25/–	9.4/–	6.25/–	86.5/–	89.6/–	1
Merion et al.	SRTR (Michigan)	2006	472/ 23598	–	–	–	–	60.5/75	–	3
Kaczmarek et al.	Newcastle	2007	11/164	0/–	0/–	45/17	9/–	–	–	–
Selk et al.	SRTR (Columbia, NY)	2008	855/21089	–	–	–	14/–	–	57/–	3
Grewal et al.	Mayo Clinic Jacksonville	2009	108/1328	3.7/1.4	0.9/1.7	8.3/1.9	14.8/9.3	71/69.1	88.1/77.2	5
Skaro et al.	Chicago	2009	32/237	3/1	9/3	53/22	22/7	53/74	74/81	3
Pine et al.	St James Hospital, Leeds	2009	39/39	5.1/0	2.5/5.1	36/10.2	2.5/0	63.6/97.4	68.2/100	3
De Vera et al.	Pittsburgh	2009	141/282	12/2	6/6	25/13	18/7	44/63	57/64	10
Busuttil et al.	UCLA	2009	47/505	2.6/5.5	5.3/4	21/9	–	66/69	70/74	5

BC: biliary complication, DBD: donor after brain death, DCD: donor after cardiac death, HAT: hepatic artery thrombosis, OLT: orthotopic liver transplantation, PNF: primary nonfunction, SRTR: Scientific Registry of Transplant Recipients

period at King's College Hospital.[33] The selective use of the best DCD organs was shown to produce good and durable graft survival in the pediatric population. A split-liver transplant was also reported in the early series as successful in the child. The right lobe was transplanted sequentially in an adult recipient with a cold ischemia time of just in excess of 14 h and failed to function, leading to retransplantation.

Segments of split or reduced or even unused whole DCD livers may be a significant source of hepatocytes. Hepatocyte transplantation is emerging as an additional modality of treatment for patients with acute liver failure or liver-based metabolic disorders. DCD hepatocytes isolated from unused segments of reduced DCD and cryopreserved were used for hepatocyte transplantation in two children: a 3-year-old girl with Crigler–Najjar syndrome Type 1 and a 4-month-old boy with inherited clotting factor VII deficiency.[34] There was a beneficial effect in terms of lowered serum bilirubin and decrease in requirement for recombinant factor VII, respectively without adverse clinical reactions. When cryopreservation of human hepatocytes from different liver tissue sources was investigated, cells isolated from a small number of DCD livers seemed to be more vulnerable to the effects of freezing in terms of lower cell viability and albumin production rates on thawing compared to hepatocytes isolated from conventional donor livers.

Assessment of graft

Assessment of the suitability of a DCD for liver donation remains difficult and somehow subjective to the experience of retrieving and implanting surgeons. Parameters reported to identify the best DCD liver donors include age <50 years, a DWIT of <20 min, cold ischemia time of <8 hours and minimal steatosis. Transplants of these ideal DCD liver grafts achieve similar results of recipients of standard DBD livers. The DCD liver seems to be more edematous than the standard DBD liver graft and the verdict of suitability of a DCD liver for transplantation is still generally made on gross appearance, ease of perfusion, degree of steatosis, and thorough evaluation of donor characteristics. Liver biopsy is of limited value and a comparison of post-reperfusion biopsies of DCD and DBD livers performed by a blinded pathologist showed essentially no differences between the two types of grafts. Other markers, including glutathione S-transferase and xanthine oxidase, have not proved to be reliable indicators of DCD liver graft quality. The relevance of hepatocyte viability with trypan blue exclusion technique was also assessed in choosing DCD liver grafts for transplantation, though it was not valuable in terms of graft selection.[13]

Recipient selection

The choice of recipient should be restricted to those not requiring long, difficult dissections, including retransplants, or patients with previous extensive upper abdominal surgery, as this extends the CIT. High-risk patients, such as those already on multi-organ support and those with severe portal hypertension, requiring robust early graft function, are not generally considered to be good candidates for DCD liver grafts.

Techniques of implantation have not been formally evaluated in clinical trials, but experience from small-for-size grafts and experimental studies suggest that mitigation of severe portal hypertension with a temporary porto-caval shunt, blood flush prior to reperfusion and arterial rather than portal reperfusion may all be of value and may extend donor criteria for DCD.

Malignancy is a good indication for DCD liver transplantation. Patients transplanted for hepatocellular carcinoma (HCC) rather than for end-stage liver disease, given their good performance status, may better tolerate the significant reperfusion injury, which follows the implantation and revascularization of DCD livers. Patients with HCC, who are suitable for and consent to DCD grafts, experience less competition whilst waiting, and are transplanted more rapidly, thus minimizing the risk of dropping out for HCC progression beyond transplant criteria.

Primary sclerosing cholangitis (PSC) should be looked at critically as a potential indication for DCD liver transplantation. DWIT-related biliary injury, specific to DCD grafts, could trigger disease recurrence in patients transplanted for PSC. Nevertheless there is currently no clear evidence suggesting that patients with PSC do worse with DCD livers and that they should not receive DCD grafts.

Similarly there is no substantive evidence that DCD livers would be more likely to be affected by severe hepatitis C recurrence in HCV recipients. Preservation and reperfusion injury of the liver are associated with hepatocyte death followed by a rapid proliferation and a marked inflammatory response. In theory, in the setting of DCD and two bouts of ischemia, HCV infection may be facilitated. A study on the HCV population including 14 DCDs and 188 DBDs showed a lower 1- and 5-year patient and graft survival in patients transplanted with DCD grafts. Despite these results, the worse outcomes were not directly associated to HCV recurrence.[35] A report from the Mayo Clinic showed an increased rate in graft loss in HCV-positive compared with HCV-negative recipients of DCD grafts, with a graft survival in HCV-positive patients at 1, 3 and 5 years of 67%, 50% and 50%, respectively.[36] On the contrary the Pittsburgh group found no difference in outcomes of DCD liver transplantation in HCV-positive vs HCV-negative recipients.[37]

High-risk recipients who anecdotally do not do well after DCD liver transplantation include those with pulmonary hypertension. The well-known severe reperfusion syndrome, at times associated with prolonged cardiovascular instability, is detrimental for these patients. For similar reasons, patients with pre-transplant renal impairment will be more exposed to acute tubular necrosis and post-transplant need for temporary filtration or dialysis. Thus in patients with weak renal function and receiving a DCD liver graft, delayed introduction of the calcineurin inhibitor after transplantation, based for example on an induction regimen with anti-IL-2 receptor, may be beneficial. On the other hand it is also debatable whether a good-risk recipient, with a quality of life indication including, for example, primary biliary cirrhosis with associated intractable pruritus or polycystic liver disease, should be offered a DCD liver, with the awareness of the inferior long-term graft survival and, if so, what should be the appropriate procedure to get the patient's consent.

It is controversial whether a recipient with a lower MELD would be disadvantaged by receiving a DCD liver graft. The expected lifetime of a liver transplant candidate offered a DCD liver should be compared with that of the same potential recipient turning down the DCD graft offer and deciding to wait longer for a DBD liver. In different terms it is likely to be better to accept a DCD liver than dying on the waiting list, but this is clearly also relative to the vast variations of the waiting list time around the world.

Higher-risk recipients have been reported to have a greater chance of survival 1 year after the time of listing, when accepting a DCD liver graft rather than remaining on the list waiting for a DBD liver transplant, supporting the hypothesis of greater transplant benefit of DCD grafts in candidates with high MELD scores.

Other issues

While economic outcomes for subsets of DCD organs have been described for renal transplantation, this is just starting to be explored for liver transplantation. Axelrod and colleagues analyzed extended-criteria donors, including DCD.[38] Using UNOS data between 2002 and 2005 they assessed the relationship between recipient MELD score, organ quality as defined by donor risk index (DRI)[25] and hospital length of stay. In the lowest recipient MELD group (<10), the difference of length of hospital stay between ideal (DRI <1.0) and very high-risk donors (DRI >2.5) was 10.6 days with an estimated incremental cost of $47 986, showing that the use of marginal liver grafts results in increased hospital costs independent of recipient risk factors. Longer ITU stay and greater costs were also reported for patients transplanted with DCD livers by the group in Pittsburgh. Such analysis did not take into account the cost of staffing retrieving teams and admitting the potential recipient when the donor does not arrest within the time limit or when the liver is deemed nontransplantable. Jay et al. estimated direct medical care costs based on inpatient and outpatient hospital costs for 28 DCD and 198 DBD liver recipients. Organ acquisition and physician costs were excluded. As expected, higher rates of graft failure and biliary complications translated into markedly increased direct medical care costs for DCD recipients.[39]

These significant financial implications should be considered in decisions regarding the use of DCD livers as they might have an impact in the near future on payment or reimbursement policies of transplant centers using a high proportion of livers from DCD.

A trend towards DCD at the expense of the numbers of brain-dead donors emerged from the Dutch experience. A similar phenomenon has been observed in the UK in the past year.[40] Possible causes include the perceived benefit of a reduction in donor stay in the, constantly under pressure for beds, Intensive Care Units, and the advantage of a more swift procedure. Such shifting donor referral pattern, however, needs to be analyzed in detail to ensure that all potential brain-dead donors are effectively tested for brain death rather than diverted to a DCD procedure with detrimental effects on the recovery of extra-renal organs.

Conclusion

Experience with hepatic transplantation from DCD has not yet reached the degree of maturity as that of renal transplantation. Only a few centers have achieved results comparable with the brain-dead donor setting using organs from controlled donors, mainly by effective and rapid organ procurement, a strict selection of organs transplanted, and reduction of CIT. The liver graft selection is still an art and at this time there is no effective algorithm to differentiate transplantable livers from those that should be discarded. Although the experience is limited, livers from uncontrolled donors do not have the same survival rate as those from controlled donors. Liver transplantation from uncontrolled DCD may have a greater potential but currently the risks of PNF and ITBS have a major impact on graft survival.

To develop safely and fully the potential of DCD, changes are needed to provide a clear legal framework in many countries, funding and training for the infrastructure and informed acceptance by the public. A trend towards a possible erosion of DCD into the brain-dead donor pool must be carefully monitored and corrected as it may eventually threaten the overall number of transplantable organs.

Additional work is required to better define which DCD organs are optimal for hepatic transplantation, the acceptable limits of DWIT, and which recipients are best served with the use of these organs. Normothermic extracorporeal membrane oxygenation has already shown a great potential to improve results in uncontrolled liver donors and may become in the near future the standard of preservation also for older controlled donors. Extracorporeal liver machine perfusion (hypothermic or normothermic) is a promising tool that may soon contribute to improve safety and outcomes of DCD liver grafts. The development of effective new means to preserve, resuscitate and assess controlled and uncontrolled DCD grafts may, in the future, see these donors challenge or surpass cadaveric heart-beating and living donation as a source of livers for transplantation.

References

1. A definition of irreversible coma. Report of the Ad Hoc Committee of the Harvard Medical School to Examine the Definition of Brain Death. JAMA 1968;205: 337–40.
2. Kootstra G, Daemen JH, Oomen AP. Categories of non-heart-beating donors. Transplant Proc 1995;27: 2893–4.
3. Casavilla A, Ramirez C, Shapiro R, et al. Experience with liver and kidney allografts from non-heart-beating donors. Transplantation 1995;59:197–203.
4. Fondevila C, Hessheimer AJ, Ruiz A, et al. Liver transplant using donors after unexpected cardiac death: novel preservation protocol and acceptance criteria. Am J Transplant 2007;7:1849–55.
5. Takada M, Nadeau KC, Hancock WW, et al. Effects of explosive brain death on cytokine activation of peripheral organs in the rat. Transplantation 1998;65: 1533–42.
6. Alvarez J, del Barrio MR, Arias J, et al. Five years of experience with non-heart-beating donors coming from the streets. Transplant Proc 2002;34:2589–90.
7. Otero A, Gómez-Gutiérrez M, Suárez F, et al. Liver transplantation from Maastricht category 2 non-heart-beating donors. Transplantation 2003;76:1068–73.
8. Quintela J, Gala B, Baamonde I, et al. Long-term results for liver transplantation from non-heart-beating donors maintained with chest and abdominal compression–decompression. Transplant Proc 2005;37:3857–8.
9. Suárez F, Otero A, Solla M, et al. Biliary complications after liver transplantation from Maastricht category-2 non-heart-beating donors. Transplantation 2008;85: 9–14.
10. Jiménez-Galanes S, Meneu-Diaz MJ, Elola-Olaso AM, et al. Liver transplantation using uncontrolled non-heart-beating donors under normothermic extracorporeal membrane oxygenation. Liver Transpl 2009;15: 1110–8.
11. Lewis J, Peltier J, Nelson H, et al. Development of the University of Wisconsin donation after cardiac death evaluation tool. Prog Transplant 2003;13:265–73.
12. DeVita MA, Snyder JV. Development of the University of Pittsburgh Medical Center policy for the care of terminally ill patients who may become organ donors after death following the removal of life support. Kennedy Inst Ethics J 1993;3:131–43.
13. Muiesan P, Girlanda R, Jassem W, et al. Single-center experience with liver transplantation from controlled non-heartbeating donors: a viable source of grafts. Ann Surg 2005;242:732–8.
14. Bernat JL, D'Alessandro AM, Port FK, et al. Report of a National Conference on Donation after cardiac death. Am J Transplant 2006;6:281–91.
15. Reich DJ, Mulligan DC, Abt PL, et al. ASTS Standards on Organ Transplantation Committee. ASTS recommended practice guidelines for controlled donation after cardiac death organ procurement and transplantation. Am J Transplant 2009;9:2004–11.
16. Abt PL, Desai NM, Crawford MD, et al. Survival following liver transplantation from non-heart-beating donors. Ann Surg 2004;239:87–92.
17. Moench C, Heimann A, Foltys D, et al. Flow and pressure during liver preservation under ex situ and in situ perfusion with University of Wisconsin solution and histidine–tryptophan–ketoglutarate solution. Eur Surg Res 2007;39:175–81.
18. Stewart ZA, Cameron AM, Singer AL, Montgomery RA, Segev DL. Histidine–tryptophan–ketoglutarate (HTK) is associated with reduced graft survival in deceased donor livers, especially those donated after cardiac death. Am J Transplant 2009;9:286–93.
19. Guarrera JV, Henry SD, Samstein B, et al. Hypothermic machine preservation in human liver transplantation: the first clinical series. Am J Transplant 2010;10: 372–81.
20. Foley DP, Fernandez LA, Leverson G, et al. Donation after cardiac death: the University of Wisconsin experience with liver transplantation. Ann Surg 2005;242: 724–31.
21. Abt P, Crawford M, Desai N, Markmann J, Olthoff K, Shaked A. Liver transplantation from controlled non-heart-beating donors: an increased incidence of biliary complications. Transplantation 2003;75: 1659–63.

22. Garcia-Valdecasas JC, Tabet J, Valero R, et al. Evaluation of ischemic injury during liver procurement from non-heart-beating donors. Eur Surg Res 1999;31:447–56.
23. Skaro AI, Jay CL, Baker TB, et al. The impact of ischemic cholangiopathy in liver transplantation using donors after cardiac death: the untold story. Surgery 2009;146:543–52.
24. Chan EY, Olson LC, Kisthard JA, et al. Ischemic cholangiopathy following liver transplantation from donation after cardiac death donors. Liver Transpl 2008;14: 604–10.
25. Feng S, Goodrich NP, Bragg-Gresham JL, et al. Characteristics associated with liver graft failure: the concept of a donor risk index. Am J Transplant 2006;6: 783–90.
26. Manzarbeitia CY, Ortiz JA, Jeon H, et al. Long-term outcome of controlled, non-heart-beating donor liver transplantation. Transplantation 2004;78:211–5.
27. Fujita S, Mizuno S, Fujikawa T, et al. Liver transplantation from donation after cardiac death: a single center experience. Transplantation 2007;84:46–9.
28. Merion RM, Pelletier SJ, Goodrich N, Englesbe MJ, Delmonico FL. Donation after cardiac death as a strategy to increase deceased donor liver availability. Ann Surg 2006;244:555–62.
29. Mateo R, Cho Y, Singh G, et al. Risk factors for graft survival after liver transplantation from donation after cardiac death donors: an analysis of OPTN/UNOS data. Am J Transplant 2006;6:791–6.
30. Lee KW, Simpkins CE, Montgomery RA, Locke JE, Segev DL, Maley WR. Factors affecting graft survival after liver transplantation from donation after cardiac death donors. Transplantation 2006;82:1683–8.
31. Selck FW, Grossman EB, Ratner LE, Renz JF. Utilization, outcomes, and retransplantation of liver allografts from donation after cardiac death: implications for further expansion of the deceased-donor pool. Ann Surg 2008;248:599–607.
32. Abt P, Kashyap R, Orloff M, et al. Pediatric liver and kidney transplantation with allografts from DCD donors: A review of UNOS data. Transplantation 2006;82:1708–11.
33. Muiesan P, Jassem W, Girlanda R, et al. Segmental liver transplantation from non-heart beating donors – an early experience with implications for the future. Am J Transplant 2006;6:1012–6.
34. Hughes RD, Mitry RR, Dhawan A, et al. Isolation of hepatocytes from livers from non-heart-beating donors for cell transplantation. Liver Transpl 2006;12:713–7.
35. Yagci G, Fernandez LA, Knechtle SJ, et al. The impact of donor variables on the outcome of orthotopic liver transplantation for hepatitis C. Transplant Proc 2008;40:219–23.
36. Nguyen JH, Bonatti H, Dickson RC, et al. Long-term outcomes of donation after cardiac death liver allografts from a single center. Clin Transplant 2009;23:168–73.
37. Tao R, Ruppert K, Cruz RJ Jr, et al. Hepatitis C recurrence is not adversely affected by the use of donation after cardiac death liver allografts. Liver Transpl 2010;16:1288–95.
38. Axelrod DA, Schnitzler M, Salvalaggio PR, Swindle J, Abecassis MM. The economic impact of the utilization of liver allografts with high donor risk index. Am J Transplant 2007;7:990–7.
39. Jay CL, Lyuksemburg V, Kang R, et al. The increased costs of donation after cardiac death liver transplantation: caveat emptor. Ann Surg 2010;251:743–8.
40. Devey L, Wigmore S. Non-heart-beating organ donation. Br J Surg 2009;96:833–5.

19 Transmission of malignancies and infection through donor organs

Aaron M. Winnick and Lewis Teperman

NYU Langone Medical Center, The Mary Lea Johnson Richards Organ Transplant Center, Department of Surgery, New York, NY, USA

Key learning points

- Donor-derived disease transmission occurs in less than 1% of all transplants.
- Early recognition and screening of the donor is essential to prevent transmission. Nucleic acid testing, though costly, is more sensitive and accurate than serologic testing; and when used appropriately can effectively identify high-risk donors.
- Prompt and aggressive treatment of any recipient of donor-derived disease is essential for patient survival. Early removal of the transplanted organ is often necessary.
- Some instances of malignancy may be acceptable for organ donation.

Introduction

The shortage of livers has prompted many centers to implement the use of extended-criteria donors (ECDs). Organs with advanced age, infections, and prior malignancy are used to try to offset this discrepancy between supply and demand. Use of these donors is not without risk. Some of the older donors will undoubtedly have a higher incidence of undiagnosed malignancy, which will potentially increase the incidence of donor tumor transmission.[1] Despite all the innovations with donor screening, there are an increasing number of reports of disease transmission (i.e. infection and malignancy) from the donor to the recipient with substantial morbidity and mortality among affected recipients. Unfortunately, until 2008, there was no formalized reporting process or standard way of monitoring transmission from donor to multiple recipients. There have been scattered reports over the years of transmission of several types of viruses and malignancies, including human immunodeficiency virus (HIV), West Nile virus (WNV), rabies, hepatitis C virus (HCV), leukemia, lymphoma and several types of carcinomas.[2] As a result, the United Network for Organ Sharing (UNOS) and Organ Procurement and Transplantation Network (OPTN) established the Disease Transmission Advisory Group in 2005 to monitor such potential transmissions, provide guidance in these cases, and analyze trends. The intention is to maximize organ allocation while minimizing untoward side effects.[3] This was later formalized as the *Ad Hoc* Disease Transmission Advisory Committee (DTAC). Several policies have since been enacted across the country, each designed to reduce the risk of potential disease transmission. There is policy in the USA mandating the routine screening of potential donors for specific pathogens, including HIV, hepatitis B virus (HBV), HCV, syphilis, cytomegalovirus (CMV), tuberculosis (TB) and Epstein–Barr virus (EBV).[4] A complete medical and social history must be obtained and communicated to the transplant center in order to obtain fully informed consent from the recipient.

Donor-derived disease transmissions are extremely rare events in solid-organ transplantation, with a reported incidence of 0.96% from deceased-donor

Medical Care of the Liver Transplant Patient, Fourth Edition. Edited by Pierre-Alain Clavien, James F. Trotter.

donations in 2007.[2] Prior to instituting better guidelines and screening for donors more efficiently, reports of malignancy transmission were often due to the use of organs from a donor with active malignancy. Currently, most cases of donor-transmitted malignancies are because either the tumor was detected at autopsy after the organs have been procured and transplanted, the living donor developed a malignancy after organ donation, or the recipient developed a malignancy that was traced back to the donor. Before the DTAC reported their findings and established a protocol for all transplant centers to report any case suspicious for transmission, disclosure was at the discretion of the transplant center. Since then, the number of potential donor-derived transmission events (PDDTEs) reported to the OPTN has increased from seven to 97 per year over the years 2005–2007. This significant increase is attributed to improved recognition and the development of a formalized reporting process.[2]

Most of the data that was collected prior to the formation of DTAC was based on voluntary registries, leading to inaccurate sampling. Data from the Israel Penn International Transplant Tumor Registry (IPITTR) represents cases over a 38-year period from 1965 to 2003. From the overall series examining nearly 300 cases of high-risk transplants using donors with known or incidentally discovered malignancies, 124 (42%) cases had a confirmed donor transmission. Liver donors comprised 38 of these, of which 14 (37%) had transmission of a malignancy.[1] Although this data is representative of a prolonged time period, it is a limited registry of occurrences and cannot give an adequate assessment of true incidence, thus the creation of the DTAC.

The key to limiting the incidence of this complication is early identification, starting with the donor. After a thorough and detailed history and physical, a careful surgical exploration of the donor is always warranted. Inspection of the thoracic and abdominal organs, with attention also given to lymph nodes, should be performed before and after the organs have been removed. Unfortunately, transmission of undiagnosed cancer will inevitably occur.

The goal of this chapter is to provide some of the most up-to-date information for many malignancies and infections that are donor derived. While it is not an exhaustive review, the focus will be on the more common and deleterious scenarios (Table 19.1).

Malignancy transmission

Transmission of donor malignancies is rare, with 18 cases from 34 933 deceased donors and three cases from 32 052 living donors being reported to UNOS from 1994 to 2001.[5]

In 2007, the Malignancy Subcommittee of the DTAC proceeded with its first data analysis.[3] From 2005 to 2007, there were 65 reports of unexpected malignancy-related events made to the OPTN. The most commonly reported malignancies included renal cell carcinoma, adenocarcinoma of the lung, glioblastoma multiforme and lymphoma. Documented transmission of malignancy from donor to recipient could be confirmed in 22% of these cases. In 2007 alone, donor-derived tumor was traced in seven recipients from four donors (four transplant recipients developed lymphoma, one glioblastoma multiforme, one small-cell lung cancer, and one hepatocellular carcinoma). There was one documented case of possible transmission of melanoma, where it could not be determined if the tumor was of donor or recipient origin. A total of five deaths were attributable to donor-derived malignancy transmissions in 2007.[2]

The practice among most transplant centers is to exclude donors with a known history of malignancy, except for those with low-grade skin cancers and certain primary tumors of the central nervous system (CNS), which is then determined on a case-by-case basis. Precautions to prevent malignancy transmission include detailed preoperative screening of donors, examination of all organs at the time of procurement (especially those not being utilized), routine biopsy of any suspicious lesions or nodules, and donor autopsy, if applicable.

CNS tumors

Gliomas are tumors arising from specialized connective tissue cells of the CNS (oligodendrocytes and astrocytes). Astrocytomas are divided into four clinical grades with the most aggressive, grade 4, referred to as glioblastoma multiforme (GBM). Data identifying the risk of glioma transmission to transplant recipients is sparse, with most coming from individual case reports. From 1987 to 2004, there were eight case reports in the literature documenting CNS cancer transmission from seven donors to 19 recipients (five cases of GBM, one medulloblastoma, and one

Table 19.1 Transmission of Malignancy and Infection through donor organs

Malignancy	Risk of Transmission	Use of Organ	Treatment if transmission found	Comments
CNS Tumors				
– Astrocytoma – Schwannoma – Non-malignant meningioma	Low	Yes		
Glioblastoma multiforme	Conflicting data- risk increased with prior surgical manipulation or radiation/chemo.	Yes- case-by-case basis		
Medulloblastoma	High	No		
Melanoma	High	No- regardless if tumor is active or occurred in past	Explant of kidney Re-transplant of heart, liver, or lung	5-year survival <5%
Renal Cell Carcinoma	Low – low grade tumor, no extracapsular or vascular invasion High- high grade tumor	Yes No		Small tumors can be excised and then kidney transplanted
Lung Cancer	High	No	If found within 1–2 weeks- emergent explant and re-transplantation	Donor organ should *NEVER* be used
Lymphoma	High	No	Explant (for kidney), chemotherapy	Donor organ should *NEVER* be used
Prostate Cancer	Low- low grade, Gleason score <6	Yes		

Infection	Risk of Transmission	Use of Organ	Treatment if transmission found	Comments
HTLV 1 and 2	Low			No longer tested as part of donor screening
HIV	High	No	HAART	
HBV	Low- anti HBs High- anti HBc High- HBsAg	Yes Used in selective cases with positive recipient	HBIg × minimum 3 days with antiviral agent. Monitor anti HBs levels, keep >500 IU/mL	
HCV	High	Only in HCV negative patients in exceptional cases. Yes- HCV positive recipients		Liver biopsy of donor suggested to evaluate for fibrosis
Tuberculosis	Low- history of / latent TB High- Active TB	Yes- with full disclosure No	Multi-drug approach with isoniazid, pyrazinamide, rifampin +/– ethambutol	Early recognition crucial. Treat for >1 year if extrapulmonary
WNV	High	No- exclude all donors with meningoencephalopathic symptoms in regions with WNV activity	No specific treatment +/– antibody therapy	

Abbreviations: *CNS- Central nervous system; HTLV- Human T-lymphotrophic virus; HIV- Human immunodeficiency virus; HBV- Hepatitis B virus; anti HBs- Hepatitis B surface antibody; anti HBc- Hepatitis B core antibody; HBsAg- Hepatitis B surface antigen; HBIg- Hepatitis B immune globulin; HCV- Hepatitis C virus; TB- Tuberculosis; WNV- West Nile virus.*

malignant meningioma).[6] Eleven recipients developed donor-transmitted malignancy, of which five died from the cancer. The only survivors were kidney recipients, who underwent transplant nephrectomy with cessation of immunosuppression. The single heart recipient and **three liver recipients** with evidence of donor-transmitted malignancy died.

There are conflicting data among the few registries regarding the transmission of CNS tumors. The UNOS Transplant Tumor Registry reported on 397 donors with a history of CNS tumor or documentation of CNS tumor as the cause of death between the years 1992 and 1999. Histologic diagnosis was only available for **30 of these donors** (7.5%), with 17 donors having GBM and two with medulloblastoma. There were no cases of donor-transmitted tumor identified in 1220 recipients over a mean follow up of 36 months.[6,7]

The Australian and New Zealand Organ Donation Registry reported on 46 donors with primary CNS tumors over the years 1989–1996, of which 28 had malignant tumors (four GBM, 10 unspecified astrocytoma, five medulloblastoma, one malignant meningioma, four unspecified glioma, and four unspecified tumors). There were no cases of donor-transmitted tumor in the 151 recipients over a mean follow up of 40 months.[8] In contrast, the IPITTR identified 46 donors with primary CNS tumors between the years 1969–1997. Of these, eight were found to have transmitted tumor to 10 of 55 possible recipients, correlating to an incidence of 17%.[9] One possible explanation for this discrepancy is that the data reported in the latter study reflects an earlier time period, and in the earlier days of transplantation, organs were used from donors with active cancer, often with local excision of the tumor. More importantly, the true denominator was not known, thus significantly underestimating the true transmission rate.

Brain tumors have been classified into categories of low, moderate or high risk for transmission according to their biological behavior. Certain CNS tumors have a very low metastatic rate, such as pilocystic astrocytomas, acoustic schwannomas, nonmalignant meningiomas, and craniopharyngiomas; patients with these tumors can often be considered as potential donors. The World Health Organization (WHO) has classified CNS tumors into four histologic grades: low-grade CNS tumors (WHO grade I or II) typically have a low risk of transmission, while high-grade tumors (WHO grade III or IV) have a high risk of transmission.[10]

One study identified an overall CNS tumor transmission rate of 23%, but found that the presence of one or more risk factors (such as high tumor grade, presence of ventriculoperitoneal shunt, prior craniotomy, chemotherapy or radiotherapy) increased the incidence of transmission to 53%. The absence of these risk factors reduced the incidence of donor transmission to 7%, which appears to be a more accurate estimate of risk.[11]

Based on the information given earlier, it is the current authors' recommendation that organs from a donor with any CNS tumor should be used with considerable caution and with duly executed informed consent. Regarding glioblastoma multiforme, the associated risk of transmission appears to increase with prior surgical manipulation of the tumor or radiation/chemotherapy. Medulloblastoma and ventricular shunts should, at present, be absolute contraindications to procurement.

Melanoma

Malignant melanoma is one of the most common donor-transmitted cancers, with some reports identifying it in more than one-quarter (28%) of all donor-transmitted tumors. It is also associated with a 5-year survival rate of less than 5%.[12,13] The treatment ranges from explant of the transplanted organ with cessation of immunosuppression (for kidneys) to re-transplantation (liver, heart, and lung grafts). There is currently not enough data on the rates of transmission for different stages of melanoma. As such, all melanoma patients should be considered high-risk donors, regardless of whether the tumor is active or occurred in the past. If there is clear documentation of in-situ melanoma, the metastatic risk is lower; but centers should proceed with optimistic caution and full disclosure to the potential recipient.[3]

Renal cell carcinoma

Renal cell carcinoma (RCC) can have a low or high risk of transmission depending on the size and/or stage of the tumor. The incidence is more prevalent with renal grafts compared to liver grafts. The ones with the most favorable prognosis, and thus the least risk of tumor transmission, are those with low-grade histology and no extracapsular or vascular invasion. In one report, 14 patients received kidneys with RCC that was identified at the time of procurement, excised ex vivo, and then implanted into the recipient. There was no evidence of tumor transmission in any of these patients. The mean tumor size was 2.1 cm with tumor grades of either Fuhrman grade I–II/IV.[14] Thus, donor kidneys with small, incidental RCC may be managed with excision and transplantation, without tumor recurrence in recipients. In another study examining 70 donors with previous or undetected RCC, donor transmission was identified in 61%, with the majority confined to the allograft.[15] Successful intervention could be implemented with early detection, especially since most tumor growth occurs from 3 to 36 months after transplantation. Higher grade or stage RCCs are regarded as being intermediate or high risk for tumor transmission, and organs from these donors should not be used.

Lung cancer

Lung cancer is the leading cause of cancer deaths in men and women in the USA. Organ donors with malignancies in the lung had a tumor transmission rate of 43% and a recipient mortality rate of 32%.[1,9] It is the authors' recommendation that any donor with a history of lung cancer, regardless of type, **should not be considered for organ transplantation**. Furthermore, any prospective donor with a significant history of smoking (i.e. 20–30 pack-years) should undergo a CT scan of the chest to evaluate for possible malignancy prior to procurement. A thorough exploration of the chest cavity is warranted in all procurement cases regardless of which organs are going to be transplanted.

If in the early period, within 1–2 weeks after transplantation, a donor is found to have lung cancer, the liver recipient should undergo an emergent explant and retransplantation.

Lymphoma

Lymphoid neoplasms are not always easy to diagnose, and can masquerade as other causes of death. Transmission in organ transplantation can have devastating consequences if not recognized early and treated aggressively. In 2007, there was transmission of anaplastic large-cell lymphoma from a 15-year-old donor to four recipients (liver, pancreas and two kidneys). The donor was thought to have partially treated bacterial meningitis, and subsequently the family consented for donation after cardiac death (DCD). It was not until 1 month post donation that biopsy results of the brain demonstrated anaplastic large cell lymphoma. At that time, the liver recipient was asymptomatic; but MRI revealed lymphomatous disease involving the liver with periportal, cardiophrenic and retroperitoneal lymphadenopathy. He underwent three cycles of chemotherapy with Cytoxan, hydroxydoxorubicin, Oncovin, and prednisone (CHOP) with no improvement. The lymphoma spread to the CSF, brain and spinal cord. The patient eventually died on postoperative day 116. The pancreas and kidney recipients all underwent resection of the transplanted organs with subsequent treatment with CHOP. The pancreas recipient died within 1 year of transplant. Both renal recipients are tumor free. The removed organs all had nodules positive for anaplastic large cell lymphoma.[16]

Any donor organ with lymphoma should never be used for transplantation. In cases where the donor was found to have lymphoma after transplant, if possible, the organs must be quickly removed and the patient started on appropriate chemotherapy. The above case also reinforces two important issues: 1) organs from donors with suspected bacterial meningitis only be transplanted after identification of the infectious organism, and 2) donation performed after cardiac death may warrant extensive scrutiny.

Prostate cancer

The incidence of prostate cancer increases with age, and thus the probability of an incidental tumor rises as more ECDs are utilized. One study looked at the prostates of 340 donors with no known prostate disease. Adenocarcinoma was found in 23% of donors aged 50–59, 35% aged 60–69, and 45% in those aged 70–81. Despite this, there has not been any correlation to date with an increase in donor-transmitted prostate adenocarcinomas.[3,17] There are currently no guidelines defining when there is a significant risk of transmission. Use of frozen-section analysis of prostate specimens at the time of organ procurement has had a low sensitivity, and is inefficient at evaluating both the Gleason score and extension into extra-prostatic soft tissue.[18] A low-grade intra-prostatic prostate carcinoma, with a Gleason score ≤6, can be viewed as not having a significantly increased risk, and may be used pending fully informed consent.[19]

Infection transmission

There is a wide range of infectious agents that cause clinically significant disease when transmitted from donors to recipients. Currently, OPTN policy requires specific serologic tests to screen for HIV, HBV, HCV, EBV, CMV, and syphilis.

There were 99 events reported between 2005 and 2007 that were related to infectious disease transmission in transplant patients. Ten of these reports were considered "expected," based solely on the positive serology of the donor (i.e. with toxoplasmosis). The remaining 89 were classified as "unexpected" and included HCV, HBV, TB, HIV, Chagas disease, toxoplasmosis and West Nile virus, among others.[2] Documented transmission of infection from donor to recipient could be confirmed in 24% of these reports.

Detection of infection in the donor is dependent on the serologic test being able to assess the donor's response to an infection, which is limited because it may not detect an infection that is newly acquired. The period of time between infection and the ability to detect antibodies to a pathogen, known as the window period, varies from 22 days for HIV, 44 days for HBV, and 70 days for HCV with standard testing. Serologic tests may be negative despite active infection in the donor if the interval between infection and procurement is less than the window period. Nucleic acid testing (NAT) shortens the window period for HIV, HCV and HBV relative to serology (6 d, 5 d, and 22 d, respectively), and therefore may be useful in decreasing the risk of transmission in serology-negative donors[20,21] (Table 19.2). Unfortunately, NAT is costly and not readily available in all organ procurement organizations (OPOs). Its routine use may lead to the unnecessary loss of uninfected organs due to false positives; however, this is offset in donors with identified behavioral risk factors, where it may actually increase organ use. Use of NAT should be guided by weighing the risks and benefits on an individual case-by-case basis.

Table 19.2 Window period estimates (in days) for infection testing

Infection	Serologic testing (days)	NAT (days)
HIV	22	6
HBV	44	5
HCV	70	22

NAT: nucleic acid testing

Human T-lymphotrophic virus

Human T-lymphotrophic virus (HTLV) 1 and 2 (HTLV-1/2) was previously part of the testing requirements, but recently has been found to lead to a greater loss of organs than disease prevention, and has since been removed from routine testing. Now there is only one assay that can be used for screening. While HTLV-1 has been associated with the very rare development of acute T-cell leukemia/lymphoma and neurologic sequela, HTLV-2 has not been convincingly associated with disease in humans. The true incidence of HTLV-1/2 is not well described, but is estimated to be between 0.03–0.5% in US organ donors.[22] There is no successful treatment for HTLV disease. To date, no proven case of disease has been reported in the USA by organ donation.

HIV

HIV is readily transmitted in solid organ transplantation, although the incidence of transmission is not known. Reports have decreased over the past 15 years due to improvements in screening protocols.[23] In fact, from 1994 until 2007 there were no reported cases of HIV transmission in solid-organ transplants. In 2007, however, four transplant recipients contracted HIV and HCV from a single donor who tested negative by serology.[24]

There is still controversy regarding transplanting HIV-positive recipients, and some centers will not consider listing these patients. To date, there are no studies examining transplanting HIV-positive organs in HIV-positive recipients. Any potential donor regarded as high risk by Centers for Disease Control (CDC) standards should undergo NAT if serology is negative. Extreme care and caution should be taken when considering transplanting organs from a high-risk patient, and, as always, full disclosure must be made to all recipient candidates. Highly active antiretroviral therapy (HAART) should be initiated if transmission has occurred.

HBV

Not too long ago, it was a contraindication to use donors who were seropositive for HBV in liver transplantation, until it was realized that there was a significant difference if the donor was positive for the hepatitis B surface antibody (anti-HBs) or positive for hepatitis B core antibody (anti-HBc). In one study, it was reported that no HBV transmission occurred after liver transplantation from an anti-HBs-positive donor to an HBV-naïve recipient; while transmission was noted in 72% of HBV-naïve recipients who received a liver graft from an anti-HBc-positive donor.[25] Recipients of livers from anti-HBc-positive donors are at higher risk for acquiring HBV infection compared to recipients of livers from anti-HBs-positive donors. Reduction of transmission and prevention of recurrence of HBV is seen with combined prophylaxis using hepatitis B immune globulin (HBIg) and an antiviral agent/nucleoside reverse transcriptase inhibitor (such as lamivudine or tenofovir).[26,27]

While it has become common practice to use anti-HBc-positive organs in patients with HBV-related liver disease, many centers are now using these donors for HBV-naïve recipients with comparable results.[28] It is the current authors' practice to treat all recipients with HBIg for a minimum of 3 consecutive days post transplant and monitor anti-HBs levels. Anti-HBs levels are then monitored postoperatively for a minimum of 6 months, with HBIg infusions given as indicated to maintain a level >500 IU/ml. A pilot trial utilizing emtricitabine/tenofovir and the discontinuation of HBIg has had excellent early results, with no recurrence of hepatitis B.[29]

Hepatitis B surface antigen (HBsAg)-positive donors have a significantly higher rate of transmission, and are typically used in selective cases where the recipient is also HBsAg positive.[23,30]

HCV

Liver grafts from HCV-positive donors practically always transmit the HCV infection to an HCV-negative recipient, which is why these grafts should only be used in HCV-negative recipients in exceptional cases.[27,31] Some studies have demonstrated no significant difference in survival comparing HCV-positive recipients who received HCV-positive grafts and those who received HCV-negative grafts.[32–34] Interestingly, an analysis of UNOS data revealed that patient survival at 2 years was significantly higher in HCV-positive recipients of HCV-positive grafts than in HCV-positive recipients of HCV-negative grafts (90% vs 77%, $P = 0.01$).[35] This is likely due to the 20% false-positive serology that is not confirmed in the absence of PCR. Additionally, donor age was found to be significant. Recipients of HCV-positive livers from donors older than 50 years of age had higher rates of graft failure and death compared to recipients of HCV-negative livers from the same age group. In addition, more advanced fibrosis was observed in HCV-positive grafts from older donors compared to HCV-positive grafts from younger donors ($P = 0.012$).[33] The use of liver biopsy prior to implantation is suggested, but there is no supporting evidence.

TB

TB is caused by *Mycobacterium tuberculosis*, and it primarily invades the lungs, although it can also be seen in the kidneys, bone, and brain. The incidence in transplant recipients is 20–74 times higher than that for the general population.[36] A standard part of the pre-transplant evaluation of potential recipients includes screening using purified protein derivative (PPD) skin testing and chest x-ray, when indicated. Donor screening, however, can be more complicated depending on time constraints and what is known about the medical history. Historical data, such as previous exposure, treatment and recent travel is often limited to information obtained from family or friends, and is not always accurate.

Establishing donor transmission is sometimes difficult since the recipient and donor may have had latent TB infection at the time of transplantation. At least 15 cases have been reported of possible, probable or proven transmission of TB after kidney, liver, heart, or lung transplants.[37] Evidence ranges from circumstantial (recipient developing TB within a few months after transplant) to proven (multiple recipients of a single donor's organs both developing TB through genotypically identical *M. tuberculosis*). In one case, the donor was a 46-year old US-born man with a history of alcoholism, homelessness, and prior incarceration who was admitted to the hospital with alcohol withdrawal seizures and aspiration pneumonitis. The liver and both kidneys were transplanted into three recipients in two states. The donor died and 3 weeks later a CSF culture sent to evaluate his fever grew *M. tuberculosis*. Subsequently, the same bacteria grew from stored donor spleen tissue. Over the 6 months prior to the donor's admission, he had been tested twice with tuberculin skin tests (for homeless shelters and jails), both of which were documented to be negative. The two kidney recipients developed fever and pancytopenia 6 and 7 weeks post transplantation, respectively, with the former dying of disseminated TB 9 weeks post transplantation. *M. tuberculosis* was cultured from the deceased recipient's blood, liver, lungs and spleen, and the polymerase chain reaction (PCR)-based genotype matched that of the donor. The latter kidney recipient had positive cultures from the blood and urine specimens, and was successfully treated with anti-TB medications. The liver recipient was asymptomatic with negative cultures, however a routine liver biopsy performed 7 months post transplantation demonstrated granulomas suggestive of mycobacterial infection. He, too, was treated with anti-TB medications. None of the cultures grew *M. tuberculosis*.[38]

Early recognition of TB in the post-transplant recipient is critical for successful outcomes. Treatment consists of a multi-drug approach, usually with isoniazid, pyrazinamide, rifampin, and sometimes ethambutol, and length of therapy can sometimes extend more than 1 year if there is extrapulmonary disease. There is great concern when using these medications, specifically since rifampin can interfere with tacrolimus and cyclosporine by lowering their levels, and pyrazinamide and ethambutol can cause hepatotoxicity.[36] However, the overall risk of not aggressively treating TB in transplant patients outweighs that of potential side effects from the medications.

Active TB is a contraindication for organ donation. A history of TB in the donor with no signs of active disease does not preclude organ donation; but full disclosure must be made to the recipient, and a decision for prophylactic treatment must be made on an individual basis.

WNV

WNV is a *Flaviviridae* virus, part of the Japanese encephalitis antigenic complex of viruses, and it is found in both tropical and temperate regions. The host animal is usually a bird or horse, and transmission is through a mosquito vector. In humans, the disease can progress to encephalitis and meningitis. The most effective method of detecting the virus is measuring immunoglobulin M (IgM) antibodies in serum or cerebrospinal fluid.[39] A few cases of human-to-human transmission after organ transplant have been reported over the past 10 years. Donor-transmission of WNV in organ transplantation was reported in 2002, when four recipients of organs from the same donor (heart, liver, and two kidneys) developed fever and neurological symptoms 15–18 d postoperatively. The donor died from severe trauma, and had received multiple blood transfusions from more than 60 different donors. Three of the transplant recipients developed encephalitis, and one subsequently died. Three recipients became seropositive for the WNV IgM antibody, and the fourth recipient had brain tissue that was positive for WNV by nucleic acid and antigen assays. Specimens from the donor prior to and immediately after blood transfusions did not show any evidence of WNV. However, serum samples from the time of procurement were positive on NAT and viral culture. It is believed that this transmission can be attributed to the transfusion of WNV-positive blood received by the donor the day before organ procurement.[40]

The first report of donor transmission of WNV not from a blood transfusion occurred in 2005, when infection was confirmed in three of four recipients of organs transplanted from a common donor (lung, liver, and two kidneys). One kidney recipient was asymptomatic, the other kidney recipient had no evidence of infection, and the lung and liver recipients, at 2 weeks post-transplant, developed high fever, severe encephalitis and flaccid paralysis with respiratory failure and subsequently died. Donor samples were positive for WNV IgM antibodies, but were negative for WNV RNA by PCR.[41]

One concern regarding the screening for WNV is that tests based on specific antibody detection are not particularly useful, since these antibodies typically appear 1–2 weeks after the infection. Also, recipients of infected organs may have prolonged WNV incubation periods, and there could be a delayed antibody response. Unfortunately, NAT is not readily available in all OPOs, and not all donors can be screened for WNV. Based on this, current recommendations include: 1) excluding potential donors with meningoencephalitic symptoms of undetermined etiology who live in regions with WNV activity, 2) screening with NAT as close to the time of procurement as possible, and 3) having a suspicion in transplant recipients with postoperative fever and/or neurologic symptoms not otherwise explained. Serologic testing of the donor and all recipients from that donor should be performed, as well as lumbar puncture as indicated. At this time, there is no specific treatment for WNV. Traditional antibody therapy and a high-titered product have been attempted for treatment and prophylaxis without proven benefit. Monitoring in an ICU setting is recommended due to the possibility of rapid progression to paralysis and respiratory failure.

Rabies

Rabies virus, which also causes acute encephalitis, is potentially fatal in unvaccinated hosts. While usually transmitted to humans from contact with saliva from infected animals, such as dogs and bats, there have been a couple of reports of transmission after solid organ transplantation. In 2004, three organs (one liver and two kidneys) and the iliac artery (used for an arterial conduit in a different patient) were procured from a common donor who died from an intracranial bleed. Routine donor screening was performed, including a thorough history and pre-mortem blood, urine and sputum cultures, none of which identified anything precluding organ donation. All four recipients developed encephalitis within 30 days of transplantation, which rapidly progressed to seizures, respiratory failure and coma. The patients died an average of 13 days after the onset of neurologic symptoms. The diagnosis of rabies transmission was only confirmed after post-mortem examination on each of the patients, and was able to be traced to the donor, who in fact had been bitten by a bat, but that information was not relayed to the OPO prior to procurement.[42] If donor transmission of rabies occurs, treatment with rabies virus vaccine and immunoglobulin must be initiated immediately.

There are currently no recommendations regarding the screening of all donors for the presence of rabies virus antibodies. Donor screening is warranted in some cases where there are questions concerning animal bites and the donors' travel history. A thorough history must be obtained from the patient's family members and friends, especially concerning exposure to bats and mammalian bites. Any potential donor with unexplained neurologic symptoms should also be evaluated for the possibility of CNS infection.

Fungal infections

While the primary concern in the immunosuppressed transplant patient is reactivation or contracting a fungal infection, there are several types of fungal infections that can be transmitted from an infected donor. A comprehensive review of all possibilities is too exhaustive for this chapter, so the focus will be on the more common ones. In all cases, if the donor resides in or has even visited areas of endemnicity, serologic screening of the respective organism is warranted.

Coccidioidomycosis is a pulmonary infection that, in immunosuppressed patients, can disseminate to any organ. *Coccidioides* species is found principally in the southwestern USA, northern Mexico, and throughout Central and South America. Reports have detailed transmission from infected donors to recipients of lung, kidney, and liver. Almost all of the cases resulted in death of the recipient due to rapid dissemination without a known diagnosis. One kidney transplant recipient was successfully treated with itraconazole, and a possible explanation for this patient's survival is the 37-hour cold ischemia time, whereby the viability of the fungal species was significantly impaired by prolonged exposure to the cold.[39]

Diagnosis is based on clinical suspicion supported by microbiologic, histopathologic or serologic evidence. Skin test reagents are no longer readily available. Treatment consists of long-term therapy with itraconazole or posaconazole with serological monitoring of efficacy.

Histoplasmosis is a soil-based fungus caused by *Histoplasma capsulatum*, which is endemic in the Mississippi and Ohio River valleys, Central America, some areas of the Mediterranean basin and Southeast Asia. It is acquired by the inhalation of mycelial fragments and microconidia, but transmission from donor to recipient via graft has been described. Detection remains problematic, with serology not reliable in immunosuppressed patients. The development of PCR for *H. capsulatum* is in progress. Definitive diagnosis can be made with growth of the organism from tissue or fluid samples, but that may take weeks to grow. Detection of antigen in body fluids can sometimes offer a rapid diagnosis in patients with diffuse pulmonary histoplasmosis and progressive disseminated histoplasmosis.[39]

Two cases of donor transmission of histoplasmosis have been reported, both in kidney recipients from separate non-endemic areas that received their organ from the same donor. They developed symptoms 8 months and 9 months post transplant. The liver transplant recipient remained asymptomatic. There was no evidence of transmission on testing.[43] Treatment should consist of itraconazole or voriconazole for at least 3 months, and sometimes up to 6 months. Prophylaxis in recipients from donors with suspected exposure or a past history of histoplasmosis is controversial. The current authors believe that prophylaxis should be offered to recipients of organs from seropositive donors for a course of at least 3 months. Involvement of the infectious disease specialists and the CDC is encouraged.

There are no reported cases of donor transmission of blastomycosis or paracoccidioidomycosis in transplant patients.[39]

Tort reform

No chapter can be complete without a short discussion on the legal ramifications and consequences of transmission. Any known donor risk factors and ambiguous or conflicting tests should be conveyed to the recipient. All CDC high-risk patients (i.e. those who engage in risky sexual behavior in or out of prison) warrant an augmented consent. The high-risk standard is being re-evaluated but is not complete at the time of this writing.

Previous tumor history should be conveyed to the recipient and documented in the patient record. Informed consent is the physician's best protection. Once a likely transmittable malignant event has occurred, the organ should be switched if it is early – within 1–2 weeks. Later liver explantation may have benefit, but two-way trafficking of malignant cells has already taken place.

The US legal system allows for errors or mistakes; unfortunately the press is less forgiving. The liver is a life-saving organ. As long as there are open and frank discussions about risk, the patient and transplant team will be protected.

More donor transmissions will be recorded as there is expansion of the donor pool and results are registered. The donor pool is on the whole safe and these transmissions account for less than 1% of all transplants.

References

1. Buell JF, Beebe TM, Trofe J, et al. Donor transmitted malignancies. Ann Transplant 2004;9:53–6.
2. Ison MG, Hager J, Blumberg E, et al. Donor-derived disease transmission events in the United States: data reviewed by the OPTN/UNOS Disease Transmission Advisory Committee. Am J Transplant 2009;9: 1929–35.
3. Nalesnik M, Woodle E, DiMaio J, et al. Donor Transmitted Malignancies in Organ Transplantation: Assessment of Clinical Risk. Report of the Ad Hoc Donor Malignancy Subcommittee of the OPTN/UNOS Disease Transmission Advisory Committee (DTAC). 2010.
4. Organ Procurement and Transplantation Network. Policy 2: Minimum Procurement Standards For An Organ Procurement Organization (OPO). Department of Health and Human Services, Health Resources and Services Administration, Healthcare Systems Bureau, Division of Transplantation, Rockville, MD; 2009.
5. United Network for Organ Sharing website. (http:www.unos.org) (accessed June 2010).
6. Collignon FP, Holland EC, Feng S. Organ donors with malignant gliomas: an update. Am J Transplant 2004;4:15–21.
7. Kauffman HM, McBride MA, Delmonico FL. First report of the United Network for Organ Sharing Transplant Tumor Registry: donors with a history of cancer. Transplantation 2000;70:1747–51.
8. Chui AK, Herbertt K, Wang LS, et al. Risk of tumor transmission in transplantation from donors with

primary brain tumors: an Australian and New Zealand registry report. Transplant Proc 1999;31:1266–7.
9. Penn I. Transmission of cancer from organ donors. Ann Transplant 1997;2:7–12.
10. Louis DN, Ohgaki H, Wiestler OD, et al. The 2007 WHO classification of tumours of the central nervous system. Acta Neuropathol 2007;114:97–109.
11. Buell JF, Trofe J, Sethuraman G, et al. Donors with central nervous system malignancies: are they truly safe? Transplantation 2003;76:340–3.
12. Penn I. Malignant melanoma in organ allograft recipients. Transplantation 1996;61:274–8.
13. Kim JK, Carmody IC, Cohen AJ, Loss GE. Donor transmission of malignant melanoma to a liver graft recipient: case report and literature review. Clin Transplant 2009;23:571–4.
14. Buell J, Beebe T, Hanaway R, Thomas M, Rudich S, Woodle E. Transplant-related malignancies. In: Busuttil RW, Klintmalm GK, editors. Transplantation of the liver. 2nd ed. Philadelphia: Elsevier Saunders; 2005: 1149–64.
15. Penn I. Primary kidney tumors before and after renal transplantation. Transplantation 1995;59:480–5.
16. Harbell JW, Dunn TB, Fauda M, John DG, Goldenberg AS, Teperman LW. Transmission of anaplastic large cell lymphoma via organ donation after cardiac death. Am J Transplant 2008;8:238–44.
17. Yin M, Bastacky S, Chandran U, Becich MJ, Dhir R. Prevalence of incidental prostate cancer in the general population: a study of healthy organ donors. J Urol 2008;179:892–5; discussion 5.
18. Falconieri G, Lugnani F, Zanconati F, Signoretto D, Di Bonito L. Histopathology of the frozen prostate. The microscopic bases of prostatic carcinoma cryoablation. Pathol Res Pract 1996;192:579–87.
19. Montalti R, Rompianesi G, Di Benedetto F, et al. Liver transplantation utilizing grafts from donors with genitourinary cancer detected prior to liver implantation. Transplant Proc 2009;41:1275–7.
20. Ison MG. The epidemiology and prevention of donor-derived infections. Adv Chronic Kidney Dis 2009;16: 234–41.
21. Humar A, Morris M, Blumberg E, et al. Nucleic acid testing (NAT) of organ donors: is the "best" test the right test? A consensus conference report. Am J Transplant 2010;10:889–99.
22. Kaul DR, Taranto S, Alexander C, et al. Donor screening for human T-cell lymphotrophic virus 1/2: changing paradigms for changing testing capacity. Am J Transplant 2010;10:207–13.
23. Singer AL, Kucirka LM, Namuyinga R, Hanrahan C, Subramanian AK, Segev DL. The high-risk donor: viral infections in solid organ transplantation. Curr Opin Organ Transplant 2008;13:400–4.
24. Grady D. Four transplant recipients contract HIV. The New York Times. 2007;November 14, (http://www.nytimes.com/2007/11/14/health/healthspecial/14hiv.html?ex=1353214800&en=0fa408520f8965e6&ei=5088&partner=rssnyt&emc=rss)(accessed15June2011).
25. Dodson SF, Issa S, Araya V, et al. Infectivity of hepatic allografts with antibodies to hepatitis B virus. Transplantation 1997;64:1582–4.
26. Hashimoto K, Miller C. The use of marginal grafts in liver transplantation. J Hepatobiliary Pancreat Surg 2008;15:92–101.
27. Gastaca M. Extended criteria donors in liver transplantation: adapting donor quality and recipient. Transplant Proc 2009;41:975–9.
28. Burton JR Jr, Shaw-Stiffel TA. Use of hepatitis B core antibody-positive donors in recipients without evidence of hepatitis B infection: a survey of current practice in the United States. Liver Transpl 2003;9:837–42.
29. Teperman L, Spivey J, Poordad F, et al. A randomized trial of HBIG withdrawal using emtricitabine/tenofovir DF in post-orthotopic liver transplant recipients. Liver Transplantation. Supplement: The International Liver Transplantation Society: 16th Annual International Congress 2010(Suppl 1):S70.
30. Perrillo RP, Eason JD. The use of HBsAg-positive organ donors: far more than meets the eye? Liver Transpl 2005;11:875–7.
31. Busuttil RW, Tanaka K. The utility of marginal donors in liver transplantation. Liver Transpl 2003;9: 651–63.
32. Ghobrial RM, Steadman R, Gornbein J, et al. A 10-year experience of liver transplantation for hepatitis C: analysis of factors determining outcome in over 500 patients. Ann Surg 2001;234:384–93; discussion 93–4.
33. Khapra AP, Agarwal K, Fiel MI, et al. Impact of donor age on survival and fibrosis progression in patients with hepatitis C undergoing liver transplantation using HCV+ allografts. Liver Transpl 2006;12: 1496–503.
34. Saab S, Ghobrial RM, Ibrahim AB, et al. Hepatitis C positive grafts may be used in orthotopic liver transplantation: a matched analysis. Am J Transplant 2003;3: 1167–72.
35. Marroquin CE, Marino G, Kuo PC, et al. Transplantation of hepatitis C-positive livers in hepatitis C-positive patients is equivalent to transplanting hepatitis C-negative livers. Liver Transpl 2001;7:762–8.
36. Munoz P, Rodriguez C, Bouza E. Mycobacterium tuberculosis infection in recipients of solid organ transplants. Clin Infect Dis 2005;40:581–7.
37. Rose G. The risk of tuberculosis transmission in solid organ transplantation: Is it more than a theoretical concern? Can J Infect Dis Med Microbiol 2005;16: 304–8.

38. Transplantation-transmitted tuberculosis – Oklahoma and Texas, 2007. MMWR Morb Mortal Wkly Rep 2008;57:333–6.
39. Martin-Davila P, Fortun J, Lopez-Velez R, et al. Transmission of tropical and geographically restricted infections during solid-organ transplantation. Clin Microbiol Rev 2008;21:60–96.
40. Iwamoto M, Jernigan DB, Guasch A, et al. Transmission of West Nile virus from an organ donor to four transplant recipients. N Engl J Med 2003;348:2196–203.
41. Teperman L, Diflo T, Fahmy A, et al. West Nile virus infections in organ transplant recipients – New York and Pennsylvania, August–September, 2005. MMWR Morb Mortal Wkly Rep 2005;54:1021–3.
42. Srinivasan A, Burton EC, Kuehnert MJ, et al. Transmission of rabies virus from an organ donor to four transplant recipients. N Engl J Med 2005;352: 1103–11.
43. Limaye AP, Connolly PA, Sagar M, et al. Transmission of *Histoplasma capsulatum* by organ transplantation. N Engl J Med 2000;343:1163–6.

20 The transplant operation

Philipp Dutkowski, Olivier de Rougemont and Pierre-Alain Clavien

Swiss HPB and Transplantation Centers, Department of Surgery and Transplantation, University Hospital Zürich, Zürich, Switzerland

Key learning points

- Abdominal donor procurement is initiated by cold flush through the aorta and portal system.
- Graft function depends on multiple factors including donor condition, procurement quality, cold ischemia, rewarming ischemia, and recipient factors.
- Liver transplantation can be done either by the classic technique including complete replacement of the retrohepatic vena cava or by the cava-preserving piggyback technique.
- Fast arterilization of the graft appears important to avoid biliary injury.

Introduction

Early graft function after orthotopic liver transplantation (OLT) is essential. Unlike in kidney, pancreas, or, to some extent, lung and heart transplantation, there is no effective artificial support for a liver transplant patient in the event of graft failure. Without rapid restoration of hepatic function, death from bleeding or cerebral edema generally occurs within 72 h. Importantly, liver function after OLT remains unpredictable *before* transplantation and ranges from immediate and full function to complete absence of any function. Although less frequent than in other organs, such as the kidney, primary graft nonfunction (PNF), defined as nonlife-sustaining function of the liver graft, leads to death or retransplantation within 7 d.[1,2] Such life-threatening complication still occurs in about 3% of cases nowadays in most centers. Delayed graft function (DGF), defined as impaired liver function responding to support therapy,[3] occurs at a much higher percentage (~10–20%), presumably in recipients, where "extended-critera" grafts are used.

One of the known causes of PNF or DGF is poor organ quality at the time of OLT, which depends however on numerous factors, such as the condition of the donor, the quality of the organ procurement, the preservation solution or method used, the length of the cold-ischemic period, and also the recipient's condition before and during OLT.[3] The development of modern preservation solutions has reduced liver injury related to the harvest and storage procedure. Euro-Collins solution has been replaced by histidine–tryptophan–ketoglutarate (HTK) solution, University of Wisconsin (UW) solution, Celsior or IGL (Institute George Lopez) solution.[4,5] Cold storage of nonsteatotic, relatively young liver grafts can be extended safely up to 15 h with these solutions. Extended criteria grafts demand a much shorter cold storage period (<8 h) or a different preservation strategy. In this context, machine liver perfusion is currently discussed as a potential alternative for improved preservation.[6]

Medical Care of the Liver Transplant Patient, Fourth Edition. Edited by Pierre-Alain Clavien, James F. Trotter.

Donor selection

Determining the quality of the donor liver in a heart-beating cadaver remains imprecise; careful attention to the circumstances of the donor's death and the function and morphologic characteristics of the organ prior to harvest is critical.[7] The ideal donor can be described as follows:
- 50 years old or younger
- No presence of liver steatosis or any other hepatobiliary disease
- Hemodynamic and respiratory stability (systolic blood pressure >100 mmHg and central venous pressure >5 cm H_2O) with low requirement of inotropic drugs and with acceptable pO_2 and hemoglobin level
- Without severe abdominal trauma, systemic infection, or cancer
- With a diuresis >50 mL/h and normal serum creatinine, without hypernatremia.

This ideal donor is far from common and many potential donors are older than 60 years with some evidence for hepatic steatosis, are hemodynamically unstable, and have been treated in the intensive care unit for more than 5 d.[8] In Switzerland, more than half of the cadaveric liver grafts are from such marginal or extended-criteria donors (ECDs).

The steady increase in number of liver transplant candidates and the dramatic rise in waiting list mortality have led to adoption of more aggressive donor selection criteria, thus introducing a greater potential risk for postoperative graft dysfunction. Accordingly, abnormal liver test function, long intensive care unit stay, hemodynamic instability (prolonged hypoxia or hypotension), donor age over 65 years old, and limited steatosis (<30% macrosteatosis) are no longer absolute contraindications for organ retrieval.[9] Furthermore, the progressive expansion of liver-splitting techniques comes with longer harvesting times and parenchymal manipulation that may influence postoperative graft recovery.

No single parameter alone defines the acceptability of a donor for organ harvest. Donor livers are usually discarded when there is a combination of factors that predicts poor function.[9] The decision to accept or reject a donor liver must also take into consideration the severity of the recipient's disease. Personal inspection of the liver and histologic examination of a liver biopsy performed by an experienced transplant surgeon and pathologist can be very helpful in reaching a decision.

Matching donor and recipient

Only donor and recipient ABO types are usually matched. Convincing data about HLA mismatch regarding liver transplantation are lacking in contrast to kidney and pancreas transplantation. An additional issue is that of size compatibility. Smaller organs are easily adapted to a large recipient. In contrast, large grafts are very difficult to implant in small recipients. Size reduction of an adult liver or the use of segments was initially implemented to overcome the need for size-matched grafts in pediatric recipients. Usually segments 2 and 3 or the left hemiliver are used, allowing up to one-tenth weight mismatch between the donor and the recipient weight.[10]

As a next step, split-liver transplantation was implemented.[11,12] This technique allows a whole liver to be divided into two allografts and therefore the total number of grafts to be increased. However, the incidence of vascular and biliary complications, as well as PNF rates, was higher than after whole-organ transplantation. The reason is that splitting of the liver is a time-consuming procedure is usually associated with a longer cold-ischemia time and with the risk of prolonged rewarming, therefore selection of high-quality organs and low-risk recipients is mandatory. Although this procedure could shorten the waiting list for transplantation, it can be performed in only a small proportion of "optimal" livers (15–20%). Splitting the liver in situ and carefully transecting the bile duct for the left liver or the left lateral segment close to the parenchyma without damaging the vasculature of the right bile duct usually helps reduce cold ischemia time and prevents biliary complications.[13]

Liver transplantation in two adults using a split-liver graft has been also performed.[11] A small recipient must be selected for the left hemiliver since only grafts with more than 1% of the liver volume/recipient body weight ratio or more than 40% of the native liver volume are considered sufficient. Transplanting less than 1% of the liver volume can be dangerous and could render an elective patient a highly urgent retransplantation candidate. The procedure must be considered very carefully and only carried out in centers with experience in major liver surgery as well as segmental graft LT. The right hemiliver of a living-related adult donor has been also increasingly used over the past few years.[14] This strategy offers an optimal graft with controlled ischemia times, but is associated with significant risk for the living donor.[15]

Procurement

The procurement of the liver should be performed by an experienced surgeon, with particular care taken to optimize organ viability of the heart-beating cadaver. Cardiovascular and respiratory instability is suggested by the necessity for vasopressor support, poor blood gas values, or other adverse findings familiar to intensive care physicians. If such donors are unstable or if the heart stops beating before the patient has been transferred to the operating room, the kidney might be the only suitable organ for transplantation. Most brain-dead donors, however, can be maintained and improved with conventional intensive care and an attempt can be made to coordinate the needs of surgeons who perform transplantation to allow multiple cadaveric organ procurement. Adequate management of the donor prior to and during the harvesting is very important to achieve immediate hepatic function after OLT. The surgeon must be aware of common problems of resuscitation including excessive use of vasopressor drugs, prolonged acidosis, hypoperfusion from hypovolemia, persistent anemia, and uncorrected hypernatremia.

A flexible procedure for multiple cadaveric organ procurement should allow excision of various organ combinations without jeopardizing any individual grafts. The guiding principle is to avoid warm ischemia to any potential graft. This is achieved by carefully timed and controlled infusion of cold solutions into anatomic regions, the limits of which are defined by preliminary meticulous surgical dissection.

Removal of thoracoabdominal organs must be coordinated with the abdominal team. The organ procurement is generally performed through a midline incision from jugular notch to pubis including median sternotomy. The long incision provides good exposure for removal of the heart, lungs, kidneys, pancreas, small bowel, and liver. The liver is inspected to be sure that its color and texture are normal. If this is in any doubt, a liver biopsy is recommended. Anomalies are looked for, of which arteries to the left liver from the left gastric artery or to the right liver from the superior mesenteric artery are the most frequent. Failure to complete the arterial revascularization of the graft due to unrecognized aberrant arterial supply is poorly tolerated after cold storage, leading to PNF or acute biliary problems in the recipient.

The abdominal procurement starts with the incision of the peritoneal reflection of the ascending colon, cecum, and distal small intestine (Cattell–Braasch maneuver). The distal part of the cava and aorta are dissected free up to the left renal vein and encircled. The inferior mesenteric artery is ligated. The inferior mesenteric vein can be ligated distally and a cannula is placed proximally for later perfusion of the portal system (not mandatory). The superior mesenteric artery (SMA) should be exposed at its origin to check for replaced or aberrant right hepatic arteries.

Mobilization of the right liver is not required as for a liver resection since a large part of the diaphragm in contact with the liver is also resected. However, the left triangular ligament of the liver is incised to expose the upper part of the abdominal aorta. The gastrohepatic ligament is divided if no aberrant left hepatic artery is present. The right diaphragmatic crus is divided and the supraceliac aorta is encircled.

Preparation of the hepatoduodenal ligament should be very limited. First, careful palpation for a right aberrant or replaced hepatic artery has to be done. Next, the common bile duct is transected distally. The gallbladder is incised and bile washed out in order to prevent autolysis of the mucosa of the biliary tract. The hepatic artery may be prepared from the gastroduodenal artery down to the splenic artery, but all branches should be kept open.

Additional cannulae are placed in the distal part of the aorta and the inferior vena cava. The clamped aortic and inferior mesenteric vein cannulae are attached to an air-free infusion system through which a chilled preservation infusion can later be infused. The clamped vena cava cannula is connected to tubing that leads to a bleeding bag on the floor. When all the teams involved in the harvesting are ready to proceed with the procurement, the supraceliac aorta is cross-clamped. The cannulae of the portal vein and inferior aorta containing the chilled preservation solution are immediately opened to perfuse intra-abdominal organs. Increased aortic perfusion pressure is associated with improved outcome (150 mmHg). The portal system is flushed by gravity (80 cm H_2O). There is no good evidence for the optimum total perfusion volume, but mostly, the graft is completely flushed by the first 2–3 L of preservation solution.

The effluent is drained out through the inferior vena cava cannula to the bag on the floor. The right atrium is also opened as an extra precaution against congestion of the liver. Anesthesiologist support is stopped. Topical ice slush is rapidly applied on the abdominal organs. Liver harvest is performed after removal of the heart and lungs and before the pancreas and kidneys.

The hepatogastric ligament is further divided in the cold. Care must be taken to prevent hepatic artery injury or portal vein transection when simultaneous pancreas harvesting is performed. The vena cava is transected below and above the liver with the surrounding cuff of the diaphragm. Particular care should be taken to prevent caval injury during cardiac retrieval. Finally, a portion of the aorta including the celiac axis and the initial part of the superior mesenteric artery is resected to complete the removal of the washed-out liver. Both iliac arteries and veins are harvested systematically in case vascular reconstruction is required.

Generally, dissection of abdominal organs for transplantation should be performed following cold perfusion and abdominal organs should be removed rapidly, preferably en bloc, and separated during back table dissection in the cold, particularly if the pancreas or intestine is included.

Preparation of the liver on the back table includes careful preparation of the supra- and infrahepatic vena cava of the portal vein up to its bifurcation, and of the hepatic artery. Aberrant or replaced hepatic arteries should be identified and can be reconstructed ex situ or later after implantation. Dissection of the hilus proximal the gastroduodenal artery should be avoided to prevent injury in the vascular supply of the bile duct. Additional back table portal and arterial flush is routinely done by many transplant surgeons.

Recipient operation

Few surgical procedures require the same fastidious attention to technical details that is necessary in OLT. Technical errors translate directly into poor liver function or infectious or biliary complications. Thus, transplantation should be performed only by surgeons proficient in the procedure. In addition, the operative environment should include experienced nursing and auxiliary support. Intraoperative management by a knowledgeable anesthesiologist with experience in OLT is critical for a successful result. The procedure presents the challenge of maintaining homeostatic temperature, circulation (including oxygen-carrying capacity and coagulation competence), gluconeogenesis, and electrolyte concentration while establishing adequate anesthesia and muscle paralysis with agents not requiring hepatic function for degradation. In cases of OLT using the standard technique with resection of the retrohepatic vena cava, the anesthesiologist should maintain an adequate preload during cava occlusion and correct metabolic abnormities after release of the congested portal circulation. In cases of OLT with preservation of the native vena cava, the hemodynamic consequences of the cross-clamping of the inferior vena cava can be avoided. The most important factor predictive of postoperative success is the stability of the patient during the operation and his or her delivery to the intensive care unit normothermic with adequate circulatory competence.

For many years, veno-venous bypass (VVB) was used to prevent congestion and minimize the release of lactate and other byproducts of gut hypoperfusion into the portal circulation. In addition, it improved venous return to the heart during implantation and thus improved hemodynamic stability during the period of caval occlusion. However, several disadvantages related to the use of VVB have been reported: longer operative time, transient hypothermia, cannula- and incision-related morbidity, hemodilution, and increment of cost.[16] Many centers employ this technique selectively in patients without portal hypertension or those with hemodynamic instability during intraoperative trial of portal vein and vena cava clamping.

From the surgical point of view, a successful organ engraftment begins with a controlled recipient hepatectomy. This can be a considerable task in individuals with severe portal hypertension and extensive collateral formation or in patients with multiple previous operations. Particular surgical challenges include patients who have undergone a previous liver resection for hepatocellular carcinoma, prior biliary repairs for biliary tract injuries, portosystemic shunts, or prior liver transplantation. To avoid blood loss it is recommendable to start the recipient hepatectomy with preparation of the hepatoduodenal ligament *before* mobilization or even touching the liver. This includes stepwise separation and ligation of the hepatic arteries and the bile duct, while the fully prepared portal vein is usually left unclamped until complete exposure of the supra- and infrahepatic vena cava. In selected cases, however, with severe portal hypertension and many adhesions on the right liver side, clamping or ligation of the portal vein at this stage may lead to much easier and faster later mobilization of the right hepatic lobe due to decreased liver volume. In addition, exposure of the infrahepatic vena cava for cava-preserving hepatectomy and piggyback liver transplantation is easier after ligation or clamping of the portal vein. If closure of the portal vein is not tolerated, particularly in patients with metabolic disease or fulminant hepatic failure who lack adequate portosystemic collateral in the splanchnic area, a portocaval shunt or VVB can be helpful.[17]

After complete preparation and division of the hepatoduodenal ligament, the liver is mobilized on both sides and the infrahepatic as well as the suprahepatic vena cava are fully exposed. If a classic liver transplantation is planned, retrocaval preparation is necessary. However, entering the retrocaval space may cause bleeding in cases with severe portal hypertension and requires careful hemostasis before implantation of the graft. Care to the right adrenal gland during caval dissection is also important to prevent bleeding.

In cases where piggyback liver transplantation is preferred, the retrocaval space remains untouched but the vena cava has to be freed up to the hepatic veins. Generally, this can be done from the left or right side, but is more time consuming than the classic hepatectomy.

In Europe, preservation of the vena cava has gained wide acceptance in many centers due to its advantages in terms of preserved caval flow and expected improved kidney function.[18] The evidence for renal protection by cava-preserving technique, however, is not very high, since there is only one randomized trial with a small case load.[19] It still remains unclear whether the protective effect of the piggyback technique is due to a reduction of blood loss or to effective decompression of the vena cava and the renal veins.

Before the new graft is placed in the recipient, the transplant surgeon should check the portal vein and hepatic artery flow. In addition, preparation of the hepatic artery to the branch of the gastroduodenal artery is recommended at this stage, but can be difficult in severe portal hypertension. If the hepatic artery is fully exposed up to the expected position of the anastomoses, a faster graft arterialization is feasible, which is important to avoid biliary injury.

The implantation technique in the classical operation begins with the suprahepatic caval anastomosis, followed by the infrahepatic caval anastomosis (Figure 20.1). If the vena cava was preserved, it is anastomosed either side-to-side or end-to-side with the recipient vena cava (Figures 20.2 and 20.3). When present, the temporary portocaval shunt is taken down. The operation then proceeds to the portal anastomosis as soon as possible. The time period to complete the caval and portal anastomosis before reperfusion (rewarming ischemia) should not exceed 45 min in order to avoid additional liver injury.

Before or during reperfusion, the liver must be washed out of the hyperkalemic and adenosine-rich Wisconsin preservation solution. Starzl et al.[20] described flushing the liver via the portal vein with lactated Ringer's solution and then allowing the liver

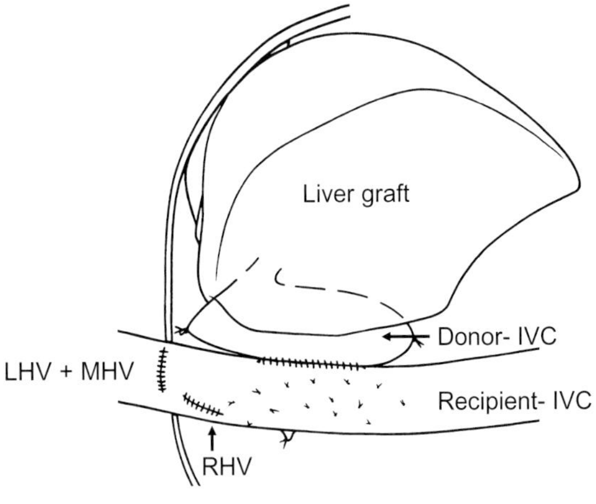

Figure 20.1 Liver transplantation using the standard technique with resection of the retrohepatic vena cava. IVC: inferior vena cava, LHV: left hepatic vein, MHV: middle hepatic vein, RHV: right hepatic vein

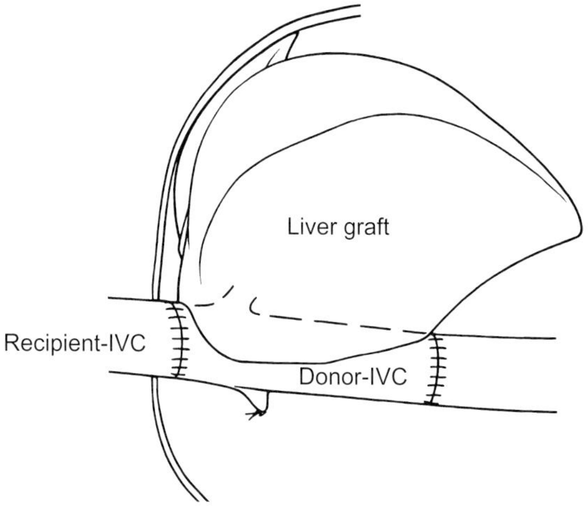

Figure 20.2 Liver transplantation with preservation of the recipient inferior vena cava: anastomosis using the middle and left hepatic vein. IVC: inferior vena cava

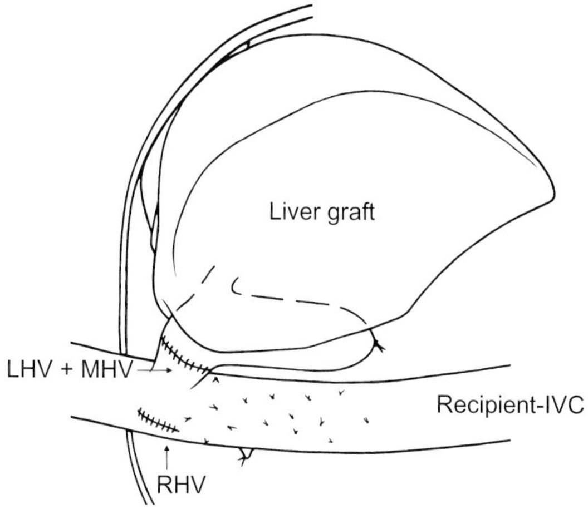

Figure 20.3 Liver transplantation with preservation of the recipient inferior vena cava: side-to-side cavocaval anastomosis. IVC: inferior vena cava, LHV: left hepatic vein, MHV: middle hepatic vein, RHV: right hepatic vein

to be reperfused with blood without venting of the vena cava. Others have advocated a 200–300 cc blood flush through the portal vein, with caval venting after all venous connections are established but with the suprahepatic cava temporally occluded.[20,21] Both techniques attempt to reduce the release of potassium in the circulation and to ameliorate the postreperfusion syndrome.[22]

The hepatic artery anastomosis is the final vascular step in the procedure. Most groups suggest anastomoses at the level of the recipient's gastroduodenal artery or proximally. A careful check of adequate arterial flow after anastomosis is mandatory. If the arterial flow rate is below 150 ml/min and does not increase by portal clamping or vasodilating agents (papaverin), more proximal anastomosis or a check for celiac trunk stenosis should be done.[23] In such cases an aortic conduit with infrarenal or supraceliac reconstruction may be preferable (see Chapter 21). Some groups advocate simultaneous arterial and venous reperfusion, arguing that it decreases reperfusion injury and late biliary strictures.[24,25] Clearly, the time period between portal reperfusion of the graft and arterialization should be kept as short as possible.

The biliary tract reconstruction can be carried out according to two main techniques. The duct-to-duct anastomosis with a cholecocholedochostomy (CC) has become the most widely employed technique of biliary reconstruction and can be performed end to end or side to side depending on the anatomic situation or surgeon preference.[26] The Roux-en-Y (RY) hepatojejunostomy is used mostly in some special situations as listed in Box 20.1.

Before suturing the bile duct, adequate vascular supply of both ends has to be verified. Electrocautery in this area should be avoided.

The CC has several advantages over RY in that it is: 1) easier to perform, 2) faster, 3) avoids an additional jejunal anastomosis, 4) preserves Oddi's sphincter function, 5) results in more physiological biliary reconstruction, and 6) provides easy access

Box 20.1 Indications for Roux-en-Y hepatojejunostomy

- Retransplantation (not mandatory)
- Insufficient length of the bile duct
- Small-size pediatric recipient
- Severe mismatch in donor and recipient common bile duct size
- Disease of the extrahepatic bile ducts
  - Primary or secondary sclerosing cholangitis
  - Biliary atresia
  - Bile duct injury
  - Cholangiocarcinoma

for subsequent biliary manipulation using an endoscopic transpapillary approach.

The surgical dictum has been to drain a biliary anastomosis. The traditional CC over a T-tube allows the evaluation of the bile flow and bile quality (color and viscosity) in the immediate post-transplant period. This approach has three additional theoretical advantages as well as a number of disadvantages:

1. The tube has the potential to divert the bile and control a biliary fistula when there is a leak in the CC.
2. The drain has the potential to stent the CC and prevent strictures at the anastomotic site.
3. The T-tube provides access for visualization of the biliary tree.[27]

Although the T-tube may prevent a biliary fistula, its placement may be associated with a leak at the T-tube insertion site in the immediate postoperative period or at the time of removal, dislodgment, or cholangitis from partial obstruction.[28] A 2001 randomized trial of CC with or without T-tube after LT showed a higher complication rate in the first group (33% vs 15%); 60% of the complications were related to the presence of the T-tube.[29] Bile leakage and cholangitis occurred more frequently in the T-tube group (10% vs 2% and 28% vs 0%, respectively); the occurrence of early and late strictures did not differ between the two groups.[29] In contrast, a recent prospective study showed that T-tubes in side-to-side choledocholedochostomy decreased the need for postoperative diagnostic and therapeutic measures.[30]

The advantage of being able to visualize the biliary tree must be weighed against the complication rate related to the T-tube and the performance of unnecessary cholangiograms. T-tube cholangiography tends to become a routine procedure, with occasional cholangitis despite the use of prophylactic antibiotics.[29,31] Access to the biliary tract with a T-tube is no longer a justification for its use given the existence of safe and effective procedures for biliary exploration (percutaneous or endoscopic).

Nowadays, in most centers, when it is feasible, the standard procedure for biliary reconstruction is the direct end-to-end CC without stenting to avoid T-tube-related biliary complications.

The intraoperative mortality rate is currently very low. Most intraoperative deaths occur in high-risk patients such as those with fulminant liver failure. Blood loss and requirement for transfusion have also decreased significantly with better selection of patients and increased experience with the procedure. Although the blood requirement can still be very high in cases with previous biliary surgery, retransplantation, or previous liver resection, most of the patients receive less than 4 IU of packed red blood cells.

Immediate postoperative management

Postoperative intensive care unit management is similar to that following any major procedure. Ventilatory support and volume replacement are standard. Isolation is not required beyond standard universal precautions. No sedation is given until extubation. For unclear reasons, postoperative pain is usually mild; any discomfort should raise suspicion of possible complications. Monitoring of serum liver test values is critical; increasing abnormalities or failure of liver test values suggests PNF or technical complications such as hepatic artery thrombosis, acute Budd–Chiari syndrome, or portal vein thrombosis. Examination of portal vein and hepatic artery flow by Doppler ultrasound is routinely indicated within the first 24 h after LT or in case of suspicion of any vascular complication. When the evaluation with ultrasound is unclear, an urgent angiogram must be done to exclude hepatic artery thrombosis. Early diagnosis with immediate surgery is the only factor separating a return to normal liver function from graft necrosis and death.

Drain management and perioperative antibiotic prophylaxis are not different in this operation from that in any other major abdominal procedure, however some transplant centers nowadays decide to omit any drains in liver transplantation.[32] If used, closed suction drains should be preferred and removed early after the threat of postoperative hemorrhage and bile leak is over. Antibiotic prophylaxis for 1 day is appropriate with an agent with adequate skin and biliary organism. Prophylaxis of infection with *Pneumocystic carini*, toxoplasmosis, cytomegalovirus, and *Candida* may be done according to each center's protocol but starts 2 weeks after transplant at the earliest. Patients with chronic hepatitis B virus infection require special treatment with gamma globulin. Two- or three-drug immunosuppression therapy is started depending on the decision of the multidisciplinary team.

Patients are discharged when they are familiar with their medication. Those patients whose homes are more than 2 h from the transplant center must stay in the vicinity of the transplant center for an additional 2–4 weeks. Close monitoring of hepatic function, immunosuppression level, and medical compliance is continued weekly for 4 weeks and then once every 3 weeks until corticoid therapy is completely stopped. After 2–3 months of outpatient control, the patient's care is remanded to their referring physician for long-term follow up. It is important to establish open lines of communication between the community physician and the transplant center to ensure early diagnosis and referral of postoperative complication and rejection.

References

1. Ploeg RJ, D'Alessandro AM, Knechtle SJ, et al. Risk factors for primary dysfunction after liver transplantation – a multivariate analysis. Transplantation 1993;55: 807–13.
2. Cavallari A, Cillo U, Nardo B, et al. A multicenter pilot prospective study comparing Celsior and University of Wisconsin preserving solutions for use in liver transplantation. Liver Transpl 2003;9:814–21.
3. Avolio AW, Agnes S, Chirico AS, et al. Primary dysfunction after liver transplantation: donor or recipient fault? Transplant Proc 1999;31:434–6.
4. Janssen H, Janssen PH, Broelsch CE. UW is superior to Celsior and HTK in the protection of human liver endothelial cells against preservation injury. Liver Transpl 2004;10:1514–23.
5. Nardo B, Beltempo P, Bertelli R, et al. Comparison of Celsior and University of Wisconsin solutions in cold preservation of liver from octogenarian donors. Transplant Proc 2004;36:523–4.
6. Guarrera JV, Henry SD, Samstein B, et al. Hypothermic machine preservation in human liver transplantation. Am J Transplant 2010;10:372–81.
7. Loinaz C, Gonzalez E. Marginal donors in liver transplantation. Hepatogastroenterology 2000;47:256–63.
8. Rull R, Vidal O, Momblan D, et al. Evaluation of potential liver donors: limits imposed by donor variables in liver transplantation. Liver Transpl 2003;9: 389–93.
9. Verran D, Kusyk T, Painter D, et al. Clinical experience gained from the use of 120 steatotic donor livers for orthotopic liver transplantation. Liver Transpl 2003;9: 500–5.
10. de Santibanes E, McCormack L, Mattera J, et al. Partial left lateral segment transplant from a living donor. Liver Transpl 2000;6:108–12.
11. Azoulay D, Castaing D, Adam R, et al. Split-liver transplantation for two adult recipients: feasibility and long-term outcomes. Ann Surg 2001;233:565–74.
12. Azoulay D, Marin-Hargreaves G, Castaing D, et al. Ex situ splitting of the liver: the versatile Paul Brousse technique. Arch Surg 2001;136:956–61.
13. Yersiz H, Renz JF, Farmer DG, et al. One hundred in situ split-liver transplantations: a single-center experience. Ann Surg 2003;238:496–505; discussion 506–7.
14. Tanaka K, Kiuchi T, Kaihara S. Living related liver donor transplantation: techniques and caution. Surg Clin North Am 2004;84:481–93.
15. Miller CM, Gondolesi GE, Florman S, et al. One hundred nine living donor liver transplants in adults and children: a single-center experience. Ann Surg 2001;234:301–11; discussion 311–12.
16. Chari RS, Gan TJ, Robertson KM, et al. Venovenous bypass in adult orthotopic liver transplantation: routine or selective use? J Am Coll Surg 1998;186: 683–90.
17. Figueras J, Llado L, Ramos E, et al. Temporary portocaval shunt during liver transplantation with vena cava preservation. Results of a prospective randomized study. Liver Transpl 2001;7:904–11.
18. Belghiti J, Ettorre GM, Durand F, et al. Feasibility and limits of caval-flow preservation during liver transplantation. Liver Transpl 2001;7:983–7.
19. Jovine E, Mazziotti A, Grazi GL, et al. Piggy-back versus conventional technique in liver transplantation: report of a randomied trial. Transplant Int 1997;10: 109–12.
20. Starzl TE, Groth CG, Brettschneider L, et al. Orthotopic homotransplantation of the human liver. Ann Surg 1968;168:392–415.
21. Fukuzawa K, Schwartz ME, Acarli K, et al. Flushing with autologous blood improves intraoperative hemodynamic stability and early graft function in clinical hepatic transplantation. J Am Coll Surg 1994;178: 541–7.
22. Brems JJ, Takiff H, McHutchison J, et al. Systemic versus nonsystemic reperfusion of the transplanted liver. Transplantation 1993;55:527–9.
23. Müller SA, Schmied BM, Nehrabi A, et al. Feasibility and effectiveness of a new algorithm in preventing hepatic artery thrombosis after liver transplantation. J Gastrointest Surg 2009;13:702–12.
24. Millis JM, Melinek J, Csete M, et al. Randomized controlled trial to evaluate flush and reperfusion techniques in liver transplantation. Transplantation 1997;63: 397–403.

25. Post S, Palma P, Gonzalez AP, et al. Timing of arterialization in liver transplantation. Ann Surg 1994;220: 691–8.
26. Davidson BR, Rai R, Kurzawinski TR, et al. Prospective randomized trial of end-to-end versus side-to-side biliary reconstruction after orthotopic liver transplantation. Br J Surg 1999;86:447–52.
27. Ascher NL. Advances in biliary reconstruction after liver transplantation. Liver Transpl Surg 1996;2: 238–9.
28. Rolles K, Dawson K, Novell R, et al. Biliary anastomosis after liver transplantation does not benefit from T tube splintage. Transplantation 1994;57:402–4.
29. Scatton O, Meunier B, Cherqui D, et al. Randomized trial of choledochocholedochostomy with or without a T tube in orthotopic liver transplantation. Ann Surg 2001;233:432–7.
30. Weiss S, Schmidt SC, Ulrich F, et al. Biliary reconstruction using a side-to-side choledochocholedochostomy with or without T-tube in deceased donor liver transplantation. Ann Surg 2009; 250:766–71.
31. Ben-Ari Z, Neville L, Davidson B, et al. Infection rates with and without T-tube splintage of common bile duct anastomosis in liver transplantation. Transpl Int 1998;11:123–6.
32. de Rougemont O, Dutkowski P, Weber M, Clavien P-A. Abdominal drains in liver transplantation: useful tool or useless dogma? A matched case–control study. Liver Transpl 2009;15:96–101.

21 Difficult surgical patients

Philipp Dutkowski, Stefan Breitenstein and Pierre-Alain Clavien

Swiss HPB and Transplantation Centers, Department of Surgery and Transplantation, University Hospital Zürich, Zürich, Switzerland

Key learning points

- Complete portal vein thrombosis is no longer a contraindication for orthotopic liver transplantation (OLT).
- Extension of splanchnic vein thrombosis should be clearly documented before OLT.
- Several options are feasible to perform OLT in the presence of portal vein thrombosis, ranging from simple thrombectomy to jump graft interposition or portocaval hemitransposition.
- Dislocated stents in the portal vein or suprahepatic vena cava can lead to extremely difficult surgical situations during liver transplantation and should be carefully diagnosed before OLT.

Introduction

Patients considered candidates for liver transplantation may vary widely in their medical condition as well as in their previous medical and surgical history. With growing success rates of liver transplantation, several transplant candidates once regarded as not or less than ideal for transplantation for technical reasons are currently evaluated for liver transplantation and frequently successfully receive a liver graft. Vascular challenges include extended portal vein or splanchnic vein thrombosis, complete occlusion of the suprahepatic vena cava, dislocated stents in the vena cava or portal vein, and stenosis or occlusion of the celiac trunk. Various techniques have been described to overcome such predictable or sometimes unpredictable conditions in liver transplantation. Most methods, however, require the transplant surgeon and center to have a high level of experience as these operations may be associated with higher intraoperative blood loss and transfusion rates. Morbidity and mortality rates are also higher in these so-called "difficult" recipients. Although a lot has been learned during the last 3 decades in liver transplantation, those cases deserve transfer to experienced centers. In general, costs usually cumulate higher than average.[1]

Portal inflow obstruction

Adequate inflow of both portal and arterial blood is essential for successful liver transplantation. About 70–80% of the normal blood flow to the liver is provided by the portal vein and the splanchnic venous circulation. Thrombosis of the portal vein develops gradually in patients with liver cirrhosis.[2,3] Although the exact mechanism of this remains unclear, it is believed to be related to decreased or reversed portal vein flow secondary to increased intrahepatic resistance. Thrombosis of the portal vein can be clinically subtle, but usually results in the development of abundant venous collaterals and ascites. In patients with a pre-existing thrombosis of the portal vein and/or of its tributaries, technical modifications are necessary to reconstitute adequate portal venous inflow to the graft during liver transplantation.[2,3] In most cases of portal vein thrombosis, however, only the main stem of the portal vein is occluded and the confluence of

Medical Care of the Liver Transplant Patient, Fourth Edition. Edited by Pierre-Alain Clavien, James F. Trotter.

the portal vein and splenic vein remains patent. In this situation, blood flow through the splenic vein is usually reversed and blood from the mesenteric veins is shunted to the systemic circulation via the splenic vein and its collaterals to the left renal vein and/or the paraesophageal venous plexus.

Based on this, preoperative knowledge of such portal vein disease appears decisive. As most transplant candidates receive color flow Doppler ultrasonography, portal vein thrombosis usually can be assessed already at the time of listing with high sensitivity. In unclear cases additional MR angiography is the preferred imaging modality. Whenever possible, the extent of portal vein thrombosis should be determined before OLT in order to obtain appropriate deceased donor organs and venous conduits. In addition, the most experienced transplant surgeon of the team should be present in the critical part of the operation.

Various surgical techniques have been described to treat portal or mesenteric vein thrombosis by liver transplantation (Box 21.1). If the portal vein is occluded only at the level of the bifurcation or intrahepatic, a classic reconstruction by end-to-end portal anastomosis is feasible. If portal vein thrombosis extends to the confluence of the superior mesenteric vein (SMV) and the splenic vein but appears relatively fresh, a successful eversion thrombectomy can be performed with consecutive regular end-to-end anastomosis. The risk of this procedure is rupture of the portal vein behind the pancreas with desperate bleeding due to an often thin-walled vessel. Therefore, if the thrombus can not easily be removed, the SMV and the splenic vein should be prepared and exposed before further manipulation. Importantly, in all cases of portal vein thromboses, the transplant surgeon should decide during hepatectomy before removal of the cirrhotic liver, whether simple thrombectomy is likely to be achieved or if an advanced reconstruction will be necessary. Pre-emptive preparation and encirculation of the vessels proximal to the thrombosis will shorten the length of the nonhepatic period or of the rewarming graft ischemia.

After thrombectomy, the endothelium of the surgically recanalized portal vein is mostly absent or at least severely injured and it is generally advised to provide anticoagulation postoperatively for 3 months to avoid rethrombosis of the portal vein.

When thrombectomy of the portal vein appears to be technically demanding due to longstanding thrombosis and calcification or fibrosis of the portal vein lumen, several other options are feasible:

1. Most patients with chronic portal vein thrombosis develop huge varices in the area of the occluded portal vein (Figure 21.1). Connection of the donor portal vein may be possible to a dilated gastroepiploic vein. Great caution should be used when controlling

Box 21.1 Surgical alternatives for portal vein reconstruction in patients with portal or mesenteric vein thrombosis

Thrombosis limited to the main stem of the portal vein
- Eversion thrombectomy
- Anastomoses to gastric varices
- Venous extension graft to the confluence of splenic and mesenteric vein
- Venous jump graft to the superior mesenteric vein

Extensive thrombosis of the portal and mesenteric venous system
- Portocaval hemitransposition
- Arterialization of the portal vein
- Anastomosis of donor portal vein with the recipient left renal vein
- Combined liver and small bowel transplantation

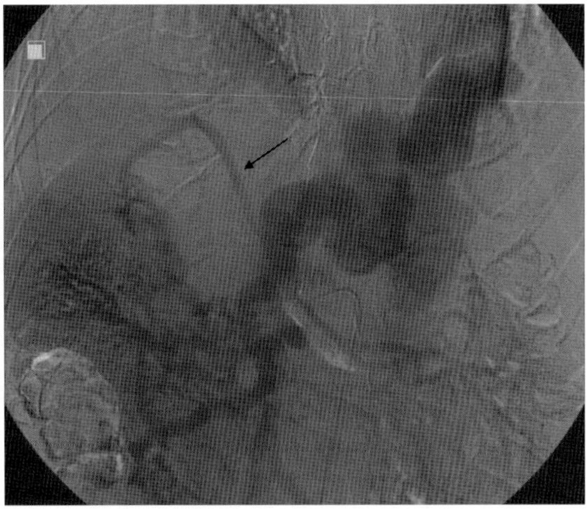

Figure 21.1 Huge gastric varix in the presence of portal vein thrombosis. The arrow marks the small and only partially perfused original portal vein

and suturing these vessels, because they are extremely fragile. Flow measurement of the connected portal vein should document more than 1000 ml/min.

2. If sufficient varices are not present or their surgical exposure appears to be too dangerous, careful preparation of the superior mesenteric vein below the pancreas is recommended. If the SMV is open, the creation of a "venous jump graft" to the superior mesenteric vein is indicated.[3–5] A segment of the iliac vein, obtained during organ procurement from the donor, can be used to extend the portal vein of the allograft. This "jump graft" can be positioned behind the pancreas in an anatomically correct position or also prepancreatic in a non-anatomical retrocolic antepyloric route. In this case the degree of angulation is important to avoid kinking of the graft. The graft should be first anastomosed to the SMV, carefully positioned in front or back of the pancreas, and afterwards anastomosed to the donor portal vein.

3. In rare cases, thrombosis of the splanchnic venous circulation is more extended and includes the portal vein, splenic vein as well as the proximal SMV (Figure 21.2), and many of its tributaries.[6] In such patients only multiple friable venous collaterals may be present without any suitable vessel for anastomosis with the portal vein of the donor liver. Some alternative surgical procedures have been described to deal with this situation. These procedures include portocaval hemitransposition, portal anastomosis with the left renal vein, arterializations of the portal vein or combined liver–small-bowel transplant.

Portacaval hemitransposition refers to a direct connection between the infrahepatic inferior vena cava (IVC) of the recipient and the portal vein of the donor liver.[7–9] The donor suprahepatic IVC is subsequently anastomosed in a "classical" end-to-end fashion with the IVC of the recipient. The anastomosis between the recipient infrahepatic IVC and the donor portal vein can be either end-to-end or end-to-side. Several groups have reported good short- and long-term outcome in these patients.[6–9] Anticoagulation is generally advised in these patients for 3 months. The shortcoming of this procedure is the persistent portal hypertension, which leads in the majority of cases to a bleeding risk from gastroesophageal varices. These bleeding problems can be treated by splenectomy, gastric devascularization, splenic artery embolization or endoscopic intervention. Ascites and lower-extremity edema can also occur after cavoportal hemitransposition although these problems tend to improve with time.

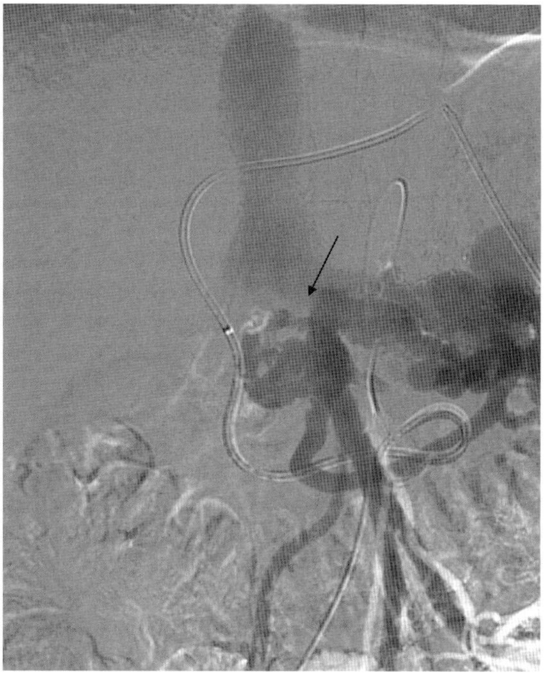

Figure 21.2 Complete portal vein thrombosis below the confluens of the SMV and splenic vein. The arrow marks the beginning of thrombosis with complete occlusion of the confluens

Arterialization of the portal vein can be an acceptable alternative.[10,11] This technique does not seem to have an effect on transplant function. The number of successful cases of portal vein arterialization reported in the literature is low, long-term follow up is lacking, and some centers have reported unfavorable results after portal vein arterialization in liver transplantation.[12] The third alternative is a direct anastomosis between the donor portal vein and the left renal vein of the recipient. This technique can be a good option in patients with portal vein thrombosis and a previous distal splenorenal shunt.[13] Combined liver and small bowel transplantation is indicated in selected patients with concomitant anatomical or functional intestinal failure and dependency on parenteral nutrition. The addition of a small bowel transplant increases the risk of postoperative morbidity and is associated with a lower long-term survival rate.[14] The main complications after small bowel transplantation are related to infectious conditions due to the direct contact between the small bowel transplant and its nonsterile contents.

Complete absence of the portal vein is a very rare congenital malformation that can be coincidentally found in liver transplant candidates.[15] These patients usually have a large congenital portosystemic shunt, but no portal hypertension and venous collaterals. Although the superior mesenteric in these patients is usually of adequate quality and diameter for direct anastomosis with the donor portal vein, the procedure may be complicated because of formation of massive edema of the viscera during cross-clamping of the superior mesenteric vein.[15]

Despite many potential technical difficulties that can be encountered during liver transplantation in patients with extensive portal or splanchnic venous thrombosis, these conditions are no longer considered an absolute contraindication for liver transplantation.[3,4] The best surgical approach may change from patient to patient and is dependent on the anatomical situation as well as on the personal preferences and experience of the surgeon. Studies comparing the various surgical techniques are lacking and most likely will never become available given the low incidence of these conditions.

Arterial inflow obstruction

Adequate arterial inflow to the grafted liver is of paramount importance to avoid ischemic injury of the bile ducts and subsequent biliary complications (see Chapter 20). In the presence of pre-existing thrombosis of the hepatic artery, or in cases with insufficient arterial flow (<150 ml/min) due to persistent celiac trunk stenosis, alternative sites should be used for arterial anastomosis with the allograft. The alternative options for hepatic artery anastomosis are summarized in Box 21.2. Most frequently, an anastomosis with the abdominal aorta will be made, either directly (if the arterial vasculature of the donor liver is of adequate length) or after extension with a donor iliac artery interposition graft.[5,16] Anastomosis with the abdominal aorta can be made either below the origin of the renal arteries (infrarenal) or cranial from the celiac trunk (supraceliac). The advantage of the anastomosis with the infrarenal aorta is that the liver can first be reperfused on the portal vein, as subsequent cross-clamping of the infrarenal aorta will not lead to a reduction of the portal vein flow. In contrast, cross-clamping of the supraceliac aorta for constructing a supraceliac anastomosis leads to reduction of the portal vein flow and additional warm-ischemic injury of the liver. On the other hand, a much shorter segment of iliac artery conduit is needed when the anastomosis is made with the supraceliac aorta, compared with the infrarenal aorta. This may facilitate long-term patency of this conduit and the hepatic artery of the graft.[16] Despite acceptable long-term patient survival in these patients, the patency of arterial conduits after liver transplantation is lower than that of direct anastomosis with the native hepatic artery.[5,16]

Box 21.2 Surgical alternatives for hepatic artery reconstruction in patients with thrombosis or severe stenosis of the native hepatic artery and celiac trunk

Iliac artery conduit to the infrarenal aorta

Indirect anastomosis with the supraceliac aorta via an iliac artery conduit

Direct anastomosis with the supraceliac aorta

Anastomosis with the splenic artery

The third alternative for hepatic artery anastomosis is an end-to-end anastomosis with the splenic artery.[17] When using this technique, the recipient splenic artery is dissected free from its origin alongside the pancreas. After obtaining adequate length, the splenic artery is subsequently ligated distally and transected. The splenic artery is then flipped ventral and toward the right side to facilitate an end-to-end anastomosis with the donor common hepatic artery or celiac trunk. A disadvantage of this technique is that it leads to a 25–40% reduction of blood flow through the portal vein, somewhat increasing the risk of postoperative portal vein thrombosis.

Venous outflow obstruction

Budd–Chiari syndrome is defined as an obstruction of venous drainage of the liver due to various causes, leading to progressive liver damage and portal hypertension.[18] Occlusion may occur at the level of the hepatic veins or the inferior vena cava (IVC) at any point between the entrance of the hepatic veins and the right atrium. Normally, the liver drains into three major hepatic veins and a variable amount of smaller caudate veins that enter directly into the IVC. Pretransplantation occlusion of the hepatic venous drainage, as in Budd–Chiari syndrome, is uncommon and is invariably associated with ascites. In about one-third of the patients no etiological factor can be identified, whereas hematological disorders are identified as the cause of venous occlusion in about 40%. The use of oral contraceptives as well as intra- or extrahepatic tumors has been reported in 10–15% of the patients.[18] Patients with Budd–Chiari syndrome may become a candidates for liver transplantation when liver insufficiency develops or ascites becomes irretractable.[19–21] The typical anatomical abnormalities underlying Budd–Chiari syndrome make liver transplantation in these patients technically more demanding and risky.[20] Much depends on the level of venous occlusion, and adequate preoperative imaging studies of the vascular anatomy are of paramount importance in these patients. Complete anatomical visualization can be obtained by venocavography or magnetic resonance imaging (MRI) or computed tomography (CT) scanning, using two-dimensional reconstructions. When the occlusion is predominantly situated at the level of the hepatic veins, leaving the IVC unaffected, liver transplantation can usually be performed in a standard fashion. Based on local and personal preference, this can be either the "classical" technique with two end-to-end anastomoses between the recipient suprahepatic and infrahepatic IVC and the donor IVC, or the "piggyback" technique with an end-to-side or side-to-side anastomosis between the recipient and donor IVC.[22]

The surgical procedure may become technically more difficult when the suprahepatic IVC is occluded. To ensure adequate venous drainage of the liver allograft a direct end-to-end anastomosis is required between the donor IVC and the right atrium of the recipient. Adequate exposure is of great importance for this procedure and the diaphragm and pericardium may need to be opened alongside the IVC. In most cases this can be achieved through the abdominal approach, and thoracotomy is rarely necessary. Dissection of the IVC, however, may be difficult and time consuming due to secondary scarring and perivascular inflammation. In addition, massive hypertrophy of the caudate lobe is found in most patients with Budd–Chiari syndrome and this may seriously hinder surgical access to the IVC.[21] Venovenous bypass may be helpful in these patients to decompress the IVC and to reduce congestion of the liver by decreasing portal blood flow through the liver. This may also reduce blood loss in these technically difficult cases. Some patients with Budd–Chiari syndrome may have had previous decompressive surgery, such as portacaval or mesocaval shunt operations.[22] This will present an additional risk factor in these patients, as will be described later. In addition, concomitant thrombosis of the portal vein has been found in up to 83% of the patients undergoing liver transplantation for Budd–Chiari syndrome, further increasing the technical challenges in these patients.[18–20,23]

In rare cases, huge collaterals in the v. azygos system may be present and allow infrahepatic cavocavostomy. The important principle of all cava reconstructions is, however, to achieve a low resistance venous drainage for the liver graft.

Postoperatively, systemic anticoagulation therapy is indicated, especially in patients with an underlying primary hypercoagulability that has led to hepatic outflow obstruction. Early series have shown a high incidence of recurrent obstruction of the hepatic veins in patients who were not treated with long-term anticoagulant therapy.[19,20] Most centers have adopted a protocol with immediate postoperative administration of heparin (either unfractioned or low-molecular-weight heparin) with subsequent conversion to long-term treatment with warfarin.

In patients with an underlying myeloproliferative disorder, long-term therapy directed toward this disease should be continued. Anticoagulant therapy is not indicated in patients with obstructing lesions of the IVC or hepatic veins, such as venous webs, which will be completely removed during transplantation and replacement of the IVC. Reported 3-year survival rates after liver transplantation in patients with Budd–Chiari syndrome range from 45 to 88%.[18–21,23] Long-term survival may be influenced by progression of the underlying hematologic disorder.[21]

Previous upper abdominal surgery or shunt procedures

It is well known that previous abdominal operations can make liver transplantation a surgically more difficult procedure due to the intra-abdominal formation of adhesions and fibrosis. In patients with portal hypertension, multiple venous collaterals may develop in the adhesive scar tissue, resulting in excessive blood loss and difficult dissection of the native liver. Most challenging situations can occur in patients with a history of previous hepatobiliary surgery or portosystemic shunt procedure.

Surgical operations in the liver hilum and/or on the liver itself lead to perihepatic adhesions and scar formation, which makes it more difficult to mobilize the native liver during a transplant procedure. This is particularly relevant after surgery of the hepatoduodenal ligament, such as cholecystectomy and portoenterostomy in children with biliary atresia.[24] Dissection of the hepatoduodenal ligament can be challenging in these children. In addition, scarring of the liver hilum leads to a higher incidence of portal vein fibrosis and subsequent thrombosis in these children. This contributes to portal hypertension and the formation of venous collaterals and neovascularization in the adhesive scar tissue. It is well recognized that blood loss is higher in children with a previous portoenterostomy. However, overall mortality and morbidity are not different for liver transplantation for biliary atresia or other indications in children, such as metabolic disorders.[24]

Similar problems of adhesion and perihepatic fibrous scar formation can be encountered in patients who had a previous partial liver resection, for example for a hepatocellular carcinoma. With growing experience and refinements in surgical technique and anesthesiological management, previous hepatobiliary surgery is certainly no longer an absolute obstacle for liver transplantation and in experienced centers the long-term outcome is not different from patients without previous surgery in the right upper quadrant of the abdomen.

Portosystemic shunt procedures, such as a splenorenal shunt or a mesocaval shunt, may be indicated in patients with complications of portal hypertension but still relatively preserved liver function.[25,26] Although these procedures are less frequently performed today due to the availability of percutaneous transjugular intrahepatic portosystemic shunts (TIPS) and better medical management of these patients, a shunt procedure may have been previously performed in a transplant candidate. Apart from the intra-abdominal adhesions due to these surgical procedures, these shunts also reduce portal blood flow to the liver. This may, at least theoretically, increase the risk of portal vein thrombosis after liver transplantation. To avoid future problems with the portal vein anastomosis during liver transplantation, an end-to-side or side-to-side portacaval shunt should best be avoided in patients with chronic liver disease. Types of portosystemic shunts that have the least impact on a possible future liver transplant are the distal splenorenal shunt and a well-positioned TIPS[25,26] Given the early occlusion rate and the need for constant surveillance, it is generally advised that TIPS should be reserved for patients with Child C classification of cirrhosis, whereas a distal splenorenal shunt is a safe, durable, and effective treatment in patients with acceptable operative risk and still good liver function.[25]

Extreme hepatomegaly

Some liver diseases, such as polycystic liver disease or large liver tumors, may be associated with extreme hepatomegaly. The presence of an extremely large liver or a large liver tumor makes it technically more difficult to mobilize the native liver, dissect the IVC, and perform the hepatectomy.

Liver transplantation may be indicated in selected patients with polycystic liver disease and disabling or life-threatening secondary complications.[27,28] Rarely, polycystic liver disease results in liver insufficiency, but progressive compression of hilar strictures, such as the portal vein or bile duct, may lead to massive ascites or jaundice. In most cases, this can be managed with a conservative medical or endoscopic management. In selected patients with areas of relatively spared normal tissue in the polycystic liver, partial liver resection may result in (partial) relief of the symptoms and complaints.[29] When complications become life threatening or when they have a significant impact on the patient's quality of life, liver transplantation can become a therapeutic option.[28,30,31] In these patients, the size of the liver may have become extraordinary and the liver may almost completely fill up the entire abdominal cavity. Liver transplantation in these patients can be technically demanding due to the difficult exposure and dissection of the hilar vascular structures as well as the IVC. Many patients have associated polycystic kidney disease, also affecting renal function. This further hampers the management of these patients. Combined liver and kidney transplantation may, therefore, become the best treatment option in selected patients with polycystic liver and kidney disease.

An extremely large liver size can also be encountered in patients with very large, rare tumors, such as hemangioendothelioma. Liver transplantation may be indicated in selected patients with hepatic hemangioendothelioma.[32,33] These patients normally have normal liver function and usually do not have coagulation abnormalities, thereby reducing the risk of major bleeding. Once the native liver has been removed, liver transplantation in these patients usually becomes a relatively straightforward procedure.

Late retransplantation

Retransplantation of the liver is indicated in selected patients with failure of their previous transplant, either acutely or chronically.[34,35] Various causes may lead to failure of a previous liver transplant, including early hepatic artery thrombosis, chronic rejection, non-anastomic biliary strictures, and recurrence of the original disease.[35] When the need for retransplantation is urgent and occurs within a few weeks after primary liver transplantation (i.e. primary nonfunction or hepatic artery thrombosis) the retransplant procedure can be relatively quick and simple. However, in case of a "late" retransplantation (>3–6 months) after primary transplantation, the original liver graft may have become firmly attached to the surrounding organs and structures due to adhesions and fibrous reaction.[34,36] This is particularly true for patients who need retransplantation for chronic rejection or intrahepatic bile duct strictures. In the latter group, patients have frequently been treated with percutaneous biliary catheters, leading to perihepatic adhesions and fibrous tissue formation. Apart from the intra-abdominal adhesions, patients may have received steroids for several years, resulting in more friable blood vessels and weakening of the tissue strength in general. This can complicate a late retransplant procedure and increases the risk for postoperative complications, such as wound-healing complications and infections.

Dislocated vascular stents in portal vein or vena cava

Several studies suggest that placement of TIPS (transjugular intrahepatic portosystemic shunts) are a safe bridge to liver transplantation, however migration of theses stents either in the portal vein or in the vena cava complicate liver transplantation. Location of the TIPS at the confluence of the SMV and splenic vein require clamping below the TIPS and thus complete exposure below the pancreas, which should be done before hepatectomy. Location of the TIPS in the right atrium requires dissection along the suprahepatic vena cava to the heart and open cardiotomy. Both procedures can be difficult and should be foreseen before transplantation.

References

1. Filipponi F, Pisati R, Cavicchini G, et al. Cost and outcome analysis and cost determinants of liver transplantation in a European National Health Service hospital. Transplantation 2003;75:1731–6.
2. Gayowski T, Marino I, Doyle H, et al. A high incidence of native portal vein thrombosis in veterans undergoing liver transplantation. J Surg Res 1996;60:333–8.
3. Yerdel M, Gunson B, Mirza D, et al. Portal vein thrombosis in adults undergoing liver transplantation: risk factors, screening, management, and outcome. Transplantation 2000;69:1873–81.
4. Lerut J, Mazza D, van Leeuw V, et al. Adult liver transplantation and abnormalities of splanchnic veins: experience in 53 patients. Transpl Int 1997;10:125–32.
5. Cappadonna C, Johnson L, Lu A, et al. Outcome of extra-anatomic vascular reconstruction in orthotopic liver transplantation. Am J Surg 2001;182:147–50.
6. Manzanet G, Sanjuan F, Orbis P, et al. Liver transplantation in patients with portal vein thrombosis. Liver Transpl 2001;7:125–31.
7. Gerunda GMR, Neri D, Angeli P, et al. Cavoportal hemitransposition: a successful way to overcome the problem of total portosplenomesenteric thrombosis in liver transplantation. Liver Transpl 2002;8:72–5.
8. Tzakis A, Kirkegaard P, Pinna A, et al. Liver transplantation with cavoportal hemitransposition in the presence of diffuse portal vein thrombosis. Transplantation 1998;65:619–24.
9. Varma C, Mistry B, Glockner J, et al. Cavoportal hemitransposition in liver transplantation. Transplantation 2001;72:960–3.

10. Charco R, Margarit C, Lopez-Talavera J, et al. Outcome and hepatic hemodynamics in liver transplant patients with portal vein arterialization. Am J Transplant 2001;1:146–51.
11. Stange B, Glanemann M, Nussler N, et al. Indication, technique, and outcome of portal vein arterialization in orthotopic liver transplantation. Transplant Proc 2001;33:1414–15.
12. Ott R, Bohner C, Muller S, et al. Outcome of patients with pre-existing portal vein thrombosis undergoing arterialization of the portal vein during liver transplantation. Transpl Int 2003;16:15–20.
13. Kato T, Levi D, DeFaria W, et al. Liver transplantation with renoportal anastomosis after distal splenorenal shunt. Arch Surg 2000;135:1401–4.
14. Brown RS, Rush SH, Rosen HR, et al. Liver and intestine transplantation. Am J Transplant 2004;4:81–92.
15. Wojcicki M, Haagsma E, Gouw A, et al. Orthotopic liver transplantation for portosystemic encephalopathy in an adult with congenital absence of the portal vein. Liver Transpl 2004;10:1203–7.
16. Muralidharan V, Imber C, Leelaudomlipi S, et al. Arterial conduits for hepatic artery revascularisation in adult liver transplantation. Transpl Int 2004;17:163–8.
17. Figueras J, Pares D, Aranda H, et al. Results of using the recipient's splenic artery for arterial reconstruction in liver transplantation in 23 patients. Transplantation 1997;64:655–8.
18. Menon K, Shah V, Kamath P. The Budd–Chiari syndrome. N Engl J Med 2004;350:578–85.
19. Klein A, Molmenti E. Surgical treatment of Budd–Chiari syndrome. Liver Transpl 2003;9:891–6.
20. Olzinski A, Sanyal A. Treating Budd–Chiari syndrome: making rational choices from a myriad of options. J Clin Gastroenterol 2000;30:155–61.
21. Srinivasan P, Rela M, Prachalias A, et al. Liver transplantation for Budd–Chiari syndrome. Transplantation 2002;73:973–7.
22. Miyamoto S, Polak W, Geuken E, et al. Liver transplantation with preservation of the inferior vena cava. A comparison of conventional and piggyback techniques in adults. Clin Transplant 2004;18:686–93.
23. Min A, Atillasoy E, Schwartz M, et al. Reassessing the role of medical therapy in the management of hepatic vein thrombosis. Liver Transpl Surg 1997;3:423–9.
24. Peeters P, Sieders E, de Jong K, et al. Comparison of outcome after pediatric liver transplantation for metabolic diseases and biliary atresia. Eur J Pediatr Surg 2001;11:28–35.
25. Abou Jaoude M, Almawi W. Liver transplantation in patients with previous portasystemic shunt. Transplant Proc 2001;33:2723–5.
26. Jenkins R, Gedaly R, Pomposelli J, et al. Distal splenorenal shunt: role, indications, and utility in the era of liver transplantation. Arch Surg 1999;134:416–20.
27. Everson G, Taylor M, Doctor R. Polycystic disease of the liver. Hepatology 2004;40:774–82.
28. Gustafsson B, Friman S, Mjornstedt L, et al. Liver transplantation for polycystic liver disease – indications and outcome. Transplant Proc 2003;35:813–14.
29. Chen M. Surgery for adult polycystic liver disease. J Gastroenterol Hepatol 2000;15:1239–42.
30. Pirenne J, Aerts R, Yoong K, et al. Liver transplantation for polycystic liver disease. Liver Transpl 2001;7:238–45.
31. Swenson K, Seu P, Kinkhabwala M, et al. Liver transplantation for adult polycystic liver disease. Hepatology 1998;28:412–15.
32. Ben-Haim M, Roayaie S, Ye M, et al. Hepatic epithelioid hemangioendothelioma: resection or transplantation, which and when? Liver Transpl Surg 1999;5:526–31.
33. Lerut J, Orlando G, Sempoux C, et al. Hepatic haemangioendothelioma in adults: excellent outcome following liver transplantation. Transpl Int 2004;17:202–7.
34. Facciuto M, Heidt D, Guarrera J, et al. Retransplantation for late liver graft failure: predictors of mortality. Liver Transpl 2000;6:174–9.
35. Sieders E, Peeters P, TenVergert EM, et al. Retransplantation of the liver in children. Transplantation 2001;71:90–5.
36. Lerut J, Bourlier P, de Ville de Goyet J, et al. Improvement of technique for adult orthotopic liver retransplantation. J Am Coll Surg 1995;180:729–32.

22 Domino and split-liver transplantation

Abhideep Chaudhary and Abhinav Humar
Thomas E. Starzl Transplantation Institute, University of Pittsburgh Medical Center, Pittsburgh, PA, USA

Key learning points

- Paramount to the success of split-liver transplantation (SLT) is appropriate donor and recipient selection.
- Split procedures can be performed *in situ* or *ex situ*; the *in situ* technique reduces cold ischemia, enhances identification of biliary and vascular structures, and reduces hemorrhage upon graft reperfusion.
- Domino liver transplantation (DLT) requires careful selection of the domino donor and domino recipient pair and is justified only for patients whose condition precludes a long time on the waiting list.
- Hepatic venous outflow is the most important technical issue for domino liver transplantation (DLT) as this vein is usually short in the graft.

Introduction

The greatest single problem facing the field of liver transplantation today remains the shortage of donor organs. This is a problem affecting all transplant centers around the world. Several innovative methods have been developed in an effort to expand the donor pool, including the techniques of split liver transplant (SLT) and domino liver transplant (DLT).

With SLT, a whole liver from a deceased donor is divided into two functioning grafts, which can be transplanted into two appropriately sized recipients. The first SLT was performed by Pichlmayr et al. in 1988.[1] Subsequently, several centers have published their SLT series. The vast majority of SLTs have been for one adult and one pediatric recipient. Usually the liver is split into a smaller portion consisting of the left lateral segment (which can be transplanted into a pediatric recipient) and the remaining larger extended right lobe (which can be transplanted into a normal-sized adult recipient). The benefits for pediatric recipients have been tremendous, including an expansion of the donor pool and a significant decrease in waiting times and mortality rates. Less common is splitting the liver for two adult recipients. Here the liver is generally split into the anatomic right and left lobe, which are then transplanted into two adult-sized recipients.

DLT, whereby a patient undergoes a liver transplant and in turn donates his liver to another recipient, has been performed since 1995.[2] Although livers from a handful of metabolic disorders cured by liver transplantation have been used for domino transplantation, livers from patients with familial amyloidotic polyneuropathy (FAP) are by far the most common source.

SLT

SLT is an attractive alternative or addition to living donation that can expand the donor pool and lower the waiting time for a deceased-donor organ. Paramount to the success of SLT is careful donor and recipient selection. SLT techniques have been restricted to ideal donors who are young, stable, and have had a relatively short period of hospitalization. Split

Medical Care of the Liver Transplant Patient, Fourth Edition. Edited by Pierre-Alain Clavien, James F. Trotter.

procedures can be performed *in situ* (splitting in a heart-beating donor) or *ex situ* (splitting performed on the back table in an ice bath after the organ is retrieved in a standard procurement fashion). The *in situ* technique reduces cold ischemia, enhances identification of biliary and vascular structures, and reduces hemorrhage upon graft reperfusion. Comparison of living-donor, *in situ*, and *ex vivo* split-liver pediatric grafts suggested a higher incidence of primary nonfunction among grafts prepared *ex vivo* vs *in situ* or living-donor techniques.[3,4]

The current challenge within the transplant community is the formulation of public policy that will realize the greatest potential from a critically limited donor pool. Split-liver transplantation is an integral mechanism to achieve this goal, however it is a technically demanding endeavor that requires additional logistic as well as personnel support. Broader application of SLT, including extension of SLT to two adults from one adult deceased-donor graft, will only be realized after the liberalization of allocation policy as well as the provision of incentives for centers that choose to invest in this effort, since benefit will be derived by all potential candidates awaiting liver transplantation.

Selection criteria

Proper recipient and donor selection are crucial in ensuring a good outcome. When selecting the recipient, important issues are graft size requirement, cause of liver failure, and severity of illness (as critically ill patients with severe portal hypertension and high MELD scores are not good candidates for SLT).[5] A graft weight/recipient weight (GW/RW) ratio of close to 0.8% should likely be the minimum when selecting appropriate recipients, but graft size is not the only criterion in selecting donors and recipients. Donors should be medically ideal to minimize the risks of primary nonfunction, especially for left lobe recipients. Young, hemodynamically stable donors with normal liver function test results, short ICU stay (<5 d) and absent or fairly short down time should be selected; with such donors, primary nonfunction for the recipients should be uncommon.

Cold ischemic time should be minimized as much as possible in all SLT recipients. For this reason, it may be preferable to do the actual transection of the parenchyma in situ in the donor. Performing the split on the back table could add up to 2–3 h of cold ischemia; there is also likely some warming of the liver on the back table, even if the split is being performed in a cold ice bath of perfusion solution.

Performing the split *in situ* also has other advantages. Significantly less bleeding occurs when the organs are reperfused. Additionally, the two liver grafts can be assessed in the donor immediately after parenchymal transection and before vascular interruption, to ensure adequate perfusion and viability.

Adult/pediatric split

This represents the most common type of SLT procedure performed today. Usually the liver is split into a smaller portion (the left lateral segment, which can be transplanted into a pediatric recipient), and a larger portion (the extended right lobe, which can be transplanted into a normal-sized adult recipient) (Figure 22.1). Results for pediatric recipients with SLTs have been very good, almost equivalent to those seen with whole-liver transplants. Benefits have included significant decreases in wait-list times, decreased wait-list mortality, and lower utilization of living donors.[6]

Technique

Prior to splitting the liver, isolation of the supraceliac and infrarenal aorta, and cannulation of the inferior mesenteric vein is done to have control in case the donor becomes hemodynamically unstable. The split procedure starts with isolation of the left hepatic artery, the left branch of the portal vein, and the extrahepatic portion of the left bile duct. This is followed by transaction of the parenchyma at about 0.5 to 1 cm to the right of the falciform ligament, yielding a left lateral graft (segments II and III) and an extended right graft (segments I, IV–VIII). The left hilar plate and bile ducts are divided sharply with scissors so as not to devascularize the duct. The left hepatic vein, the entire length of the celiac axis, and the left portal vein are generally retained with the left lateral segment while the middle hepatic vein, the main portal vein, common bile duct, and vena cava are retained with the extended right graft.

Adult/adult split

The vast majority of SLTs have been performed between an adult and a pediatric recipient. The

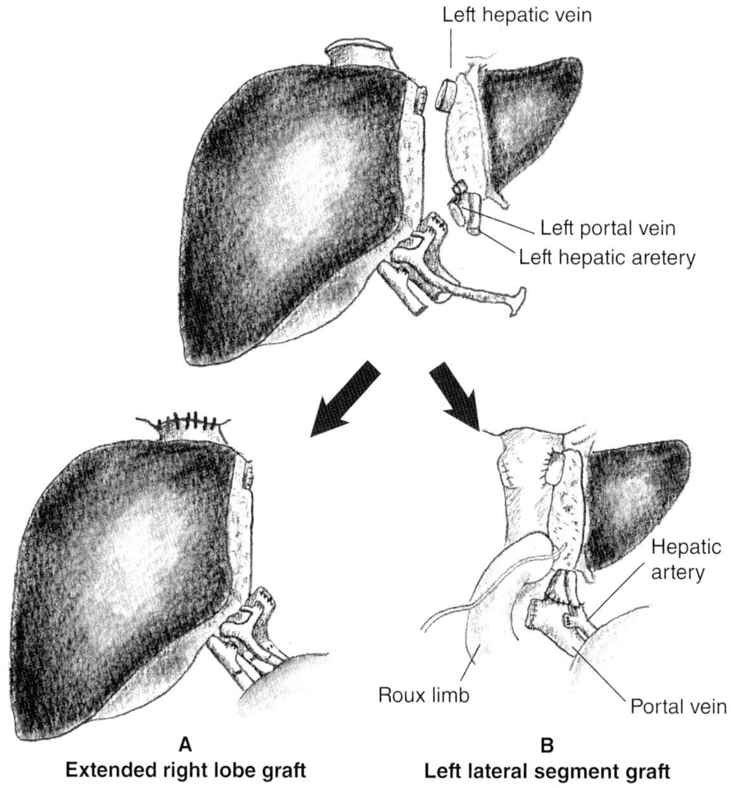

Figure 22.1 Adult/pediatric split. The liver is split into the left lateral segment, which can be transplanted into a pediatric recipient and an extended right lobe, which can be transplanted into a normal-sized adult recipient

benefits for pediatric recipients have been tremendous, with a significant decrease in waiting times and mortality rates. Splitting an adult liver for pediatric recipients has no negative impact on the adult donor pool, but it does not increase it either. Yet adults now account for 96% of patients dying on the waiting list; in 1988, they accounted for only 70%. If SLTs are to have a significant impact on waiting list time and mortality, they must be performed so that the resulting two grafts can also be used in two adult recipients.

Division of the liver at the falciform ligament will generate a left lateral segment, which would be inadequate in liver volume for the majority of adult recipients. Transection in the midplane of the liver divides it into the anatomic right lobe (60% of the liver) and the left lobe (40% of the liver); this will usually generate grafts of sufficient size for two adult recipients. The minimum amount of liver mass needed to sustain life immediately post transplant is unclear. Some experience with living-donor liver transplants suggests that a GW/RW ratio of 0.8% is the minimum. For deceased donors, the minimum amount of liver mass may also be influenced by such factors as donor hemodynamic stability and cold ischemic time.

Technical aspects

Several technical points need emphasis regarding the donor operation, which is somewhat similar to right lobe liver procurement from a living donor. The transection plane should stay to the right of the middle hepatic vein, so that this structure is retained with the left lobe (Figure 22.2). Segment IV makes up a crucial part of the left lobe, and hence the middle hepatic vein should be preserved with the left lobe to ensure there is no congestion. Loss of the middle hepatic vein may affect drainage of segments V and

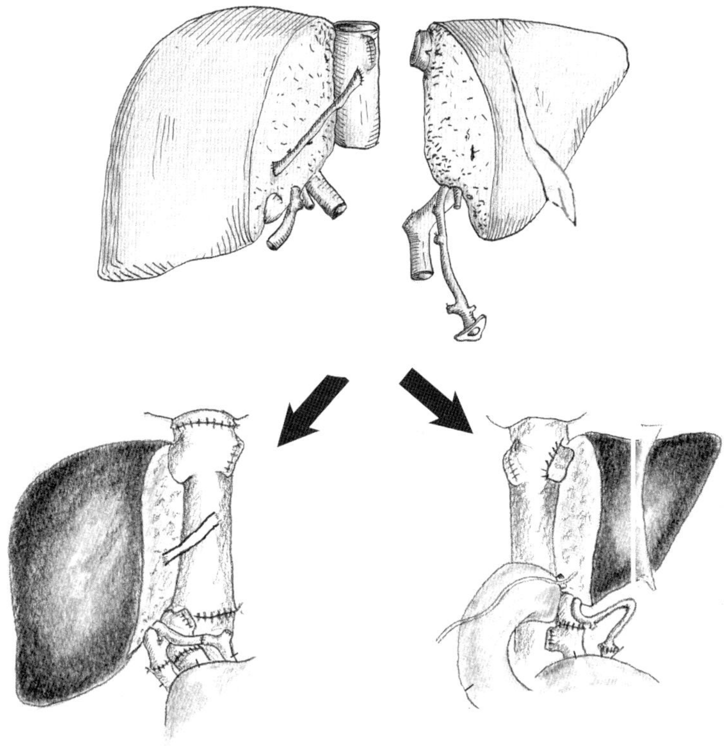

Figure 22.2 Adult/adult split. The liver is split into the left lobe, which can be transplanted into a smaller adult and a right lobe, which can be transplanted into a normal-sized adult recipient. The middle hepatic vein is maintained with the left lobe graft and important tributaries draining segments 5 and 8 of the right lobe are reconstructed with venous interposition grafts

VIII in the right lobe graft. If significant draining vessels are identified they can easily be reconstructed on the back table using vascular conduits from the deceased donor. Regarding the dissection in the hilum, the current authors' preference has been to leave the full length of the hilar vascular structures intact with the left lobe. The right-sided hilar structures are usually larger than the left-sided structures. Therefore, leaving the main vessels intact with the left lobe makes that transplant easier. The common bile duct is left maintained with the right lobe graft though so that there is a greater chance of ending up with a single bile duct orifice to reconstruct on both the right and left lobe grafts. One crucial technical point for the recipient operation is ensuring adequate venous outflow of the grafts to prevent congestion. Preserving the cava with the right lobe graft helps to maximize outflow by preserving all inferior hepatic veins. This also allows for back-table reconstruction of any segment V and VIII veins draining from the right lobe to the middle hepatic vein.

Results

The initial series of adult/pediatric SLT until the mid1990s showed a poor recipient and graft survival of 50%.[7,8] It was in 1995 when first large series of European split-liver registry with 96 patients undergoing SLT showed a 6-month patient and graft survival similar to that for whole-liver transplant.[9] In a North American series, Reyes et al. reported an overall 1-year patient and graft survival of 85 and 72%, respectively.[10] On comparing the split techniques it was found that patient survival was somewhat worse with *ex vivo* (74%) as compared with the *in situ* splitting group (96%; $P = 0.06$), as was graft survival in *ex vivo* (61%) vs *in situ* (81%) splitting ($P = 0.15$). The pediatric population benefited most from the in situ technique, with a 1-year patient survival rate of 100% with the *in situ* technique vs the *ex vivo* technique survival rate of 64% at 1 year ($P = 0.02$). The 1-year graft survival comparing these two techniques was 83% for the *in situ* group vs 45% for the *ex vivo* group.[10]

Hong et al. recently reported their 10-year experience of SLT and compared the results with whole-liver transplant and living-donor transplant. There were differences in outcomes between adults and children when compared separately by graft types. In adults, 10-year patient survival was significantly lower for the split extended right-liver graft compared with the adult whole-liver and living-donor right liver graft (57% vs 72% vs 75%, respectively, $P = 0.03$). Graft survival for adults was similar for all graft types. Retransplantation, recipient age >60 years, donor age >45 years, split extended right-liver graft, and cold ischemia time >10 h were predictors of diminished patient survival outcomes. In children, the 10-year patient and graft survival rates were similar for all graft types but there was a higher frequency of primary graft nonfunction in SLTs because of increased use in urgent and redo transplantations. The overall biliary and vascular complication rate in adults and children were 2.7 and 4.2%, and 9.2 and 4.2%, respectively.[11]

Lee et al. reviewed the United Network for Organ Sharing/Organ Procurement and Transplantation Network (UNOS/OPTN) data from 1996 to 2006 to analyze factors affecting graft survival in adult/child split cases. In multivariate analysis, recipient medical condition (hospitalization), status 1 assignment, ABO incompatibility, donor age (>40 years), donor body weight (≤40 kg), calculated whole-graft volume to recipient body weight ratio (cGRWR ≤ 1.5%) and no sharing between centers were significant risk factors in adult recipients. Recipient diagnosis of tumor, dialysis prior to transplant, recipient body weight (≤6 kg), donor age (>30 years), donor history of cardiac arrest after declaration of death and cold ischemia time (CIT >6 h) increased the risk of graft failure in pediatric recipients. Transplanting livers from young donors showed comparable outcomes to whole-organ deceased-donor liver transplantation when other transplant-related risk factors were minimized in adult recipients. Reducing CIT is important to obtain comparable outcomes to living-donor LT in pediatric recipients.[12]

SLT for two adults is less frequently performed due to technical difficulties and hence less data is available. Azoulay et al. reported their outcomes of transplantation with right and left split-liver grafts and also compared these with those of whole-liver transplants.[13] For whole-liver, right and left split-liver grafts, respectively, the patient survival rates were 88%, 74%, and 88% at 1 year and 85%, 74%, and 64% at 2 years. Graft survival rates were 88%, 74%, and 75% at 1 year and 85%, 74%, and 43% at 2 years. Patient survival was adversely affected by graft steatosis and recipients' inpatient status before transplantation. Graft survival was adversely affected by steatosis and a graft-to-recipient body weight ratio of <1%. Primary nonfunction occurred in three left split-liver grafts. The rates of arterial (6%) and biliary (22%) complications were similar to published data from conventional transplantation for an adult and a child. SLT for two adults increased the number of recipients compared with whole-liver transplantation and was logistically possible in 16 of the 104 (15%) optimal-cadaver donors.

Humar et al. reported their experience of *in situ* splitting of livers from six cadaver donors, and transplanting them in 12 adult recipients. The patient and graft survival rates were 80% each and arterial and biliary complications occurred in 16 and 25% of recipients, respectively.[14] Analysis of the SLT suggested a time-dependent learning curve, which was applicable to surgical splitting technique, implantation, and recipient selection.

Ethics of splitting

Surgical complications are probably more common in SLT (vs whole-graft) recipients, related to the cut surface of the liver, smaller vessels for anastomosis, and more complicated biliary reconstruction. Therefore, one important aspect of the recipient selection process is to adequately inform the potential recipient of the splitting procedure and obtain informed consent.

Split potential

More data is needed to better define donor and recipient selection criteria, which are crucial to success. It is difficult to estimate how much impact adult SLTs will have on the donor pool. About 25% of all deceased donors in the USA are between 15 and 35 years of age. In many of these cases, livers could be used for splits; the number of liver transplants could potentially increase by 20 to 25%, or by close to 1000. With better preservation techniques, more livers may be amenable to splitting. In the near future, this technique will likely become part of every major liver transplant center's repertoire, in order to provide the maximum advantage for their candidates on the waiting list.

DLT

In 1995 a new transplant technique – sequential transplant or "domino liver transplant" (DLT) – was developed by Furtado et al. (Portugal) in which potential liver donors consisted of some selected liver recipients whose own native explanted liver, in turn, could be considered for transplantation into another patient.[2] Today, DLT is performed all over the world, as shown by the many centers reporting to the Domino Liver Transplant Registry (DLTR).[15] The domino approach can be considered in patients with some genetic or biochemical disorders that are treated by liver transplantation. The rationale behind this approach is that such livers are otherwise normal.

Selection criteria

DLT requires careful selection of the domino donor (DD) and domino recipient (DR) pair based on blood type, size, anatomy, and indication for transplant.

Domino donor

Familial Amyloid Polyneuropathy (FAP) patients are most often used as domino donors, but some with other selected genetic or metabolic disorders are also considered.[16]

1. FAP: an autosomal dominant, debilitating and ultimately fatal condition is caused by a point mutation in protein transthyretin, one of the prealbumins. As the liver is the main source of the circulating mutant form of transthyretin, a liver transplant is a potentially curative treatment for FAP. The main rationale for using FAP livers for transplantation are:

A. FAP livers show no abnormal functioning other than producing variant transthyretin.

B. The anatomy of the FAP liver is normal.

C. The FAP domino donor is a relatively young individual, a characteristic which, in combination with a short cold ischemia time, allows excellent conditions for the liver to be used as a graft.

D. Only a proportion of all patients with the mutation will develop clinical disease. The disorder normally requires a minimum of 15 years for the development of disease symptoms in genetically affected individuals. It is assumed that when these liver grafts are given to genetically unaffected patients, a long time will be needed for the development of symptoms or, at best, the disease may never manifest itself.

2. Primary hyperoxaluria (PH): DLT from PH donors is a rescue option for carefully selected patients. This is no longer regarded as a good indication for DLT, however, as the alanine-glyoxylate aminotransferase (AGT) enzyme is located exclusively in the liver, and hyperoxaluria will inevitably occur in the domino transplant recipient after a DLT. There are a few case reports of domino recipients developing renal failure early after transplantation.[17]

3. Maple syrup urine disease (MSUD): MSUD is an autosomal recessive disorder characterized by impaired activity of the branched-chain alpha-keto acid dehydrogenase complex resulting in accumulation of branched-chain L-amino acids and alpha-keto acids, which exert neurotoxic effects. DLT from patients with MSUD is feasible as branched-chain alpha-keto acid dehydrogenase is expressed widely, with a minority of the body's distribution being hepatic, so that the metabolic effects in the domino recipient would be at least substantially attenuated.[18]

4. Homozygous familial hypercholesterolemia (HFH): HFH is a metabolic disease caused by a defect in the gene that encodes the synthesis of the cellular receptor for low-density lipoprotein receptors (LDL-Rs). A high plasma level of cholesterol is present from birth and leads to severe atherosclerosis in childhood. The liver contains approximately 50–75% of the total body LDL-Rs, therefore liver transplantation has been carried out to treat this metabolic disorder effectively. The rationale for using an HFH liver for a domino graft is that the absence of functional LDL-Rs in the liver may be compensated for by the extra-hepatic LDL-Rs. Therefore, an HFH liver can possibly be used as a domino graft for a recipient with a normal plasma cholesterol level before transplantation.[19]

5. Other hepatic disorders used in domino situations:
   A. Protein C deficiency
   B. Citrullinemia
   C. Native liver of a recipient of a multivisceral graft.[20]

Domino recipient

The domino procedure is justified for potential recipients whose condition precludes a long time on the waiting list, elderly patients with life expectancy shorter than the time needed to develop disease symptoms from the domino graft, and patients for whom palliative treatment rather than long-term cure remains the only option.[16] Examples of such patient categories are:

- Age >60 years
- Malignancies such as hepatocellular carcinoma (HCC), hepatoblastoma and neuroendocrine tumors
- Hepatitis C patients in whom the risk of developing FAP symptoms can be assumed to be smaller than the risk of clinically relevant recurrent hepatitis in the new liver
- Domino livers can also be used as interim liver transplants.

Ethics

DLT raises ethical issues in terms of safety of the domino donor and the risk of transferring the metabolic disease to the domino recipient. It is important, therefore, that the following conditions are fulfilled when debating the domino liver procedure:

1. The technique to remove the liver should not significantly increase the risk for the domino donor.
2. The liver to be transplanted must be fully functional and anatomically normal, apart from the existing metabolic disorder.
3. The existing genetic abnormality should not be expected to develop into a manifest disease within a too-short latency time period
4. Absolute necessity to maintain close life-long monitoring, consisting of clinical, laboratory, and metabolic tests, in the domino liver transplant recipient.

Technique

DLT can be whole-organ liver transplant or split-liver transplant. The choice of procedure depends on graft size, recipient size and transplant center preference. There are a few reports suggesting that from a technical perspective, whole-liver DLT is superior to a partial-liver graft due to the complexity of multiple vascular and biliary anastomoses in the latter.

Domino donor hepatectomy

For whole-organ DLT, the technique is somewhat similar to a hepatectomy performed for the live donor recipient, preserving sufficient length of vascular and biliary structures. The portal vein and hepatic artery are usually shorter than in the conventionally procured deceased-donor liver. This is seldom a problem; however, the donor and the recipient share a relatively short segment of the suprahepatic vena cava that needs particular attention (this length can be increased by opening the diaphragm slightly in the donor). Most centers prefer to leave a long enough segment of this vein in the donor to avoid any venous reconstruction in the domino donor.

Domino recipient technique

In the domino recipient, the technique of native hepatectomy is similar to hepatectomy performed for the live-donor recipient, preserving the entire length of the vascular and biliary structures. The domino graft is usually implanted in a piggyback fashion. Hepatic venous outflow is the most important technical issue for DLT as this vein is usually short in the graft, often needing some kind of reconstruction to make a proper cuff for the implantation of the domino liver in the recipient. The reconstruction of the domino suprahepatic vena cava is usually performed by using a vein graft from the deceased donor.

Results

Transplant centers all over the world can report their experience of DLT to the DLTR, an international registry that was created in 1999 as an extension of the already existing Familial Amyloidotic Polyneuropathy World Transplant Registry. The register records data on livers used for transplantation from patients with various metabolic disorders. Livers from FAP donors make up the majority of those reported to the DLTR. By December 31, 2009, a total of 902 domino transplantations on 883 patients were registered. They were reported from 57 different hospitals in 21 countries.[15]

Data from the registry shows that the mean DD and DR age at the time of transplant was 41.2 ± 11.5 years (range 21–72 years) and 54.9 ± 9.1 years (range 3–74 years), respectively. Donor and recipient data showed that 56% of DDs and 75% of DRs were male. The majority of DDs are FAP patients. The metabolic disease spectrum of DDs is as described earlier.

Primary hepatic malignancy, cirrhosis due to hepatitis C and B, and alcohol cirrhosis are the three most common indications for DLT, accounting for 41%, 20 and 18% of the domino recipients, respectively. Other less common indications included primary biliary cirrhosis, Wilson's disease, primary sclerosing cholangitis, and hemochromatosis.

The overall 1-year, 5-year, and 8-year graft survival rates in DLT recipients were 79.9%, 65.3%, and 61.6%, respectively. The main causes of DR death are tumor recurrence (23%), septicemia (17%), cardiac-related deaths (7%), and preoperative deaths (6%).

Transthyretin amyloidosis developing 7–8 years after transplant in the domino recipients has been reported,[21] thus some centers recommend retransplant if DRs survive more than 5 years after DLT. Owing to early renal failure developing after DLT from PH donors, Saner et al. suggested DLT using donors with PH should not be recommended for transplantation unless preventive strategies have been identified.[22]

Conclusion

In conclusion, using livers for transplantation from patients with hepatic metabolic disorders or splitting livers from suitable deceased donors represent useful methods to expand the donor pool and thereby to reduce the existing liver graft shortage. Both procedures benefit patients by either decreasing the waiting time or increasing the chances of a patient receiving a life-saving transplant.

References

1. Pichlmayr R, Ringe B, Gubernatis G, et al. Transplantation of a donor liver to 2 recipients (splitting transplantation) – a new method in the further development of segmental liver transplantation. Langenbecks Arch Chir 1988;373:127–30.
2. Furtado A, Tomé L, Oliveira FJ, et al. Sequential liver transplantation. Transplant Proc 1997;29:467–8.
3. Goss JA, Yersiz H, Shackleton CR, et al. In situ splitting of the cadaveric liver for transplantation. Transplantation 1997;64:871–7.
4. Rogiers X, Malagó M, Gawad K, et al. In situ splitting of cadaveric livers. The ultimate expansion of a limited donor pool. Ann Surg 1996;224:331–9.
5. Renz JF, Emond JC, Yersiz H, et al. Split-liver transplantation in the United States: outcomes of a national survey. Ann Surg 2004;239:172–81.
6. Busuttil RW, Goss JA. Split liver transplantation. Ann Surg 1999;229:313–21.
7. Emond JC, Whitington PF, Thistlethwaite JR, et al. Transplantation of two patients with one liver. Analysis of a preliminary experience with "split-liver" grafting. Ann Surg 1990;212:14–22.
8. Broelsch CE, Emond JC, Whitington PF, et al. Application of reduced-size liver transplants as split grafts, auxiliary orthotopic grafts, and living related segmental transplants. Ann Surg 1990;212: 368–75.
9. de Ville de Goyet J. Split liver transplantation in Europe – 1988 to 1993. Transplantation 1995;59:1371–6.
10. Reyes J, Gerber D, Mazariegos GV, et al. Split-liver transplantation: a comparison of ex vivo and in situ techniques. J Pediatr Surg 2000;35:283–9.
11. Hong JC, Yersiz H, Farmer DG, et al. Longterm outcomes for whole and segmental liver grafts in adult and pediatric liver transplant recipients: a 10-year comparative analysis of 2,988 cases. J Am Coll Surg 2009;208: 682–9.
12. Lee KW, Cameron AM, Maley WR, et al. Factors affecting graft survival after adult/child split-liver transplantation: analysis of the UNOS/OPTN data base. Am J Transplant 2008;8:1186–96.
13. Azoulay D, Castaing D, Adam R, et al. Split-liver transplantation for two adult recipients: feasibility and long-term outcomes. Ann Surg 2001;233:565–74.
14. Humar A, Ramcharan T, Sielaff TD, et al. Split liver transplantation for two adult recipients: an initial experience. Transplant 2001;1:366–72.
15. Domino Liver Transplant Registry. Systemic but asymptomatic transthyretin amyloidosis 8 years after domino liver transplantation. J Neurol Neurosurg Psychiatry

(http://www.fapwtr.org/ram_domino.htm) 2010; 9 Oct (Accessed 23-6-11).

16. Wilczek HE, Larsson M, Yamamoto S, et al. Domino liver transplantation. J Hepatobiliary Pancreat Surg 2008;15:139–48.
17. Donckier V, El Nakadi I, Closset J, et al. Domino hepatic transplantation using the liver from a patient with primary hyperoxaluria. Transplantation 2001;71: 1346–8.
18. Barshop BA, Khanna A. Domino hepatic transplantation in maple syrup urine disease. New Engl J Med 2005;353:2410–1.
19. Popescu I, Simionescu M, Tulbure D, et al. Homozygous familial hypercholesterolemia: specific indication for domino liver transplantation. Transplantation 2003;76: 1345–50.
20. Tzakis AG, Nery JR, Raskin JB, et al. "Domino" liver transplantation combined with multivisceral transplantation. Arch Surg 1997;132:1145–7.
21. Conceição I, Evangelista T, Castro J, et al. Acquired amyloid neuropathy in a Portuguese patient after domino liver transplantation. Muscle Nerve 2010;42: 836–9.
22. Saner FH, Treckmann J, Pratschke J, et al. Early renal failure after domino liver transplantation using organs from donors with primary hyperoxaluria type 1. Transplantation 2010;90:782–5.

23 Surgical aspects of living-donor transplantation

Kelvin K.C. Ng and Sheung Tat Fan

Department of Surgery, The University of Hong Kong, Queen Mary Hospital, Pokfulam, Hong Kong, China

Key learning points

- To overcome the critical organ shortage in Asian countries, there is a drive for surgical innovations of liver transplantation, which includes living-donor liver transplantation (LDLT). LDLT is technically demanding and involves complicated manpower and more logistical issues such as donor selection and safety.
- An adequate graft size is essential to ensure satisfactory early graft function and recipient survival after LDLT. Graft-to-body size mismatch and the resulting small-for-size syndrome is still the major problem in adult-to-adult LDLT. The minimum requirement of a small-for-size graft for predictable recipient success is set to range from 30 to 40% of the estimated standard liver volume.
- LDLT using the right liver graft is the preferred procedure if there is donor-to-recipient body weight mismatch. The importance of good venous drainage of the right liver graft remains the fundamental issue to ensure adequate graft function. Different approaches have been adopted in Asian transplantation centers to ensure venous drainage of the anterior sector of a right liver graft.
- The incidence of biliary complication remains high (up to 67%) after LDLT. This complication has significantly affected the quality of life of LDLT recipients and occasionally causes graft and patient loss. The ischemia of the right hepatic duct and the high incidence of anatomical variation of the right duct system may account for this high complication rate.

Introduction

Orthotopic liver transplantation (OLT) is currently the treatment of choice for chronic liver diseases, acute liver failure, and selected patients with early-stage unresectable hepatocellular carcinoma (HCC). With advances in perioperative management and immunosuppression, the outcome of OLT recipients has much improved, with a 5-year survival rate of 80% and a good quality of life.[1] Nonetheless, the number of deceased donors per million of population among the Asian transplantation centers remains low, ranging from 0.07 to 6.5 in the year 2005. Such deceased organ donation rates were far below those of western countries (35.1 per million population in Spain and 25.2 per million population in the USA). The critical shortage of deceased organs in Asia is mainly related to the cultural and religious barriers of organ donation among the general population. The advent of living-donor liver transplantation (LDLT) and other surgical innovations has arisen to overcome this problem in Asian countries. In addition to the technical demands of LDLT, complicated manpower and more logistical issues such as donor selection and safety go hand in hand with this surgery.

The history of LDLT originally started in western countries. Smith proposed the idea of liver transplantation using a liver graft from a living donor in 1969.

Medical Care of the Liver Transplant Patient, Fourth Edition. Edited by Pierre-Alain Clavien, James F. Trotter.

The first attempt of LDLT was made by Raia in Brazil in 1988 and the first successful LDLT from adult to child was performed by Strong in Australia in 1989. In Asia, the first LDLT was performed by Nagasue of Shimane University in Japan in 1989. Since then, this operation has been rapidly taken up and propagated among Asian transplantation centers. Many technical refinements have taken place to optimize its benefits for patients. Initial LDLT programs involved transplanting a segment II/III graft from a parent donor to a pediatric patient. To suit the demand of adult patients, frontiers of the Shinshu group in Japan modified the operation by using an extended left liver graft and reported the first successful adult-to-adult LDLT using the left liver in 1993. The recipient suffered from primary biliary cirrhosis and the donor was her son.

Even with a left liver graft, the minimal graft volume for sustaining the patient's survival might not be reached if there was body size mismatch between the recipient and donor. In such an instance, the use of a right liver graft could solve the problem of graft-to-body size mismatch.

In 1993, the Kyoto group reported a case of unplanned adult-to-child LDLT using the right liver to avoid the difficult arterial anatomy of the donor's left liver. Subsequently, the first successful adult-to-adult LDLT using the right liver graft including the middle hepatic vein (MHV) was performed at the authors' center in 1996.[2] Further advances in the techniques of LDLT were then reported by other Asian centers, including addition of the caudate liver to a left liver graft and the use of right lateral sector graft in Japan, and the dual grafts from two donors for one recipient in Korea. To minimize donor morbidity, the practice of minimally invasive surgery was applied to the donor operation,[3] but was not yet widely practiced.

General principles of LDLT

Minimal graft size

Adequate graft size is essential to ensure satisfactory early graft function and recipient survival after LDLT. Graft-to-body size mismatch and the resulting small-for-size syndrome is still the major problem in adult-to-adult LDLT. The clinical manifestation of small-for-size syndrome includes cholestasis, intractable ascites, encephalopathy, and eventual mortality. The histopathologic features of small-for-size graft injury include hepatocyte ballooning, steatosis, apoptosis, sinusoidal congestion, endothelial denudation, and parenchymal cholestasis.

An experimental study has demonstrated that the minimal graft weight for successful OLT was 25% of the original liver weight.[4] In a retrospective study on 276 patients with LDLT, Kiuchi et al.[5] found that the use of small-for-size liver graft of <1% of the recipient body weight resulted in a significantly poor graft survival. This observation is related to the small-for-size graft injury and the reduced metabolic and synthetic capacity of the small-for-size liver graft. Using mathematic formulation, the estimated standard liver volume (ESLV) of the recipient could be accurately derived.[6] The minimal requirement of a small-for-size graft for predictable recipient success was then set to range from 30 to 40% of the ESLV.[7] Portal hyperperfusion in the presence of relative outflow obstruction is the major contributing factor for hepatocyte damage in a small-for-size graft. Various procedures have been reported to modulate superfluous portal vein flow in order to alleviate small-for-size graft damage. These included: hemiportocaval shunt, mesocaval shunt, splenic artery ligation, splenectomy, and pharmacologic modulation. The use of heat shock protein inducer has been shown to suppress inflammatory response and improve survival after massive hepatectomy in a rat model, and this may become a new treatment strategy for the small-for-size liver graft.[8]

Venous drainage of anterior sector of right liver graft

LDLT using the right liver graft is the preferred procedure if there is donor-to-recipient body weight mismatch. The adequate graft size can be achieved with the use of a right liver graft. Nevertheless, the importance of good venous drainage of the right liver graft remains the fundamental issue to ensure adequate graft function. The detrimental effects of impaired venous drainage of the anterior sector (segments V and VIII) of a right liver graft include venous congestion and hepatic necrosis of that part of the liver graft. This is frequently observed when the MHV tributaries from the anterior section are ligated in case the MHV is not included in the right liver graft. The recipient may manifest the small-for-size syndrome, and the risk of hepatic artery thrombosis increases due to poor hepatic venous outflow. The impaired graft regeneration is unavoidable due to the elevating sinusoidal pressure and disrupted sinusoidal endothelium.[9]

Different approaches have been adopted in Asian transplantation centers to ensure venous drainage of the anterior sector of a right liver graft. The Korean group[10] advocated the application of a "modified right liver graft" by reconstruction of hepatic venous drainage of the anterior sector directly into the inferior vena cava, using an interposition vein graft. Satisfactory survival outcome was reported by the same group using this modified graft. The Tokyo group[11] adopted the selective reconstruction of venous drainage of the anterior sector based on the presence of dominant segment V and VIII hepatic veins by intraoperative ultrasonography and perfusion of the anterior sector when the right hepatic artery and MHV were clamped in the donor operation. The prominent segment V and VIII hepatic veins were anastomosed to the recipient MHV and left hepatic vein using interposition vein grafts in selected recipients. The Kyoto group[12] included the MHV with the right liver graft when the graft is MHV dominant, or the graft-to-recipient weight ratio is <1%, and the remnant donor left liver volume is 35% in all cases. The Taiwan group[13] also used similar criteria to include the MHV with the right liver graft when the graft weight is <50% of the ESLV of the recipient, or the graft is MHV dominant.

It has been demonstrated by the current authors' center that routine inclusion of the MHV with the right liver graft resulted in uniformly good venous drainage of the liver graft and thus favorable operative outcomes were achieved.[14] This approach was considered to be crucial for patients with high metabolic demands and poor functional reserve, such as patients with fulminant hepatic failure or acute decompensation of chronic liver disease. In addition, the authors' center proposed the technique of hepatic venoplasty by joining the MHV to the right hepatic vein (RHV) of the liver graft to form a single cuff on the back-table to further enhance the outflow capacity of the liver graft.[15] With routine inclusion of the MHV with the right liver graft, special care is necessary to preserve the segment IVb hepatic vein with the donor liver remnant to safeguard donor safety.[16] There has been some concern about donor safety in harvesting the MHV with the right liver graft. Up until now, there has been insufficient evidence supporting the direct relationship between donor morbidity and the absence of MHV in the donor liver remnant. Donor safety in terms of low morbidity and early liver remnant regeneration after right hepatectomy with inclusion of the MHV has been reported.[17]

Biliary reconstruction

The incidence of biliary complications remains high (up to 67%) after LDLT.[18,19] This complication has significantly affected the quality of life of LDLT recipients and occasionally causes graft and patient loss. The ischemia of right hepatic duct and the high incidence of anatomical variation of the right duct system may account for this high complication rate. To avoid ischemia of the right hepatic duct, it is mandatory to preserve the blood supply of the bile duct. As the arterial supply of the right hepatic duct originates from the right hepatic artery and hilar plate, it is necessary to avoid dissection into the area between the right hepatic duct and right hepatic artery beyond the point of right hepatic duct division in the donor operation.[20] In addition, sufficient liver tissue around the right hepatic duct should be preserved to ensure adequate venous drainage for the right hepatic duct. High-quality cholangiogram by fluoroscopy helps to delineate the complicated right hepatic ductal system if anatomical variation exists.

Hepaticojejunostomy (HJ) was the preferred biliary reconstruction technique in an early series of LDLT,[21] however it was associated with a long operating time, contamination of the operation field due to opening of the small bowel, and delay in return of gastrointestinal function. In contrast, duct-to-duct reconstruction has the advantages of avoidance of contamination of the operation field and early return of bowel function. Since the function of sphincter of Oddi is preserved in duct-to-duct reconstruction, enteric reflux to the biliary system and the resulting ascending infection can be potentially avoided. In addition, this reconstruction technique allows subsequent intervention by endoscopic retrograde cholangiopancreatography if necessary. The feasibility of duct-to-duct biliary reconstruction has been reported and there was no proven difference in the incidence of biliary complications between HJ and duct-to-duct reconstruction from retrospective studies. In a study by Liu et al.,[19] the outcomes of 41 LDLT recipients who underwent duct-to-duct reconstruction were compared with those of 71 LDLT recipients who underwent HJ. There was no significant difference in biliary complications between the duct-to-duct group (24%) and the HJ group (31%).

In an attempt to lower the biliary complication rate following duct-to-duct reconstruction, Ishiko et al.[18] advocated the practice of continuous suture combined with external stent. Possible factors reported to be associated with increased risk of biliary complications after duct-to-duct reconstruction included multiple ductal openings and high preoperative Model for End-stage Liver Disease (MELD) score (≥35).[19] Whether continuous or interrupted sutures, and stent or no stent make any significant difference in preventing biliary complications requires a higher level of clinical evidence by randomized, controlled trials for validation.

Donor operation

The donor needs to be regarded as a patient once he or she is put on the operating table. All surgical maneuvers and techniques deserve full attention to minimize donor damage and to maximize the functional quality of the liver graft in order to maintain the best results of LDLT.

A high-quality operative cholangiogram is an essential step in the success of the operation.[20] During the procedure, the cystic duct is freed and cannulated by a Fr 3.5 catheter. At the liver hilum, gentle dissection is made to identify the confluence of the hepatic ducts. For right liver donor operation, a large-sized metal clip is applied to the liver capsule at the point of division of the right hepatic duct. The location of the metal clip in relation to the right hepatic duct is studied on fluoroscopic images. Counterclockwise rotation of the x-ray tube to the right side of the donor can produce a clear picture of the anatomic relationship between branches of the right hepatic duct and left hepatic duct. In some instances, the metal clip is re-positioned until the most appropriate position of the duct division is determined. Using this technique, the most appropriate site of bile duct division can be defined so as to avoid multiple hepatic duct openings in the graft and injury to the confluence of the hepatic ducts.[20]

For right liver donor operation, dissection of the right hepatic artery should not be made beyond the left side of the common hepatic duct and into the tissue plane between the right hepatic duct and right hepatic artery. This maneuver is to preserve the blood supply to the common hepatic duct and right hepatic duct, which is crucial in avoiding bile duct stricture of the liver graft after biliary reconstruction. The segment IV hepatic artery arising from the right hepatic artery must be preserved to prevent ischemic necrosis of segment IV. For dissection of the right portal vein, sufficient length of this vein is preferred for the subsequent anastomosis. To achieve this, caudate branches must be divided and ligated. Any branch that enters the right posterior portal fissure must be preserved as it may be the early branch of segment VI portal vein.

For left liver donor operation, hilar dissection starts with dissection of the left hepatic artery. Gentle dissection until the junction of left hepatic artery with the main trunk is made to ensure maximum length of the artery, but the part near to the umbilical fissure should not be dissected to avoid ischemic injury to the left hepatic duct. Then, the left portal vein is dissected until the junction with the main trunk is seen. The caudate branches near the junction of the left and right portal veins should be ligated and divided to ensure adequate length of the left portal vein. The aberrant left hepatic artery within the lesser omentum should be inspected, palpated, and preserved.

Special attention should be paid to the venous drainage of the liver graft during donor operation.

For the right liver donor operation, apart from the main RHV and/or MHV, the inferior (draining segment VI) or middle RHV (draining segment VII) should be preserved for subsequent reconstruction. Sometimes, small hepatic veins (<5 mm in diameter) can be sacrificed, but it would be good practice to occlude the vein and observe for a color change of the corresponding liver segment before ligation. For a right liver graft with inclusion of the MHV, separation of the caudate liver from the inferior vena cava by dividing the caudate hepatic veins should be carried out to the left side to facilitate liver transection. For a left liver graft with caudate liver, the caudate hepatic vein should preferably be preserved

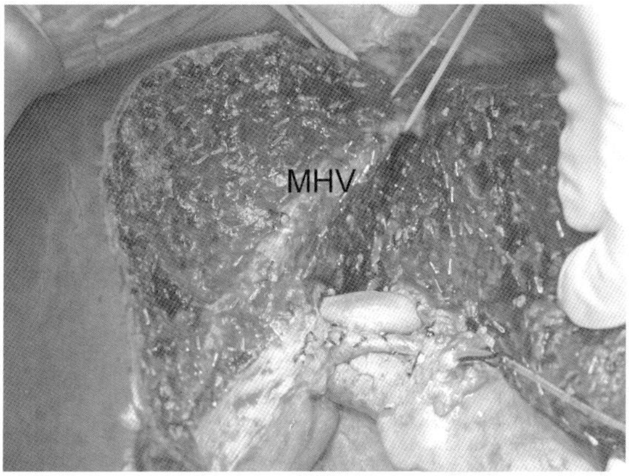

Figure 23.1 The MHV is exposed on the left side in the donor operation of right liver graft with inclusion of the MHV

for subsequent implantation to ensure adequate venous drainage of the liver graft.

The liver transection plane varies according to the different liver graft types.[22] The general principle is to minimize the amount of necrotic liver tissue both in the graft and donor, otherwise the necrotic tissue predisposes to infection in the recipient and systemic inflammatory response in the donor. For a right or left liver graft, liver transection is at the midplane of the whole liver marked on the surface by temporary occlusion of the ipsilateral inflow blood vessels. Whether including the MHV to the liver graft or not, it should be a good practice to expose the MHV, which will serve as a correct landmark for guidance on the liver transection plane (Figure 23.1) and the amount of necrotic liver tissue left to either the donor or the recipient can be minimized.

For a segment II/III liver graft, the liver transection plane is on the right side of the falciform ligament. At this transection plane, an umbilical vein draining into the left hepatic vein should be preserved to improve venous drainage of segment III.[23] The segment IV in the donor may become dusky due to venous congestion, but the ischemic area could be reduced by preserving an independent segment IV hepatic artery at the hilar dissection.

Liver transection is carried out using the ultrasonic dissector, which could identify the major hepatic branches clearly. Apart from the meticulous surgical technique using ultrasonic dissector, methods to reduce bleeding from the major hepatic veins include lowering the central venous pressure and intermittent inflow vascular occlusion.[24] Although a brief period of inflow vascular occlusion may be beneficial for recovery of the liver graft, prolonged ischemia is definitely harmful to the liver graft. The liver will not tolerate accumulated ischemic time of intermittent inflow vascular occlusion of more than 120 min.[25] Nonetheless, with standard surgical techniques, liver transection can be performed safely without inflow vascular occlusion in the donor operation and the volume of blood loss can be kept to a minimum.

The techniques of liver graft retrieval have changed much during the evolution of LDLT. Cannulation of the right or left portal vein for flushing of the liver graft by preservation solution before graft retrieval has no longer been practiced, as this may shorten the length of portal vein available. Instead, the liver graft is retrieved without cannulation in the donor's abdominal cavity.

At the back-table, the graft portal vein is pinched with a cannula *in situ* for uniform flushing of the liver graft with preservation solution. Sometimes the cannula is pushed into the right anterior or posterior portal vein for efficient right liver graft flushing. Heparin is not routinely necessary for flushing of the liver graft. The issue of hepatic artery flushing by preservation solution is debatable. On the one hand, cannulation of the hepatic artery may cause intimal damage as the lumen of the artery is small. Meanwhile, communication between the hepatic artery and portal vein may exist and the flushing solution may readily traverse to the artery by portal vein flushing.

It is not known whether the lack of hepatic artery flushing is responsible for the high incidence of biliary complications in LDLT. At the current authors' center, hepatic artery flushing is a routine procedure. In a liver graft that includes the MHV, it is preferred to perform venoplasty of the RHV/MHV (Figure 23.2) or the MHV/left hepatic vein to form a large triangular orifice for implantation to the inferior vena cava of the recipient. By using this maneuver, adequate venous drainage of the liver graft is ascertained to ensure good graft function.[20] For a right liver graft without the MHV, the venous drainage of segments V and VIII needs to be restored by the vascular conduits.[11,26,27]

Before wound closure in the donor operation, a second dose of IV antibiotics is necessary to prevent

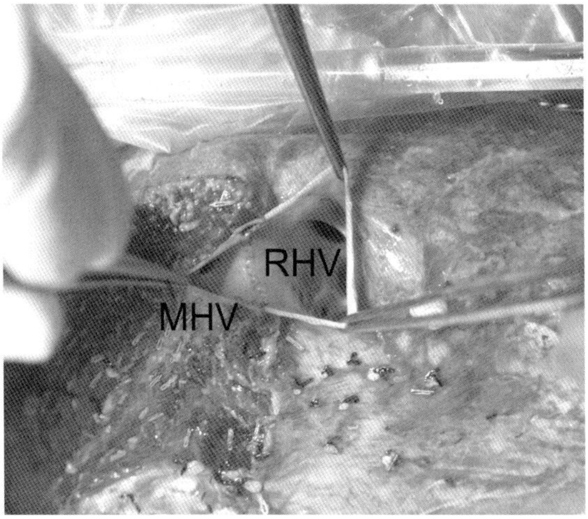

Figure 23.2 Venoplasty of the RHV and MHV at the back-table of right liver donor operation

wound infection, which may predispose to late incision hernia. Identification of possible sites of bile leakage by flushing of the bile duct using a cannula inserted into the cystic duct is crucial so that meticulous suturing of the site of bile leakage is carried out to ensure donor safety. Bile leakage may occur on the liver surface, hepatic duct stump, hilar plate, and caudate process. In case of right liver donor operation, the left liver remnant should be anchored to the anterior abdominal wall to prevent its rotation into the right subphrenic cavity causing venous outflow obstruction of the remnant liver.[28] The right subphrenic space will be occupied by the hepatic flexure of the colon. Attention must be paid to avoid the small bowel migrating into the right subphrenic space causing twisting of the small bowel and subsequent obstruction. An abdominal drain is routinely not deployed.[29]

Recipient operation

In the case that LDLT is performed on patients with nonmalignant liver diseases, donor and recipient operations are carried out simultaneously. If the recipient has HCC or has undergone multiple abdominal operations, it is preferable to start the recipient operation first to rule out any possible reasons that prohibit LDLT.

The recipient hepatectomy in LDLT differs from the deceased graft operation in that the maximal lengths of the hepatic artery, portal vein, common hepatic duct, and the entire inferior vena cava have to be preserved. The hepatic artery branches are temporarily controlled by the atraumatic microvascular clamp before division. The common hepatic duct is left open after division near the hilar plate and then the right and left portal veins are freed for subsequent anastomosis or lengthening of the MHV of the liver graft.

During implantation of the liver graft, the practice of inferior vena cava occlusion varies among different centers. Some centers prefer side-clamping of the inferior vena cava to maintain venous return to the heart,[30] whereas other centers prefer cross-clamping the entire inferior vena cava to allow creation of a large hepatic vein anastomosis.[31] It has been shown that cross-clamping of the inferior vena cava for 45–60 min is well tolerated without the conventional veno-venous bypass.[32] At the authors' center, venoplasty is routinely performed for the RHV/MHV in the right liver graft and for the MHV/left hepatic vein in the left liver graft. Direct anastomosis is constructed between the large triangular hepatic vein orifice of the liver graft and the recipient's inferior vena cava.

In the case of venous conduit draining prominent segments V and VIII hepatic veins of the liver graft, it is anastomosed to the recipient MHV stump or inferior vena cava. The long-term patency of this venous conduit is questionable, and it may be occluded for a short period of time after LDLT due to compression by the regenerated liver graft. Nevertheless, the patency of this venous conduit contributes to the satisfactory graft function in the early postoperative period.

For portal vein anastomosis, attention should be focused on the possibility of tension, redundancy, and disorientation of the donor and recipient portal veins. In the case of the presence of double portal veins in the liver graft, the two portal veins could be joined together as a single cuff for subsequent anastomosis.[20] Hepatic artery anastomosis is preferably performed under the operating microscope. Since hepatic artery anastomosis is so important that graft survival is jeopardized if the anastomosis fails, the exact technique is needed and anastomosis under the operating microscope by experienced microvascular surgeons is mandatory.

Upon completion of all the vascular anastomoses, Doppler ultrasonography is necessary to assess the patency of these anastomoses. The color flow signal across the anastomosis is the best indicator for a perfect anastomosis to be created. In particular, a more important criterion of full patency of hepatic venous anastomosis is the triphasic pulsatility spectral waveform, which is present in a normal liver. Using the Doppler signal, it is possible to define partial occlusion as a low flow rate and absent pulsatility waveform, and complete occlusion as an absent flow signal.[20] For left liver and pediatric LDLT, Doppler ultrasonography is even more important because the blood flow in the portal vein and hepatic vein may be jeopardized by different graft positions.[33]

Special issues of LDLT

Right lateral-sector graft and dual grafts

LDLT using the right liver graft has imposed a potentially higher surgical risk on the donor, who may have a relatively small liver remnant. The authors' center has suggested that a liver remnant of at least 30% should be preserved to ensure donor safety.[34] To accommodate this safety limit, a right lateral-sector graft and dual grafts from two donors have been developed as the variant grafts for LDLT.

Utilization of the right lateral-sector graft (segments VI and VII) in LDLT was first advocated by the Tokyo group.[35] This variant graft was chosen under the conditions that the donor left liver volume was <30% of the estimated total liver volume, and the estimated volume of the right lateral-sector graft being larger than that of donor left liver. The successful use of the right lateral-sector graft has been reported in six recipients by the same group.[36] However, harvesting of this kind of liver graft was highly technically demanding and the associated bile leakage rate was reported to be as high as 50%. Hence, this variant graft has not been widely adopted in other transplant centers.

Lee et al.[37] invented the use of dual liver grafts from two donors for LDLT. The usual grafts chosen were the left liver or segment II/III graft. Implantation of this variant graft was complex. The first graft was implanted orthotopically, while the second graft was rotated 180 degrees and implanted heterotopically in the right upper quadrant of the recipient. Technical modification was required for implantation of the second graft, in which biliary reconstruction was performed prior to anastomoses of the portal vein and hepatic artery. This dual graft technique carried unwelcome ethical issues concerning two major operations in two healthy donors, with the associated potential morbidities and mortalities for one recipient. Again, this variant liver graft is not widely performed around the world, but it could be used in a situation when both potential donors have fatty liver.

Donor safety

Donor safety is crucial in the application and expansion of LDLT. Never in the history of surgery does a healthy person undergo a major operation like hepatectomy. The balance between recipient success and donor risk should always be considered when LDLT comes into clinical practice. In one survey of 1508 living liver donors receiving hepatectomy in five Asian transplantation centers from 1990 to 2001, the overall donor complication rate was 15.8%, and 1.1% of donors required re-operation.[38] The complication rate of right liver donors was higher than that of left liver donors (28 vs 7.5%). In particular, right liver donors had experienced more serious complications, such as cholestasis, bile leakage, biliary stricture, portal vein thrombosis, intra-abdominal bleeding, and pulmonary embolism. There was no hospital mortality but one late donor death was reported 3 years after operation. The cause of that donor death was unknown. The authors' center has reported another late donor death, which occurred 10 weeks after surgery as a result of duodenocaval fistula formation from a chronic duodenal ulcer. The overall donor mortality rate was 0.5%.[17]

In Japan, the first donor death occurred in a hypertensive woman who died from liver failure after right liver donation with a residual left liver of 28% of the total liver volume.[39] With more than 12 000 living donor operations performed worldwide, the mortality rates for right liver donors and left liver donors approached 0.5 and 0.1%, respectively.[40] There are two recent large Asian series reporting the living donor outcomes. Umeshita et al.[41] have evaluated 1853 donors in 46 liver transplant centers in Japan.

Postoperative complications occurred in 12% of donors and the complication rate was significantly higher in right liver donors than left liver donors. In another study of 1162 living donors by Hwang et al.[42] from Korea, there was no donor mortality and only 3.2% of donors experienced major complications. The donor complication rate could be reduced to 1.3% when the donor liver remnant exceeded 35%, especially for young donors with no hepatic steatosis. Hence, careful donor selection and meticulous donor operation by experienced transplant surgeons should be vigilantly adhered to in order to maintain or decrease donor mortality and morbidity.

Ethical issues

The number of LDLTs performed has grown exponentially out of that of deceased-donor liver transplantation (DDLT) in Asia, because of the scarce supply of liver grafts in the deceased-donor pool. From an international survey on liver transplantation in Asia conducted in 2006, the number of DDLTs in Asia has remained static (80–140 cases per year) over the past decade. Meanwhile, there was a resurgence in the number of LDLTs performed since the 1990s, when LDLT using the right liver was introduced. The annual number has increased from <50 cases in 1999 to 1387 cases in 2005. The proportion of patients receiving LDLT exceeded 90% among patients undergoing liver transplantation in the year 2005.

With such a high proportion of LDLTs performed in Asian transplant centers, ethical justification for using living-donor liver grafts for transplantation should be clearly established. The risk–benefit ratio for both the donor and recipient should be well balanced, and not underestimated. Patient selection in terms of recipient and donor selection plays a crucial role in the ethical justification of LDLT. The expected recipient benefits, potential donor risks (see earlier) and recipient risks ought to be assessed in great detail on both medical and psychological grounds. In general, living organ donation must be absolutely voluntary, with consent given on the basis of unbiased information and chosen only when the option for DDLT is practically nil. Only if the donor operation can be performed with minimal risk by experienced surgeons, the indications are clear, and the living donor gives voluntarily informed consent, is LDLT justified.

LDLT for HCC

LDLT can theoretically provide an unlimited source of liver grafts for HCC patients whose tumor status is within the selection criteria. The uncertainty of prolonged waiting time on the list and the risk of drop-out can virtually be eliminated by LDLT. There were two decision analyses that support the application of LDLT for HCC. These hypothetical studies concluded that LDLT is superior to DDLT for patients with HCC within the Milan criteria when the waiting time for a deceased liver graft exceeds 6 months.[43,44] The unaffected donor pool of organs for patients with nonmalignant liver disease is another crucial advantage of LDLT because the living-donor graft is a dedicated gift directed exclusively to the recipient. The role of LDLT and its intention-to-treat survival benefit over DDLT in patients with early HCC has been demonstrated by the current authors' center. Lo et al.[45] found that patients who opted for LDLT had significantly better survival outcomes compared with those who waited for DDLT.

Caution should be taken when assuming the superiority of LDLT over DDLT in some aspects. Firstly, donor voluntarism and donor selection criteria form the main frame determining the availability of living-donor liver grafts. The current authors' center[45] has reported that >50% of patients with transplantable HCC might not have suitable voluntary donors. Secondly, there is a tendency toward a higher rate of tumor recurrence following LDLT when compared with DDLT for HCC. A multicenter LDLT cohort study (A2ALL) from the West[46] has reported a significantly higher 3-year tumor recurrence rate after LDLT (29%) compared with that after DDLT (0%). Similar results were obtained from the current authors' center.[47] Some of the possible contributing factors for the high tumor recurrence after LDLT are selection bias for patients with aggressive tumor behaviors, elimination of natural selection during the waiting period, and enhancement of tumor growth and invasiveness by small-for-size graft injury and regeneration.

Extending the tumor selection criteria to include patients with more advanced HCC to receive LDLT is an attractive option, because a living-donor graft is not subject to the system of equitable allocation. The Kyoto group[48] has adopted the extended criteria that included any size or numbers of tumors provided that there was no gross vascular involvement or distant metastasis. They reported a 4-year overall patient survival rate of 64% in all HCC patients and 59% in patients whose tumors were beyond the Milan criteria. In another study from 49 transplant centers in Japan on 316 HCC patients receiving LDLT, the Milan criteria was adopted in one-third of the transplantation programs. The overall survival and recurrence-free survival rates at 3 years were significantly worse when the Milan criteria were not met (60.4 vs 78.7 and 52.6 vs 79.1%). The preoperative alphafetoprotein level, tumor size, vascular invasion, and bilobar distribution were identified as independent risk factors for recurrence after LDLT.[49] Similar results were also reported by Hwang et al.[50] based on four transplantation programs in Korea. Hence, the policy of extended criteria of liver transplantation for HCC is yet to be further validated by large-scale studies.

Conclusion

LDLT has been widely practiced in Asia to counteract the problem of organ shortage. Balancing the recipient benefits and donor risks should be vigilantly considered in LDLT. Issues of minimal graft weight, side of liver to donate and inclusion of the MHV with graft or donor are still debatable and associated technical innovations and refinements are ongoing. Vascular complications in the recipient have been reduced but not the biliary complications, which sometimes require retransplantation. Owing to the high incidence of viral hepatitis, HCC is a growing indication for liver transplantation in Asia. LDLT would act as the dominant strategy in this respect. For HCC patients with preserved liver function, primary hepatectomy and salvage transplantation for recurrence is an attractive approach. Whether to extend the selection criteria based on the autonomy of the decision of donor and recipient in LDLT is still poorly defined.

References

1. Roberts MS, Angus DC, Bryce CL, Valenta Z, Weissfeld L. Survival after liver transplantation in the United States: a disease-specific analysis of the UNOS database. Liver Transpl 2004;10:886–97.
2. Lo CM, Fan ST, Liu CL, et al. Extending the limit on the size of adult recipient in living donor liver transplantation using extended right lobe graft. Transplantation 1997;63:1524–8.
3. Koffron AJ, Kung R, Baker T, Fryer J, Clark L, Abecassis M. Laparoscopic-assisted right lobe donor hepatectomy. Am J Transplant 2006;6:2522–5.
4. Shirakata Y, Terajima H, Mashima S, et al. The minimum graft size for successful orthotopic partial liver transplantation in the canine model. Transplant Proc 1995;27:545–6.
5. Kiuchi T, Kasahara M, Uryuhara K, et al. Impact of graft size mismatching on graft prognosis in liver transplantation from living donors. Transplantation 1999;67:321–7.
6. Urata K, Kawasaki S, Matsunami H, et al. Calculation of child and adult standard liver volume for liver transplantation. Hepatology 1995;21:1317–21.
7. Lo CM, Fan ST, Liu CL, et al. Minimum graft size for successful living donor liver transplantation. Transplantation 1999;68:1112–16.
8. Oda H, Miyake H, Iwata T, Kusumoto K, Rokutan K, Tashiro S. Geranylgeranylacetone suppresses inflammatory responses and improves survival after massive hepatectomy in rats. J Gastrointest Surg 2002;6:464–72.
9. Man K, Fan ST, Lo CM, et al. Graft injury in relation to graft size in right lobe live donor liver transplantation: a study of hepatic sinusoidal injury in correlation with portal hemodynamics and intragraft gene expression. Ann Surg 2003;237:256–64.
10. Lee SG, Park KM, Hwang S, et al. Adult-to-adult living donor liver transplantation at the Asan Medical Center, Korea. Asian J Surg 2002;25:277–84.
11. Sugawara Y, Makuuchi M, Sano K, et al. Vein reconstruction in modified right liver graft for living donor liver transplantation. Ann Surg 2003;237:180–5.
12. Tanaka K, Yamada T. Living donor liver transplantation in Japan and Kyoto University: what can we learn? J Hepatol 2005;42:25–8.
13. de Villa VH, Chen CL, Chen YS, et al. Right lobe living donor liver transplantation-addressing the middle hepatic vein controversy. Ann Surg 2003;238:275–82.
14. Liu CL, Fan ST, Lo CM, et al. Live-donor liver transplantation for acute-on-chronic hepatitis B liver failure. Transplantation 2003;76:1174–9.
15. Liu CL, Zhao Y, Lo CM, Fan ST. Hepatic venoplasty in right lobe live donor liver transplantation. Liver Transpl 2003;9:1265–72.
16. Chan SC, Lo CM, Liu CL, Wong Y, Fan ST, Wong J. Tailoring donor hepatectomy per segment 4 venous drainage in right lobe live donor liver transplantation. Liver Transpl 2004;10:755–62.

17. Chan SC, Fan ST, Lo CM, Liu CL, Wong J. Toward current standards of donor right hepatectomy for adult-to-adult live donor liver transplantation through the experience of 200 cases. Ann Surg 2007;245:110–17.
18. Ishiko T, Egawa H, Kasahara M, et al. Duct-to-duct biliary reconstruction in living donor liver transplantation utilizing right lobe graft. Ann Surg 2002;236: 235–40.
19. Liu CL, Lo CM, Chan SC, Fan ST. Safety of duct-to-duct biliary reconstruction in right-lobe live-donor liver transplantation without biliary drainage. Transplantation 2004;77:726–32.
20. Fan ST. Living donor liver transplantation. Shenzhen: Takungpao Publishing; 2007.
21. Lo CM, Fan ST, Liu CL, et al. Adult-to-adult living donor liver transplantation using extended right lobe grafts. Ann Surg 1997;226:261–9.
22. Kokudo N, Sugawara Y, Imamura H, Sano K, Makuuchi M. Tailoring the type of donor hepatectomy for adult living donor liver transplantation. Am J Transplant 2005;5:1694–1703.
23. Couinaud C. Liver anatomy: portal (and suprahepatic) or biliary segmentation. Dig Surg 1999;16:459–67.
24. Imamura H, Kokudo N, Sugawara Y, et al. Pringle's maneuver and selective inflow occlusion in living donor liver hepatectomy. Liver Transpl 2004;10:771–8.
25. Man K, Lo CM, Ng IO, et al. Liver transplantation in rats using small-for-size grafts: a study of hemodynamic and morphological changes. Arch Surg 2001;136: 280–5.
26. Cattral MS, Greig PD, Muradali D, Grant D. Reconstruction of middle hepatic vein of a living-donor right lobe liver graft with recipient left portal vein. Transplantation 2001;71:1864–6.
27. Kornberg A, Heyne J, Schotte U, Hommann M, Scheele J. Hepatic venous outflow reconstruction in right lobe living-donor liver graft using recipient's superficial femoral vein. Am J Transplant 2003;3:1444–7.
28. Ogata S, Kianmanesh R, Belghiti J. Doppler assessment after right hepatectomy confirms the need to fix the remnant left liver in the anatomical position. Br J Surg 2005;92:592–5.
29. Liu CL, Fan ST, Lo CM, Chan SC, Yong BH, Wong J. Safety of donor right hepatectomy without abdominal drainage: a prospective evaluation in 100 consecutive liver donors. Liver Transpl 2005;11:314–19.
30. Tanaka K, Uemoto S, Tokunaga Y, et al. Surgical techniques and innovations in living related liver transplantation. Ann Surg 1993;217:82–91.
31. Marcos A, Ham JM, Fisher RA, Olzinski AT, Posner MP. Surgical management of anatomical variations of the right lobe in living donor liver transplantation. Ann Surg 2000;231:824–31.
32. Fan ST, Yong BH, Lo CM, Liu CL, Wong J. Right lobe living donor liver transplantation with or without venovenous bypass. Br J Surg 2003;90:48–56.
33. Lo CM, Liu CL, Fan ST. Correction of left hepatic vein redundancy in paediatric liver transplantation. Asian J Surg 2005;28:55–7.
34. Fan ST, Lo CM, Liu CL, Yong BH, Chan JK, Ng IO. Safety of donors in live donor liver transplantation using right lobe grafts. Arch Surg 2000;135:336–40.
35. Sugawara Y, Makuuchi M, Takayama T, et al. Liver transplantation using a right lateral sector graft from a living donor to her granddaughter. Hepatogastroenterology 2001;48:261–3.
36. Sugawara Y, Makuuchi M, Takayama T, Imamura H, Kaneko J. Right lateral sector graft in adult living-related liver transplantation. Transplantation 2002;73:111–14.
37. Lee S, Hwang S, Park K, et al. An adult-to-adult living donor liver transplant using dual left lobe grafts. Surgery 2001;129:647–50.
38. Lo CM. Complications and long-term outcome of living liver donors: a survey of 1,508 cases in five Asian centers. Transplantation 2003;75:S12–15.
39. Akabayashi A, Slingsby BT, Fujita M. The first donor death after living-related liver transplantation in Japan. Transplantation 2004;77:634.
40. Barr ML, Belghiti J, Villamil FG, et al. A report of the Vancouver Forum on the care of the live organ donor: lung, liver, pancreas, and intestine data and medical guidelines. Transplantation 2006;81:1373–85.
41. Umeshita K, Fujiwara K, Kiyosawa K, et al. Operative morbidity of living liver donors in Japan. Lancet 2003;362:687–90.
42. Hwang S, Lee SG, Lee YJ, et al. Lessons learned from 1,000 living donor liver transplantations in a single center: how to make living donations safe. Liver Transpl 2006;12:920–7.
43. Cheng SJ, Pratt DS, Freeman RB Jr, Kaplan MM, Wong JB. Living-donor versus cadaveric liver transplantation for non-resectable small hepatocellular carcinoma and compensated cirrhosis: a decision analysis. Transplantation 2001;72:861–8.
44. Sarasin FP, Majno PE, Llovet JM, Bruix J, Mentha G, Hadengue A. Living donor liver transplantation for early hepatocellular carcinoma: A life-expectancy and cost-effectiveness perspective. Hepatology 2001;33: 1073–9.
45. Lo CM, Fan ST, Liu CL, Chan SC, Wong J. The role and limitation of living donor liver transplantation for hepatocellular carcinoma. Liver Transpl 2004;10: 440–7.
46. Fisher RA, Kulik LM, Freise CE, et al. Hepatocellular carcinoma recurrence and death following living and

deceased donor liver transplantation. Am J Transplant 2007;7:1601–8.
47. Lo CM, Fan ST, Liu CL, Chan SC, Ng IO, Wong J. Living donor versus deceased donor liver transplantation for early irresectable hepatocellular carcinoma. Br J Surg 2007;94:78–86.
48. Kaihara S, Kiuchi T, Ueda M, et al. Living-donor liver transplantation for hepatocellular carcinoma. Transplantation 2003;75:S37–40.
49. Hirohashi K, Yamamoto T, Shuto T, et al. Multifocal hepatocellular carcinoma in patients undergoing living-related liver transplantation. Hepatogastroenterology 2003;50:1617–20.
50. Hwang S, Lee SG, Joh JW, Suh KS, Kim DG. Liver transplantation for adult patients with hepatocellular carcinoma in Korea: comparison between cadaveric donor and living donor liver transplantations. Liver Transpl 2005;11:1265–72.

24 Anesthesia

Beatrice Beck-Schimmer
Swiss HPB and Transplantation Centers, Institute of Anesthesiology, University Hospital Zürich, Zürich, Switzerland

Key learning points

- The reader should know the anesthesia-relevant disturbances induced by hepatic failure, which can include the following pathologies: hyperdynamic circulation, portopulmonary hypertension, hepatopulmonary syndrome, hepatorenal syndrome, encephalopathy, coagulation disorders, and electrolyte imbalance. Patients might also suffer from coronary heart disease, which has an extremely negative impact on postoperative outcome, and therefore has to be carefully evaluated and if possible treated in the preoperative phase.
- Expanded monitoring of anesthesia is recommended for liver transplantation, including invasive measurement of arterial and central venous pressure. Volume management and evaluation of cardiac function can be performed using a pulmonary artery catheter or transesophageal echocardiography.
- The intraoperative phases of the pre-anhepatic (phase 1), anhepatic (phase 2), and neo-hepatic (phase 3) period are crucial with regard to hemodynamic changes. Phase 1 can be associated with hypovolemia due to drainage of ascites and/or bleeding after mobilization of the liver. Phase 2 is determined by a decrease of the cardiac output up to 50%, initiated by clamping of the hepatic vessels and the inferior vena cava. At the beginning of phase 3, reperfusion syndrome can be observed with prolonged arterial hypotension.
- Intraoperative volume management should follow a rather restrictive strategy to avoid further portal hyperemia as well as hemodilution-induced aggravation of an existing coagulopathy.

Introduction

In the last decade patients present with more advanced disease for liver transplantation. This is due to a nearly stagnant supply of organs in many countries that cannot accommodate an increasing number of transplant candidates, as well as to the implementation of the Model for End-stage Liver Disease (MELD) score as indication for transplantation.[1] This implies that not only surgery but also anesthesia for liver transplantation becomes more and more challenging. A profound understanding of the pathophysiology and pharmacology is thereby crucial to provide distinct knowledge and skill requirements for organ transplantation in severely compromised patients. Another important factor is the interdisciplinary work: the anesthesiologist has to be part of a team of surgeons and intensivists, and also has to collaborate with partner specialties including hepatology, cardiology, pneumology, nephrology, infectious disease, and psychiatry.[2]

Preoperative evaluation

Deterioration of liver function has an impact on virtually all other organ systems. All these organs need to be evaluated before surgery and have to be protected during liver transplantation.

Patient history

The cause of impaired liver function is important for several reasons. Liver cirrhosis due to former excessive alcohol abuse might be accompanied

Medical Care of the Liver Transplant Patient, Fourth Edition. Edited by Pierre-Alain Clavien, James F. Trotter.

by deficiency of vitamin B12 with compromised neurologic peripheral and autonomous function, the latter leading to gastropathy with increased risk of reflux during induction of anesthesia. Patients with viral infections as an underlying disease for liver dysfunction are potentially contagious. Optimal protection of the transplant team members requires particular attention to prevent injuries during invasive procedures.

Hepatic dysfunction

In patients with hepatic dysfunction pharmacokinetics and pharmacodynamics can differ from healthy patients for several reasons:

1. With impaired hepatic production of proteins, serum albumin concentration is diminished. Upon administration of a drug, the active unbound fraction is increased with potentially aggravated effects of these compounds.
2. As the volume of distribution is increased in end-stage liver disease, elimination of certain drugs is prolonged. Owing to the larger volume of distribution the initial dose of a compound might have to be increased.
3. Dysfunction of the hepatic detoxication system with impaired metabolism leads to limited systemic clearance. All these deteriorations are responsible for an accentuated duration of action and an accumulation of certain drugs. This implies that the use and dosage of these drugs have to be considered accordingly.

Cardiovascular system

Elevated cardiac output and arteriolar vasodilatation due to a hyperdynamic state occurs in 70% of patients with end-stage liver disease. A study performed in cirrhotic animals showed that vasoactive substances such as endocannabinoids are involved in cardiovascular changes.[3] Another reason for the hemodynamic alterations is the release of nitric oxide from necrotic liver tissue, increasing activity of guanosine 3′-5′-cyclic monophosphate (cGMP), which contributes to the decrease of vascular tone.[4] With a cirrhotic cardiomyopathy the hemodynamic situation is less stable due to various factors: 1) cardiac output is increased but systolic contractile response to stress is blunted, 2) diastolic function is impaired, 3) electrophysiologic abnormalities might be present such as prolonged QT interval. The hemodynamic situation may improve after transplantation, but persistence has also been observed for several years.

Many patients on the transplantation list suffer from non-ischemic cardiomyopathy, which has been associated with alcoholic liver disease, hemochromatosis, and Wilson's disease. A preoperative assessment of the ejection fraction by echocardiography is mandatory, and improvement through appropriate pharmacologic treatment should be established. The presence of valvular cardiomyopathy with preserved left ventricular function is not a contraindication for liver transplantation. Successful transplantations have also been reported in recipients with hypertrophic cardiomyopathy with left ventricular outflow obstruction.[5]

Owing to a more liberal indication for liver transplantations in older recipients, ischemic cardiomyopathy with coronary heart disease needs to be considered as an important possible pre-existing factor that determines adverse outcome.[6,7] In the presence of coronary heart disease, perioperative morbidity and mortality rates increase up to 81 and 50%, respectively, and the 3-year mortality rate is as high as 45%.[8] Negative diagnosis for coronary heart disease, however, correlates with a good perioperative prognosis regarding cardiac events,[9] therefore routine screening with stress echocardiography, stress thallium nuclear imaging or stress single-photon emission computed tomographic (SPECT) imaging is essential for patients undergoing liver transplantation. If inconclusive, a coronary arteriography will be necessary. Alternatively, coronary computer tomography angiography might be an elegant alternative in the future.[10]

Another important evaluation is the right ventricular function of patients on the waiting list, as patients with terminal liver failure often suffer from portopulmonary hypertension (PPH) (see Chapter 5). The diagnostic criteria for PPH include portal hypertension, mean pulmonary artery pressure (PAP) >25 mmHg, and pulmonary vascular resistance >240 dyn × s × cm^{-5} in the presence of normal pulmonary capillary wedge pressure (<15 mmHg). PPH is found in 1% of patients with portal hypertension. The screening test is estimation of right ventricular systolic pressure determined by Doppler echocardiography. If it reaches cut-off values of 35–50 mmHg, right heart catheterization is recommended for confirmation, as the systolic right ventricular pressure might not only be increased in PPH but also in situations of high flow.[11] While mean PAP values of 25–35 mmHg do not raise concerns for liver transplantation, mean PAP values higher than 35 mmHg have been shown to be correlated with an increased mortality rate, mostly due to right ventricular failure during surgery.[12] Mortality in these patients is as high as 30–50%.[12,13] Patients with a mean PAP >50 mmHg with right ventricular dysfunction carry a mortality risk higher than 50%, so that liver transplantation may become contraindicated.[12] Treatment with epoprostenol might improve the pulmonary hemodynamic situation, but data demonstrating an improvement of prognosis are missing.[14] Echocardiography should be repeated every 6 months as PPH may also appear after listing a patient, or mild PPH rapidly progresses to severe levels.

Another pulmonary complication is hepatopulmonary syndrome (HPS), defined as a triad of liver disease, arterial deoxygenation, and pulmonary vascular dilatation with anatomical shunt due to ventilation-perfusion abnormalities, leading to refractory hypoxemia.[15] A real treatment is not available apart from symptomatic therapy with permanent application of oxygen. Other causes leading to ventilation–perfusion mismatch should be eliminated. HPS disappears after successful transplantation, but is correlated with increased mortality rate.[13,16] Hypoxemia associated with HPS should be evaluated by complete pulmonary function testing, high-resolution chest computed tomographic scanning, radionuclide lung scanning contrast (technetium-99m-labelled, 99mTc; macroaggregated albumin perfusion scanning) and pulmonary angiography in patients without response to 100% inspired oxygen.[17]

In conclusion, cardiac and pulmonary vascular evaluation is performed with the help of echocardiography to determine myocardial contractility and function of the valves, to diagnose coronary heart disease (stress echocardiography), and to detect pulmonary hypertension (Doppler echocardiography).

Pulmonary system

Beside PPH and HPS affecting primarily the vascular compartment, several other pulmonary complications can be found in patients with terminal liver failure, leading to ventilation–perfusion mismatch. A common condition is restrictive lung disease as a result of pleural effusion and ascites leading to the formation of atelectasis. Fluid removal might be a successful treatment in such situations. Pulmonary restriction is also observed in patients with primary biliary cirrhosis with interstitial lung disease. Patients with cystic fibrosis often suffer from bronchial obstruction. All these pulmonary problems result in ventilation–perfusion mismatch, leading to various degrees of hypoxemia.

Preoperative evaluation with assessment of lung function and eventually by echocardiography is mandatory to determine the risk related to the pulmonary situation and to define a preoperative therapeutic strategy such as inhaled corticosteroids and bronchodilatators for obstruction.

Renal status

Patients with end-stage liver disease frequently have concomitant renal dysfunction. Acid–base disturbance as well as pre-renal hypovolemia, induced by long-term use of diuretics, are common causes for compromised renal function. Hypovolemia can be corrected preoperatively. Whether natural or artificial colloids are superior to crystalloids is not clear. Another cause for renal failure is hepatorenal syndrome, which is the consequence of chronic hypoperfusion of the kidneys due to splanchnic vasodilatation. Preoperative treatment consists of vasoconstrictors such as terlipressin, inducing splanchnic vasoconstriction and increasing systemic blood pressure, thereby improving renal blood flow, in combination with intravenous administration of albumin.[18]

Gastrointestinal tract

Patients with terminal liver failure most often suffer from esophageal varices, as a consequence of portal hypertension. Repetitive bleeding is frequently observed, leading to potentially severe anemia. In such cases intraoperative transesophageal echocardiography is a relative contraindication. The presence of extensive ascites inducing delayed gastric emptying has to be considered as an aspiration risk, which leads to important precautions regarding the management of induction of anesthesia.

Cerebral status

End-stage liver disease can lead to encephalopathy of varying degrees. The majority of patients undergoing liver transplantation have a subclinical encephalopathy, however patients with fulminant liver failure may present with acute cerebral edema, increased intracranial pressure (ICP) and subsequent brain herniation. Owing to compromised hepatic clearance of toxins, accumulation of ammonium and manganese leads to impaired function of cerebral transmitters such as gamma-aminobutyric acid (GABA), glutamate, and nitric oxide. A recent guideline of the US Acute Liver Failure Study Group recommends ICP monitoring in patients with grade III–IV encephalopathy (somnolence or coma),[19] although a retrospective analysis was unable to show improved outcome in the presence of invasive monitoring of ICP.[20] Notably, 10% of these patients developed intracranial hemorrhage. Placement of an ICP probe therefore requires aggressive correction of coagulopathy as well as initiation of antibiotic therapy. Monitoring with non-invasive methods such as transcranical Doppler ultrasonography and jugular venous oximetry is still under evaluation.

Coagulation

Another unbalanced system in liver failure is the coagulation system – not only the number and function of platelets, but also the coagulation factors are quantitatively compromised. Sequestered platelets in the spleen result in thrombocytopenia, which can further be accentuated by a decreased production of blood cells in the bone marrow. Impaired function of platelets is possible, although the detailed mechanism leading to this dysfunction is not known. Synthesis of vitamin K-dependent clotting factors is reduced, and therefore the level of vitamin K-dependent clotting factors is diminished (factors II, VII, IX, and X), which can be assessed by determination of prothrombin time (PT). Decreased levels of fibrinogen and factor VIII indicate the presence of fibrinolysis or disseminated intravascular coagulation (DIC). Another cause of fibrinolysis may be inadequate clearance of tissue plasminogen activator and low levels of antiplasmin. Summarized, the balance between pro- and anti-coagulatory systems is severely impaired. Preoperative corrections with blood products have to be considered carefully and are discussed in Chapter 25.

Electrolytes

Patients with liver cirrhosis often present with electrolyte abnormalities due to the preoperative use of diuretics and the secondary hyperaldosteronism, resulting in a low potassium level. If potassium is increased up to values >5.5 mmol/L due to concomitant renal insufficiency, preoperative hemofiltration should be considered. Sodium is often reduced due to retention of excess water, loss of sodium with a thiazide therapy, or a mixture of water excess and solute deficit.[21] Partial correction of existing hyponatremia might be achieved by fluid restriction and discontinuation of all diuretics. Rapid correction of hyponatremia has been reported to be associated with central pontine myelinolysis/extrapontine myelinolysis (CPM/EPM).[22] Clinical manifestations of CPM/EPM are postoperative delirium, pseudobulbar palsy, and spastic quadriplegia. While previous studies have mainly focused on preoperative serum sodium values, further data reveal that other factors such as pretransplant hepatic encephalopathy, severe preoperative liver dysfunction, and intraoperative electrolyte imbalances may trigger CPM/EPM as well.[23] Preoperative values <126 mmol/L have been described as a strong independent predictor of increased mortality.[24]

Potential disorders of different organ systems in patients with end-stage liver disease are summarized in Box 24.1, based on work from Ozier et Klinck[25] and Steadman et al.[26,27]

Intraoperative considerations

Monitoring

In addition to basic monitoring such as with ECG and pulse oximetry, invasive hemodynamic monitoring for continuous blood pressure measurements requires an **arterial line**, which is preferentially placed in the radial or femoral artery. At the same time, an arterial line allows easy access for blood gas analysis. In severe hypotension, radial arterial pressure measurement might provide less accurate blood pressure values, usually underestimating aortic arterial pressure. The difference between the radial and femoral values becomes even more pronounced with the use of vasoconstrictors. In such conditions,

Box 24.1 Possible disturbances in homeostasis in various organ systems in patients with end-stage liver disease

Cardiovascular: systemic

Hyperdynamic circulation (increased cardiac output)

Cirrhotic cardiomyopathy (increased cardiac output with suboptimal stress response)

Coronary heart disease

Cardiomyopathy (alcohol, amyloid, Wilson's disease, hemochromatosis)

Cardiovascular: pulmonary

Portopulmonary hypertension

Hepatopulmonary syndrome (HPS)

Lungs

Restrictive lung disease (ascites, pleural effusion, intrapulmonary shunting flow – related or due to HPS, interstitial lung disease such as primary biliary cirrhosis)

Obstructive lung disease (cystic fibrosis, asthma)

Kidneys

Hepatorenal syndrome

Renal tubular acidosis

Prerenal insufficiency (ascites, diuretics)

Acute tubular necrosis

Tacrolimus/cyclosporin-induced renal impairment

Central and peripheral nervous system

Encephalopathy

Cerebral edema

Autonomic neuropathy

Hematology/coagulation

Anemia

Thrombocytopenia, platelet dysfunction

Reduced vitamin K-dependent factors

Hyperfibrinolysis

Electrolytes

Hyponatremia

Hyperkalemia

Hypomagnesemia

measurements based on radial pressure values have to be interpreted with particular caution. Patients undergoing liver transplantation need a **central venous line** for central venous pressure assessment, which is most often combined with the insertion of a **pulmonary artery catheter** (PAC), which is used for advanced hemodynamic assessment.

Central filling pressures, reflecting major fluid shifts during surgery as well as possible cardiac dysfunction upon reperfusion of the liver, are monitored, directly measuring right atrial and ventricular as well as pulmonary artery systolic and diastolic pressures, cardiac output, and mixed venous oxygen saturation. The use of ultrasound guidance during insertion of the central lines is recommended in patients with compromised coagulation to ensure avoidance of a carotid puncture. A special requirement for invasive monitoring is prevention of infections by taking sterile precautions with the placement and management of the lines. Patients with liver failure with portal hypertension and mesenteric congestion have a higher incidence of infections and systemic inflammatory response syndrome.[28]

Transesophageal echocardiography (TEE) is a suitable alternative to the pulmonary catheter to monitor fluid status as well as cardiac function. In many centers, TEE, a less invasive monitoring tool, has replaced the PAC as evidence of improved outcome in using a PAC is missing,[29] and PAC-induced ventricular (up to 30% of ventricular tachycardia) or atrial arrhythmias can pose significant risk to the already compromised patient. With the use of TEE, information about preload as well as contractility is continuously provided. In addition, embolization of peripheral thrombus material or air embolism can be detected immediately and treated accordingly.[30] TEE offers significant advantages, but it requires training and also experience in performing and correctly interpreting TEE.

Bispectral index (BIS) is a newer tool used to assess and monitor the depth of anesthesia. It allows the anesthesiologist to optimally adjust the amount of anesthetic agent to the needs of the patient, and at the same time might reduce the incidence of intraoperative awareness.

Hypothermia is another risk factor for the liver transplant patient and the control of body temperature and avoidance of this pathologic condition is essential.

Anesthetics

Premedication with a sedative such as midazolam should be avoided if the patients show signs of hepatic encephalopathy. Anesthesia is induced by an IV anesthetic such as propofol, thiopental or etomidate. In patients who are not fasted and/or carry other risk factors for aspiration such as ascites, active or recent gastrointestinal bleeding, known gastroesophageal reflux or hepatic encephalopathy, rapid sequence induction with administration of propofol or thiopental and succinylcholine is the appropriate procedure. In a situation of impaired hemodynamic status, the use of etomidate is recommended as anesthetic for induction. Patients with a contraindication for the use of succinylcholine such as high serum potassium levels and/or absolute immobility might benefit from the application of rocuronium as the application of this depolarizing neuromuscular blocker could further increase potassium levels. The effect of the various anesthetic techniques on the outcome of the patient is unknown. Most centers administer anesthesia with a volatile anesthetic and fentanyl. Historically, isoflurane has been the anesthetic of first choice.[31] Total IV anesthesia with propofol and fentanyl is possible as well. Dosage of propofol has to be monitored as blood levels are theoretically expected to increase during the anhepatic phase, concomitant with a fall in BIS. No studies exist so far demonstrating a better outcome with the use of volatile anesthetics compared to propofol. Volatile anesthetics applied in a pre- or postconditioning setup, however, might render the transplanted liver less vulnerable to ischemia–reperfusion injury as previously shown in situations of hepatic ischemia–reperfusion for liver resection.[32] Muscle relaxation with cisatracurium is advantageous for the anesthesia for liver transplantation as its elimination is independent of renal or hepatic function. In contrast, the duration of muscle relaxation might be affected by the impaired liver function when using rocuronium, which is eliminated by the liver and the kidneys. It should be monitored using a transcutaneous nerve stimulator, which allows titration of this muscle relaxant.

In view of its risks, it is not clear if a regional anesthesia is indicated. The benefit of a thoracic epidural anesthesia (TEA) in this type of surgery is to provide postoperative analgesia. Neuroaxial guidelines are therefore important to define contraindications, which are defined in the guidelines of the American Society of Regional Anesthesia and Pain Medicine (ASRA),[33] however, possible changes in the coagulation profile after liver transplantation are not considered in these guidelines. The presence of large venous collaterals can be associated with increased risk of vessel penetration and hematoma formation. Prior to the placement of an epidural catheter any neurologic deficit should be documented by a specialist. Administration of immunosuppressive drugs might result in an increased risk of local infections related to the placement of the catheter. Therefore, a decision to perform a TEA in liver transplantation surgery is an individual benefit–risk consideration for each recipient.

Operative procedure

Pre-anhepatic phase

This first phase of a liver transplantation starts with the surgical incision of the skin and ends with the clamping of the portal vein, inferior vena cava and hepatic artery. Signs of hypovolemia might occur after incision and drainage of the abdominal cavity, if the patient suffers from ascites. Mobilization and dissection of the liver can lead to significant blood loss and subsequent hypovolemia.

Anhepatic phase

After the occlusion of the vascular inflow of the liver, the anhepatic and ischemic phase begins. It ends with the reperfusion of the graft. Owing to the occlusion of the inferior vena cava and portal vein ("cross-clamping"), venous return is diminished, decreasing cardiac output by 40–50%. In this operative phase fibrinolysis might arise as a risk factor, because of the unopposed action of tissue plasminogen activator, which cannot be inhibited by hepatic counteraction by a plasminogen activator inhibitor.

Neo-hepatic phase

Reperfusion of the liver leads to an abrupt increase in preload and at the same time a decrease of systemic blood pressure. In extreme situations hypotension, bradycardia, supraventricular and ventricular arrhythmias, and variable cardiac output, eventually with cardiac arrest, are observed.

Hemodynamic changes and management

As outlined earlier, rapid hemodynamic changes are observed upon cava clamping, hepatic reperfusion, and sudden blood loss. The fall of cardiac output due to clamping of the inferior vena cava and the portal vein can be controlled by using a veno-venous bypass, which limits the decline in cardiac output to only 20–30%. This extracorporal circuit returns blood from the infrahepatic inferior vena cava and the splanchnic area to more centrally located veins, improves preload of the heart and renal perfusion, and decreases splanchnic congestion. Another elegant way to overcome a pronounced drop in cardiac output is the use of a piggyback technique: instead of complete clamping of the inferior vena cava the vessel is side-clamped, still allowing partial backflow to the heart. This may also be considered in patients with poor cardiac reserve.[34] While both approaches improve the hemodynamic situation they also carry risks. Implanting cannulae for establishment of the extracorporal circuit can be accompanied by potentially lethal complications such as air or thrombus embolism, or perforation of vessels. Evidence that the use of a veno-venous bypass and/or the piggyback technique result in an improved short- or long-term clinical outcome is still missing.

Hemodynamic instability due to reperfusion is a commonly observed phenomenon, called post-reperfusion syndrome. It is defined as a 30% decrease of mean systemic blood pressure for more than 1 min during the first 5 min following graft reperfusion. Desaturated blood, accumulated with high amounts of potassium, protons and metabolites as well as inflammatory mediators from the graft induces decreased peripheral vascular tone, reduced heart rate, and impaired myocardial contractility, leading to arterial hypotension. Pulmonary capillary wedge pressure, central venous pressure, and pulmonary artery pressure usually increase. Therapy with vasoactive substances might be necessary as well as procedures to decrease hyperkalemia such as application of calcium chloride or calcium gluconate, or sodium bicarbonate to avoid potassium-induced arrhythmia. Post-reperfusion syndrome is attenuated in the presence of the piggyback technique or by an initial arterial reperfusion of the graft with more gradual reperfusion.

A special concern during liver transplantation is the presence of cirrhotic cardiomyopathy. Owing to chronotropic incompetence, these patients are prone to acute heart failure with pulmonary edema upon the onset of physiologic stress. Careful hemodynamic monitoring is mandatory and fast volume shift should be avoided. No "gold standards" have been defined, however preload optimization as well as avoidance of cardiac volume overload are special cornerstones.

Volume management

Over the last decades, there has been a conventional approach to minimize preload changes in the intraoperative setting by generously loading the patient with fluids, mostly colloids. Several centers advocate more restrictive fluid therapy due to the following reasons.[35,36] Patients with portal hypertension have an altered blood and volume distribution with venous pooling in the splanchnic circulation. If these patients' blood volume is expanded rapidly by aggressive fluid administration, splanchnic congestion increases as well as portal hyperemia, which is correlated with an increased risk of blood loss. Another problem of aggressive volume therapy might be an aggravation of coagulopathy by hemodilution. These apparent benefits, however, need to be balanced with inherent risks of fluid restriction. There is also a marked risk of systemic and especially renal hypoperfusion if volume is administered restrictively and vasopressors are used liberally. A recent retrospective study showed renal failure to occur more often in patients after intraoperative restrictive volume management compared to a liberal fluid regimen.[37] The decision which regimen is favored needs to be taken according to the patients' need and specific condition. Regular urine output should be maintained.

Improvement of surgical and anesthesiologic management together with a refined understanding of the coagulation system, has decreased the use of blood products over the last years. Several factors might have contributed to this result:

1. Implementation of the piggyback technique and the use of a veno-venous bypass are important approaches to reduce application of blood
2. Increasing evidence that the number of applied blood products is associated with graft survival and clinical outcomes of the recipient[38,39]
3. Many centers modify their coagulation management by incorporating the administration of anti-fibrinolytics.

Renal function

Long-term hypotension can induce or aggravate renal dysfunction. Although administration of mannitol, furosemide and dopamine has been tested in operative settings, clear evidence for a measurable benefit in preventing postoperative acute renal failure is missing.[40,41] A balanced approach with appropriate control of blood pressure and volume management as outlined earlier is recommended.

Intracranial pressure management

During liver transplantation in patients with acute liver failure, the anhepatic period is the most critical phase for a potential increase in ICP. A head-up position of 30 degrees as well as hyperventilation to a low normal $PaCO_2$ value (4–4.5 kPa) are common non-invasive strategies to lower ICP. According to the US Acute Liver Failure Study Group, ICP of higher than 25 mmHg should be treated in a more aggressive way:[19] osmotic therapy with mannitol is recommended. An equivalent alternative is the application of hyertonic saline (30%).[42,43] In the presence of renal failure, the use of osmotic agents is very limited. In patients with hypotension, hypovolemia needs to be corrected prior to the administration of vasopressors.[19]

Electrolytes

Potassium and sodium are the most important electrolytes, which should be carefully monitored during surgery. Hyperkalemia most often is observed during reperfusion, but may also result from red blood cell transfusion.[44] In a retrospective analysis, further predictors for hyperkalemia were high baseline potassium, organ donation after cardiac death, long warm ischemia time, long donor hospital stay, low intraoperative urine output as well as the use of a veno-venous bypass.[45] High potassium levels should be treated aggressively before reperfusion. For this immediate treatment, administration of insulin-glucose, salbutamol (endotracheally and/or intravenously applied) or furosemide should be considered. Patients might undergo liver transplantation with hypokalemia in the prehepatic phase of transplantation, in combination with metabolic alkalosis, however, in contrast to the more aggressive treatment of relevant hyperkalemia, potassium supplementation in hypokalemia should always be performed deliberately. Hypokalemia observed in the late neohepatic phase is induced by aggressive uptake of potassium by the grafted liver, even more accentuated in pediatric patients.[46]

Hyponatremia should not be corrected too fast due to the risk of CPM/EPM.[42] Calcium chloride must be administered in the absence of a functioning liver to avoid citrate intoxication with ionized hypocalcemia, resulting from application of citrate-rich blood products. Hypomagnesemia should be included in the differential diagnosis in case of arrhythmias during transplantation with or without massive transfusion, which could also be induced by citrate-rich infusions.

Living related transplantations: anesthesia for donor

The anesthetic management for a living related transplantation is challenging as well, even though the patient is not compromised in state of health. Owing to that fact that this is a major invasive medical procedure, rules rather than exceptions have to be implemented in this field. It is essential to choose an organ-protective anesthesia regimen with a stable hemodynamic situation throughout the entire surgical procedure, which allows optimal liver perfusion. Reasonably low central venous pressure (CVP) during parenchymal transection is desirable, which might reduce bleeding. Intraoperative cell salvage, preoperative autologous blood donation, and intraoperative hemodilution are proposed procedures to reduce transfusion of red blood cells.[47] Postoperative pain can be controlled by local anesthetics, applied through an epidural catheter.

References

1. Trotter JF. Impact of the Model for Endstage Liver Disease score on liver transplantation. Curr Opin Organ Tranplant 2007;12:294–7.
2. Walia A, Schumann R. The evolution of liver transplantation practices. Curr Opin Organ Transplant 2008;13: 275–9.
3. Batkai S, Jarai Z, Wagner JA, et al. Endocannabinoids acting at vascular CB1 receptors mediate the vasodilated state in advanced liver cirrhosis. Nat Med 2001;7:827–32.
4. Schneider F, Lutun P, Boudjema K, Wolf P, Tempe JD. In vivo evidence of enhanced guanylyl cyclase activation during the hyperdynamic circulation of acute liver failure. Hepatology 1994;19:38–44.

5. Aniskevich S, Shine TS, Feinglass NG, Stapelfeldt WH. Dynamic left ventricular outflow tract obstruction during liver transplantation: the role of transesophageal echocardiography. J Cardiothorac Vasc Anesth 2007;21: 577–80.
6. Carey WD, Dumot JA, Pimentel RR, et al. The prevalence of coronary artery disease in liver transplant candidates over age 50. Transplantation 1995;59: 859–64.
7. Tiukinhoy-Laing SD, Rossi JS, Bayram M, et al. Cardiac hemodynamic and coronary angiographic characteristics of patients being evaluated for liver transplantation. Am J Cardiol 2006;98:178–81.
8. Plotkin JS, Scott VL, Pinna A, Dobsch BP, De Wolf AM, Kang Y. Morbidity and mortality in patients with coronary artery disease undergoing orthotopic liver transplantation. Liver Transpl Surg 1996;2:426–30.
9. Donovan CL, Marcovitz PA, Punch JD, et al. Two-dimensional and dobutamine stress echocardiography in the preoperative assessment of patients with end-stage liver disease prior to orthotopic liver transplantation. Transplantation 1996;61:1180–8.
10. Schroeder S, Achenbach S, Bengel F, et al. Cardiac computed tomography: indications, applications, limitations, and training requirements: report of a Writing Group deployed by the Working Group Nuclear Cardiology and Cardiac CT of the European Society of Cardiology and the European Council of Nuclear Cardiology. Eur Heart J 2008;29:531–56.
11. Krowka MJ, Swanson KL, Frantz RP, McGoon MD, Wiesner RH. Portopulmonary hypertension: Results from a 10-year screening algorithm. Hepatology 2006;44:1502–10.
12. Ramsay MA. Perioperative mortality in patients with portopulmonary hypertension undergoing liver transplantation. Liver Transpl 2000;6:451–2.
13. Krowka MJ, Mandell MS, Ramsay MA, et al. Hepatopulmonary syndrome and portopulmonary hypertension: a report of the multicenter liver transplant database. Liver Transpl 2004;10:174–82.
14. Fix OK, Bass NM, De Marco T, Merriman RB. Long-term follow-up of portopulmonary hypertension: effect of treatment with epoprostenol. Liver Transpl 2007;13: 875–85.
15. Hoeper MM, Krowka MJ, Strassburg CP. Portopulmonary hypertension and hepatopulmonary syndrome. Lancet 2004;363:1461–8.
16. Arguedas MR, Abrams GA, Krowka MJ, Fallon MB. Prospective evaluation of outcomes and predictors of mortality in patients with hepatopulmonary syndrome undergoing liver transplantation. Hepatology 2003;37: 192–7.
17. Krowka M. Hepatopulmonary syndrome and liver transplantation. Liver Transpl 2000;6:113–5.
18. Gines P, Schrier RW. Renal failure in cirrhosis. N Engl J Med 2009;361:1279–90.
19. Stravitz RT, Kramer AH, Davern T, et al. Intensive care of patients with acute liver failure: recommendations of the US Acute Liver Failure Study Group. Crit Care Med 2007;35:2498–508.
20. Vaquero J, Fontana RJ, Larson AM, et al. Complications and use of intracranial pressure monitoring in patients with acute liver failure and severe encephalopathy. Liver Transpl 2005;11:1581–9.
21. Castello L, Pirisi M, Sainaghi PP, Bartoli E. Hyponatremia in liver cirrhosis: pathophysiological principles of management. Dig Liver Dis 2005;37:73–81.
22. Wszolek ZK, McComb RD, Pfeiffer RF, et al. Pontine and extrapontine meylinolysis flollowing liver transplantation. Relationship to serum sodium. Transplantation 1989;48:1066–12.
23. Lee EM, Kang JK, Yun SC, et al. Risk factors for central pontine and extrapoontine myelinolysis following orthotopic liver transplantation. Eur Neurol 2009;62: 362–8.
24. Biggins SW, Rodriquez HJ, Bacchetti P, Bass NM, Roberts JP, Terrault NA. Serum sodium predicts mortality in patients listed for liver transplantation. Hepatology 2005;41:32–9.
25. Ozier Y, Klinck JR. Anesthetic management of hepatic transplantation. Curr Opin Anaesthesiol 2008;21:391–400.
26. Steadman RH. Anesthesia for liver transplant surgery. Anesthesiology Clin N Am 2004;22:687–711.
27. Steadman RH, Van Rensburg A, Kramer DJ. Transplantation for acute liver failure: perioperative management. Curr Opin Organ Transplant 2010;15: 368–73.
28. Rolando N, Wade J, Davalos M, Wendon J, Philpott-Howard J, Williams R. The systemic inflammatory response syndrome in acute liver failure. Hepatology 2000;32:734–9.
29. Gwak MS, Kim JA, Kim GS, et al. Incidence of severe ventricular arrhythmias during pulmonary artery catheterization in liver allograft recipients. Liver Transpl 2007;13:1451–4.
30. Burtenshaw AJ, Isaac JL. The role of trans-oesophageal echocardiography for perioperative cardiovascular monitoring during orthotopic liver transplantation. Liver Transpl 2006;12:1577–83.
31. Carton EG, Plevak DJ, Kranner PW, Rettke SR, Geiger HJ, Coursin DB. Perioperative care of the liver transplant patient: Part 2. Anesth Analg 1994;78: 382–99.
32. Beck-Schimmer B, Breitenstein S, Urech S, et al. A randomized controlled trial on pharmacological preconditioning in liver surgery using a volatile anesthetic. Ann Surg 2008;248:909–18.

33. Horlocker TT, Wedel DJ, Benzon H, et al. Regional anesthesia in the anticoagulated patient: defining the risks (the second ASRA Consensus Conference on Neuraxial Anesthesia and Anticoagulation). Reg Anesth Pain Med 2003;28:172–97.
34. Moreno C, Sabate A, Figueras J, et al. Hemodynamic profile and tissular oxygenation in orthotopic liver transplantation: Influence of hepatic artery or portal vein revascularization of the graft. Liver Transpl 2006;12:1607–14.
35. Reyle-Hahn M, Rossaint R. Coagulation techniques are not important in directing blood product transfusion during liver transplantation. Liver Transpl Surg 1997;3:659–63; discussion 63–5.
36. Massicotte L, Lenis S, Thibeault L, Sassine MP, Seal RF, Roy A. Effect of low central venous pressure and phlebotomy on blood product transfusion requirements during liver transplantations. Liver Transpl 2006;12: 117–23.
37. Schroeder RA, Collins BH, Tuttle-Newhall E, et al. Intraoperative fluid management during orthotopic liver transplantation. J Cardiothorac Vasc Anesth 2004;18: 438–41.
38. Ramos E, Dalmau A, Sabate A, et al. Intraoperative red blood cell transfusion in liver transplantation: influence on patient outcome, prediction of requirements, and measures to reduce them. Liver Transpl 2003;9: 1320–7.
39. de Boer MT, Christensen MC, Asmussen M, et al. The impact of intraoperative transfusion of platelets and red blood cells on survival after liver transplantation. Anesth Analg 2008;106:32–44.
40. Swygert TH, Roberts LC, Valek TR, et al. Effect of intraoperative low-dose dopamine on renal function in liver transplant recipients. Anesthesiology 1991;75: 571–6.
41. Reddy VG. Prevention of postoperative acute renal failure. J Postgrad Med 2002;48:64–70.
42. Murphy N, Auzinger G, Bernel W, Wendon J. The effect of hypertonic sodium chloride on intracranial pressure in patients with acute liver failure. Hepatology 2004;39: 464–70.
43. Wendon J, Lee W. Encephalopathy and cerebral edema in the setting of acute liver failure: pathogenesis and management. Neurocrit Care 2008;9:97–102.
44. Nakasuji M, Bookallil MJ. Pathophysiological mechanisms of postrevascularization hyperkalemia in orthotopic liver transplantation. Anesth Analg 2000;91: 1351–5.
45. Xia VW, Ghobrial RM, Du B, et al. Predictors of hyperkalemia in the prereperfusion, early postreperfusion, and late postreperfusion periods during adult liver transplantation. Anesth Analg 2007;105:780–5.
46. Xia VW, Du B, Tran A, et al. Intraoperative hypokalemia in pediatric liver transplantation: incidence and risk factors. Anesth Analg 2006;103:587–93.
47. Lutz JT, Valentin-Gamazo C, Gorlinger K, Malago M, Peters J. Blood-transfusion requirements and blood salvage in donors undergoing right hepatectomy for living related liver transplantation. Anesth Analg 2003;96:351–5.

25 Coagulation and blood transfusion management

Herman G.D. Hendriks, Ton Lisman and Robert J. Porte
University Medical Center Groningen, University of Groningen, the Netherlands

Key learning points

- Abnormalities in routine hemostatic tests such as the prothrombin time (PT) or platelet count do not accurately reflect the hemostatic status in patients with liver disease.
- The hemostatic system in patients with liver disease is in a "rebalanced" status as a result of concomitant reductions in pro- and antihemostatic pathways.
- Routine correction of hemostasis by FFP or platelet concentrates prior to liver transplantation is not required.
- Maintenance of temperature, pH, and electrolyte status is important to support hemostasis during liver transplantation.
- A restrictive transfusion policy combined with maintenance of a low CVP appears to reduce blood loss during liver transplantation.

Introduction

The first human orthotopic liver transplantation was performed in 1963 by Starzl. Unfortunately, as Starzl stated, "He bled to death as we worked desperately to stop the hemorrhage."[1] Today liver transplantation is the treatment of choice in patients with acute or chronic end-stage liver disease.

Despite improvements during the last decades in surgical technique, anesthesiologic management and organ preservation, transfusion-free transplantations are achieved in only a minority of patients. Blood loss and subsequently the administration of blood products have a negative impact on outcome, even in centres where blood loss is low. Not only the administration of red blood cell concentrates (RBC) but also the administration of fresh–frozen plasma (FFP) and platelet concentrates (PC) have deleterious effects on outcome;[2,3] therefore, every measure to reduce blood loss is an important objective to improve morbidity and mortality after liver transplantation.

Management of hemostatic defects requires an understanding of coagulation, not only to reduce blood loss but equally important also to prevent thromboembolic events.

Hemostatic alterations in cirrhosis

Traditionally, blood loss during liver transplantation was ascribed to profound deficits in the hemostatic system of patients with liver disease. It was reasoned that alterations in primary and secondary hemostasis and fibrinolysis led to a bleeding tendency in these patients that resulted in inevitable blood loss if corrections were not made. Today a substantial proportion of transplant procedures are performed without correction of the underlying defects in hemostasis, and more importantly without the need for any blood products, even in patients with laboratory evidence of a coagulopathic state such as a prolonged PT and a reduced platelet count.[4] This observation

Medical Care of the Liver Transplant Patient, Fourth Edition. Edited by Pierre-Alain Clavien, James F. Trotter.

has challenged the concept of a bleeding tendency in cirrhotic patients. Evidence is growing that since hemostatic alterations not only concern prohemostatic pathways but also antihemostatic pathways, patients with end-stage liver disease have a rebalanced hemostatic system. Although the rebalanced hemostatic system is not reflected in routine laboratory tests such as the PT and platelet count, more sophisticated laboratory tests such as thrombin generation testing and platelet function measurements under physiologic flow conditions indicate adequate hemostatic capacity.[4,5] This balance, however, is delicate and a slight disturbance may result in a bleeding state but also in a hypercoagulable state, which may be associated with thromboembolic complications.[6] Figure 25.1 is a schematic representation of the hemostatic changes in cirrhotic patients.

As illustrated in Figure 25.1, cirrhotic patients are in a delicate hemostatic balance and will not necessarily bleed if they undergo an operation, however this balance can easily be disturbed leading to a bleed, but equally important may also lead to thrombotic complications. With current hemostatic tests that not only include the PT and platelet count, but also more global or sophisticated tests such as thromboelastography or thrombin generation measurements, it is not yet possible to predict which patients can undergo liver transplantation without any hemostatic complication and which patients will experience severe bleeding or thrombosis.

Clinical evidence for a bleeding diathesis in patients undergoing liver transplantation is represented by those patients who bleed profusely during the procedure, requiring transfusion of blood products. The success of antifibrinolytic therapy in reducing intraoperative blood loss also indicates that these patients may be in a relative hypocoagulable status. On the other hand, clinical evidence for prothrombotic status in patients with end-stage liver disease has recently emerged from a number of studies showing that patients with liver disease can experience venous thrombosis. One study has even demonstrated that patients with liver disease have a substantially increased risk of venous thromboembolism compared to population controls.[7] During and after liver transplantation thrombotic complications may also occur:

- Intraoperative pulmonary embolism or intracardiac thromboses are rare, but may be related to excessive coagulation activation.[8]
- Occurrence of hepatic artery thrombosis after liver transplantation may be related to hypercoagulability as evidenced by the success of thromboprophylaxis with aspirin.[9]
- Patients transplanted for familial amyloidotic polyneuropathy have a substantially increased risk for hepatic artery thrombosis.[10] Since these patients have a normal preoperative coagulation profile, it appears that hepatic artery thrombosis is not just a surgical complication, but that coagulation activation plays a prominent role as well.

Hemostasis monitoring

Interpretation of the results of hemostasis testing in patients with liver disease is difficult. Coagulation tests such as the PT and activated partial thromboplastin time (APTT) are performed on plasma only and provide no information about interactions of blood cells and plasmatic hemostasis. Importantly, the PT and APTT are only sensitive for levels of procoagulants and not for levels of anticoagulants, and pro- and antifibrinolytic factors. Since patients with end-stage liver disease have deficiencies in both pro- and anticoagulant proteins, the PT and APTT do not reflect hemostatic capacity in these patients, and are therefore poorly suited to predict bleeding or to guide hemostatic therapy. Consequently, there is no link between coagulation defects and bleeding or the required amount of RBC or plasma transfusions.[11] Based on these data, and on the observation that a large proportion of patients can undergo liver transplant surgery without requiring a blood transfusion, there is little evidence to support correction of coagulation defects before or during the liver transplant procedure if there are no signs of overt bleeding. Routine prophylaxis with FFP, platelets and/or procoagulants should therefore be reconsidered.

Thromboelastography is used to assess hemostasis and enables evaluation of the whole clotting process from its initiation, and the structural characteristics and stability of the formed clot.

Thromboelastography

There are two coagulation monitors that measure viscoelastic changes: thromboelastography (TEG) (Hemoscope, Niles, IL, USA) and thromboelastometry (RoTEM) (Pentapharm, Munich, Germany). The

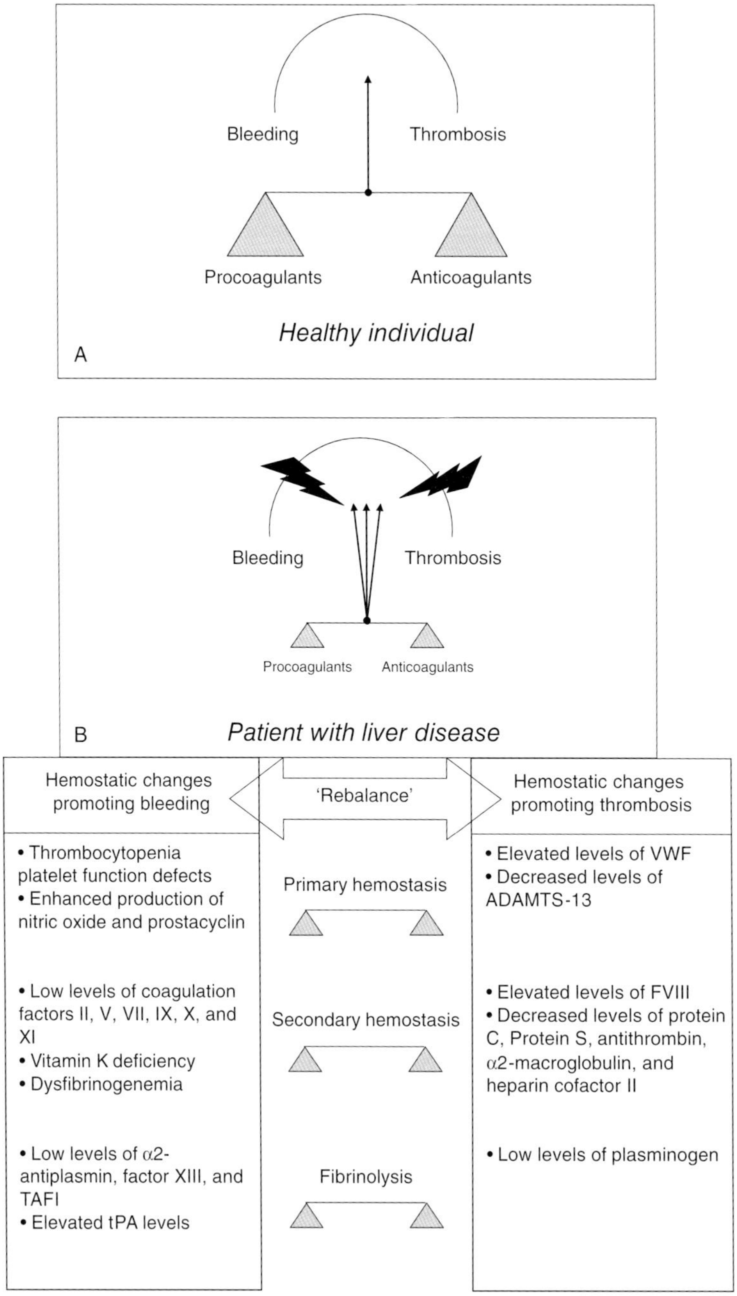

Figure 25.1 Schematic representation of the balance between pro- and anticoagulant factors in a healthy individual (**A**) and in a patient with liver disease (**B**). In a patient with liver disease both sides of the balance are functionally reduced, resulting in a delicate rebalance. This balance is easily disturbed, leading to a bleeding tendency or leading to a thrombosis. FVIII: factor VIII, TAFI: thrombin activatable fibrinolysis inhibitor, tPA: tissue-type plasminogen activator, VWF: von Willebrand factor. Part of this figure has been used with permission from Wolters Kluwer Health. Warnaar, N. The two tales of coagulation in liver transplantation. Curr Opin Organ Transpl (2008)13:298–303

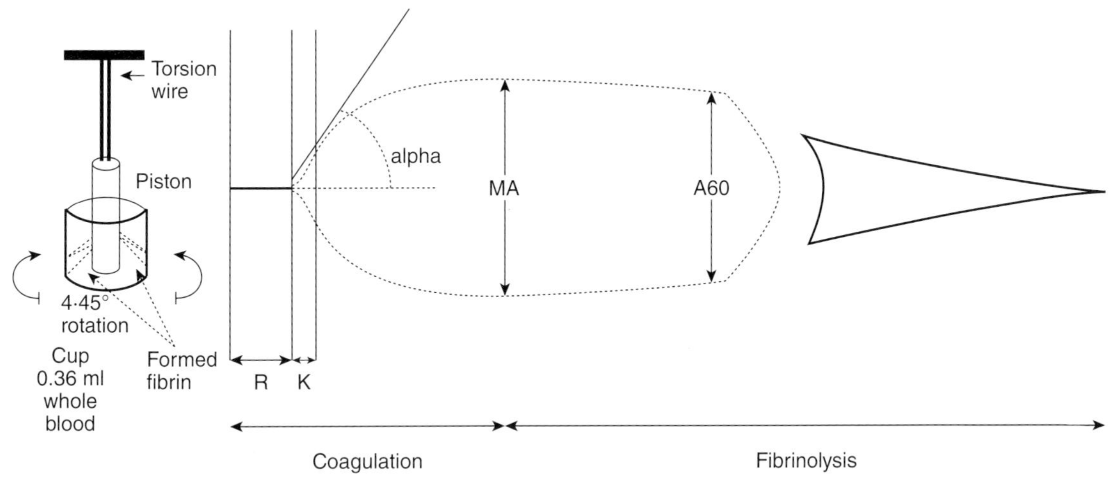

Figure 25.2 Diagram of the thromboelastograph and its tracing. The TEG cup contains 0.36 ml whole blood and is oscillated at an angle of 4°45' every 5 s. Fibers composed of fibrin and platelets attach to the cup and pin, affecting the rotation of the freely suspended piston. Liquid whole blood does not transmit torque from cup to piston, resulting in a straight line on the tracing. A strong clot moves the piston directly in phase with the cup, producing a huge magnitude in the tracing. Lysis results in a diminished transfer motion of the cup with consequent reduced tracings. In the RoTEM system, the cup (sample volume 0.34 ml) remains stationary and the pin is oscillated at an angle of 4°45' every 6 s. The measured variables are: **TEG reaction time (r)/RoTEM clotting time (CT)**: representing the time from initiating the test to the initial fibrin formation (defined as tracing amplitude of 2 mm). Prolongation indicates coagulation deficiencies or a heparin effect. **TEG kinetic time(k)/RoTEM clot formation time (CFT)**: represents the time from clot initiating (amplitude 2 mm) until the amplitude reaches 20 mm. **TEG/RoTEM α angle (α)**: the tangent of the curve made as the k is reached and represents the speed of clot forming. **TEG maximal amplitude (MA)/RoTEM maximum clot formation (MCF)**: the greatest amplitude of the trace. It reflects the absolute clot strength. A low MA/MCF indicates a decreased platelet number (or function) and/or decreased plasma fibrinogen level (or function). **TEG A_{60} /RoTEM clot lysis CL60**: the extension of *fibrinolysis* measured 60 min after MA/MCF – represents the stability of the clot

RoTEM is based on thromboelastographic principles and generates a similar trace to TEG. The test results are available more rapidly compared to the conventional coagulation testing offering the possibility of timely interventions, which is important in the rapidly changing coagulation profiles of patients during liver transplantation.

Figure 25.2 represents the principles of the thromboelastography and its tracing including the definitions of its variables. There are however several differences between the two systems affecting the results of the measurements. As shown in Figure 25.2, in TEG the cup rotates, and in the RoTEM the suspended wire rotates. Furthermore, the TEG cup contains a larger blood volume (0.36 ml) compared to the RoTEM cup (0.34 ml) and the latter cup is composed of a plastic with greater surface charge. Most important are the different activators used: in TEG kaolin is commonly used as activator of the coagulation process, whereas in RoTEM either partial thromboplastin/phospholipid (inTEM) or thromboplastin (exTEM) is used. The differences in the two systems may generate significant differences in hemostatic data.[12] As a consequence, the measured variables are not interchangeable and for clinical interpretation it is important to realize which activator is used.[12,13]

Figure 25.3 depicts four TEG-tracings from liver transplant patients with corresponding treatment options.

As seen in Figure 25.3 hypercoagulability can easily be differentiated from hypocoagulability, which is

	Thromboelastographic tracing	*Diagnosis*	*Treatment option*
1	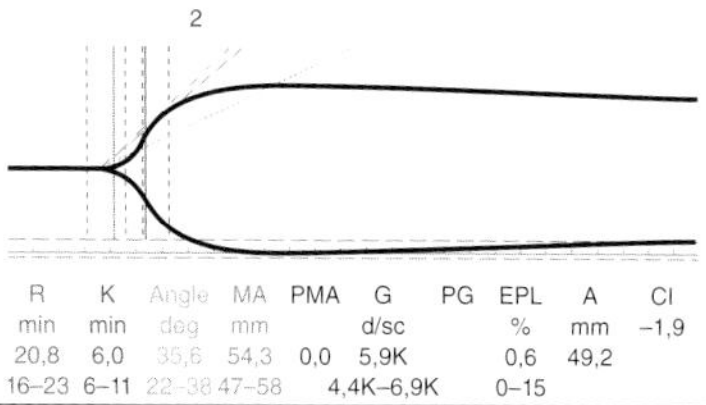	*Normal tracing.*	No intervention If bleeding is overt consider a surgical origin.
2	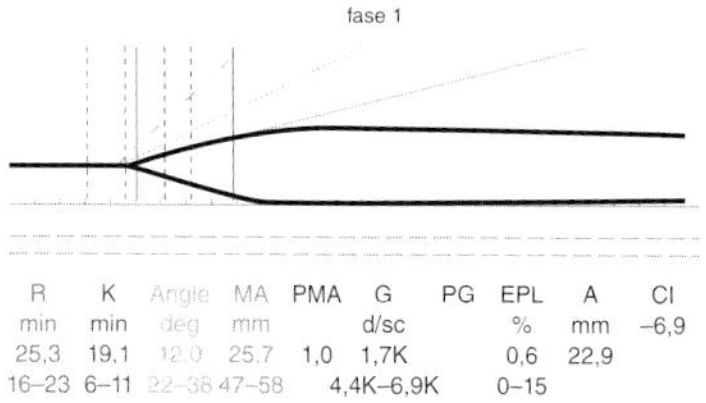	*Hypocoagulability* in a patient with hepatitis C at the start of transplantation. Prolonged r and k, small α and MA, no fibrinolysis.	If bleeding is nonsurgical consider prolonged r and k : FFP small MA: deficit in platelets *and/or* fibrinogen concentration (see text)
3	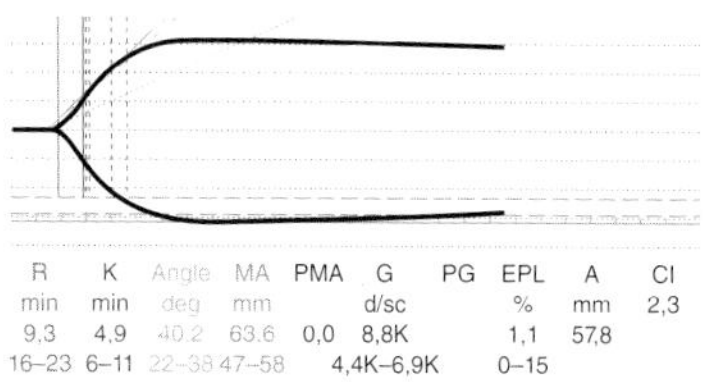	*Hypercoagulability* at the start of transplantation in a patient with primary biliary cirrhosis Short r and k, large α and MA, no fibrinolysis:	Consider anticoagulation therapy during or immediately after the liver transplantation procedure.
4	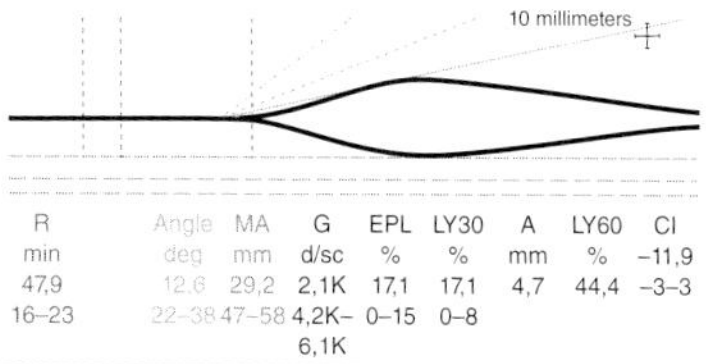	*Fibrinolysis* after reperfusion in a child with biliary atresia.	Consider antifibrinolytics: ε-aminocaproic acid or tranexamic acid

Figure 25.3 Four TEG tracings of liver transplant patients with the subsequent diagnosis and treatment options

impossible with PT and aPTT results, which are frequently prolonged during liver transplantation and may not give an accurate indication of the hemostatic status in these patients.[14] The clinical consequence is important: in patients with evidence of hypercoagulability, anticoagulants during or immediately after the transplant procedure are warranted and prohemostatic agents should be administered very cautiously. Based on TEG, hypercoagulability is often seen in patients with primary biliary cirrhosis (28%) and primary sclerosing cholangitis (43%) compared to noncholestatic cirrhosis (5%).[13] Patients with biliary liver disease are thus more prone to overt hypercoagulation and hence for thrombosis of the hepatic artery and portal vein.

Hypocoagulability is the most common finding in liver transplant patients, however hypocoagulation on TEG/RoTEM does not necessarily mean that the patient will bleed. If there is no bleeding it is our policy not to administer blood products or prohemostatic agents. When there is bleeding of a nonsurgical origin, depending on its cause, it can be treated with FFP, platelets and/or fibrinogen. RoTEM fib-monitoring, a qualitative test of fibrinogen concentration and fibrin polymerization, provides specific guidance for both fibrinogen and platelet administration. TEG differentiates between a platelet and a coagulation defect by using modified thromboelastography with ReoPro®, which eliminates platelet function from the TEG tracing. The MA will then become a function of fibrinogen activity. Plasma fibrinogen concentration and platelet count may also help to guide hemostatic treatment but these conventional tests do not reflect a decline in function of platelets. If fibrinolysis is detected, treatment with ε-aminocaproic acid (EACA) or tranexamic acid is indicated if bleeding is overt and nonsurgical.

TEG and RoTEM are influenced by the presence of heparin or heparinoids, which prolong the r/CT, and to a lesser extend k/CFT with a small MA/MCF. Heparinase reagents, antagonizing both the effect of heparin and heparinoids, are used in TEG (hep-TEG) and RoTEM (hep-TEM) and show the relative contribution of heparin and heparinoids. After hepatic graft reperfusion, a heparin-like effect is often seen and hep-TEG/RoTEM may guide protamine sulphate administration if there is nonsurgical bleeding, although the efficacy of protamine for reversal of bleeding associated with a heparin-like effect is only based on individual case reports.

Unfortunately, standardized transfusion algorithms for TEG, RoTEM and conventional coagulation tests are lacking.[15]

General measures to reduce blood loss

Transfusion guidelines

The use of blood products differs substantially from center to center, which may in part be due to the variety of transfusion protocols and transfusion thresholds that are currently being used.[16] There is no consensus regarding transfusion policy: prospective, multicenter studies are simply lacking.[17] Roughly speaking there are two strategies: a conventional transfusion policy and a restrictive transfusion policy. In the conventional strategy blood products are administered according to the results of coagulation tests. It is common for instance to administer FFP if the aPTT or PT is 2× prolonged compared to reference values, and platelets are often administered if the platelet count is $<50 \times 10^9$/L. In the restrictive transfusion policy, however, the results of coagulation testing are not used to administer blood products. Transfusion only occurs in the presence of clinically overt bleeding. The results of coagulation tests are then used to tailor the therapy in a bleeding patient and do not serve as a trigger to start the transfusion. There is increasing evidence that a restrictive transfusion policy leads to a reduction in blood loss.

Central venous pressure

With the introduction of the "piggyback" implantation technique it became possible to reduce the intraoperative fluid load. With this technique the inferior vena cava of the recipient is preserved and the upper caval cuff of the donor is anastomosed either to a common orifice in the hepatic veins or to a longitudinal incision in the inferior vena cava of the recipient. In contrast to a classical implantation, especially when a veno-venous bypass technique is used, the piggyback technique enables the anesthetist to aim for a low central venous pressure (CVP). A low CVP in the pre-anhepatic phase has been shown to reduce intraoperative bleeding during liver transplantation.[18] An important benefit of a low CVP (<5 mmHg) during liver transplantation is the reduced venous bleeding during hepatectomy. A low CVP can be achieved by different techniques. Restriction of fluid replacement is advocated in the current authors' center, but phlebotomy, and/or the use of vasodilatators is effective as well. In addition, the intraoperative CVP measurement changes as a result of the pressure of surgical retractors, mechanical ventilation, ascites, and table positioning, by which an objective CVP measure often is an illusion.

Volume restriction often requires the use of vasopressors to normalize blood pressure and results in the risk of renal hypoperfusion. In a previous study, two centers with different fluid management strategies were compared retrospectively with respect to postoperative renal complications. The center using volume restriction was successful in lowering blood transfusion requirements but observed a higher rate of postoperative renal failure, compared to a center with a more liberal infusion policy.[19] A patient with pre-existing severely reduced kidney function is probably not the ideal candidate for a restrictive volume strategy.

A recent publication, however, with 86 patients randomly divided into a low CVP group and a control group found again that a low CVP during the pre-anhepatic phase reduced intraoperative blood loss significantly, protected liver function and had no detrimental effects on renal function.[20] Evidence is growing that a low CVP reduces intraoperative blood loss and hence improves the results of liver transplantation.

Temperature

Since temperature drop has a negative impact on hemostasis, every measure must be taken to prevent intraoperative hypothermia. All fluids should be administered at 39°C and each patient should be covered with a warming blanket device. On each side of the patient, plastic bags can be attached to collect fluids (such as ascites, blood loss, and irrigation water). Fluid contact with the patient's body with subsequent temperature drop by evaporation is prevented with this method.

Calcium

FFPs and to a lesser degree RBCs contain citrate, which is used during blood collection to bind ionized calcium to prevent coagulation activation. Infusion with these citrated blood products results in hypocalcemia. Serum ionic calcium (Ca^{++}) is routinely monitored and corrected to obtain a serum Ca^{++} ≥1 mmol/L to prevent ventricular hypocontractility and to prevent dysfunctional hemostasis, since a number of coagulation reactions require calcium ions.

Acid–base balance

In a study with artificial acidification of blood it was shown that acidosis causes significant impairment of clot formation and clot strength as demonstrated by thromboelastography.[21] Hypothermia has the same effects, but to a lesser extent. Alkalization and temperature rise did not affect the thromboelastographic variables. These findings emphasize the need for correction of acidosis and again, to avoid hypothermia to normalize hemostasis. The intraoperative acidosis can be treated with sodium bicarbonate (BIC) or tris-hydroxymethyl aminomethane (THAM). BIC infusion will result in an increase in carbon dioxide production, while THAM reduces the carbon dioxide output. Mechanical ventilation can be adapted during infusion of these buffer solutions. The effect on carbon dioxide however is transient. It should be noted however that there is no hard evidence that intraoperative acidosis correction with buffers will lead to improved outcome. Prevention and correction of the underlying cause of acidosis therefore remain the pillars of treatment.

Pharmacologic strategies to minimize blood loss

Antifibrinolytics

Increased fibrinolytic activity has been demonstrated during liver transplantation, in particular following reperfusion, and these observations have provided a scientific base to administer fibrinolysis inhibitors. Aprotinin, a serine protease inhibitor with potent antifibrinolytic activity, has been shown to substantially reduce intraoperative blood loss, and has been used routinely in many centers.[22] In 2007, however, this antifibrinolytic was withdrawn from the market after serious concerns were raised by the use of aprotinin in thoracic surgery.[23] EACA and tranexamic acid are lysine analogues and their antifibrinolytic activity is caused by competitive inhibition of the binding of plasminogen to fibrin. High-dose tranexamic acid was effective compared with placebo in reducing blood loss and transfusion requirements by 46 and 31%, respectively.[24] In another study a positive effect of EACA on blood transfusion was not found but in the same study the red blood cell requirement was 36% lower in the tranexamic acid group, compared to placebo.[25]

As antifibrinolytics promote coagulation, this drug should be cautiously used in patients with pre-existing thrombotic conditions such as portal vein thrombosis, Budd–Chiari syndrome, and inherited protein C or S deficiency. The current authors do not administer tranexamic acid routinely in their center but administration is guided by the results of the thromboelastography and a hypercoagulable state (defined as the presence of at least three variables of the TEG indicating a hypercoagulable state) is considered a contraindication for the administration of antifibrinolytics. If >5% lysis on the other hand is detected after 60 min (A_{60} >5%), an IV bolus of 1000 mg tranexamic acid is administered. This dose can be repeated if necessary.

Recombinant factor VIIa (rFVIIa)

rFVIIa is a prohemostatic drug developed for patients with inhibitor-complicated hemophilia, and it is also registered for patients with factor VII deficiency and Glanzmann thrombasthenia. Massive off-label use has suggested the drug to be effective in a variety of hemostatic disorders, however two large placebo-controlled multicenter trials showed that rFVIIa was not effective when it was prophylactically administered during OLT.[26,27] So far no studies justify the routine use of rFVIIa in liver transplantation, but there may be a place for it in liver transplantation as a rescue agent, i.e in patients in whom bleeding occurs and are not responding to conventional therapy. Considering the potential prothrombotic effect, especially at sites of vascular anastomosis, administration of the drug should be performed with great caution.

General measures to reduce thromboembolic events

As noted earlier, hypercoagulability and thromboembolism may cause fatal complications during and after OLT. Patients with primary sclerosing cholangitis, primary biliary cirrhosis, and hepatocellular carcinoma seem to be at risk for thromboembolic complications. Several other factors have been associated with an increased risk, including a low portal blood flow velocity. Until now hard evidence of which factors play a crucial role is lacking. Thromboelastography has potential benefits, but its application in this specific setting needs to be validated in properly designed controlled clinical trials. Until this time the current authors can only make some recommendations.

Hematocrit

Rheologic factors may be important in the development of thrombosis. A raised hematocrit level increases blood viscosity and subsequently may reduce blood flow. Raised viscosity, such as in patients with polycythemia vera is associated with thrombotic episodes. A low hematocrit level may help to reduce thrombotic events, especially hepatic artery thrombosis (HAT), during and after liver transplantation. A hematocrit level below 30% might decrease the incidence of HAT and thus lower the post-transplant mortality. A raised hematocrit level is sometimes caused by the minimal blood loss during transplantation but more often by overtransfusion of red blood cells. If at the end of the transplant procedure the hematocrit is above 30%, the current authors consider a phlebotomy and replace the tapped volume with saline 0.9%.

Blood pressure

During the hepatectomy, mild hypotension can be accepted to avoid blood loss. After recirculation, hypotension should be avoided in order to prevent compromising the donor liver. Furthermore, because the result of systolic hypotension is decreased flow, making it more susceptible to thrombosis, low blood pressure should not be accepted.

Conclusion

In conclusion, in liver transplantation there is no standard approach in anesthetic management, surgical technique, hemodynamic and coagulation monitoring, and transfusion threshold.

Even patients with the same underlying disease differ in their coagulation profiles as expressed in differences in Child–Pugh score and MELD score at the time of transplantation. At this moment there is still not enough evidence to point out best practise. Adherence to a transfusion algorithm reduces blood loss and as long as there is no gold standard the current authors believe that every liver transplant center should adhere to their local transfusion algorithm and evaluate this on a regular basis.

There is mounting evidence for the negative effects on outcome if blood products are administered, therefore it is important for every practitioner involved in liver transplantation to take measures to reduce operative blood product use. There is accumulating evidence that prophylactic administration of blood products (e.g. FFP or platelet concentrates) is not effective and does not lead to a reduction in blood loss and transfusion requirements. Emerging results indicate that maintaining relative hypovolemia and restrictive use of blood products are keystones to strategies to reduce intraoperative blood loss. There is accumulating evidence that liver transplant patients are at risk of developing thromboembolic complications. This stresses a careful approach not only with the administration of blood products but also with the administration of procoagulant drugs. The anesthetic approach should be tailored to the individual patient.

References

1. Starzl TE. The puzzle people. Memoires of a transplant surgeon. Pittsburgh: University of Pitsburgh Press; 1992.
2. Boer MT, Christensen MC, Amussen M, et al. The impact of intraoperative transfusion of platelets and red blood cells on survival after liver transplantation. Anesth Analg 2008;106:32–44.
3. Massicotte L, Sassine MP, Lenis S, Seal RF, Roy A. Survival rate changes with transfusion of blood products during liver transplantation. Can J Anaesth 2005;52:148–55.
4. Lisman T, Porte RJ. Rebalanced hemostasis in patients with liver disease: evidence and clinical consequences. Blood 2010;116:878–85.
5. Tripodi A, Salerno F, Chantarangkul V, et al. Evidence of normal thrombin generation in cirrhosis despite abnormal conventional coagulation tests. Hepatology 2005;41:553–8.
6. Warnaar N, Lisman T, Porte RJ. The two tales of coagulation in liver transplantation. Curr Opin Organ Transplant 2008;13:298–303.
7. Søgaard KK, Horváth-Puhó E, Grønbæk H, Jepsen P, Vilstrup H, Sørensen HT. Risk of venous thromboembolism in patients with liver disease: a nationwide population-based case-control study. Am J Gastroenterol 2009;104:96–101.
8. Warnaar N, Molenaar IQ, Colquhoun SD, et al. Intraoperative pulmonary embolism and intracardiac thrombosis complicating liver transplantation: a systematic review. J Thromb Haemostasis 2008;6:297–302.
9. Vivarelli M, La Barba G, Cucchetti A, et al. Can antiplatelet prophylaxis reduce the incidente of hepatic artery thrombosis alter liver transplantation? Liver Transpl 2007;13:651–4.
10. Bispo M, Marcelino P, Freire A, Martins A, Mourão L, Barosso E. High incidence of thrombotic complications early alter liver transplantation for familial amyloidotic polyneuropathy. Transpl Int 2009;22:165–71.
11. Massicotte L, Beaulieu D, Thibeault L, et al. Coagulation defects do not predict blood product requirements during liver transplantation. Transplantation 2008;85: 956–62.
12. Nielsen VG. A comparison of the thrombelastograph and the ROTEM. Blood Coagul Fibrinolysis 2007;18: 247–52.
13. Ben-Ari Z, Panagou M, Patch D, et al. Hypercoagulability in patients with primary biliary cirrhosis and primary sclerosing cholangitis evaluated by thromboelastography. J Hepatol 1997;26:554–59.
14. Lisman T, Porte RJ. Rebalanced hemostasis in patients with liver disease: evidence and clinical consequences. Blood 2010;116:878–85.
15. Venema LF, Post WJ, Hendriks HGD, Huet RCG, Wolf de JThW, de Vries AJ. An assessment of clinical interchangeability of TEG and RoTEM thromboelastographic variables in cardiac surgical patients. Anesth Analg 2010;111:339–44.
16. Coakley M, Reddy K, Mackie I, Mallet S. Transfusion triggers in orthotopic liver transplantation: a comparison of the thromboelastometry analyzer, the thromboelastogram, and conventional coagulation tests. J Cardiothorac Vasc Anesth 2006;20:548–53.
17. Lopez-Plaza I. Transfusion guidelines and liver transplantation: time for consensus. Liver Transpl 2007;13: 1630–2.
18. Massicotte L, Lenis S, Thibeault L, Sassine MP, Seal RF, Roy A. Effect of low central venous pressure and phlebotomy on blood product transfusion requirements during liver transplantations. Liver Transpl 2006;12: 117–23.
19. Schroeder RA, Collins BH, Tuttle-Newhall E, et al. Intraoperative fluid management during orthotopic liver transplantation. J Cardiothorac Vasc Anesth 2004;18: 438–41.
20. Feng ZY, Xu X, Zhu SM, Bein B, Zheng SS. Effects of low central venous pressure during preanhepatic phase on blood loss and liver and renal function in liver transplantation. World J Surg 2010;34:1864–73.
21. Ramaker AJDWR, van der Meer J, Struys MMRF, Lisman T, van Oeveren W, Hendriks HGD. Effects of acidosis, alkalosis, hyperthermia and hypothermia on haemostasis: results of point-of-care testing with the thromboelastography analyser. Blood Coagul Fibrinolysis 2009;20:436–9.
22. Boer de MT, Molenaar IQ, Hendriks HGD, Slooff MJH, Poerte RJ. Minimizing blood loss in liver transplantation: progress through research and evolution of techniques. Dig Surg 2005;22:265–75.
23. Mangano DT, Tudor IC, Dietzel C. Multicenter study of perioperative ischemia research group; ischemia research and education foundation. N Engl J Med 2006;354:353–65.
24. Boylan JF, Klinck JR, Sandler AN, et al. Tranexamic acid reduces blood loss, transfusion requirements, and coagulation factor use in primary orthotopic liver transplantation. Anesthesiology 1996;85:1043–8.

25. Dalmau A, Sabaté A, Acosta F, et al. Tranexamic acid reduces red cell transfusion better than epsilon-aminocaproic acido or placebo in liver transplantation. Anesth Analg 2000;91:29–34.
26. Planinsic RM, van der Meer J, Testa G, et al. Safety and efficacy of a single bolus administration of recombinant factor VIIa in liver transplantation. Liver Transpl 2005:11:895–900.
27. Lodge JP, Jonas S, Jones RM, et al. Efficacy and safety of repeated perioperative doses of recombinant factor VIIa in liver transplantation. Liver Transpl 2005:11:973–9.

26 Critical care of the liver transplant recipient

Markus Béchir[1], *Erik Schadde*[2] *and Philipp Dutkowski*[2]

Swiss HPB and Transplantation Centers, Section of Intensive Care Medicine[1], and Department of Surgery[2], University Hospital Zürich, Zürich, Switzerland

Key learning points

- Early extubation and careful assessment of pulmonary hypertension minimize pulmonary morbidity.
- Persistent acidosis, lack of liver function and persistent transaminitis should trigger immediate evaluation of the hepatic artery and raise concern about primary nonfunction or initial poor graft function.
- Estimation of renal risk based on preoperative assessment, judicious use of simultaneous liver–kidney transplantation and use of nephroprotective intraoperative strategies help to reduce renal dysfunction.
- Delirium is the most common psychiatric complication and its etiology includes infection, calcineurin inhibitors, and pre-existing encephalopathy.
- Biliary complications have to be recognized early to reduce infectious complications.
- Hepatic artery thrombosis (HAT) is the most feared surgical complication and HAT within the first days requires retransplantation.
- Most donor and recipient scoring systems for prediction of morbidity after liver transplantation (LT) are unreliable.

Introduction

LT is a highly standardized operative procedure and has been recognized as a valuable treatment option for many patients with end-stage liver disease. In spite of numerous improvements in organ procurement, preservation, and implantation techniques, one key factor for reliable outcome after LT remains professional intensive care treatment in the direct postoperative course. Because artificial liver support is still not reliable as a bridge for transplant failure, recipients are dependent on immediate graft function after transplantation. While a liver transplant recipient with a low Model of End-stage Liver Disease (MELD) score and a standard liver graft usually will develop sufficient liver metabolism already shortly after transplantation and thus only needs a short stay in an intensive care unit (ICU), the requirement of advanced intensive care is high in those liver transplant recipients who are already extremely sick before transplantation. This risk appears to be even more increased if extended-criteria donor (ECD) liver grafts are used, as is often necessary today due to the severe shortage of organs. The most feared complications in such cases are septic in nature and deserve careful evaluation. This chapter will summarize the current methods for assessment of graft function after LT, list management of common medical and surgical complications and of nutrition, and review the currently available prediction models for risk evaluation before LT.

Assessment of graft function

The function of a transplanted liver depends on graft quality, procurement and storage conditions, and

Medical Care of the Liver Transplant Patient, Fourth Edition. Edited by Pierre-Alain Clavien, James F. Trotter.

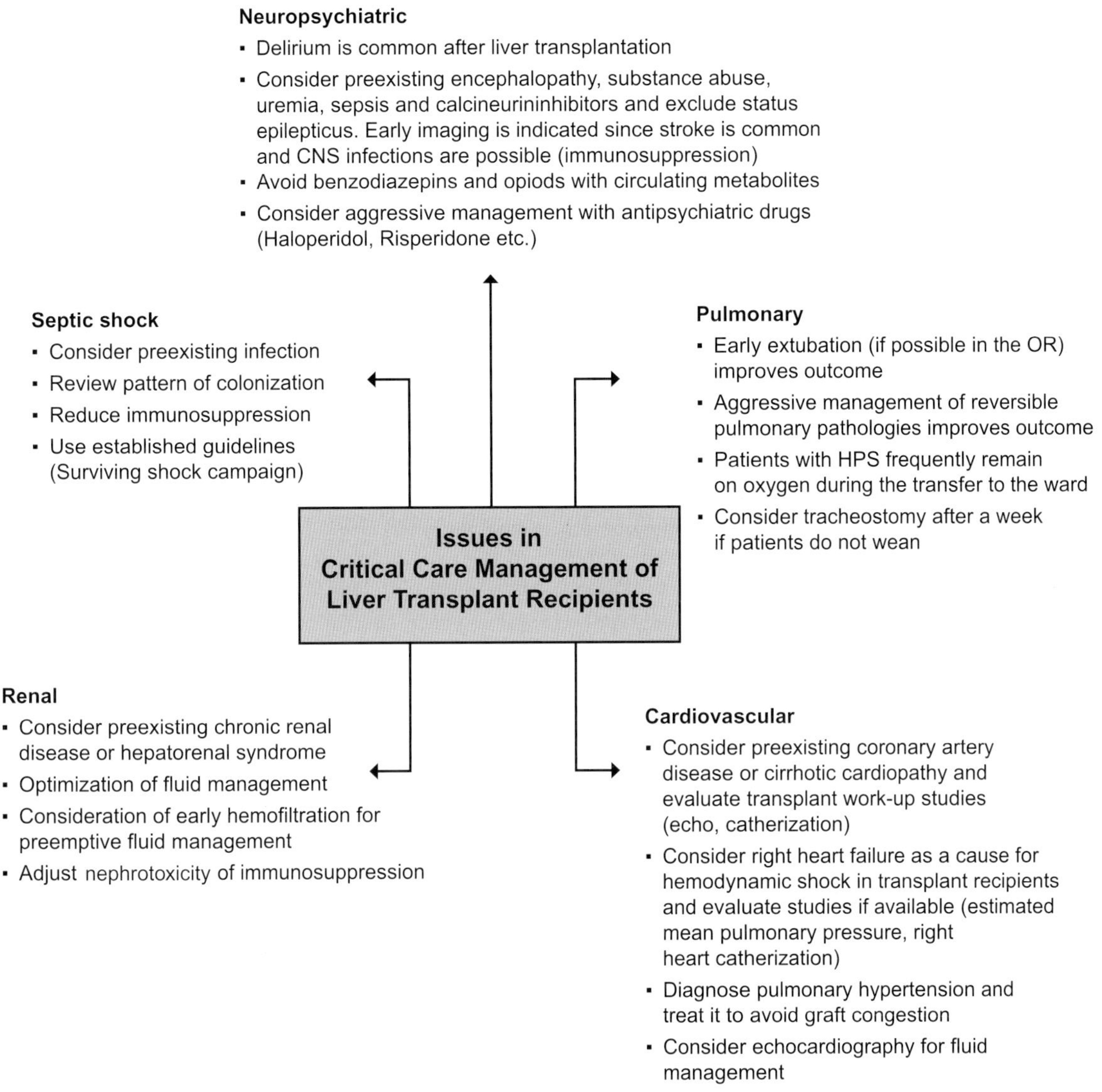
Neuropsychiatric
▪ Delirium is common after liver transplantation
▪ Consider preexisting encephalopathy, substance abuse, uremia, sepsis and calcineurininhibitors and exclude status epilepticus. Early imaging is indicated since stroke is common and CNS infections are possible (immunosuppression)
▪ Avoid benzodiazepins and opiods with circulating metabolites
▪ Consider aggressive management with antipsychiatric drugs (Haloperidol, Risperidone etc.)
Septic shock
▪ Consider preexisting infection
▪ Review pattern of colonization
▪ Reduce immunosuppression
▪ Use established guidelines (Surviving shock campaign)
Pulmonary
▪ Early extubation (if possible in the OR) improves outcome
▪ Aggressive management of reversible pulmonary pathologies improves outcome
▪ Patients with HPS frequently remain on oxygen during the transfer to the ward
▪ Consider tracheostomy after a week if patients do not wean
Issues in Critical Care Management of Liver Transplant Recipients
Renal
▪ Consider preexisting chronic renal disease or hepatorenal syndrome
▪ Optimization of fluid management
▪ Consideration of early hemofiltration for preemptive fluid management
▪ Adjust nephrotoxicity of immunosuppression
Cardiovascular
▪ Consider preexisting coronary artery disease or cirrhotic cardiopathy and evaluate transplant work-up studies (echo, catherization)
▪ Consider right heart failure as a cause for hemodynamic shock in transplant recipients and evaluate studies if available (estimated mean pulmonary pressure, right heart catherization)
▪ Diagnose pulmonary hypertension and treat it to avoid graft congestion
▪ Consider echocardiography for fluid management

Figure 26.1 Multidisciplinary aspects after liver transplantation

recipient factors. Feng et al. performed an analysis on donor risk factors in LT and found that 1-year mortality depends on seven donor risk factors, including: 1) age, 2) race, 3) height, 4) cause of death, 5) donation after cardiac death status, 6) cold ischemia, and 7) partial graft status, resulting in a comprehensive donor risk index (DRI) for liver grafts.[1] Along the lines of the increased mortality and morbidity, a prolonged stay in the ICU can be expected. However, evidence-based guidelines for the recognition of graft dysfunction in LT do not exist. One of the first indications of graft function is the hepatic bile flow during implantation, often documented by the surgeons. Another point is the clearance of anesthetic agents in the immediate postoperative period by clinical neurologic assessment. It is important to withhold sedation until the patient's liver function is established in the ICU. While some degree of preservation injury and elevated liver enzymes are observed in every liver transplant, coagulation parameters and transaminases (alanine aminotransferase (ALT) and aspartate aminotransferase (AST)) should improve continuously after LT. However, the level of liver enzymes does not correlate with liver function at all, therefore most centers rely on assessment of INR and factor V, analyzed every 6h after transplantation within the first 2d. Coagulation threshold values for the definition of primary nonfunction or delayed graft function do not exist, but generally primary nonfunction has been defined as the combination of poor bile production, hypoglycemia, coagulopathy, encephalopathy, renal dysfunction, elevated transaminases and shock, leading to retransplantation or death within 7d after transplantation. Any lack of neurologic stability, increasing hemodynamic instability and noncorrection of the INR and or factor V in the presence of patent vascular supply by ultrasound is suspicious for primary nonfunction and the patient might have to be relisted. The application of fresh–frozen plasma or coagulation factor concentrates bears a risk of masking the actual liver synthetic function and can only be recommended once the definitive decision for retransplantation is made.

Liver assist devices are rarely available and generally worsen coagulopathy. If the patient becomes more unstable and cannot be managed with conventional means, the patient may need an allograft hepatectomy and portal-caval shunt in order to preserve his candidacy for retransplantation.

Even more difficult is the recognition of those cases with delayed graft function, where no retransplant is necessary due to the fact that liver graft function recovers after 2–3 d. The distinction between primary nonfunction and delayed graft function requires, therefore, repeated assessment of all biochemical and clinical parameters. Ploeg et al. defined delayed graft function by the combination of serum AST >2000U/L, prothrombin time <16s and amomonia >50 μmol/L during the postoperative days 2–7.[2] A more recent definition from 2010 is based on the presence of least one of the following parameters 7d after LT: serum bilirubin ≥10 mg/dl, INR ≥1.8 or ALT >2000 U/L.[3]

Beside static tests of liver function, such as serum activities of liver enzymes, protein synthesis and bilirubin, several dynamic tests have been developed to better stratify risk candidates for graft failure. In general, dynamic liver tests are related to the ability of the liver to metabolize or eliminate defined substance. For example, the capability of the liver to exclusively eliminate indocyanine green (ICG) into the bile without enterohepatic recirculation can be analyzed. Importantly, the plasma disappearance rate (ICG-PDR) is not only dependent on biliary excretion but also on blood flow and hyperbilirubinemia, and short-term changes in ICG-PDR may reflect changes in blood flow rather than hepatocellular function.[4]

Another dynamic liver test is the monoethylglycinexylidine test (MEGX), based on the hepatic conversion of lidocaine to MEGX, which is related to the cytochrome P450 system. In contrast to ICG-PDR, the MEGX test does not allow beside assessment since it requires immunoassays or chromatograhic analysis. The results have to interpreted in relation to other substances that interfere with the cytochrome P 450 system like antibiotics, immunosuppressive agents or antidepressants.[4]

The LiMAx test is a newly developed bedside test based on the hepatocyte-specific metabolism of the C^{13}-labelled substrate (methocetin) by the cytochrome P450 IA2 isoenzyme.[5] Recently, initial graft performance measured by the LIMAx test at day 1 was closely associated with early post-transplant outcome.[6] Clear threshold values for reliable separation of primary nonfunction and delayed graft function, however, are not yet available.

Medical complications

Sepsis

Patients undergoing LT may have undetected previous infections, therefore all previous antibiotics and colonization patterns should be investigated prior to transplantation. In high-risk patients, as for example in cholestatic liver diseases (primary sclerosing cholangitis (PSC), primary biliary cirrhosis (PBC)), or retransplantations, a culture of the cut surface of the bile duct at the time of transplant is helpful to guide further antibiotic administration. Since bacterial translocation is a possible etiology for bacteremia, some investigators have proposed that probiotic therapy prevents infections in liver transplant recipients. In this context Rayes et al. reported that early enteral nutrition supplemented by lactobacillus and fiber reduces bacterial infection rates following LT.[7] Deep surgical space infections and biliary infection are other common bacterial infections.[8] As a rule, all potential sites for infection should be explored and, if possible, eliminated (catheters, hematoma, or abscess-suspicious fluid collection). The threshold for surgical re-exploration is therefore low, if the source of infection cannot be determined by imaging and culture.

There are data supporting the use of activated protein C in liver transplant patients with septic shock. There is currently no good algorithm guiding management of immunosuppression in infection and septic shock, however patients will likely die from infection, not from rejection. Consequently, calcineurin and mTOR inhibitors and antiproliferative agents have to be reduced in severe sepsis.

While the risk of bacterial infections remains high after LT, the risk of fungal infections is <5%[8] in the standard case. This is different if small bowel perforation or biliary leaks occur, which generally require antifungal treatment. The majority of fungal infections are due to *Candida* species. A recent meta-analysis recommends prophylaxis for subgroups of patients who have been shown to be at high risk for fungal infection including those: 1) with acute liver failure, 2) who have undergone re-transplantion, 3) who experience large blood loss, 4) with acute renal failure, 5) requiring hemodialysis, and 6) requiring re-operations for complications. Because infections occur mainly in the first months after transplantation, prophylaxis should be continued for 2–6 weeks after transplantation. In most centers, prophylaxis for *Candida* species with fluconazole at a prophylactic dose will be considered sufficient. However if fluconazole-resistant *Candida* species are proven or even an *Aspergillus* infection is detected, either liposomal amphotericin-B solutions or echinocandins such as micafungin should be used.

Renal dysfunction

The incidence of acute renal failure after LT varies largely in the literature, ranging between 27 and 67%. The Acute Dialysis Quality Inititative workgroup has proposed a multilevel classification system for acute kidney injury (AKI) using the acronym RIFLE (Risk, Injury, Failure, Loss of kidney function, and End-stage kidney disease).

The most important risk factor for postoperative renal dysfunction is pretransplant dysfunction. The Model for End-stage Liver Disease (MELD) score includes kidney function (creatinine) as an important parameter along with international normalized ratio (INR) and bilirubin. Because liver grafts are currently allocated by the MELD system in many countries, numerous candidates for liver transplantation present today with impaired kidney function already before transplant. The differentiation between chronic kidney disease and acute pre-transplant renal injury due to hepatorenal syndrome and acute tubular necrosis can be difficult and involves ultrasound, urinary electrolytes, urinary sediment analysis, and biopsy. Biopsy data have demonstrated that chronic structural changes are seen in liver transplant patients with normal creatinine, and are more common than suspected at least in the large group of patients with hepatitis C.[9] In patients needing hemodialysis for more than 8 weeks prior to LT, a combined liver–kidney transplantation should be discussed.

It has been assumed that the prevention of early AKI begins in the operating room. Meticulous surgery with avoidance of blood loss, short anhepatic phase, and minimization of adrenergic agents may mitigate renal injury. Some studies have further suggested that using partial caval clamping (i.e. "piggyback technique") has less risk of hemodynamic instability and AKI, but evidence by larger randomized studies is clearly lacking.[10] Renal risk is likely additive in the postoperative period and the use of known nephrotoxins (e.g. aminoglycosides) should be avoided. There is no clear consensus whether the use of drugs such as prostaglandin E1, intraoperative diuretics, N-acetylcysteine, sodium bicarbonate, or fenoldopam have a nephroprotective effect during or after surgery. Randomized studies will be needed to test pharmacologic intervention to protect renal function.

Postoperative AKI may be reduced by limiting reoperations and early recognition of infections. Calcineurin inhibitors for immunosuppression can be decreased by the combination with interleukin 2 inhibitors and/or mTOR inhibitors. In spite of the fact that LT may correct hepatorenal syndrome, temporary renal replacement therapy (RRT) is currently needed in many cases because impaired kidney function already exists pre transplantation in numerous recipients. Most kidneys recover with time after LT and only a small percentage of patients will develop long-term kidney failure.

If necessary, renal replacement therapy should be initiated early, before fluid overload or hyperkalemia are dominant after LT. In spite of this fact, there is little data available on the value of intraoperative RRT, although some centers find it useful in managing the fluid status intraoperatively.

Cardiovascular complications

Liver transplant centers perform risk stratification for patients by evaluating their pre-transplant cardiac performance by using a dobutamine stress echocardiogram or myocardium scintigraphy to detect critical coronary artery stenosis. If there are questions based on these screening tests, cardiologic consultation should be obtained. It has been acknowledged that non-alcoholic steatohepatitis (NASH), a history of previous coronary artery disease, and peripheral vascular disease in asymptomatic patients are strong risk predictors in patients with liver disease, as are hypertension, diabetes, hyperlipidemia, age >50, and obesity.[11] Programs with a higher percentage of patients with NASH should pursue a more aggressive screening strategy.

Specific attention should be paid to patients who have a positive stress test but a negative catheterization. It has been demonstrated that there are more postoperative deaths in patients with positive stress tests even if their catheterization was negative.[12] Patients with impaired cardiac performance may present in the ICU with myocardial depression and insufficient cardiac reserve, especially in the face of bleeding or sepsis.[13] At baseline, liver transplant patients have a high cardiac output state, low systemic vascular resistance, and a chronic inflammatory condition. The procedure of LT constitutes severe physiologic stress with a wide range of changes in oxygen requirement by the myocardium. Plaque rupture and coronary thrombosis may occur in patients who have normal stress tests and subcritical stenoses (<50% occlusions). Whether subcritical stenoses should be treated in preparation for LT or whether patients at high risk with negative stress tests should nevertheless undergo coronary catheterization are currently areas of debate. Reports have shown that myocardial infarction may occur in liver transplant recipients with as little as 30% of vessel occlusion.[12]

A low cardiac index after LT with signs of systemic hypoperfusion (reduced glomerular filtration, acidosis, delirium, liver graft dysfunction) could also be due to cirrhotic cardiomyopathy or to the cardiomyopathies associated with alcohol, hepatitis or hemochromatosis. Preoperatively cardiac decompensation is often absent because the cardiac workload is reduced through systemic vasodilation associated with advanced liver disease.

The majority of low cardiac output states in the ICU after LT are most likely caused by postoperative pulmonary hypertension with or without a component of right heart dysfunction. This condition is especially problematic since it adds to venous graft congestion and dysfunction, the hemodynamic problem of low cardiac output, and arterial hypoperfusion of the transplanted liver. The experience from the Baylor Transplant Center and Mayo Clinic Rochester confirmed that mortality after LT for patients with mean pulmonary pressures of >35 mmHg ("moderate pulmonary hypertension") is prohibitive.[14,15] The authors of this chapter follow the Baylor algorithm, which dictates that these patients should be treated with epoprostenol therapy. These patients may be active on the list as long as mean estimated pulmonary arterial pressure (PAP) on screening echocardiography remains <35 mmHg. These patients should be called in for liver transplantation with a backup. Intra-operative vasodilator therapy with epoprostenol, inhaled nitric oxide and restrictive volume management are usually initiated to improve cardiopulmonary flow and avoid right heart decompensation, especially during the reperfusion phase. This treatment needs to be continued on ICU.

Recently the liver transplant anesthesia consortium (LTrAC) surveyed international and US transplant programs and found that 85% of US programs and 65% of international programs use the pulmonary artery catheter (PAC, Swan–Ganz catheter) for monitoring, whereas intraoperative transesophageal echocardiography (TEE) is less common at 45 and 35%, respectively.[16] Owing to the ease of the PAC in the ICU postoperatively, and the lack of availability of TEE in most ICUs, PAC remains the most commonly used modality. Major complications associated with PAC have been reported to occur in 4–5% of insertions. Intermittent transcutaneous echo requires a lot of resources and is most likely only applicable in settings where

Echocardiograms are performed by physicians themselves. Preliminary data suggest that this technique overestimates the cardiac output in subjects with low peripheral vascular resistance.[17] Many studies have demonstrated that central venous pressure measurement is a poor volume guide for intravascular volume and adequate resuscitation.

Oliguria should prompt TTE to improve cardiac filling with bolus colloids. If there is no fluid responsiveness to fluid bolus, no more fluids should be given to avoid over-resucitation based on central venous pressure (CVP), urinary output or pulmonary artery wedge pressure (PAWP) numbers.

Despite early reports that low-CVP resuscitation strategies result in more acute tubular necrosis (ATN) and decreased survival, more recent reports support the concept for restrictive fluid and transfusion management.[18,19] Whereas Massicotte et al. demonstrate that there is no need for albumin, fresh–frozen plasma (FFP) and platelet transfusion after LT, a problem of their study is the low mean MELD score of their patient population and the lack of a subgroup analysis with chronic renal disease.[18] Feng et al. confirmed in a randomized prospective trial that low CVP during the pre-anhepatic phase results in about a 50% reduction in blood loss and transfusion requirements without any adverse effects on mortality or renal function.[19]

Respiratory complications

There is good evidence that extubation of patients who have had cardiac surgery and major abdominal surgery reduces length of ICU and hospital care without a negative impact on morbidity and mortality. A recent multicenter study confirmed that fast-track management with extubation of liver transplant patients in the operating room can be achieved with only a 7.7% risk of adverse advents.[20] Non-invasive ventilation (NIV) is a possibility to avoid re-intubation if aspiration precautions are taken.

In order to assess the patient's ability to be extubated early, pre-existing lung pathologies need to be known. All patients undergoing LT should have screening spirometry. Structural lung disease might be an exclusion criterium for LT. Most programs do not transplant patients with severe chronic obstructive pulmonary disease (COPD) (FEV1 <50%). There is no study to date defining postoperative respiratory morbidity in liver transplant recipients with different grades of COPD. Reversible pulmonary pathologies like pleural effusions due to hepatic hydrothrorax, lobar collapse, and pneumothorax secondary to vascular access procedures or surgical injury to the diaphragm or phrenic injury as well as reduced ventilatory volume due to restriction from postoperative ascites may easily be identified on chest x-ray. In the current authors' experience, reversible pathologies should be aggressively addressed with interventional procedures. Not resolving pleural effusions after LT, especially in conjunction with mild graft dysfunction, warrant thorough workup of right heart function and pulmonary arterial pressures.

Hepatopulmonary syndrome (HPS) is defined by the triad of liver dysfunction or portal hypertension, abnormal gas exchange and evidence of pulmonary vascular shunts. The latter is diagnosed by echocardiography with the use of air bubbles or macroaggreated albumin perfusion scanning. Patients with HPS have an increased length of stay in ICU (median 4 d) and hospital (median of 39 d). The median time to cessation of oxygen is 4.5 months in some series.[21]

Faenza et al. found that the PaO2/FiO2 ratio of <300 (an element of the definition of acute lung injury) at the end of a liver transplant predicts the need for prolonged mechanical ventilation in liver transplant patients.[22] There is no evidence that the mode of ventilation should be different in liver transplant patients compared to other post-surgical patients to improve graft outcomes. The current authors recommend that standard low-tidal ventilation is used to avoid ventilator-induced lung injury. Despite contrary reports in animal models,[23–25] there is no conclusive evidence that positive end expiratory pressure (PEEP) up to 15 cmH_2 impairs liver outflow or systemic hemodynamics in liver transplant patients.[26] As long there is no dilatation of the right ventricle, PEEP does not influence hepatic outflow.

Patients cared for in the ICU prior to transplant are at risk for prolonged ventilation due to pre-existing ventilation and concomitant loss of muscle mass. Patients intubated postoperatively for more than 5–7 d should most likely undergo a tracheotomy. Waller at al. demonstrated that percutaneous dilatational tracheotomy with direct bronchoscopic guidance can safely be performed in liver transplant recipients, even in the face of coagulation abnormalities.[27] Early tracheotomy provides the ability to reduce sedation, aggressively wean from mechanical ventilator support, improve patient comfort, enhance participation in physical therapy, and improve overall patient care.

Transient severe pulmonary edema might occur due to transfusion-related lung injury (TRALI). TRALI has been reported in LT and may occur due to transfusion of packed red blood cells, FFP or platelets. It has been linked to anti-neutrophile or anti-HLA antibodies contained in the transfusion volume. TRALI generally follows a transfusion incident and needs to be carefully differentiated from other causes of sudden de-oxygenation (pulmonary embolism, myocardial infarction, and acute respiratory distress syndrome (ARDS)). Sometimes temporary extra-corporal gas exchange may become necessary (extracorporal membrane oxygenation (ECMO)).

Neuropsychiatric complications

Neuropsychiatric complications occur in up to 30% of liver transplant patients and require extensive management in the ICU. Chiu et al. reported that after LT the three equally most common reasons for psychiatric consultation were delirium, anxiety disorders, and depression.[28]

The liver transplant population contains a high percentage of patients with substance abuse problems involving nicotine, alcohol, IV drugs, marihuana, medications for chronic pain, benzodiazepines and sometimes long-term methadone use to treat dependency states. Patients might have a pre-existing history of seizure disorder, sometimes due to past cerebral hemorrhage due to falls. During their liver transplant work-up, patients are found to have varying degrees of hepatic encephalopathy and if accompanied by renal insufficiency, a component of uremic encephalopathy. Both tacrolimus and cyclosporine have neuropsychiatric side effects ranging from coma and cognitive impairment to seizures, delirium, and neuropathies.[29,30] Susceptibility to calcineurin inhibitor (CNI) change during the transplant course might be related to changes in the blood–brain barrier permeability to circulating CNI due to improving liver function and the evolving ischemia reperfusion injury from the new graft.[28] The stroke risk is increased in post-LT patients compared to other post-surgical populations. Patients with hyponatremia are at risk for central pontine myelinolysis and patients with fulminant hepatic failure have increased intracerebral pressures. Doppler ultrasound for the evaluation of elevated ICP might be helpful.

The early extubation group generally receives pain management with short-acting opiates like fentanyl based on pain level assessed by ICU nurses. Fast-track patients are cooperative in the operating room before they reach the ICU. Any change in their mental status should be carefully evaluated. A common reason for change in mental status in this patient population is the effect of starting calcineurin inhibitors. The current authors routinely employ a "calcineurin holiday" and use induction agents to bridge the time period of observation. If there are any neurologic focal deficits or the patient suddenly becomes unconscious, a computed tomography (CT) of the head needs to be obtained to rule out a stroke. If mental changes go along with signs of systemic infections like fever and elevated white blood counts, systemic infection needs to be ruled by blood cultures. If central nervous system (CNS) infection is suspected as a source, contrast-enhanced magnetic resonance imaging (MRI) of the brain and then possibly spinal tap are indicated. If both sepsis and calcineurin inhibitors are excluded as the source, frequent symptomatic treatment and expectant management is indicated. Treatment of delirium and combative states with benzodiazepines frequently results in a long setback of stupor and coma. Aggressive therapy with antipsychotic medications is much more effective. Haloperidol, risperidone, olanzepine and quetiapine are successfully used depending on the route of administration and at low starting doses. Risperidone and olanzapine are available in a quick-dissolving tablet that may be given to ICU patients who have not yet been started on an oral regimen. Nevertheless, potential interactions must be considered. Later, after the transplant course, but sometimes during their ICU stay, patients might develop anxiety disorders and insomnia. There is again a temptation to treat this with benzodiazepines. If benzodiazepines are used, short-acting medications with no active metabolites (e.g. lorazepam) and the shortest possible course are recommended. The current authors have found, however, that most states of anxiety and insomnia are better treated with non-addicting agents like selective serotonin-uptake inhibitors (fluoxetine, paroxetine, sertraline, and citalopram). Fluvoxamine and nafzodone have significant interactions with calcineurin inhibitors and should be avoided. Psychiatric consultation is strongly indicated in these patients.

The patient population arriving in the ICU intubated may be more challenging. Patients with pre-existing, albeit remote, dependency disorders are sometimes not cooperative enough to be extubated in the operating room. Generally normalization of intracerebral pressure is fast in patients with fulminant failure and an eventual intracranial pressure (ICP) monitor should be discontinued within the first 72 h. If graft function is good but there is a history of hepatic encephalopathy or substance dependence, a combative, noncooperative patient who is difficult to extubate despite good pulmonary function is common. In patients with prolonged neurologic deficit, neurologic consultation should be obtained, and status epilepticus ruled out by electroencephalogram (EEG). Even if there are no signs of systemic infections, fungal infections should be considered, especially in the debilitated patient population (those with severe prolonged liver disease, re-transplantation).

Surgical complications

Despite standardization and technical advances in LT, technical complications occur during the stay in the ICU. The most feared surgical complication is HAT. Today the incidence should be <2–3%, albeit higher in pediatric recipients. Of these patients, 30% develop signs of acute hepatic necrosis with high transaminases, sepsis, mental status changes and coagulopathy, but some courses are more subacute with progressive biliary infections and hepatic dysfunction. Suspicion of HAT should trigger immediate Doppler ultrasound potentially confirmed by an arteriogram. CT angiograms or MRIs have been shown to be appropriate substitutes for conventional angiography. In many organ procurement systems, HAT within the first week after OLT is an absolute indication for the relisting of the recipient with urgent status.

Portal vein thrombosis in the ICU is also a rare vascular complication and is diagnosed by Doppler ultrasound. Graft failure due to portal vein thrombosis has been reported, but is infrequent and the majority of cases will present with manifestation of portal hypertension like massive ascites and possibly gastrointestinal bleeding. If the diagnosis is made during the ICU stay, the patient will generally be re-explored and thrombectomized.

Graft congestion due to outflow obstruction at the suprahepatic vena cava anastomosis results in initially delayed graft function and possibly bleeding from hepatic congestion. Doppler ultrasound might give a hint but definite diagnosis needs to be obtained by conventional cavography. Surgical correction has been described, but is not always possible and patients frequently take a subacute course until balloon dilatation can be performed after a few weeks. Stent placement will sometimes be necessary.

Biliary complications remain frequent after LT with varying incidence between 1.6–18% for leaks and 3–23% for strictures. Multiple risk factors have been identified for biliary complications including technical issues, graft ischemia, and immunologic factors. Early bile leaks should be suspected in any patients with constant abdominal pain after liver transplant or unclear fever. Most leaks occur from anastomosis and present early; many require surgical repair although endoscopic stenting may be successful. Late bile leaks (after 30 d) are rare, while late strictures are the most frequent cause of biliary complications after LT, often associated with recurrent cholangitis. Treatment of anastomostic strictures usually requires endoscopic stenting; intrahepatic strictures are more complex and may lead to retransplantation.

Postoperative hypotension resulting from hypovolemia, decreasing hematocrit and/or bleeding from operative drains requires immediate return to the operating room to control bleeding. In most patients who are returned to the operating room for bleeding, no definite source of bleeding can be detected. Bleeding in these cases may be associated with fibrinolysis and diffuse oozing from multiple raw surfaces, especially at the retrohepatic (bare) area. A rule of 6 U transfused in the immediate postoperative period mandates re-exploration for control of bleeding and removal of hematoma. Delay in re-exploration can lead to renal injury, increased risk of infection, and sometimes ischemia of the graft due to under resuscitation and overuse of vasoactive agents.

There are no evidence-based transfusion algorithms available and adaptation of trauma algorithms is not recommended. Resuscitation of bleeding coagulopathic patients is largely based on absolute numbers of cells, prothrombin time/internationalized normalized ratio (PT/INR), and fibrinogen levels. Thrombo-elastography (TEG) has successfully reduced transfusion requirements and blood loss in cardiac surgery and the algorithms tested in those patients have been used in other patient populations. Antifibrinolytic therapy with aminocaproic acid may be initiated based on evidence of hyperfibrinolysis on TEG.

Nutritional management

Half of the patients undergoing LT are found to be malnourished by subjective global nutritional assessments and the presence of malnutrition is an independent risk factor for the length of stay in the ICU. Oral feeding should start as soon as possible after LT. A protein-rich diet is recommended as the liver patient needs 1.5–2 g protein per kg body weight per day. If oral intake is not sufficient, post-pyloric feeding through a tube should be instituted without delay. Glutamine-containing formulae have shown positive effects on outcome in critically ill patients and the current authors recommend their use in liver transplant recipients. Parenteral nutrition should be initiated if tube feeding is ineffective within 1 week.

Few centers routinely place a nasojejunal feeding tube to provide enteral feeding immediately postoperatively while the patient has a gastric and colonic ileus. In a randomized study of enteric tube feeding vs control, Hasse et al. have convincingly demonstrated that tube-fed patients had a better nitrogen balance, less viral infections, and a trend towards fewer bacterial infections when undergoing tube feeding within 12 h after LT.[32]

Peptic ulcer prophylaxis is important, especially in patients with gastro esophageal reflux or pre-existing variceal bleeding. Normally proton pump inhibitors (PPIs) are the first choice. In a sufficiently enterally fed patient, PPIs can be discontinued.

Due to the use of steroids tight glucose control may be challenging in liver transplant recipients. The current authors have applied the protocols of tight glucose control in ICU patients[31] to the liver transplant population and aim at keeping the plasma glucose levels between 5 and 9 mmol/L.

Prediction of risk

Survival models have been developed to help with patient and donor selection for LT but they may also serve as a surrogate to the intensive care specialist to estimate the morbidity of patients who are admitted after LT. Targeted management of risk arising from co-morbidities helps to decrease complications by addressing them early in the recipients' postoperative course.

Importantly, the outcome of LT today is dominated by two recent developments: the introduction of the MELD score in many transplant systems worldwide and the aggressive allocation of grafts with extended criteria to expand the donor pool and decrease time to transplantation for recipients. Several attempts have therefore been undertaken to better predict post-transplant outcome before the transplantation procedure (Table 26.1). They include models either considering donor (donor risk index, DRI[1] or recipient factors alone (survival after LT, Survival After Liver Transplantation (SALT) score),[33] or others that combine two dominant factors in donors and recipients (donor age and recipient MELD, D-MELD)[34] or even an extensive list of donor and recipient parameters (survival outcome following LT, Survival Outcome Following liver Transplantation (SOFT)).[35] Both strategies have disadvantages, as for example the selection of only one donor and recipient factor (D-MELD) implies no possibility to balance high donor age in high MELD recipients. On the other side, inclusion of numerous covariates (SOFT score) results in wide extension of the score range.

Based on the large United Network for Organ Sharing (UNOS) database, an extended analysis of 37.255 patients between March 2002 and September 2010 identified the six strongest predictors of post-transplant survival: 1) recipient MELD score, 2) cold ischemia time, 3) recipient age, 4) donor age, 5) previous OLT, and 6) life support dependence prior to transplant. A new balance of risk (BAR) score was suggested, based on these parameters, to stratify recipients in terms of patient survival. The BAR system provides a simple and reliable tool to detect unfavorable combinations of donor and recipient factors, and is readily available prior to decision making of accepting or not an organ for a specific recipient. This score may offer great potential for better justice and utility, as it appears to be superior to other recently developed prediction scores.[36]

Table 26.1 Currently available prediction models for survival (prediction of risk)

Name of risk model	End point	Parameters entering into model	Score range Score cut-off
MELD	Recipient survival on waiting list at 3 months	bilirubin INR creatinine	6 to >40
DRI	Recipient survival	Donor age Donor height Donation after cardiac death Split liver donors Race Donor cause of death from cerebrovascular accident Cold ischemia time	1 to >2
SALT	Recipient survival at 12 months	Recipient age Cholinesterase	
D-MELD	Overall survival	Race MELD	20 to >2000
SOFT	Recipient survival at 3 months	Age, BMI, Retransplant, previous abdominal surgery, albumine, dialysis, ICU status, Admitted to hospital, MELD, life support, encephalopathy, portal vein thrombosis, Ascites, portal bleed 48 hours prior, donor age, donor cause of death, donor creatinine, national allocation, CIT	0 to >40
BAR	Recipient survival at 3 months	MELD Recipient age Donor age Previous OLT, Life support prior to transplant CIT	0–27

References

1. Feng S, Goodrich NP, Bragg-Gresham JL, et al. Characteristics associated with liver graft failure: the concept of a donor risk index. Am J Transplant 2006;6: 783–90.
2. Ploeg RJ, D'Alessandro AM, Knechtle SJ, et al. Risk factors for primary dysfunction after liver transplantation – a multivariate analysis. Transplantation 1993;55: 807–13.
3. Guarrera JV, Henry SD, Samstein B, et al. Hypothermic machine preservation in human liver transplantation: the first clinical series. Am J Transplant 2010;10:372–81.
4. Sakka SG. Assessing liver function. Curr Opin Crit Care 2007;13:207–14.
5. Stockmann M, Lock JF, Riecke B, et al. Prediction of postoperative outcome after hepatectomy with a new bedside test for maximal liver function capacity. Ann Surg 2009;250:119–25.
6. Stockmann M, Lock JF, Malinowski M, et al. How to define initial poor graft function after liver transplantation? – a new functional definition by the LiMAx test. Transpl Int 2010;23:1023–32.
7. Rayes N, Seehofer D, Theruvath T, et al. Supply of pre- and probiotics reduces bacterial infection rates after liver transplantation–a randomized, double-blind trial. Am J Transplant 2005;5:125–30.
8. Sun HY, Cacciarelli TV, Singh N. Identifying a targeted population at high risk for infections after liver transplantation in the MELD era. Clin Transplant.
9. McGuire BM, Julian BA, Bynon JS, Jr., et al. Brief communication: Glomerulonephritis in patients with hepatitis C cirrhosis undergoing liver transplantation. Ann Intern Med 2006;144:735–41.

10. Nishida S, Nakamura N, Vaidya A, et al. Piggyback technique in adult orthotopic liver transplantation: an analysis of 1067 liver transplants at a single center. HPB (Oxford) 2006;8:182–8.
11. Mandell MS, Lindenfeld J, Tsou MY, et al. Cardiac evaluation of liver transplant candidates. World J Gastroenterol 2008; 14:3445–51.
12. Tsutsui JM, Mukherjee S, Elhendy A, et al. Value of dobutamine stress myocardial contrast perfusion echocardiography in patients with advanced liver disease. Liver Transpl 2006;12:592–9.
13. Guckelberger O, Byram A, Klupp J, et al. Coronary event rates in liver transplant recipients reflect the increased prevalence of cardiovascular risk-factors. Transpl Int 2005;18:967–74.
14. Ramsay MA, Simpson BR, Nguyen AT, et al. Severe pulmonary hypertension in liver transplant candidates. Liver Transpl Surg 1997;3:494–500.
15. Krowka MJ, Plevak DJ, Findlay JY, et al. Pulmonary hemodynamics and perioperative cardiopulmonary-related mortality in patients with portopulmonary hypertension undergoing liver transplantation. Liver Transpl 2000;6:443–50.
16. Walia A, Stoner T, Mandell S, et al. LTrAC 101 – Looking for Evidence. ILTS Meeting, Paris, 2008 (http://www.iltseducation.com/documents/LTrAC101_ABSTRACT-12-20-07-AW.pdf).
17. Biais M, Nouette-Gaulain K, Cottenceau V, et al. Cardiac output measurement in patients undergoing liver transplantation: pulmonary artery catheter versus uncalibrated arterial pressure waveform analysis. Anesth Analg 2008;106:1480–6, table of contents.
18. Massicotte L, Lenis S, Thibeault L, et al. Effect of low central venous pressure and phlebotomy on blood product transfusion requirements during liver transplantations. Liver Transpl 2006;12:117–23.
19. Feng ZY, Xu X, Zhu SM, et al. Effects of low central venous pressure during preanhepatic phase on blood loss and liver and renal function in liver transplantation. World J Surg 2010;34:1864–73.
20. Mandell MS, Stoner TJ, Barnett R, et al. A multicenter evaluation of safety of early extubation in liver transplant recipients. Liver Transpl 2007;13:1557–63.
21. Gupta S, Castel H, Rao RV, et al. Improved survival after liver transplantation in patients with hepatopulmonary syndrome. Am J Transplant 2010;10:354–63.
22. Faenza S, Ravaglia MS, Cimatti M, et al. Analysis of the causal factors of prolonged mechanical ventilation after orthotopic liver transplant. Transplant Proc 2006;38:1131–4.
23. Bredenberg CE, Paskanik AM. Relation of portal hemodynamics to cardiac output during mechanical ventilation with PEEP. Ann Surg 1983;198:218–22.
24. Brienza N, Revelly JP, Ayuse T, et al. Effects of PEEP on liver arterial and venous blood flows. Am J Respir Crit Care Med 1995;152:504–10.
25. Fujita Y. Effects of PEEP on splanchnic hemodynamics and blood volume. Acta Anaesthesiol Scand 1993;37: 427–31.
26. Saner FH, Olde Damink SW, Pavlakovic G, et al. How far can we go with positive end-expiratory pressure (PEEP) in liver transplant patients? J Clin Anesth 2010;22:104–9.
27. Waller EA, Aduen JF, Kramer DJ, et al. Safety of percutaneous dilatational tracheostomy with direct bronchoscopic guidance for solid organ allograft recipients. Mayo Clin Proc 2007;82:1502–8.
28. Bechstein WO. Neurotoxicity of calcineurin inhibitors: impact and clinical management. Transpl Int 2000;13: 313–26.
29. DiMartini A, Crone C, Fireman M, et al. Psychiatric aspects of organ transplantation in critical care. Crit Care Clin 2008;24:949–81, x.
30. Chiu NM, Chen CL, Cheng AT. Psychiatric consultation for post-liver-transplantation patients. Psychiatry Clin Neurosci 2009;63:471–7.
31. Hasse JM, Blue LS, Liepa GU, et al. Early enteral nutrition support in patients undergoing liver transplantation. JPEN J Parenter Enteral Nutr 1995;19:437–43.
32. van den Berghe G, Wouters P, Weekers F, et al. Intensive insulin therapy in the critically ill patients. N Engl J Med 2001;345:1359–67.
33. Weismuller TJ, Prokein J, Becker T, et al. Prediction of survival after liver transplantation by pre-transplant parameters. Scand J Gastroenterol 2008;43:736–46.
34. Halldorson JB, Bakthavatsalam R, Fix O, et al. D-MELD, a simple predictor of post liver transplant mortality for optimization of donor/recipient matching. Am J Transplant 2009;9:318–26.
35. Rana A, Hardy MA, Halazun KJ, et al. Survival outcomes following liver transplantation (SOFT) score: a novel method to predict patient survival following liver transplantation. Am J Transplant 2008;8:2537–46.
36. Dutkowski P, Oberkofler C, Slankamenac K, et al. Are there better guidelines for allocation in liver Transplantation – a novel score targeting justice and utility in the MELD Era. Ann Surg 2011 (in press).

27 Rejection and immunosuppression trends in liver transplantation

James F. Trotter
Annette C. and Harold C. Simmons Transplant Institute, Baylor University Medical Center, Dallas, TX, USA

Key learning points
- Acute cellular rejection is a common complication of liver transplantation, but it has no negative impact on long-term patient survival.
- Chronic rejection occurs in <5% of recipients and may lead to progressive graft loss.
- The most common immunosuppressive regimen for liver transplant recipients at the time of discharge is tacrolimus, mycophenolate mofetil (MMF), and prednisone.
- Chronic renal failure is a common complication of long-term immunosuppression and avoidance of calcineurin inhibitors is one strategy to attempt to minimize this problem.
- Two new classes of immunosuppressive drugs used in liver transplant recipients are the biologics and inhibitors of the mammalian target of rapamycin (mTOR).

Introduction

Immunosuppressive therapy has progressively advanced since the inception of liver transplantation. The calcineurin inhibitor (CNI) tacrolimus (TAC) remains the backbone of the immunosuppressive regimen. New agents with better side-effect profiles, however, have taken a more prominent role in the immunosuppressive regimen of current liver transplant recipients to minimize complications in these vulnerable patients.

Despite the development of highly effective immunosuppressive agents over the past several decades, acute cellular rejection (ACR) remains an important problem after liver transplantation. Although less common, chronic rejection is frequently progressive and often leads to graft failure requiring consideration for re-transplantation. The goal of this chapter is to discuss the different types of rejection that may occur and their treatment as well as to review the current immunosuppressive protocols for liver transplantation.

Rejection

Allograft rejection is the response of the recipient's immune system against the donor organ and is most common within the first several months after transplantation. In general, rejection may take on two forms recognized as "acute" and "chronic," which have specific clinical and histologic characteristics. The treatment and outcomes of acute and chronic rejection are also quite different. At the current author's center, 56% of liver recipients are treated for biopsy-proven rejection at some point after transplantation. Rejection is most likely to occur in the first few months after transplantation with half of the episodes of biopsy-proven rejection occurring within 6 weeks of the operation.

Medical Care of the Liver Transplant Patient, Fourth Edition. Edited by Pierre-Alain Clavien, James F. Trotter.

The diagnosis of ACR requires vigilance by the clinical team and is primarily suspected based on elevations in the liver function tests (LFTs), primarily the aspartate aminotransferase (AST) and alanine aminotransferase (ALT). In almost all cases, ACR is asymptomatic, unless the problem remains undetected for weeks or months, at which time jaundice, itching, or fever may develop.

Once suspected, confirmation of ACR requires a liver biopsy, which may reveal the classic findings of portal lymphocytic infiltrate, endothelialitis and biliary duct damage. (The histologic findings are reviewed in greater detail in Chapter 29). Aside from verifying ACR, the liver biopsy is also important in ruling out other common causes of LFT abnormalities including recurrent hepatitis C (HCV), cholangitis, ischemia or cytomegalovirus infection. Patients with suspected rejection should undergo other diagnostic testing, usually an hepatic Doppler ultrasound, to rule out hepatic artery thrombosis, hepatic abscess or biliary obstruction. The grade of rejection is important to determine, because it dictates the type and duration of treatment. The most popular grading scheme is the Banff criteria, which classifies rejection as mild (grade 1), moderate (grade 2) or severe (grade 3).[1]

The clinical scenario is also important to consider in the diagnosis and treatment of ACR. Specifically, the pattern of LFT changes, recent immunosuppression levels, and underlying liver disease are important points to consider, particularly in HCV patients, where the distinction between ACR and recurrent hepatitis may be difficult because many of the histologic features are similar.[2] Features associated with recurrent HCV include, slow and mild elevations in AST and ALT (over several weeks or months), high HCV viral loads and adequate immunosuppressive therapy. Findings associated with ACR include recent rapid and marked increases in AST and ALT, low immunosuppression levels and absence of hepatitis C. Because the differentiation between ACR and recurrent HCV may be difficult and anti-rejection therapy with pulse corticosteroids may substantially worsen the clinical course of HCV, patients with indeterminate histologic findings may require a second biopsy after a short interval to confirm the diagnosis rather than suffer the problems associated with empiric treatment. While almost all centers require a liver biopsy prior to the treatment of ACR, a few do not, especially in the immediate perioperative period, when ACR is most common and the risk of liver biopsy may be greater due to persistent ascites and coagulopathy.

Treatment and follow up

The treatment of ACR depends upon the severity of rejection and response to treatment. For all grades of rejection, the most common treatment is a short course (usually three doses) of high-dose IV corticosteroids. The specific protocol varies between centers, but is usually three daily doses of 500–1000 mg of IV methylprednisolone. In some cases of mild rejection (Banff 1), however, treatment may be successful without IV corticosteroid pulses. In these instances, mild rejection may be controlled with an increase in the baseline immunosuppression or a "recycle" of oral corticosteroids, which is typically a tapering dose from 200 mg/d to 20 mg/d over 7 d. The response to treatment is an important determinant in duration and extent of therapy. Over 80% of patients treated with ACR rapidly respond to corticosteroid treatment with a brisk reduction in LFTs within in 24 h and normalization in the clinical laboratories over a few days. The change in AST is perhaps the best measure of treatment and a reduction of 50% may occur following the first dose of methylprednisolone. The reduction in ALT usually lags behind the AST, normalizing in 1 week or longer. In patients undergoing treatment for rejection with a persistent LFT elevation, however, a repeat liver biopsy is required to confirm the presence and severity of persistent rejection and to rule out other causes of liver test abnormalities. In fact, some centers routinely perform a repeat liver biopsy after completion of rejection therapy to ensure complete histologic resolution of the episode. In cases where rejection persists despite IV corticosteroid therapy, the term "steroid-resistant rejection" is applied. In these cases, a biologic agent, either anti-thymocyte globulin or OKT3, is indicated to treat ongoing rejection. The biologic agents are discussed in further detail later.

Because of their importance in the diagnosis of ACR, LFTs must be monitored at least daily in the immediate perioperative period and then at least twice weekly during the first month after transplantation. Thereafter, the interval may be increased to weekly or monthly, depending on the patient's specific clinical situation. The protocol for long-term monitoring of LFTs varies between transplant centers. Some centers require strict follow up with monthly LFTs for all patients. Other centers are more lenient and may lengthen the interval to 3 or 4 times a year, especially in patients many years from transplant who have remained clinically stable. Ongoing surveillance in long-term liver transplant recipients is important, because ACR may occur even in these patients. In such cases a recent change in immunosuppression or noncompliance are common occurrences.

The long-term consequences of ACR are important to understand. Unlike renal transplantation, where rejection is associated with a long-term loss of graft function, the occurrence of ACR in liver transplant recipients may improve outcomes. Patients experiencing rejection within the first 6 weeks after transplant have a significantly higher long-term survival rate compared to patients not experiencing rejection.[3] One possible explanation for this phenomenon is that recipients with rejection may experience "clonal deletion," whereby recipient clones of immune cells directed against the graft are expended during the early rejection episode. This may lead to better immunologic acceptance of the graft with a correspondingly lower requirement of immunosuppression and improved survival.[4] In HCV-infected liver recipients, however, the treatment of rejection may significantly worsen the clinical course of post-transplant hepatitis. In fact, the administration of multiple courses of IV corticosteroid therapy and OKT3 in the treatment of steroid-resistant rejection are associated with acceleration of recurrent HCV.[5–8] Therefore, these therapies should be administered very cautiously in patients with HCV.

Occurring in <5% of liver recipients at 5 years post transplantation, chronic rejection is an uncommon complication after liver transplantation;[9] however because frequent progression leads to graft loss, chronic rejection has ominous implications. Historically, the rates of chronic rejection were much higher in the early recipients of liver transplantation, occurring in up to 20% of patients. However, with improved recognition of the condition and its risk factors along with development of more effective immunosuppressive agents and management, the current incidence is much lower.[10,11] Specifically, the risk factors for chronic rejection include refractory ACR, prolonged noncompliance with maintenance immunosuppressive therapy, a pediatric recipient, and treatment with immune-activating drugs (including interferon as therapy for recurrent hepatitis C). In addition, chronic rejection is likely to be less common in patients receiving TAC compared to cyclosporine (CSA).[12]

The diagnosis of chronic rejection is suspected in patients with elevated LFTs, although the pattern and course are different from ACR. The classic pattern of chronic rejection is that of a cholestatic picture with elevations in the alkaline phosphatase and total bilirubin. The clinical course of chronic rejection is usually more protracted than ACR and typically evolves over weeks or months. Confirmation of the diagnosis requires a liver biopsy whose histologic findings are very different from ACR.[9,13] There is minimal or mild portal inflammation with bile duct inflammation, leading to atrophy and loss of all bile ducts. The biopsy may also rule out other common causes of chronic cholestasis, which may clinically simulate chronic rejection including cytomegalovirus (CMV) infection, drug toxicity, and cholangitis due to biliary obstruction, ischemia, or recurrent primary sclerosing cholangitis (PSC). The differentiation between chronic rejection and drug reaction is relatively easy based on the histologic findings and in the case of CMV, immunohistochemical stains and systemic viral levels. The histologic findings are helpful in differentiating chronic rejection from recurrent PSC, recurrent primary biliary cirrhosis, and biliary obstruction. Separating cholangitis from chronic rejection, however, can be more difficult, especially regarding ischemic cholangitis, which may mimic chronic rejection since both conditions have the absence of microscopic biliary ducts and intrahepatic strictures. Consequently, other diagnostic tests including hepatic Doppler ultrasound, cross-sectional imaging and cholangiography are required to evaluate the patient with suspected chronic rejection.

The treatment of chronic rejection is difficult and may be ineffective. IV corticosteroids and biologic agents are not usually effective in the treatment of chronic rejection, unless ACR is present concurrently, which sometimes occurs in patients who have stopped immunosuppression due to noncompliance or other reasons. For patients who have been noncompliant, reinstitution of immunosuppression is mandatory. For compliant patients, an increase or change in immunosuppression may be useful. There is evidence that chronic rejection is less likely for patients on TAC. Therefore, patients on CSA who develop chronic rejection may benefit from conversion to TAC.[14,15]

Immunosuppression

Since the first liver transplant, immunosuppression has always required a careful balance between the benefit of organ preservation vs the risk of medication side effects.[16,17] During the early years of transplantation, the array of immunosuppressive agents was limited to drugs with nontargeted effects, such as azathioprine and prednisone. The broad immunosuppressive effects of these agents combined with their poor side-effect profile contributed to the marginal outcomes of early liver transplant recipients. One of the most important developments in the successful evolution of liver transplantation was the discovery of CSA, which targeted the T-cell, the prime agent of acute cellular rejection. The enhanced efficacy and relatively limited side-effect profile of CSA led to a marked improvement in post-transplantation outcomes. As a result, the introduction of CSA in 1984 ushered in the modern era of liver transplantation during which time the procedure has been widely applied with remarkably successful outcomes.

Over the subsequent quarter century, the progression of immunosuppressive therapy has continued with the development of new drugs with greater potency and less toxicity. According to statistics from the Scientific Registry of Transplant Recipients, the occurrence of ACR has dropped by approximately 50% in the past 10 years. In 1993, approximately half of liver transplant recipients experienced acute cellular rejection and this number dropped to only 25% by 2002.[18] Consequently, rejection is rarely a cause of graft loss for liver recipients due to the introduction of newer and more efficacious immunosuppressive drugs, primarily TAC, MMF and biologic agents (see discussion later).

Changes in the demographics of liver transplant recipients over the past quarter century have also impacted the management of immunosuppression. Perhaps the most important trend is the increasing prevalence of HCV-infected patients. In the early phases of liver transplantation, HCV was present in <25% of recipients, however this proportion has increased to the extent that at most liver transplant centers in the world, HCV is the most common indication for transplant, often more common than all other indications combined (>50%). Patients infected with HCV at the time of transplantation invariably remain infected after surgery, when the virus attacks the new organ. The severity of damage caused by the virus is directly related to the level of immunosuppression. Suppression of the natural immunity against HCV leads to increased HCV viral replication, liver damage and ultimately loss of the graft and patient. Specifically, the administration of high levels of immunosuppression for the treatment of ACR with OKT3 and IV corticosteroid boluses significantly increases the rate of patient and graft loss, as will be described later. Therefore, immunosuppressive strategies that reduce the occurrence of ACR and overall immunosuppressive exposure may help to reduce the severity of HCV recurrence after transplantation.

Another important change in demographics is the increasing age and severity of illness in patients at the time of transplantation. In the 1990s, the mean age of recipients was only 44 years compared to 48 years currently. In addition, the proportion of patients who are over the age of 50 has increased nearly 50% from 42% in 1997 to 64% in 2006.[18] These older recipients pose new problems related to immunosuppression management. Older patients are more likely to suffer the common ailments of aging such as hypertension, diabetes, hypercholesterolemia, and renal insufficiency compared to their younger counterparts, therefore the selection of immunosuppressive agents should favor drugs with a side-effect profile that would minimize these problems.

Aside from advanced age, recipients are much sicker at the time of transplant compared to 15 years ago. This is due in large part to changes in the liver allocation system based on the Model for End-stage Liver Disease (MELD) score, which substantially increased the severity of illness in liver transplant recipients. Prior to the institution of MELD-based organ allocation, transplant recipients were less sick with a mean MELD score 14, whereas the current MELD score is approximately 22. The severity of renal complications has become particularly relevant, because the MELD score utilizes serum creatinine as one of its determinants. Specifically, the number of liver recipients with renal insufficiency has increased and the proportion of recipients whose renal function is sufficiently poor to require combined liver–kidney transplantation has increased threefold from 2% in 2001 to over 6% currently.[18]

Finally, the cohort of liver transplantation recipients is aging, due in large part, to the overall success of the procedure. Early in the experience of liver transplantation, patients and their physicians were pleased to achieve 3- or 5-year survival. Outcomes have improved to the extent that current liver recipients have an anticipated 10-year survival rate of 60% or more. As a result, the cohort of liver transplant recipients in the USA now exceeds 30 000.[18] As these patients age, the risk of hypertension, diabetes, hypercholesterolemia and renal disease increases due to the combined effects of aging as well as the long-term exposure to immunosuppressive drugs, in particular the calcineurin-inhibitors TAC and CSA. Therefore, the selection of immunosuppressive drugs with a side-effect profile that minimizes these complications is one of the most important long-term management strategies.

The current immunosuppressive regimen has developed based on the careful assessment of drugs in randomized, controlled trials. The most common immunosuppressive regimen for liver transplantation is TAC administered along with MMF and corticosteroids.

CNIs

Intracellularly, the CNIs activate their binding proteins (cyclophilin or FK-506 binding protein, respectively) and block the function of calcineurin, which has serine/threonine phosphatase activity. This prevents the production of interleukin-2 and the activation of T-cells, which are the prime agents of rejection. The standard dosage of TAC is approximately 0.1–0.15 mg/kg/d (or 7–10 mg/d in an average male) administered twice daily. While IV formulations are available, the drug is given almost exclusively via the oral route, where it is rapidly absorbed from the gastrointestinal tract. Peak levels occur 1–3 h after ingestion and clearance occurs primarily in the liver through the cytochrome $P450_{3A4}$ system with a half-life of approximately 12 h. Dose adjustments must therefore be made in patients receiving medications that augment or inhibit cytochrome $P450_{3A4}$ activity or in patients with marked impairment in hepatic function. Drug levels are measured at their trough, which occurs 12 h after ingestion and the dose of TAC is adjusted based on targeted blood levels. Because the immunosuppression requirements are highest in the immediate perioperative period, the TAC levels are the highest at this time. Thereafter, drug levels are run at a much lower level. While varying between centers, TAC levels are targeted between 8 and 12 ng/ml within the first 90 d, then lowered to 5–8 ng/ml between 90 and 365 d and in stable, long-term liver recipients, TAC levels may be run as low as 3–5 ng/ml. The pharmacokinetics of CSA are very similar to TAC, with rapid oral absorption and hepatic clearance through the cytochrome $P450_{3A4}$ system. The standard starting dosage of CSA is 5–7 mg/kg (or 350–500 mg/d in an average male) administered twice daily. Typical drug levels of CSA within the first 90 d of transplant are 200–300 ng/ml and decreased to 100–200 ng/ml between 90 and 365 d after surgery. Long-term stable recipients may run levels of only 50–100 ng/ml. There is some evidence that targeted drug levels of CSA based on samples measured 2 h after oral ingestion (C2) may help to minimize the toxicity of CSA and improve patient outcomes, however this practice has not been widely adopted.[19,20]

The side effects of the CNIs are discussed in Chapter 31 ("Medical problems after liver transplantation"), but deserve mention here. The most important side effect of CNIs is renal toxicity. This is caused by renal arterial vasoconstriction, which in the short term causes a drop in glomerular filtration rate and is reversible with a dose reduction.[21] Long-term vasoconstriction leads to the irreversible loss of glomeruli, renal fibrosis and ultimately renal failure. The renal side effects of CSA are likely worse than those of TAC, since CSA is associated with a significantly higher risk (relative risk = 1.25) of chronic renal failure.[22] As previously mentioned, the changing demographics of the liver transplant candidates and recipients towards an older and sicker cohort accentuate this problem. Common strategies to avoid renal toxicity after liver transplantation include reduction in the dose and level of CNI, conversion to a nonCNI drug and the delayed introduction of CNI in the immediate postoperative period, when renal function is most impaired (see discussion later). Table 27.1 shows the other common side effects of CNIs, the most important of which include hyperlipidemia (with CSA), diabetes, and hypertension.

Tacrolimus has demonstrated greater efficacy in three head-to-head comparison trials with CSA.[23–25]

Table 27.1 Side effects of immunosuppressant agents

Agent	DM	Htxn	Renal	Lipids	Renal	Cytopenia	GI	Other
Cyclosporine	+	++	++	++	++	0	0	Hirsutism
Tacrolimus	++	+	+	0	+	0	0	Alopecia
Mycophenolate mofetil	0	0	0	0	0	++	+	0
Mycophenolic acid	0	0	0	0	0	++	?	0
Sirolimus	0	0	0	++	0	+	0	*
Azathioprine	0	0	0	0	0	+	+	0
Corticosteroids	++	+	0	++	0	0	0	Weight gain
Biologic agents	0	0	0	0	0	†	0	0

*hepatic artery thrombosis, impaired wound healing, pneumontitis, proteinuria.
†anti-thymocyte globulin associated with leukopenia and thrombocytopenia. DM: diabetes, GI: gastrointestinal, Htxn: hypertension

In the US registration trial, which was similar to the European study, TAC + corticosteroids were compared to CSA + corticosteroids + azathioprine (AZA).[23,24] Patients receiving the TAC-based immunosuppression, experienced significantly less acute cellular rejection (by approximately 15%) and steroid-resistant rejection (by approximately 50%). A study evaluating the long-term outcomes of these patients substantiated the initial findings and further reported a significant survival advantage in HCV patients receiving TAC.[26] A subsequent study by O'Grady was a direct comparison of the new microemulsified formulation of CSA (which is the current formulation) and TAC. This study compared TAC + AZA + corticosteroids to CSA + AZA + corticosteroids and found improved outcomes in the patients receiving TAC.[25] Specifically, the primary combined outcome (of death, retransplantation, or treatment failure) was reached in significantly fewer TAC patients (21%) vs CSA (32%), $P = 0.001$. A long-term analysis of the participants in this trial showed better outcomes for patients receiving TAC.[27] Because of its superiority over CSA, TAC has become the predominant CNI and is administered to almost all liver transplant recipients (87%) at the time of discharge from the hospital. CSA is largely relegated to those few patients who are intolerant of TAC.[18]

MMF

MMF was approved for the prevention of acute cellular rejection in liver transplantation in 2000, although the drug was available prior to that time related to its use in renal transplantation. Following ingestion, MMF is rapidly absorbed and hydrolyzed to form MPA, which is its active metabolite. MPA is a potent and reversible inhibitor of inosine monophosphate dehydrogenase (IMPDH), which inhibits the *de novo* pathway of guanosine nucleotide synthesis. While other cell types can utilize salvage pathways, T- and B-lymphocytes are dependent for their proliferation on *de novo* synthesis of purines. As a result, the immunosuppressive effects of MPA are related to its potent cytostatic effects on lymphocytes. MPA itself has recently become available as an enteric-coated, delayed-release agent (EC-MPA). Unlike most other immunosuppressive drugs, the dose of MMF and MPA-EC are not based on drug levels. While there is some evidence the therapeutic drug monitoring may be beneficial in liver transplant recipients, the practice has not been widely accepted largely due to the fact that toxicity is poorly correlated with drug levels.[28–30] Therefore, patients typically receive the maximum tolerated or required dose. Although MMF is available in an IV formulation, the predominant means of its administration is oral. While MMF was approved for use in liver transplant recipients at 3 g/d, most patients are intolerant of this dose and the typical daily dosage is between 1–2 g and 720–1440 mg for EC-MPA. Peak blood levels are reached 1–2 hours after ingestion and after absorption MPA is glucuronidated in the liver to its inactive compound MPAG, which is largely excreted in the urine. Some enterohepatic circulation of MPAG occurs, but is of little clinical consequence. Dose adjustments are infrequently required in patients with renal or hepatic impairment.

The side effects of MMF are important to consider, because their occurrence often limits the administration of the drug, as shown in Table 27.1. The two most common side effects include cytopenia (leucopenia, thrombocytopenia, and anemia) followed by gastrointestinal symptoms of nausea and diarrhea. Frequently, these problems can be managed with a dose reduction, although some patients require discontinuation of the drug. In fact, many patients are discontinued from MMF due to side effects. While most (73%) patients leave the hospital on MMF at the time of their transplant, by 1 and 2 years after transplantation, only 47 and 42% of patients, respectively, remain on the drug.[18] In the MMF registration trial, 45% of patients were withdrawn from the medication due to side effects, the two most common of which were gastrointestinal problems and cytopenia.

One of the greatest advantages of MMF, compared to the CNIs, is that it does not cause diabetes, hypertension, or renal toxicity. Given the serious problem of renal insufficiency in liver transplant recipients, as discussed earlier, MMF is administered in many patients to allow reduction or discontinuation of CNIs.

MMF received its indication in liver transplantation following demonstration of increased efficacy compared to azathioprine. In a randomized, controlled trial the regimen of CSA + corticosteroids + MMF was compared to CSA + corticosteroids + AZA using a combined endpoint (biopsy-proven and treated rejection or graft loss at 6 months).[31] MMF was demonstrated to be a more efficacious therapy since significantly fewer patients on MMF (39%) reached this endpoint compared to those receiving AZA (48%). There are two other notable comments about this study. As noted earlier, 45% of patients randomized to MMF had to discontinue the drug (as noted earlier) due to side effects. In addition, although the drug was approved for use with CSA, MMF is almost always administered with TAC. In fact, 73% of US liver transplant recipients are discharged from the hospital on MMF or MPA-EC, making this class the second most prescribed drug for liver transplant recipients.[18] Therefore, the most commonly used immunosuppressive regimen used (at the time of discharge from transplantation) (TAC + MMF + corticosteroids) has never been evaluated directly for its efficacy in a randomized trial. This has created problems in the registration of new immunosuppressive drugs, because the Food and Drug Administration (FDA) requires new regimens to be compared to control patients receiving only FDA-approved regimens. The only approved regimens (CSA + MMF + corticosteroids) and (TAC + corticosteroids without any other agent) are virtually never used in current liver recipients, therefore utilizing these anachronistic regimens as the required reference regimen in a control group creates difficulty in analyzing the true efficacy of new regimens.[32]

There are many studies demonstrating the benefit of CNI reduction in the perioperative as well as maintenance phase of immunosuppression. One of the largest randomized trials evaluating the benefit of early CNI reduction in the immediate postoperative period compared (groups A) standard-dose TAC (target levels > 10 ng/ml) + corticosteroids vs (group B) MMF (2 g/d) + reduced dose TAC group B (target levels <8 ng/ml) + corticosteroids vs (group C) daclizumab induction + MMF + reduced-dose TAC delayed until the fifth day post transplant + corticosteroids.[33] The primary study outcome was renal function and favorable results were found with early CNI avoidance. The estimated GFR at 1 year decreased by 23, 21 and 13 ml/min in groups A, B and C, respectively (A vs C, $P = 0.012$; A vs B, P = ns). The rate of ACR was 28, 29 and 19%, respectively, and patient and graft survival rates were similar. Therefore, delayed and reduced TAC introduction with daclizumab induction + MMF + corticosteroids was associated with less nephrotoxicity than standard immunosuppressive therapy with no difference in safety of efficacy.

Three other randomized trials have shown the benefit of MMF in mitigating the side effects of CNIs from the time of transplant.[34–36] There are also multiple small studies evaluating the benefit of converting chronic liver recipients with chronic renal insufficiency to MMF, which allows lowering the dose of the nephrotoxic CNIs.[37–41] All of these studies demonstrate a benefit in renal function following conversion to MMF. There is very little data on EC-MPA in liver transplant recipients, although this drug may have the additional benefit of less gastrointestinal distress compared to MMF.[42,43]

Corticosteroids

Corticosteroids have been a mainstay of maintenance immunosuppression since the inception of liver transplantation. Their mechanism of action in the prevention of ACR includes myriad effects on the immune system including reduction of circulating T-cells as well as inhibition of leukocyte adhesion and inflammatory mediators. The side effects of corticosteroids are widely recognized by most clinicians and are noted in Table 27.1. In recent years, the use of corticosteroids has declined in liver transplant recipients. Because of the poor side-effect profile of corticosteroids, investigators began to study the effects of their discontinuation from the immunosuppressive regimen of liver transplant recipients. The first studies were performed in long-term, stable patients in whom the discontinuation of corticosteroids was associated with a significant reduction in hypertension, diabetes, and hypercholesterolemia without an increase in ACR.[44] As a follow up to these initial positive results, the same group showed that early withdrawal of corticosteroids immediately after transplant (within 14 d of surgery) was safe.[45] Numerous other studies have demonstrated that corticosteroid avoidance is at least as effective or more effective than their continuation. A recent meta-analysis found that corticosteroid avoidance was associated with a significantly lower incidence of hypercholesterolemia and diabetes with a trend toward less hypertension without any decrement in death or graft loss.[46] Therefore, corticosteroid avoidance has been widely adopted by the liver transplant community. At the time of transplant, only 78% patients are currently discharged on corticosteroids now compared to 95% in 1997. By 1 year after transplant, only 38% of patients remain on the drug. However, in some patients corticosteroids cannot be stopped. Typically, younger patients and those with autoimmune liver disease or recurrent ACR are less likely to be successfully withdrawn from corticosteroids.[47] These patients may require low-dose maintenance corticosteroids indefinitely.

Biologic agents

Although anti-thymocyte globulin has been around since the inception of liver transplantation, other agents have recently been developed in this class of immunosuppressive agents called biologics. As shown in Table 27.2, these drugs, which are antibodies to the T-cell or one of its surface receptors, include: alemtuzumab, anti-thymocyte globulin, basiliximab, dacluzimab and OKT3. The mechanism of action of these agents is related to inhibition of the respective T-lymphocyte cell receptor as shown in Table 27.2. In the case of anti-thymocyte globulin and OKT3, complement–mediate T-cell lysis occurs. Each of these drugs requires intermittent IV administration over a period of several days or up to 2 weeks, although their immunosuppressive effects may last for weeks or even months. Currently, none of these drugs is used in the chronic phase of immunosuppression due to their high cost and requirement of IV administration. The two primary indications for the biologics are: 1) treatment of steroid-resistant rejection, and 2) induction therapy. Currently, anti-thymocyte globulin is the most commonly administered biologic agent in the treatment of steroid-resistant rejection (62%)

Table 27.2 Biologic agents

Agent	Mechanism	FDA licensed purpose
OKT3	Murine monoclonal Ab against CD3 T-cell receptor	Renal ACR Renal, hepatic SRR
Thymoglobulin	Rabbit immuneglobulin against human thymocytes	Treatment of renal ACR
Basiliximab	Murine/human monoclonal Ab to IL-2 receptor (CD25)	Renal ACR prophylaxis with CSA + steroids
Daclizumab	Humanized monoclonal Ab to IL-2 receptor (CD25)	Renal ACR prophylaxis with CSA + steroids
Alemtuzumab	Humanized monoclonal Ab against T-cell glycoprotein, CD52	Treatment of B-cell CLL

ACR: acute cellular rejection, CLL: chronic lymphocytic leukemia, CSA: cyclosporine, IL-2: interleukin 2, SRR: steroid-resistant rejection compared to OKT3 (24%).[18] This distribution has changed from 10 years prior, when >90% of cases of steroid-resistant rejection were treated with OKT3. The dosing of these agents in the treatment of steroid-resistant rejection varies from center to center, but is typically administered up to 14 d, depending on the severity and persistence of rejection. OKT3 is given at 5–10 mg/d and thymoglobulin 1.5 mg/kg/d.

Cytokine release syndrome may occur with any biologic agent, but is likely to be more common with OKT3. This syndrome is caused by the release of cytokines from lysed T-cells and may be manifest by hypotension, pulmonary edema and fever. To protect patients from this syndrome, pre-medication with antihistamine and corticosteroids may be beneficial. In addition, both agents cause lymphopenia due to their mechanism of action and thymoglobulin may cause significant thrombocytopenia requiring a dose adjustment.

The biologic agents alemtuzumab, basiliximab, dacilzumab and thymoglobulin are also used as induction therapy. Because they do not cause hypertension, diabetes, hypercholesterolemia or renal insufficiency, the biologics are administered in conjunction with other immunosuppressive drugs in the perioperative period, as induction immunosuppressive therapy, when avoidance of renal toxicity is paramount and IV administration of agents is the easiest. The use of biologic agents as induction agents has increased dramatically over the past 10 years, largely as a result of the increasing prevalence of renal dysfunction that is present in liver transplant recipients. In 1997, only 7.1% of liver recipients received a biologic agent as induction therapy, whereas in 2006 that number had increased nearly fourfold to 26%.[18] The most commonly administered biologic agents used as induction therapy are anti-thymocyte globulin (8.9%), basiliximab (6.5%) and daclizumab (5.7%).

Most of the biologic agents have been carefully evaluated in liver transplantation. OKT3 was studied more than 20 years ago as an induction agent and found to demonstrate no long-term benefit compared to CSA + AZA + corticosteroids.[48,49] Daclizumab was compared to a TAC+ corticosteroid regimen and at 90 d was found to have no difference in rejection, but significantly reduced the rate of steroid-resistant rejection by 55%, diabetes by 62% and viral infection by 55%.[50] Similarly, basiliximab + CSA + corticosteroids compared to CSA + corticosteroids, demonstrated a significantly lower rate of ACR (18%) and combined endpoint of graft loss/rejection/death (17%).[51]

There is limited data on anti-thymocyte globulin administered with TAC + MMF compared to TAC + MMF + corticosteroids. One study showed that a steroid-free regimen with anti-thymocyte globulin was associated with significantly lower rates of rejection and CMV with no difference in patient or graft survival.[52] Another study evaluated the addition of anti-thymocyte globulin to TAC + MMF + corticosteroids and found no measurable benefit from the addition of the biologic agent in terms of patient or graft survival, incidence of rejection or complications including nephrotoxicity.[53] The data on alemtuzumab in liver transplantation is quite sparse, reflecting its very limited use in liver transplantation.[54] Alemtuzumab is particularly potent and its biologic effects may last up to several months after a single administration.[55,56] Consequently, the dosing of other immunosuppressants must be done carefully to avoid overimmunosuppression. In fact, a clinical trial evaluating the effects of alemtuzumab in the induction of tolerance was stopped early due to an increased incidence of side effects and severe recurrent HCV has been associated with the drug. As a result, only 1% of liver transplant recipients receive this drug.

mTOR inhibitors

The final class of immunosuppressants used in liver transplantation is the inhibitors of the mammaliam target of rapamycin (mTOR). The two agents available for clinical use are sirolimus (SIR) and everolimus (EVR). SIR has been more extensively studied and utilized in liver transplantation.[57] EVR was not available for clinical use in the US until 2010, so fewer liver recipients have received this drug. Sirolimus binds intracellularly to the FK binding protein and inhibits lymphocyte proliferation through inhibition of the mTOR pathway, which impacts a variety of relevant biologic functions in liver transplant recipients. More than any other immunosuppressive, SIR has demonstrated potentially important positive effects in terms of the prevention of neoplasia and hepatic fibrosis.[58] SIR is also clearly associated with other deleterious effects including thrombosis, increased wound complications and hyperlipidemia. Sirolimus is available only as an oral agent and is rapidly absorbed from the gastrointestinal tract.

While a loading dose for 1 d of 6 mg is recommended, most programs initiate therapy at 2 mg/d. The oral dose of SIR is dose-adjusted to achieve targeted blood levels, although the range is much wider than with the CNIs. Therapeutic levels of SIR are similar to TAC and range between 4 and 12 ng/ml, depending on the use of other immunosuppressants and the time after transplant. The metabolism of SIR is predominantly hepatic and dose reductions are required in patients with hepatic impairment or receiving other drugs that interfere with the cytochrome P450 pathway. The side effects of SIR are listed in Table 27.1 including hyperlipidemia, cytopenia and wound healing problems. Perhaps the greatest attribute of the drug is it absence of associated diabetes, hypertension, and renal insufficiency. As a result, it is frequently used as a means to reduce these important side effects related to the CNIs.

SIR is a particularly controversial drug in liver transplantation. Two randomized, controlled trials have shown an increased risk of hepatic artery thrombosis, graft loss and patient death.[59] Consequently, SIR is not approved in liver transplantation and, in fact, carries a "black box" warning from the FDA against its use in this population. An additional warning was released by the FDA in 2009 regarding conversion from a CNI to SIR in stable liver transplant recipients. Patients on SIR experienced a possible increased mortality rate as well as an increased rate of treatment failure (acute rejection), drug discontinuation due to adverse events including mouth ulcers and hyperlipidemia.[60] Despite these problems, SIR is still available for clinical use (because of its approved indication in renal transplantation) and continues to be administered to a surprisingly large number of liver patients. Only 1.8% of liver recipients received the drug at the time of transplant, but 1 year after surgery 11.9% of liver recipients were on SIR.[18] This difference in administration likely reflects the risks and potential benefits of the drug. Immediately after transplant, when the risk of hepatic artery thrombosis is highest, SIR is rarely used, however during the maintenance phase of immunosuppression SIR is utilized to avoid the renal toxicity associated with CNIs.

The potential benefit of converting liver recipients with renal insufficiency to SIR has been evaluated in a number of studies with disappointing results. Multiple uncontrolled studies have suggested a renal sparing effect of SIR in patients with CNI-induced nephrotoxicity converted to either SIR alone or SIR used in conjunction with a low-dose CNI regimen.[61–68] Small but more carefully controlled trials have shown variable findings with no change in glomerular filtration rate or unsustained improvements in GFR.[68–71] Therefore, it must be concluded that despite a strong physiologic rationale, at the present time, there is no convincing evidence that SIR improves long-term renal outcomes in liver recipients.[72,73] Based on the current data, if there is any effect it is likely small and therefore a large number of patients would be required to detect any benefit. Unfortunately, the large multicenter trial evaluating this question was discontinued due to a higher rate of death and complications in patients undergoing SIR conversion, as discussed earlier.

The evolution of immunosuppression is constantly changing, including the development of new drugs. Two of the newest agents are belatacept and sotrastaurin. Belatacept is an intravenously administered co-stimulatory inhibitor that acts by binding to CD80/86 on the T-cell.[74] Preliminary studies in renal transplantation have demonstrated improved long-term renal function despite higher rates of rejection compared to standard therapy.[75] Studies are currently underway in liver transplantation. Sotrastaurin is an oral agent that blocks T-cell activation through inhibition of protein kinase C. This drug has the advantage in that it does not seem to cause diabetes, renal insufficiency, or hypertension. The major side effect is gastrointestinal symptoms. Preliminary studies in renal transplantation have demonstrated some efficacy and investigations in liver transplantation are ongoing.[76]

Tolerance

While new immunosuppressive agents are an area of active investigation, on the other end of the spectrum is the study of the active withdrawal of all immunosuppression from selected liver recipients. This work is based on the observation that some recipients who stopped all immunosuppression (for a variety of reasons) suffered no ill effects.[77] Such patients are noted to be "tolerant" of their transplanted organs without the requirement for immunosuppression. There have been several published reports of the successful weaning of between 11–38% of liver transplant recipients from immunosuppression.[78] These observations led to investigations of operational tolerance (defined as long-term stable graft function without immunosuppression) in liver transplantation. The two main areas of clinical interest are: 1) whether specific immune markers could be identified to select patients who would be likely to undergo successful weaning,[79] and 2) whether there are any specific immunosuppressive regimens that would be more likely induce tolerance in liver recipients.[80,81] Studies are currently underway to answer these questions, however at the time of this writing, there are no reliable immune markers or immunosuppressive regimens that have been linked to operational tolerance.

References

1. Anonymous. Banff schema for grading liver allograft rejection: an international consensus document. Hepatology 1997;25:658–63.
2. Demetris AJ, Eghtesad B, Marcos A, et al. Recurrent hepatitis C in liver allografts: prospective assessment of diagnostic accuracy, identification of pitfalls, and observations about pathogenesis. Am J Surg Pathol 2004;28: 658–69.
3. Wiesner RH, Demetris AJ, Belle SH, et al. Acute hepatic allograft rejection: incidence, risk factors, and impact on outcome. Hepatology 1998;28:638–45.
4. Starzl TE, Fung JJ. Themes of liver transplantation. Hepatology 2010;51:1869–84.
5. Wiesner RH, Sorrell M, Villamil F. International Liver Transplantation Society Expert Panel. Report of the first International Liver Transplantation Society expert panel consensus conference on liver transplantation and hepatitis C. Liver Transpl 2003;9:S1–9.
6. Fong TL, Valinluck B, Govindarajan S, Charboneau F, Adkins RH, Redeker AG. Short-term prednisone therapy affects aminotransferase activity and hepatitis C virus RNA levels in chronic hepatitis C. Gastroenterology 1994;107:196–9.
7. Gane EJ, Naoumov NV, Qian KP, et al. A longitudinal analysis of hepatitis C virus replication following liver transplantation. Gastroenterology 1996;110:167–77.
8. Sheiner PA, Schwartz ME, Mor E, et al. Severe or multiple rejection episodes are associated with early recurrence of hepatitis C after orthotopic liver transplantation. Hepatology 1995;21:30–4.
9. Banff Working Group. Liver biopsy interpretation for causes of late liver allograft dysfunction. Hepatology 2006;44:489–501.
10. Wiesner RH, Ludwig J, van Hoek B, Krom RA. Current concepts in cell-mediated hepatic allograft rejection leading to ductopenia and liver failure. Hepatology 1991;14:721–9.
11. Neuberger J. Incidence, timing, and risk factors for acute and chronic rejection. Liver Transpl Surg 1999;5: S30–6.
12. Stanca CM, Fiel MI, Kontorinis N, Agarwal K, Emre S, Schiano TD. Chronic ductopenic rejection in patients with recurrent hepatitis C virus treated with pegylated interferon alfa-2a and ribavirin. Transplantation 2007;84: 180–6.
13. Demetris AJ, Murase N, Lee RG, et al. Chronic rejection. A general overview of histopathology and pathophysiology with emphasis on liver, heart and intestinal allografts. Ann Transplant 1997;2:27–44.
14. Cholongitas E, Shusang V, Germani G, et al. Long-term follow-up of immunosuppressive monotherapy in liver transplantation: tacrolimus and microemulsified cyclosporin. Clin Transplant 2010;Aug 16 [epub ahead of print].
15. Jain A, Mazariegos G, Pokharna R, et al. The absence of chronic rejection in pediatric primary liver transplant patients who are maintained on tacrolimus-based immunosuppression: a long-term analysis. Transplantation 2003;75:1020–5.
16. Fung J, Kelly D, Kadry Z, Patel-Tom K, Eghtesad B. Immunosuppression in liver transplantation: beyond calcineurin inhibitors. Liver Transpl 2005;11:267–80.
17. Starzl TE, Fung JJ. Themes of liver transplantation. Hepatology 2010;51:1869–84.
18. (http://optn.transplant.hrsa.gov/data/annualreport.asp) (accessed September 1 2010).
19. Shenoy S, Hardinger KL, Crippin J, et al. A randomized, prospective, pharmacoeconomic trial of neoral 2-hour postdose concentration monitoring versus tacrolimus trough concentration monitoring in de novo liver transplant recipients. Liver Transpl 2008;14:173–80.
20. Levy G, Grazi GL, Sanjuan F, et al. 12-month follow-up analysis of a multicenter, randomized, prospective trial in de novo liver transplant recipients (LIS2T) comparing cyclosporine microemulsion (C2 monitoring) and tacrolimus. Liver Transpl 2006;12:1464–72.
21. Naesens M, Kuypers DR, Sarwal M. Calcineurin inhibitor nephrotoxicity. Clin J Am Soc Nephrol 2009;4: 481–508.
22. Ojo AO, Held PJ, Port FK, et al. Chronic renal failure after transplantation of a nonrenal organ. N Engl J Med 2003;349:931–40.
23. The US Multicenter FK506 Liver Study Group. A comparison of tacrolimus (FK 506) and cyclosporine for immunosuppression in liver transplantation. The U.S. Multicenter FK506 Liver Study Group. N Engl J Med 1994;331:1110–5.

24. European FK506 Multicentre Liver Study Group. Randomised trial comparing tacrolimus (FK506) and cyclosporin in prevention of liver allograft rejection. European FK506 Multicentre Liver Study Group. Lancet 1994;344:423–8.
25. O'Grady JG, Burroughs A, Hardy P, Elbourne D, Truesdale A. UK and Republic of Ireland Liver Transplant Study Group. Tacrolimus versus microemulsified ciclosporin in liver transplantation: the TMC randomised controlled trial. Lancet 2002;360:1119–25.
26. Wiesner RH. A long-term comparison of tacrolimus (FK506) versus cyclosporine in liver transplantation: a report of the United States FK506 Study Group. Transplantation 1998;66:493–9.
27. O'Grady JG, Hardy P, Burroughs AK, Elbourne D. UK and Ireland Liver Transplant Study Group. Randomized controlled trial of tacrolimus versus microemulsified cyclosporin (TMC) in liver transplantation: poststudy surveillance to 3 years. Am J Transplant 2007;7:137–41.
28. Van Gelder T. Mycophenolate blood level monitoring: recent progress. Am J Transpl 2009;9:1495–9.
29. Pisupati J, Jain A, Burckart G, et al. Intraindividual and interindividual variations in the pharmacokinetics of mycophenolic acid in liver transplant patients. J Clin Pharmacol 2005;45:34–41.
30. Tredger JM, Brown NW, Adams J, et al. Monitoring mycophenolate in liver transplant recipients: Toward a therapeutic range. Liver Transpl 2004;10:492–502.
31. Wiesner R, Rabkin J, Klintmalm G, et al. A randomized double-blind comparative study of mycophenolate mofetil and azathioprine in combination with cyclosporine and corticosteroids in primary liver transplant recipients. Liver Transpl 2001;7:442–50.
32. Vincenti F, Klintmalm G, Halloran PF. Open letter to the FDA: new drug trials must be relevant. Am J Transpl 2008;8:733–4.
33. Neuberger JM, Mamelok RD, Neuhaus P, et al. Delayed introduction of reduced-dose tacrolimus, and renal function in liver transplantation: the 'ReSpECT' study. Am J Transplant 2009;9:327–36.
34. Jain A, Kashyap R, Demetris AJ, Eghstesad B, Pokharna R, Fung JJ. A prospective randomized trial of mycophenolate mofetil in liver transplant recipients with hepatitis C. Liver Transpl 2002;8:40–6.
35. Otero A, Varo E, de Urbina JO, et al. A prospective randomized open study in liver transplant recipients: daclizumab, mycophenolate mofetil, and tacrolimus versus tacrolimus and steroids. Liver Transpl 2009;15: 1542–52.
36. Yoshida EM, Marotta PJ, Greig PD, et al. Evaluation of renal function in liver transplant recipients receiving daclizumab (Zenapax), mycophenolate mofetil, and a delayed, low-dose tacrolimus regimen vs. a standard-dose tacrolimus and mycophenolate mofetil regimen: a multicenter randomized clinical trial. Liver Transpl 2005;11:1064–72.
37. Pageaux GP, Rostaing L, Calmus Y, et al. Mycophenolate mofetil in combination with reduction of calcineurin inhibitors for chronic renal dysfunction after liver transplantation. Liver Transpl 2006;12:1755–60.
38. Reich DJ, Clavien PA, Hodge EE. MMF Renal Dysfunction after Liver Transplantation Working Group. Mycophenolate mofetil for renal dysfunction in liver transplant recipients on cyclosporine or tacrolimus: randomized, prospective, multicenter pilot study results. Transplantation 2005;80:18–25.
39. Cicinnati VR, Yu Z, Klein CG, et al. Clinical trial: switch to combined mycophenolate mofetil and minimal dose calcineurin inhibitor in stable liver transplant patients – assessment of renal and allograft function, cardiovascular risk factors and immune monitoring. Aliment Pharmacol Ther 2007;26:1195–208.
40. Nashan B, Saliba F, Durand F, et al. Pharmacokinetics, efficacy, and safety of mycophenolate mofetil in combination with standard-dose or reduced-dose tacrolimus in liver transplant recipients. Liver Transpl 2009;15: 136–47.
41. Schlitt HJ, Barkmann A, Böker KH, et al. Replacement of calcineurin inhibitors with mycophenolate mofetil in liver-transplant patients with renal dysfunction: a randomised controlled study. Lancet 2001;357: 587–91.
42. Sollinger HW. Enteric-coated mycophenolate sodium – current and future use in transplant patients. Expert Rev Clin Immunol 2005;1:203–11.
43. Dumortier J, Gagnieu MC, Salandre J, et al. Conversion from mycophenolate mofetil to enteric-coated mycophenolate sodium in liver transplant patients presenting gastrointestinal disorders: a pilot study. Liver Transpl 2006;12:1342–6.
44. Stegall MD, Everson GT, Schroter G, et al. Prednisone withdrawal late after adult liver transplantation reduces diabetes, hypertension, and hypercholesterolemia without causing graft loss. Hepatology 1997;25: 173–7.
45. Stegall MD, Wachs ME, Everson G, et al. Prednisone withdrawal 14 days after liver transplantation with mycophenolate: a prospective trial of cyclosporine and tacrolimus. Transplantation 1997;64:1755–60.
46. Segev DL, Sozio SM, Shin EJ, et al. Steroid avoidance in liver transplantation: meta-analysis and meta-regression of randomized trials. Liver Transpl 2008;14: 512–25.
47. Trouillot TE, Shrestha R, Kam I, Wachs M, Everson GT. Successful withdrawal of prednisone after adult liver

transplantation for autoimmune hepatitis. Liver Transpl Surg 1999;5:375–80.
48. Millis JM, McDiarmid SV, Hiatt JR, et al. Randomized prospective trial of OKT3 for early prophylaxis of rejection after liver transplantation. Transplantation 1989;47:82–8.
49. McDiarmid SV, Busuttil RW, Levy P, Millis MJ, Terasaki PI, Ament ME. The long-term outcome of OKT3 compared with cyclosporine prophylaxis after liver transplantation. Transplantation 1991;52: 91–7.
50. Boillot O, Mayer DA, Boudjema K, et al. Corticosteroid-free immunosuppression with tacrolimus following induction with daclizumab: a large randomized clinical study. Liver Transpl 2005;11:61–7.
51. Neuhaus P, Clavien PA, Kittur D, et al. Improved treatment response with basiliximab immunoprophylaxis after liver transplantation: results from a double-blind randomized placebo-controlled trial. Liver Transpl 2002;8:132–42.
52. Eason JD, Nair S, Cohen AJ, Blazek JL, Loss GE Jr. Steroid-free liver transplantation using rabbit antithymocyte globulin and early tacrolimus monotherapy. Transplantation 2003;75:1396–9.
53. Boillot O, Seket B, Dumortier J, et al. Thymoglobulin induction in liver transplant recipients with a tacrolimus, mycophenolate mofetil, and steroid immunosuppressive regimen: a five-year randomized prospective study. Liver Transpl 2009;15:1426–34.
54. Marcos A, Eghtesad B, Fung JJ, et al. Use of alemtuzumab and tacrolimus monotherapy for cadaveric liver transplantation: with particular reference to hepatitis C virus. Transplantation 2004;78:966–71.
55. Agarwal A, Shen LY, Kirk AD. The role of alemtuzumab in facilitating maintenance immunosuppression minimization following solid organ transplantation. Transpl Immunol 2008;20:6–11.
56. Weaver TA, Kirk AD. Alemtuzumab. Transplantation 2007;84:1545–7.
57. Neuhaus P, Klupp J, Langrehr JM. mTOR inhibitors: an overview. Liver Transpl 2001;7:473–84.
58. Trotter JF. Sirolimus in liver transplantation. Transplant Proc 2003;35S:193S–200S.
59. Fung J, Marcos A. Rapamycin: friend, foe, or misunderstood? Liver Transpl 2003;9:469–72.
60. Food and Drug Administration. (http://www.fda.gov/Safety/MedWatch/SafetyInformation/SafetyAlertsforHumanMedicalProducts/ucm171828.htm) (accessed September 1 2010).
61. Fairbanks KD, Eustace JA, Fine D, Thuluvath PJ. Renal function improves in liver transplant recipients when switched from a calcineurin inhibitor to sirolimus. Liver Transpl 2003;9:1079–85.
62. Cotterell AH, Fisher RA, King AL, et al. Calcineurin inhibitor-induced chronic nephrotoxicity in liver transplant patients is reversible using rapamycin as the primary immunosuppressive agent. Clin Transplant 2002;16:49–51.
63. Nair S, Eason J, Loss G. Sirolimus monotherapy in nephrotoxicity due to calcineurin inhibitors in liver transplant recipients. Liver Transpl 2003;9:126–9.
64. Maheshwari A, Torbenson MS, Thuluvath PJ. Sirolimus monotherapy versus sirolimus in combination with steroids and/or MMF for immunosuppression after liver transplantation. Dig Dis Sci 2006;51:1677–84.
65. Sanchez EQ, Martin AP, Ikegami T, et al. Sirolimus conversion after liver transplantation: improvement in measured glomerular filtration rate after 2 years. Transplant Proc 2005;37:4416–23.
66. Morard I, Dumortier J, Spahr L, et al. Conversion to sirolimus-based immunosuppression in maintenance liver transplantation patients. Liver Transpl 2007;13: 658–64.
67. Neff GW, Montalbano M, Slapak-Green G, et al. Sirolimus therapy in orthotopic liver transplant recipients with calcineurin inhibitor related chronic renal insufficiency. Transplant Proc 2003;35:3029–31.
68. Watson CJE, Gimson AES, Alexander GJ, et al. A randomized controlled trial of late conversion from calcineurin inhibitor (CNI)-based to sirolimus-based immunosuppression in liver transplant recipients with impaired renal function. Liver Transpl 2007;13: 1694–1702.
69. Shenoy S, Hardinger KL, Crippin J, et al. Sirolimus conversion in liver transplant recipients with renal dysfunction: a prospective, randomized, single-center trial. Transplantation 2007;83:1389–92.
70. Campbell MS, Rai J, Kozin E, et al. Effects of sirolimus vs. calcineurin inhibitors on renal dysfunction after orthotopic liver transplantation. Clin Transplant 2007;21:377–84.
71. Dubay D, Smith RJ, Qiu KG, Levy GA, Lilly L, Therapondos G. Sirolimus in liver transplant recipients with renal dysfunction offers no advantage over low-dose calcineurin inhibitor regimens. Liver Transpl 2008;14:651–9.
72. Jensen GS, Wiseman A, Trotter JF. Sirolimus conversion for renal preservation in liver transplantation: not so fast. Liver Transpl 2008;14:601–3.
73. Asrani SK, Leise MD, West CP, et al. Use of sirolimus in liver transplant recipients with renal insufficiency: a systematic review and meta-analysis. Hepatology 2010;52:1360–70.
74. Vincenti F, Larsen C, Durrbach A, et al. Costimulation blockade with belatacept in renal transplantation. N Engl J Med 2005;353:770–81.

75. Vincenti F, Charpentier B, Vanrenterghem Y, et al. A phase III study of belatacept-based immunosuppression regimens versus cyclosporine in renal transplant recipients (BENEFIT study). Am J Transpl 2010;10:535–46.
76. Budde K, Sommerer C, Becker T, et al. Sotrastaurin, a novel small molecule inhibiting protein kinase C: first clinical results in renal-transplant recipients. Am J Transplant 2010;10:571–81.
77. Starzl TE. Chimerism and tolerance in transplantation. Proc Natl Acad Sci USA 2004;101:14607–14.
78. Orlando G, Soker S, Wood K. Operational tolerance after liver transplantation. J Hepatol 2009;50: 1247–57.
79. Martínez-Llordella M, Lozano JJ, Puig-Pey I, et al. Using transcriptional profiling to develop a diagnostic test of operational tolerance in liver transplant recipients. J Clin Invest 2008;118:2845–57.
80. Shaked A, Feng S, Abecassis M, et al. (http://clinicaltrials.gov/ct2/show/NCT00135694?term=immune±tolerance±network&rank=6) (accessed May 8 2010).
81. Benítez CE, Puig-Pey I, López M, et al. ATG-Fresenius treatment and low-dose tacrolimus: results of a randomized controlled trial in liver transplantation. Am J Transplant 2010;10:2296–304.

28 Vascular complications after liver transplantation

Goran Klintmalm[1] *and Srinath Chinnakotla*[2]

[1]Annette C. and Harold C. Simmons Transplant Institute, Baylor University Medical Center, Dallas, TX, USA, and [2]University of Minnesota Medical School, University of Minnesota Amplatz Children's Hospital, Minneapolis, MN, USA

Key learning points

- Vascular complications of liver transplantation threaten outcomes for patients and allografts. Detailed pre-transplant evaluation of the liver transplant recipient, careful planning and execution of the operation, early diagnosis of the complications, and prompt intervention can significantly reduce the incidence and morbidity of vascular complications.
- Hepatic artery thrombosis (HAT) is the most common vascular complication after liver transplantation. Common factors associated with HAT include technical imperfections with anastomosis, dissection of the hepatic arterial wall, and unrecognized celiac stenosis or compression by the median arcuate ligament.
- Doppler examination is a useful screening test for diagnosis of HAT. Operative exploration or selective celiac angiography is the gold standard for the diagnosis of HAT.
- Treatment of HAT is dependent on the clinical status of the patient. Patients who present with fulminant hepatic failure are best served by expeditious retransplantation. Recipients with early HAT who are asymptomatic or mildly symptomatic candidates detected on the routine Doppler ultrasound (DUS) done on the immediate postoperative day are candidates for graft salvage with operative exploration and arterial reconstruction.

Introduction

Vascular complications of liver transplantation threaten outcomes for patients and allografts.[1] Although bleeding, stenosis, and thrombosis can arise at any of the vascular anastomoses (suprahepatic and infrahepatic, portal vein, and hepatic artery), hepatic artery thrombosis (HAT) and portal vein thrombosis (PVT) are the most common.[2] HAT and PVT interrupt the allograft's blood supply and produce early graft loss, long-term dysfunction, or patient death, making these surgical complications life threatening. Considering the ongoing scarcity of hepatic allografts, vascular complications can have a profound impact on the application of liver transplantation. Detailed pre-transplant evaluation of the liver transplant recipient, careful planning and execution of the operation, early diagnosis of the complications, and prompt intervention can significantly reduce the incidence and morbidity of the vascular complications. This chapter discusses the diagnosis and treatment of vascular complications after liver transplantation.

Vascular considerations in the recipient

The liver has a dual vascular supply from the hepatic artery and portal vein. The hepatic artery provides 25% of the blood supply of the liver and about half the oxygen supply. The hepatic artery is the primary

Medical Care of the Liver Transplant Patient, Fourth Edition. Edited by Pierre-Alain Clavien, James F. Trotter.

vascular supply to the bile ducts. The portal vein supplies 75% of the hepatic blood flow and about half the oxygen. The liver drains into three major hepatic veins and 10–50 smaller caudate veins that open into the inferior vena cava. Knowledge of the hepatic vein anatomy is critical for the preparation of reduced size, split, and living related grafts. The goal of pre-transplant imaging is adequate visualization of the anatomy of all hepatic vessels.

A non-invasive and relatively inexpensive method of evaluating the hepatic vasculature preoperatively is duplex ultrasonography. This technique evaluates the portal vein for patency, direction of flow and the presence of a thrombus. The hepatic veins, inferior vena cava (IVC) and hepatic arteries are also examined. However, the bodily habitus of the patient and overlying bowel gas may cause inadequate evaluation of the hepatic vasculature by duplex ultrasonography, most frequently of the portal vein and proximal hepatic artery. For this reason the current authors recommend all patients also receive magnetic resonance imaging (MRI) with arterial imaging.

Arterial anomalies

Arcuate ligament syndrome

The median arcuate ligament is formed by fusion of the diaphragmatic crura on either side of the aortic hiatus posterior to the origin of the celiac axis. During embryogenesis, the celiac trunk migrates caudally, thereby resulting in a variable origin from the level of the 11th thoracic vertebra to the 1st lumbar vertebra. Consequently, a high celiac axis take off relative to the median arcuate ligament may result in a variable degree of celiac axis arterial compression[3,4] (Figure 28.1). The incidence of this anatomy varies from 1.6 to 10% in transplant recipients. The superior imaging modality is now MRI and magnetic resonance arteriography, which provide excellent visualization of the hepatic vasculature and accurate assessment for presence of median arcuate ligament syndrome. Presence of the median arcuate ligament is an indication for placement of an aortoceliac graft during the liver transplant.[5]

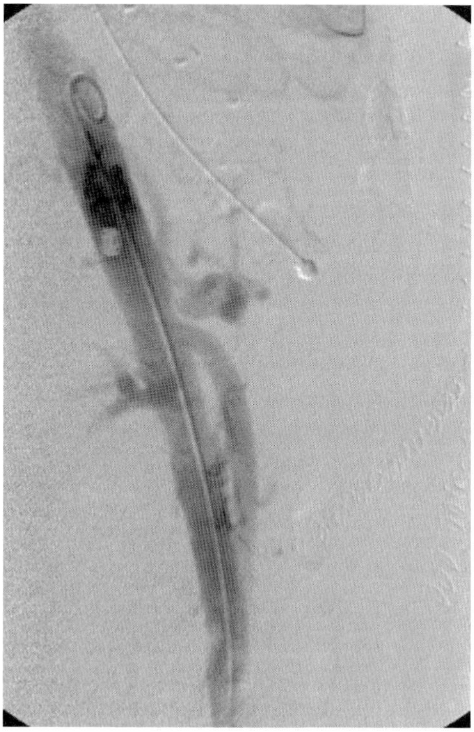

Figure 28.1 Contrast injection during an aortogram demonstrating a celiac artery stenosis due to arcuate ligament syndrome

Portal vein anomalies

Portal vein thrombosis is a well-recognized complication of end-stage liver disease and its incidence is estimated to range from 2 to 19%, reaching as high as 39% in certain patient populations.[6] Recipients with end-stage liver disease secondary to cryptogenic cirrhosis and Laennec's cirrhosis have a higher incidence.[6] If a portal vein thrombosis is suspected, either in the Duplex ultrasonography or MRI, the patient should undergo superior mesenteric angiography with a portal venous phase to evaluate the anatomy of the superior mesenteric vein, portal vein, and splenic vein. If there is a partial thrombus in the portal vein or even with a complete thrombus in the portal vein, thromboendvenectomy can be performed and flow restored in the portal vein during the time of transplant.[6] If that technique fails, placement of a venous conduit between the superior mesenteric vein and the donor portal vein may be the only option, hence it is crucial to know the anatomy of the superior mesenteric vein prior to listing the patient for transplant.

Back-table reconstruction of the donor arteries

Arterial variation occurs in 17–35% of all liver donors.[7] The most common are the accessory left hepatic artery arising from the left gastric followed by the right hepatic artery arising from the superior mesenteric artery. These variations are most efficiently addressed during the back-table dissection. The goal of arterial reconstruction is to establish a single source of inflow to the arterial graft. The most common arterial variant requiring reconstruction is a replace/accessory right hepatic artery originating from the superior mesenteric artery. In this situation the current authors' practice is to anastomose the artery to the gastroduodenal stump of the donor during the recipient operation after reperfusion of the main artery using interrupted 7-0 Prolene sutures. The reason for this sequence is to prevent the almost invariable malrotation of the replaced right hepatic artery that can occur if the reconstruction is performed on the back-table.[8] Carefully reconstructed arteries should not result in increased incidence of postoperative stenosis or thrombosis.

Vascular flow measurements

After the hepatic allograft is implanted, there should be good inflow into the new liver and also good outflow. It is a practice at the current authors' transplant center to measure arterial, portal venous flows, and pressures after implantation of the liver allograft. The hepatic arterial pressures are measured using an electromagnetic flow meter. The hepatic arterial flow should be at least 400 ml/min with a good waveform similar to an arterial line trace.[9] If the flow is less than that, the cause could be vasospasm within the liver, for which intra-arterial papaverine is injected and should increase the blood flow. Sometimes the portal vein flow is higher than normal and this could cause a compensatory decrease in the flow within the hepatic artery; in that case temporarily occluding the portal vein should increase the flow in the hepatic artery. If the flows continue to be low and if they are below 200 ml/min the current authors strongly recommend redoing the arterial anastomosis or the placement of an arterial conduit.[10] The portal vein flow should be at least 1 L/min. If the flows are lower than that, it is possible the patient may have extensive retroperitoneal collaterals that are diverting the blood away from the hepatic allograft. In that case, the current authors ligate the coronary vein and inferior mesenteric vein to increase prograde flow to the liver. The pressures are measured in the portal vein, hepatic vein and the right atrium or the IVC above the anastomosis. The pressure gradient between the hepatic vein and right atrium should be <5 mmHg unless there is a technical problem and the anastomosis needs to be revised. Paying careful attention to the details given earlier has greatly reduced the vascular complications.

HAT

HAT is the most common vascular complication after liver transplantation and the most common technical complication requiring retransplantation.[11,12] The incidence of HAT and to a lesser degree the mortality and morbidity attributable to HAT have decreased in recent years. Contemporary reviews demonstrate the incidence to be between 1.6 and 4% in adult recipients and 12% in pediatric recipients. A recent review of 71 publications describing 843 patients reported an incidence of 4.4% (children 8.3% and adults 2.9%).[13] Depending on the interval after liver transplantation, symptoms at initial evaluation, and the mode of therapy, mortality rates now range from 11 to 35% for adults.[13] Unfortunately HAT still carries an overall mortality rate of nearly 40% in the pediatric population.[13]

Factors associated with HAT include dissection of the hepatic arterial wall, technical imperfections with anastomosis, unrecognized celiac stenosis or compression by the median arcuate ligament, aberrant donor or recipient arterial anatomy, complex back-table arterial reconstructions of the allograft, and high-resistance microvascular arterial outflow caused by rejection or severe ischemia reperfusion injury.[2] With the use of transarterial chemoembolization as treatment for hepatocellular carcinoma (HCC), the hepatic artery can be traumatized, resulting in increased periarterial inflammation, friability, and a predisposition to HAT.[14] Gentle handling of arterial tissues is of paramount importance in hepatic arterial anastomosis. In addition, up to 20% of liver transplants are now performed for HCC, a malignancy associated with a generalized hypercoagulable state. So although technical precision is foremost in microvascular hepatic arterial reconstruction, other concomitant factors may predispose to HAT.

Clinical features

Acute, subacute, or chronic symptoms develop in patients with HAT, with the type of symptoms generally dependent on the time interval between OLT and the development of HAT. HAT occurring within 4 weeks is classified as early HAT and that occurring after 4 weeks is classified as late.[15] The most dramatic manifestation is fulminant hepatic ischemic necrosis, which occurs in one-third of the patients with HAT.[16] Patients often demonstrate rapid onset of hepatic decompensation with sepsis, fever, altered mental status, hypotension, and coagulopathy. Laboratory values are significantly elevated liver tests with aspartate aminotransferases and alanine aminotransferases in the thousands range. Another third of patients present subacutely in the early or late period with progressive symptoms related to ischemic bile duct injury.[17] Although adequate vascular collateralization may have occurred to prevent extensive hepatocyte necrosis, it has been demonstrated that collateralization may be insufficient to prevent ischemic bile duct injury.[17] Interruption of the singular blood supply to the biliary anastomosis may be manifested as transaminitis, leucocytosis, cholangitis, or sepsis syndrome with microscopic or macroscopic hepatic abscesses seen pathologically or radiographically. Symptoms may progress from an initial period of indolent postoperative fever of unknown origin to relapsing bacteremia, acute cholangitis, and subsequently, intrahepatic biliary necrosis. The remaining third of HAT patients may remain mildly symptomatic or asymptomatic. The diagnosis is usually made serendipitously while evaluating the patient for an unrelated condition or for transient mild transaminitis to rule out problems such as acute cellular rejection, hepatitis, or recurrence of primary disease. The significance of lack of specific symptoms is unclear; however, serious morbidity may develop over time if HAT is left untreated.

Diagnosis

Although the diagnosis of HAT is often suspected postoperatively, only through imaging studies or operative exploration, or both, can the diagnosis be confirmed. Most centers use duplex Doppler examination for screening purposes. It is difficult to ascertain the accuracy of ultrasound for HAT because not every patient is subjected to the test with the highest sensitivity necessitating operative exploration. The radiographic gold standard for the diagnosis of HAT is selective celiac angiography.

Treatment

Treatment of HAT is dependent on the clinical status of the patient. Patients who present with fulminant hepatic failure are best served by expeditious retransplantation. Recipients with early HAT who are asymptomatic or mildly symptomatic candidates detected on the routine DUS done on the immediate postoperative day are candidates for graft salvage with operative exploration and arterial reconstruction. The choice of the technique for hepatic arterial revascularization is critical. If the inflow from the recipient celiac axis inflow is adequate, thrombectomy with revision of the offending segment, whether it is the hepatic artery anastomosis or reconstructed, replaced graft vasculature is an option. Revision may require foreshortening of a segment of donor artery to prevent kinking and recurrence of HAT. If the celiac inflow is inadequate, an interposition iliac aorto-hepatic conduit is used. The current authors' preference is to use the infrarenal aorta. The operation is not complete until flows of >400 ml/min are demonstrated in the hepatic artery, otherwise the current authors perform an on-table angiogram to demonstrate the anatomy. Patients in whom late HAT develops and who have biliary sepsis as a consequence are also best served by retransplantation. Although new technologies have made non-operative intervention an option to deal with this complication,[18] the current authors' experience with catheter-directed therapies have not been encouraging, with most of the patients eventually requiring retransplantation.

Hepatic artery stenosis

Hepatic artery (HA) stenosis is an uncommon complication after liver transplantation with an incidence described as 4–5%.[10,19] Untreated, HA stenosis usually progresses to complete occlusion as a result of slow flow. HA stenosis has been demonstrated in patients following poor surgical technique, clamp injury and allograft rejection.

Clinical features

The clinical presentation of HA stenosis varies ranging from graft failure secondary to ischemia or necrosis to no influence in liver function.

The common clinical presentation is elevation of liver function tests.[10] The association of biliary complications with HA stenosis is well established. In patients with HA stenosis, the development of biliary complications has a significant impact on both graft and patient survival. Ideally, HA stenosis should be diagnosed and treated before the development of biliary complications. In case of biliary complications, conversion to Roux-en-Y choledochojejunostomy, graft loss or even patient loss may ensue. In some patients, hepatocellular drop-out noted on a liver biopsy and serendipitous discovery during a routine DUS may lead to the diagnosis of hepatic artery stenosis.[10] The median time to occurrence from transplant is 75–100 d.

Diagnosis

The DUS examination is a non-invasive method for the diagnosis of HA stenosis, showing a hepatic artery resistive index (peak systolic flow/end-diastolic flow/ peak systolic flow) of <50%. However DUS also carries a significant incidence of false-negative results. The gold standard for diagnosis is hepatic angiography. Narrowing of more that 50% or mean pressure gradient across the lesion of more than 10 mmHg is considered significant hepatic artery stenosis. The most common site of stenotic segment is the region of the arterial anastomosis followed by the donor artery.[10]

Treatment

The treatment method of HA stenosis mainly depends on the location and length of the stenotic segment, adequacy of the flow in the conduit artery and the experience of the surgeon.[20] For stenosis of short segments, excision of the stenosis and end-to-end re anastomosis appears to be the most appropriate method of arterial reconstruction.[10] If the blood flow is not sufficient in the recipient hepatic artery or if the stenosis is too long to enable primary anastomosis, the current authors prefer to do an aorto-hepatic iliac artery graft (Figure 28.2). The current authors' preference is to use a banked donor iliac artery graft (artificial (prosthetic) grafts only if banked vessels are not available) and radiologically placed stents. They avoid surgical reconstructions in patients with a primary diagnosis of hepatitis C, as they have noticed there is accelerated recurrence of hepatitis C after surgical clamping of the hepatic artery.

Portal vein thrombosis

Portal vein thrombosis complicates 3–7% of liver transplants and similar to HAT, can be fatal for both the allograft and the patient.[12] Factors associated with post-transplant portal vein thrombosis include technical issues (redundancy), pre-existing portal vein thrombosis requiring thromboendovenectomy at the time of transplant, small portal vein size (<5 mm), earlier splenectomy, and use of vein conduits for portal vein reconstruction.[2] The clinical presentation included fulminant presentation with elevated transaminases and graft failure, portal hypertension, ascites, encephalopathy, and gastrointestinal bleeding.

Diagnosis can be made on Doppler ultrasonography. Treatment when noted acutely is emergent exploration, and thrombectomy. The author's preference is to place a catheter in the inferior mesenteric vein and perform an on-table angiogram to ensure all the thrombi are removed. The same catheter can be used to infuse tissue plasminagin activator locally as well. In patients who present with graft failure, a liver biopsy is also performed at the time of exploration and if the biopsy shows >50% hepatic necrosis, the patient should be emergently retransplanted. Chronic portal vein thrombosis presents with gastrointestinal bleeding and ascites. Some patients may benefit from a surgical shunt.

Portal vein stenosis

Portal vein stenosis is an uncommon complication diagnosed in <1% of patients after liver transplantation. It is more commonly seen after living-donor liver transplantation in children.[21] The clinical presentation includes gastrointestinal bleeding, ascites, and

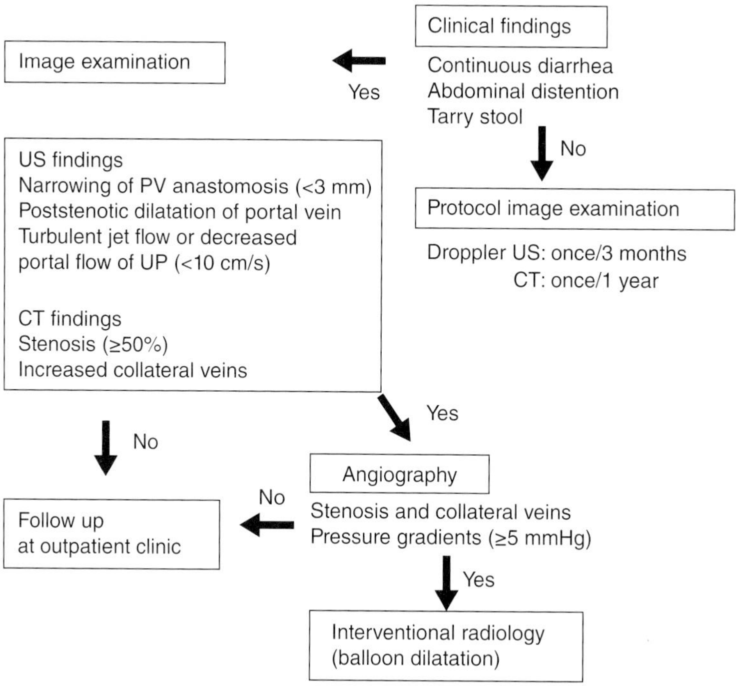

Figure 28.2 Management of HA stenosis. Based on reference[10]

continuous diarrhea. Diagnosis is by DUS and confirmation is by angiography.[22] Treatment is indicated if there is >50% narrowing or a pressure gradient of >5 mmHg, or there is narrowing with poststenotic dilatation. The first line of treatment is balloon dilatation by interventional radiology.[23,24]

Venacaval stenosis

Partial or complete obstruction of the inferior vena cava due to anastomotic stenosis or thrombosis leading to hepatic outflow obstruction, is a recognized but uncommon complication after liver transplantation with an overall incidence of <2%.[25,26] Early stenosis is often due to technical issues such as tight anastomosis, donor–recipient size mismatch, torsion of the IVC and/or intimal flap. Late anastomotic stenosis is more likely to be secondary to perivascular fibrosis, intimal hyperplasia, or external compression by a hypertrophied liver graft.[25]

Signs and symptoms of IVC and hepatic vein stenosis are often nonspecific and similar to those of portal hypertension. Ascites, increasing abdominal girth, peripheral edema, and laboratory findings of hepatic dysfunction are common findings. Computed tomography (CT), magnetic resonance imaging (MRI), or DUS scan can be used to diagnose anastomotic stenosis or thrombosis, but venography and pressure measurements are considered the gold standard, with a gradient of >10 mmHg commonly used as a diagnostic threshold for significant stenosis.[25]

Non-operative modalities for delayed IVC stenosis include balloon angioplasty with or without stenting.[27] Balloon dilatation is associated with a significant risk of re-stenosis. IVC stenoses are more resistant to angioplasty than hepatic vein stenosis. Surgical repair is technically difficult because of the short length of the suprahepatic cava and potential hepatic injury due to clamping of the hepatic outflow (and inflow). Surgical techniques include placement of a polytetrafluoroethylene patch, using a long synthetic graft and donor aortic patch, all of which are some form of refashioning the anastomosis.[28] The results of these procedures are variable and some patients eventually require retransplantation.

Splenic artery steal syndrome

This is a rare complication following liver transplantation, characterized by relative hypoperfusion of the liver graft. A prerequisite for this phenomenon is an enlarged spleen with a very prominent splenic artery. This structural rarity causes preferential blood flow to the spleen and results in detrimental hypoperfusion of the hepatic graft. The clinical diagnosis may be difficult, since it presents with elevations of transaminases, which may resemble the pattern of an acute rejection episode. A liver biopsy may show signs of ischemia and celiac axis angiography is essential for diagnosis. The treatment options include radiologic embolization of the splenic artery, splenectomy or aortohepatic vascular graft.[29] The author's preference is splenic artery embolization, which is quite successful and stops the diversion of blood flow to the spleen and prevents ischemic damage to the liver allograft.

Conclusion

Vascular complications after liver transplantation threaten the outcomes for patients and allografts, and can have a profound impact on the application of liver transplantation. HAT and PVT are the most common complications. Technical precision, especially in hepatic arterial reconstruction, is the foremost in preventing vascular complications. This becomes more important in the recent era, where 20% of all transplants are performed for HCC, and most patients receive transarterial chemoembolization (TACE), and the hepatic artery can be traumatized, resulting in increased peri-arterial inflammation, friability, and a predisposition to hepatic artery thrombosis. Early recognition of the vascular complications and intervention can save some of the allografts, however, when there is irreversible damage to the allograft or graft failure, expeditious retransplantation should be performed to save the patient's life.

References

1. Starzl TE, Porter KA, Brettschneider L, et al. Clinical and pathologic observations after orthotopic transplantation of the human liver. Surg Gynecol Obstet 1969;128:327–39.
2. Duffy JP, Hong JC, Farmer DG, et al. Vascular complications of orthotopic liver transplantation: experience in more than 4,200 patients. J Am Coll Surg 2009;208: 896–903.
3. Jurim O, Shaked A, Kiai K, Millis JM, Colquhoun SD, Busuttil RW. Celiac compression syndrome and liver transplantation. Ann Surg 1993;218:10–12.
4. Fukuzawa K, Schwartz ME, Katz E, et al. The arcuate ligament syndrome in liver transplantation. Transplantation. 1993;56:223–4.
5. Nikitin D, Jennings LW, Khan T, et al. Twenty years of follow-up of aortohepatic conduits in liver transplantation. Liver Transpl 2008;14:1486–90.
6. Molmenti EP, Roodhouse TW, Molmenti H, et al. Thrombendvenectomy for organized portal vein thrombosis at the time of liver transplantation. Ann Surg 2002;235:292–6.
7. Settmacher U, Haase R, Heise M, Bechstein WO, Neuhaus P. Variations of surgical reconstruction in liver transplantation depending on vasculature. Langenbecks Arch Surg 1999;384:378–83.
8. Klintmalm GB, Busuttil RW. The recipient hepatectomy and grafting. In: Busuttil RW, Klintmalm GB, editors. Transplantation of the liver 2nd ed. Philadelphia: Elsevier Saunders; 2005:575–87.
9. Molmenti EP, Levy MF, Molmenti H, et al. Correlation between intraoperative blood flows and hepatic artery strictures in liver transplantation. Liver Transpl 2002;8: 160–3.
10. Abbasoglu O, Levy MF, Vodapally MS, et al. Hepatic artery stenosis after liver transplantation – incidence, presentation, treatment, and long term outcome. Transplantation 1997;63:250–5.
11. Wozney P, Zajko AB, Bron KM, Point S, Starzl TE. Vascular complications after liver transplantation: a 5-year experience. AJR Am J Roentgenol 1986;147: 657–63.
12. Charco R, Fuster J, Fondevila C, Ferrer J, Mans E, García-Valdecasas JC. Portal vein thrombosis in liver transplantation. Transplant Proc 2005;37:3904–5.
13. Bekker J, Ploem S, de Jong KP. Early hepatic artery thrombosis after liver transplantation: a systematic review of the incidence, outcome and risk factors. Am J Transplant 2009;9:746–57.
14. Yao FY, Kinkhabwala M, LaBerge JM, et al. The impact of pre-operative loco-regional therapy on outcome after liver transplantation for hepatocellular carcinoma. Am J Transplant 2005;5(Pt 1):795–804.
15. Drazan K, Shaked A, Olthoff KM, et al. Etiology and management of symptomatic adult hepatic artery thrombosis after orthotopic liver transplantation (OLT). Am Surg 1996;62:237–40.
16. Shaked A, McDiarmid SV, Harrison RE, Gelebert HA, Colonna JO 3rd, Busuttil RW. Hepatic artery

thrombosis resulting in gas gangrene of the transplanted liver. Surgery 1992;111:462–5.
17. Northover J, Terblanche J. Bile duct blood supply. Its importance in human liver transplantation. Transplantation 1978;26:67–9.
18. Pinna AD, Smith CV, Furukawa H, Starzl TE, Fung JJ. Urgent revascularization of liver allografts after early hepatic artery thrombosis. Transplantation 1996;62: 1584–7.
19. Mondragon RS, Karani JB, Heaton ND, et al. The use of percutaneous transluminal angioplasty in hepatic artery stenosis after transplantation. Transplantation 1994;57:228–31.
20. Ueno T, Jones G, Martin A, et al. Clinical outcomes from hepatic artery stenting in liver transplantation. Liver Transpl 2006;12:422–7.
21. Kawano Y, Mizuta K, Sugawara Y, et al. Diagnosis and treatment of pediatric patients with late-onset portal vein stenosis after living donor liver transplantation. Transpl Int 2009;22:1151–8.
22. Cheng YF, Chen CL, Huang TL, et al. 3DCT angiography for detection of vascular complications in pediatric liver transplantation. Liver Transpl 2004;10:248–52.
23. Funaki B, Rosenblum JD, Leef JA, et al. Portal vein stenosis in children with segmental liver transplants: treatment with percutaneous transhepatic venoplasty. AJR Am J Roentgenol 1995;165:161–5.
24. Woo DH, Laberge JM, Gordon RL, Wilson MW, Kerlan RK Jr. Management of portal venous complications after liver transplantation. Tech Vasc Interv Radiol 2007;10:233–9.
25. Darcy MD. Management of venous outflow complications after liver transplantation. Tech Vasc Interv Radiol 2007;10:240–5.
26. Settmacher U, Nüssler NC, Glanemann M, et al. Venous complications after orthotopic liver transplantation. Clin Transplant 2000;14:235–41.
27. Pfammatter T, Williams DM, Lane KL, Campbell DA Jr, Cho KJ. Suprahepatic caval anastomotic stenosis complicating orthotopic liver transplantation: treatment with percutaneous transluminal angioplasty, Wallstent placement, or both. AJR Am J Roentgenol 1997;168: 477–80.
28. Saeb-Parsy K, Jah A, Butler AJ, et al. Use of a donor aortic interposition allograft to treat stenosis of the suprahepatic inferior vena cava after liver transplantation. Liver Transpl 2009;15:662–5.
29. Geissler I, Lamesch P, Witzigmann H, Jost U, Hauss J, Fangmann J. Splenohepatic arterial steal syndrome in liver transplantation: clinical features and management. Transpl Int 2002;15:139–41.

29 Biliary complications following liver transplantation

Sanna op den Dries, Robert C. Verdonk and Robert J. Porte
Department of Surgery, University Medical Center Groningen, University of Groningen, Groningen, The Netherlands

Key learning points

- The two main types of biliary reconstruction used in liver transplantation today are choledochocholedochostomy and hepatico-jejunostomy using a Roux-Y jejunal loop.
- The use of a biliary drain in liver transplant recipients remains controversial. Probably the only remaining argument to use a drain is to allow accurate monitoring and easy access to the biliary tree in high-risk liver grafts.
- Bile leaks and bile duct strictures (anastomotic or non-anastomotic) are the most common types of biliary complications after liver transplantation. Of these, non-anastomotic strictures (NAS) are the most troublesome and difficult to treat.
- Transplantation of a liver graft derived from a donation after cardiac death (DCD) donor, living donor, or a split liver carries an increased risk of developing biliary complications.
- Although ischemia of the bile ducts is a main risk factor for the development of NAS, other mechanisms, such as immune-mediated injury and bile salt toxicity play a role in the pathogenesis as well.

Introduction

Biliary complications are a major cause of morbidity and graft failure after liver transplantation. Although advances in the surgical technique of liver transplantation have led to a better overall outcome and fewer surgical complications, biliary complications still occur in 10–40% of recipients and are associated with mortality rates of 8–15%.[1,2] The continuing high biliary complication rate in liver transplantation can at least partially be explained by the increasing diversity of liver grafts used for transplantation in recent years. Besides livers derived from donation after brain death (DBD) donors, livers from DCD donors are increasingly used for transplantation, and these grafts are associated with a higher risk of biliary complications.[3] The use of these and other extended-criteria donor livers, however, is inevitable in an attempt to scale down the worldwide shortage of organs. In order to expand the pool of potential donors, split-liver transplantation and living donors have also evolved as surgical alternatives and numbers have increased in recent years, providing particularly young children with an opportunity to receive a graft in time. In western countries, both split- and living-donor transplantation currently account for about 10% of all liver transplantations, although there are large variations among countries. Some countries in Asia might even reach a living-donor liver transplantation rate of almost 100%. Yet, both surgical variants of liver transplantation carry an increased risk of biliary complications. Diversity in the quality and type of transplanted organs, variations in recipient risk factors, and variations in the applied surgical technique lead to a diversity in biliary complications that may occur after liver transplantation.

Of all biliary complications, bile leaks and bile duct strictures (anastomotic or non-anastomotic) are the

Medical Care of the Liver Transplant Patient, Fourth Edition. Edited by Pierre-Alain Clavien, James F. Trotter.

Box 29.1 Biliary complications after liver transplantation

Ischemic biliary complications due to HAT or stenosis
- Stricture
- Leak
- Bile collection (biloma)
- Biliary abscess

Technical biliary complications
- Anastomotic stricture
- Anastomotic leak
- T-tube related
- Parenchymal cut surface leak*
- Kinking of redundant bile duct
- External compression (cystic duct mucocele or hepatic lymphoma)

Ischemic-type biliary lesions / non-anastomotic strictures
- Ischemia-reperfusion injury
- Immune-mediated injury
- Bile salt cytotoxic injury

Infectious biliary complications/cholangitis

Uncommon biliary complications
- Sphincter of Oddi dysfunction
- Biliary stones, sludge, and casts

*Living-donor or split-liver grafts. HAT: hepatic artery thrombosis

most common types. These and other less frequent biliary complications are summarized in Box 29.1 and will be discussed in this chapter. First, surgical aspects of bile duct reconstruction that are relevant for the development of biliary complications will be covered, followed by a discussion of diagnostic and imaging methods and a description of the pathogenesis, clinical presentation, and management of the various types of biliary complications after liver transplantation.

Surgical technique in relation to biliary complications

Biliary reconstruction

The two main types of biliary reconstruction used in liver transplantation today are: 1) choledochocholedochostomy, also called the duct-to-duct anastomosis (using either an end-to-end anastomosis or a side-to-side anastomosis), and 2) a hepatico-jejunostomy using a Roux-Y jejunal loop. The use of one type of reconstruction instead of the other largely depends on the anatomical situation of the recipient's extrahepatic bile ducts and sometimes the surgical preference.

In case of a duct-to-duct choledochocholedochostomy, an anastomosis is created between donor and recipient choledochal ducts (common bile duct). An end-to-end anastomosis is generally easier to perform than a side-to-side anastomosis, and the former is therefore used more frequently. In a prospective, randomized trial comparing end-to-end anastomosis with side-to-side anastomosis, no major differences in outcome between the two techniques were found.[4] An end-to-end reconstruction restores the physiologic anatomical situation and does not carry the risk of bile sludge or cast formation as can occur in the dead ends of a side-to-side anastomosis.

In case of a Roux-Y hepatico-jejunostomy, an end-to-side anastomosis is constructed between the donor hepatic duct and a Roux-Y jejunal loop created in the recipient. Roux-Y hepatico-jejunostomy is mainly used in patients whose native extrahepatic bile duct is not suitable for anastomosis with the bile duct of the donor liver. The main indications for using a Roux-Y loop for biliary reconstruction are primary sclerosing cholangitis with involvement of the extrahepatic bile duct, biliary atresia, significant size discrepancy between the donor and recipient choledochal duct, and retransplantation.[1,2] Although a hepatico-jejunostomy may be a safe alternative when duct-to-duct anastomosis is not feasible, the disadvantage is that it creates an open connection between the intrahepatic bile ducts of the graft and the bowel lumen. This may result in reflux of small bowel content into the bile ducts and subsequently ascending bacterial migration and (recurrent) cholangitis. An additional advantage of using a choledochocholedochostomy is easier access for diagnostics and therapy compared with a Roux-Y hepatico-jejunostomy. It is, therefore, generally agreed that the preferred method of biliary reconstruction in liver transplantation should be a choledochocholedochostomy whenever possible.

Few centers have advocated and reported on the use of a direct connection between the donor bile duct and the recipient duodenum (so-called choledochoduodenostomy) as a safe alternative to a hepatico-jejunostomy.[5]

Use of a biliary drain

When reconstructing the biliary system in a liver transplant recipient, this can be done either with or without the insertion of a biliary drain. A biliary drain can be either a T-tube or a straight (open tip) catheter. A T-tube is a flexible tube that is inserted in the choledochal duct in the proximity of the end-to-end anastomosis in case of a choledochocholedochostomy. This tube allows the bile to drain in two directions: towards the duodenum and outward of the body. Alternatively, a straight catheter can be used, with the advantage of a lower risk of bile leakage upon removal of the drain as it results in a smaller hole in the bile duct after extraction.

Choledochocholedochostomy reconstructions over T-tubes have been the subject of controversy for many years, but it has nevertheless remained common practice in some transplant centers. Yet, with increasing surgical experience, many centers have begun to abandon the routine use of biliary drains in their liver transplant recipients.[6,7]

The benefits of using a biliary drain include direct visual evaluation of the quality of bile produced by the recently implanted graft and easy access to the biliary tree for radiologic imaging. Especially in liver grafts that contain a higher risk of developing biliary complications (e.g. livers from DCD donors) this could be an advantage. Some studies have suggested that placement of a T-tube may reduce the incidence of anastomotic strictures.[8] In addition a T-tube may result in adequate decompression of the biliary tree and a reduction of the intraductal pressure, which may subsequently contribute to a lower rate of intrahepatic biliary stricture and leakage.

The main drawback of using T-tubes is their association with an increased rate of biliary complications, especially bile leakage at the site of the drain insertion after its removal occurring in 5–15% of patients.[1] In addition, the use of a T-tube increases the risk of ascending cholangitis and peritonitis, due to an open connection of the choledochal duct with the exterior. In a recent systematic review and meta-analysis of studies focusing on the use of biliary drains in liver transplantation it was concluded that biliary drains such as T-tubes should be abandoned.[6] Although this meta-analysis showed lower rates of anastomotic and NAS in patients with a T-tube, the incidence of interventions was not diminished in comparison to patients without a T-tube. Patients without a T-tube had fewer episodes of cholangitis and fewer episodes of peritonitis. Yet, patients with or without a T-tube had equivalent outcomes with respect to anastomotic bile leaks or fistulas, the need for biliary interventions, incidence of hepatic artery thrombosis, retransplantation rate, and mortality due to biliary complications.

The use of alternative devices, like internal stents, have been reported by some centers, but these stents have been associated with increased rates of serious complications, including obstruction, migration, and erosion with hemobilia.[9]

The use of biliary drains such as a T-tube in liver transplant recipients, therefore, remains controversial. Probably the only remaining argument to use a T-tube is to allow accurate monitoring and easy access to the biliary tree in liver grafts that carry an increased risk of biliary complications, such as livers from DCD donors.

Relevance of donor/back-table procedure

Efforts to minimize the risk of biliary complications after liver transplantation should start with proper surgical and preservation techniques during the donor procedure. Aspects of liver procurement and preservation that have been demonstrated to reduce the risk of biliary complications include: 1) efforts to minimize ischemic injury of the bile ducts, 2) preservation of the vasculature of the extrahepatic bile duct by avoiding dissection too close to the bile duct, 3) thorough rinsing of the bile duct lumen to remove toxic bile, and 4) adequate arterial perfusion of the liver with preservation fluid to preserve the peribiliary capillary plexus. These aspects are relevant as biliary epithelial cells (cholangiocytes) are very sensitive to ischemia/reperfusion injury.[10] In addition to primary preservation-related ischemic injury, ischemic damage of the peribiliary plexus will result in secondary ischemic injury of the biliary epithelium. The strong relationship between ischemia and bile duct injury is illustrated by studies demonstrating an association between both cold and warm ischemia time and the development of NAS. As long as the cold ischemia time is kept below 10 h, the incidence of NAS is not increased, however more prolonged cold ischemia is clearly associated with a higher risk of such strictures.[11–13] Warm ischemia time, on the other hand, has been identified as a risk factor in several studies. The relevance of warm ischemia is also illustrated by the high incidence of NAS after transplantation of livers from DCD donors, which suffer an inevitable period of warm ischemia prior to organ procurement.[13,14]

During organ procurement, surgeons should avoid "stripping" of the extrahepatic bile duct, which will damage its microvascularization. The extrahepatic bile duct should always remain surrounded by an adequate amount of tissue to ensure sufficient blood supply.

Preservation injury results in increased arterial resistance and may cause circulatory disturbances in small capillaries, such as the biliary plexus. Since the blood supply to the biliary tract is solely dependent on arterial inflow, disturbances in the blood flow through the peribiliary plexus may result in insufficient oxygenation and subsequent damage of the biliary epithelium.

Gentle retrograde flushing of the bile ducts with preservation fluid is considered an important method to remove bile from the bile duct lumen. Bile contains bile salts, which are cytotoxic due to their detergent properties. Several studies have shown that bile salts may contribute to toxic damage of the biliary epithelium both during liver preservation and after liver transplantation.[15,16]

University of Wisconsin (UW) solution has been recognized as the gold standard preservation solution.[17] Although some studies have suggested that highly viscous preservation solutions such as the UW solution may result in an incomplete flush-out of the small donor peribiliary arterial plexus, resulting in a higher incidence of NAS,[11,18] this could not always be confirmed in other studies.[17] Therefore, it remains debatable whether low viscosity preservation fluids are associated with a lower incidence of biliary complications. Adequately powered randomized, controlled trials with long-term follow up are needed to determine whether the type of preservation fluid has an impact on biliary complications after liver transplantation.

One method to overcome inadequate flush-out and preservation of the peribiliary plexus is the application of high pressure arterial infusion of preservation fluid either *in vivo* during procurement or immediately afterwards on the back-table. Several studies have shown that additional flushing of the peribiliary plexus by controlled arterial back-table pressure perfusion may result in a considerable reduction in the incidence of NAS.[19]

Better flush-out and preservation of the peribiliary capillary plexus may also be achieved by machine preservation. Although machine preservation of organs for transplantation is receiving increasing attention and is the subject of intensive research, it remains to be established whether this technique will result in a reduction of biliary complications after liver transplantation.

Diagnostic modalities

In most cases, the suspicion of a biliary complication will arise after an increase in liver enzymes is noted. There is no specific pattern to reliably distinguish a biliary complication from other causes of graft dysfunction, although an increase in serum bilirubin, alkaline phosphatase and/or gamma-glutamyl transferase has been suggested to be most specific. Alternatively, patients can present with upper abdominal pain or bacterial cholangitis. In many instances of liver enzyme disturbances, a liver biopsy will be performed after gross biliary congestion and bile duct dilatation have been excluded by ultrasonography. The presence of specific pathologic features such as centrilobular cholestasis and portal changes including edema, predominantly neutrophil polymorph infiltration, ductular proliferation and cholangiolitis may be indicative of the presence of a biliary complication.[20] These findings, however, are not very specific and can be absent. In addition, biopsy findings are not informative with regard to the type and severity of biliary abnormalities.

The diagnostic work-up of an increase in liver enzymes will always depend on clinical context such as primary disease, time after transplantation, local experience, and information on the biliary anatomy. A general algorithm is provided in Figure 29.1.

Transabdominal ultrasonography

Transabdominal ultrasonography is a useful primary diagnostic tool when a biliary complication is suspected. Allograft vascularization can be assessed (especially patency of the hepatic artery), fluid collections can be identified, the liver parenchyma can

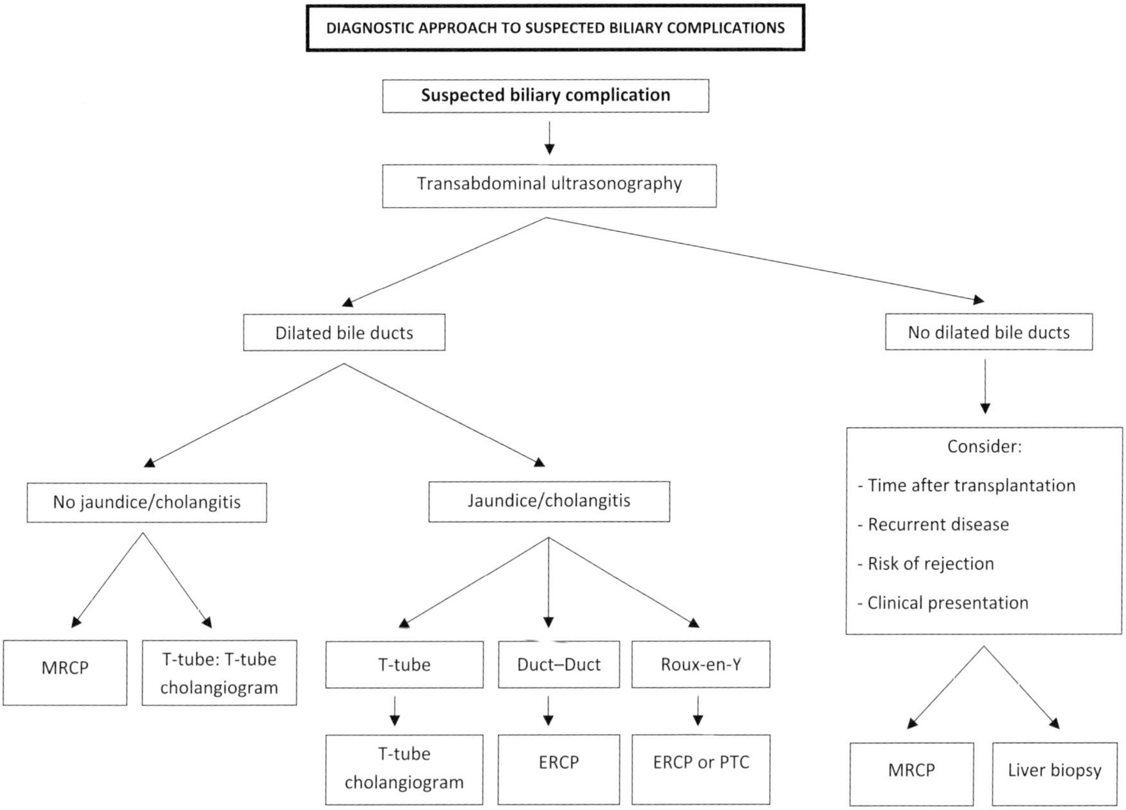

Figure 29.1 Schematic presentation of the clinical decisions and diagnostic steps in the work-up of a liver transplant recipient with a suspected biliary complication

be studied, and dilatation of bile ducts can be identified. It should be noted that the transplanted liver behaves differently from a normal liver, in that the biliary system does not dilate as easily in the presence of a biliary obstruction as in normal livers.[21] This leads to a limited sensitivity of approximately 60% of transabdominal ultrasonography to detect biliary strictures.[21,22] The predictive value of transabdominal ultrasonography to detect non-anastomotic biliary strictures is rather low. Therefore, normal ultrasonography of the liver graft in a patient with clinical or biochemical evidence of biliary pathology warrants further investigation.

Magnetic resonance cholangiography and computed tomography

Magnetic resonance cholangiography (MRC) is a rapidly emerging diagnostic tool for the detection of biliary abnormalities. It has the strong advantage of providing excellent anatomic information without being invasive. In the present era, every transplant centre should be able to offer MRC and have an expert radiologist in the transplant team. MRC is useful in the detection of both leakages and strictures. The use of an additional magnetic resonance imaging or magnetic resonance angiography scanning protocol can also provide information about the liver parenchyma and vasculature. The reported sensitivity and specificity of MRC for the detection of biliary complications is well over 90%.[23] After ultrasonography, MRC is the preferred diagnostic tool when a biliary complication is suspected. Recently, also computed tomography (CT) scanning has been suggested to be of value for the detection of post-transplant biliary complications – it has a higher spatial resolution compared to MRC. However, the experience with CT cholangiography after liver transplantation is very limited: 1) it can only be performed using a contrast medium, 2) it is associated with significant radiation, and 3) it is less reliable in the presence of biliary obstruction or high serum bilirubin levels. The use of CT cholangiography to detect a biliary complication should still be considered experimental.

Direct cholangiography

Direct cholangiography, either percutaneously or through endoscopic retrograde cholangiopancreaticography (ERCP), is the gold standard for the detection of biliary abnormalities. It has the inherent advantage of biliary access to facilitate therapeutic measures. Since the use of a biliary drain (e.g. T-tube) is no longer routine practice in most transplant centers, ERCP will be the most frequently used method to detect biliary complications. There is no data to suggest that ERCP after liver transplantation is associated with more complications than the use of ERCP in the general population. Considering the safety, diagnostic yield, and therapeutic potential of ERCP, this should be considered the preferred invasive method. In the presence of altered biliary anatomy, such as a Roux-Y hepatico-jejunostomy, ERCP is more difficult to perform. In these cases, percutaneous transhepatic cholangiography (PTC) or PTC drainage is a good alternative method to obtain adequate imaging of the bile ducts. In several series successful ERCP in the presence of a Roux-Y reconstruction has been reported using either a normal duodenoscope or double-balloon endoscopes.[24,25] PTC is most easily obtained in the presence of dilated bile ducts. In experienced hands, however, this can be a safe procedure also with undilated bile ducts.[26] It not only allows adequate imaging of the bile ducts, but also provides access for therapeutic interventions such as balloon dilatation (see later).

Hepatobiliary scintigraphy

Hepatobiliary scintigraphy can be used as a diagnostic tool to detect post-transplant biliary obstruction and leakage. It has a sensitivity of approximately 60% for these indications.[27] The main advantage is its non-invasive nature; its main disadvantage is low resolution and lack of direct visualization of the biliary anatomy. The sensitivity of hepatobiliary scintigraphy to detect NAS is not known. With the increasing use and availability of MRC, scintigraphy is today rarely used to detect biliary strictures. It could be of value in those patients in whom an obstruction at the level of the Roux-Y jejunal loop is suspected or when MRC is not possible (i.e. presence of a pacemaker).

Other diagnostic tools

Endoscopic ultrasonography is an emerging tool for the detection of hepatobiliary diseases. It has excellent diagnostic properties for the distal bile duct. Endoscopic intraductal ultrasonography can be used for the characterization of intraductal abnormalities. Use of these techniques in liver transplant recipients is still anecdotal. A potentially more valuable tool is direct cholangioscopy. With this technique, a small endoscope (cholangioscope) can be advanced through a normal duodenoscope to directly visualize the bile ducts. This can provide information about the biliary epithelium and the presence of stones, sludge and strictures. It can also be a therapeutic tool to advance guide wires or to remove bile duct stones. The number of indications for these highly specialized techniques, however, is still limited.

Pathogenesis, clinical presentation, and management

The most common types of biliary complication after liver transplantation are bile duct strictures and bile leaks. Strictures at the site of the bile duct anastomosis are often referred to as "anastomotic strictures." Strictures occurring at any other location in the biliary tree of the liver are called "NAS."

Anastomotic strictures

Pathogenesis and clinical presentation
Isolated strictures at the site of the bile duct anastomosis, so-called anastomotic strictures, are reported in 4–9% of patients after liver transplantation.[28] In general, anastomotic strictures do not remain subclinical and are detected after the occurrence of cholestatic laboratory liver function tests, jaundice, or cholangitis.[28] Anastomotic strictures are thought to result mainly from surgical technique and/or local ischemia, leading to fibrotic scarring of the

anastomosis. Surgical factors include inadequate mucosa-to-mucosa adaptation at the anastomosis and damage of microvascularization due to dissection too close to the bile duct.[29] To minimize the risk of local ischemia at the distal end of the donor choledochal duct, the bile duct should therefore remain surrounded by an adequate amount of tissue. Generalized hepatic ischemia due to hepatic artery thrombosis can also result in anastomotic stricturing. Other risk factors for the development of anastomotic structures are anastomotic bile leakage after transplantation and a sex mismatch between donor and recipient.[28,30]

Liver transplantation using a split graft or a liver derived from a living donor is associated with a higher risk of developing an anastomotic bile duct stricture, because of the frequent discrepancy between the diameter of the hepatic duct of the graft and choledochal duct in the recipient. In addition, vascularization of the hepatic duct can be compromised when a partial graft is derived from a living donor or split liver. These and other surgical aspects of living-donor and split-liver transplantation are discussed in more detail in Chapters 22 and 23.

Management

The most frequently used therapeutic approach to an anastomotic stricture is endoscopic balloon dilatation and stenting of the stenosis. This treatment has been widely studied and is both safe and effective. Technical success is obtained in 90–100%, and long-term resolution of the stricture in 70–100% of cases.[31] Although disputed by some, most centers obtain the best results with a protocol of progressive stenting every 8–12 weeks with increasing numbers and diameters of stents until resolution of the stenosis is obtained.[32] In some cases, the stenosis recurs despite effective initial therapy. Some centers have used a covered expandable metal stent to treat a refractory biliary stenosis after transplantation. This, however, is not routine practice. Presentation of an anastomotic stricture more than 6 months after transplantation and previous bile leakage at the site of the anastomosis are risk factors for difficult-to-manage strictures.[28] When an anastomotic stenosis does not respond to repeated dilatation and stenting, surgical revision or conversion to a Roux-en-Y hepatico-jejunostomy anastomosis is a good alternative with excellent long-term success.[28] Incidentally, narrowing at the anastomosis can be detected while it remains unclear whether this is a clinically relevant stricture. In such cases, a short trial of stenting can be of value.[33]

In the presence of a hepatico-jejunostomy, where the anastomosis is not accessible by endoscopy, percutaneous transhepatic treatment by balloon dilatation and temporary stenting is usually successful. This approach can also be used after split-liver or living-donor liver transplantation, although results are not as good, possibly because compromised microvascularization and local ischemia are more frequently the underlying cause.[31,34]

NAS

Pathogenesis and clinical presentation

Non-anastomotic biliary strictures are strictures at any location in the biliary system other than the anastomosis. Biliary strictures may be confined to the hepatic bifurcation, but may also present as a more diffuse type including narrowing of the more peripheral bile ducts in the liver. NAS can be accompanied by intraductal sludge or cast formation. This type of bile duct stricture is regarded as the most troublesome biliary complication as the strictures are often resistant to therapy and one of the most frequent indications for retransplantation.[31,35] The clinical presentation of patients with NAS is often not specific; symptoms may include fever due to cholangitis, abdominal complaints, and increased cholestatic liver function tests, either with or without clinical jaundice.

The reported incidence of NAS after liver transplantation varies between different studies, ranging from 1–20%,[1,2,13] which can partly be explained by variations in the definition of non-anastomotic biliary strictures used in different studies. About half of all NAS occur within 1 year after transplantation, and the remainder can be detected up to several years after transplantation.[31,35] In livers obtained from DCD donors, the incidence of NAS is about 10% higher and they may occur earlier than in livers obtained from DBD donors.[31,35]

NAS were first described after liver transplantation in association with hepatic artery thrombosis. In case of hepatic artery thrombosis occurring early after transplantation, the biliary tree (which is entirely dependent on the arterial blood supply from the hepatic artery) becomes ischemic and eventually necrotic, resulting in a typical cholangiographic image of biliary strictures, dilatations, and intraductal cast formation. Such cholangiographic abnormalities of strictures and dilatations, however, can also be seen in patients who do not have hepatic artery thrombosis. The name first given to this last group of strictures was "ischemic-type biliary lesions," because the appearance was similar to cholangiographic bile duct abnormalities seen in patients with hepatic artery thrombosis. Other names used in the literature for this condition are "ischemic cholangiopathy" or the more general term "NAS." In this chapter the latter will be used.

Knowledge about the pathogenesis of NAS is slowly emerging from clinical and experimental studies. Several risk factors for this type of biliary complication have been identified, strongly suggesting a multifactorial origin. In general, the mechanisms underlying NAS can be grouped into three categories: 1) preservation or ischemia related, 2) cytotoxic injury induced by hydrophobic bile salts, and 3) immune-mediated injury.

In one large clinical study in which patients were grouped based on the time interval between transplantation and the occurrence of biliary strictures, it was suggested that ischemia-mediated mechanisms are mainly responsible for the development of biliary strictures within the first year after transplantation, whereas immune-mediated mechanisms play a more important role in the pathogenesis of strictures occurring beyond the first year.[11]

The radiologic similarities between the bile duct abnormalities of NAS and bile duct abnormalities seen in the presence of hepatic artery thrombosis strongly suggest an ischemic factor in the origin of these strictures. The relevance of adequate blood supply and the impact of ischemia on the bile ducts have been discussed in more detail on page 321–322 (Relevance of donor/back-table procedure).

Another relevant factor in the pathogenesis of bile duct injury after liver transplantation is toxicity caused by hydrophobic bile salts. Hydrophobic bile salts have potent detergent properties towards cellular membranes of hepatocytes and biliary epithelial cells. Under physiological circumstances the toxic effects of bile salts are prevented by complex formation with phospholipids and cholesterol (mixed micelle). However, early after liver transplantation, the balance in biliary excretion of these three components is disturbed, leading to the formation of more toxic bile.[15] Evidence for a pivotal role of bile salt-mediated toxicity in the pathogenesis of bile duct injury and subsequent bile duct stricturing has gradually emerged during the last decade. Both experimental animal studies and clinical studies have demonstrated that biliary bile salt toxicity early after transplantation is associated with the development of microscopic as well macroscopic bile duct injury.[15] Bile salt toxicity acts synergistically with ischemia-mediated injury of the biliary epithelium.[16] Despite increasing evidence that bile salts play a role in the pathogenesis of bile duct injury and subsequent biliary structuring, it remains to be established whether the administration of nontoxic hydrophilic bile salts (e.g. ursodeoxycholic acid) to liver transplant recipients results in a reduction of the incidence of this type of biliary complication.

Several studies have provided evidence for an immunologic component in the pathogenesis of NAS. NAS have been associated with various immunologically mediated processes, such as ABO-incompatible liver transplantation, pre-existing diseases with a presumed autoimmune component (such as primary sclerosing cholangitis and autoimmune hepatitis), cytomegalovirus infection, chronic rejection, and finally with a genetic polymorphism in one of the CC chemokine receptors.[13] Recurrent primary sclerosing cholangitis may be another cause of NAS occurring late (>6–12 months) after transplantation.[11] The true clinical relevance of immune-mediated bile duct injury in the pathogenesis of NAS after liver transplantation remains to be established and this is an area that requires further research.

Management

Contrary to anastomotic strictures, non-anastomotic structures are much more heterogeneous in localization and severity. General recommendations regarding management are hard to make, and good-quality prospective studies are rare. In every case, adequate vascularization of the biliary system of the allograft should be obtained. In the case of diffuse and severe biliary strictures with progressive jaundice and bacterial cholangitis or biliary cirrhosis, usually re-transplantation is the most favorable option. In most patients, the strictures are more localized and cirrhosis has not yet developed. Many cases are amenable to endoscopic therapy. In endoscopic therapy, repeated endoscopies with balloon dilatation and multiple stents are used. With this approach, success rates are 50–75%.[31] As in anastomotic strictures, PTC can be used when endoscopic access is not feasible. In the case of NAS that are confined to the extrahepatic bile ducts, surgical resection of the diseased part and construction of a hepatico-jejunostomy should be considered. In case of recurrent cholangitis, maintenance antibiotics may result in long-term relief of symptoms. Although widely used, there is no clinical evidence that supports the use of ursodeoxycholic acid.

Similar approaches can be used with NAS after split- and living-donor liver transplantation, but (as with anastomotic structures) with success rates that are significantly lower than after full-size liver transplantation.

While most types of biliary complications can usually be managed successfully (either surgically or by endoscopic techniques) or run a self-limiting course, NAS remain the most challenging type of biliary complication as they are frequently therapy resistant and frequently associated with long-term sequelae. Up to 50% of patients with NAS either die or require retransplantation. Mortality rates differ markedly among studies.[2]

Bile leakage

Pathogenesis and clinical presentation

Bile leakage after liver transplantation is reported in 1–25% of recipients. The incidence of bile leakage is the highest after transplantation of a split liver or a graft from a living donor due to the hepatic resection surface.[1,2] Bile leakage can either be symptomatic or asymptomatic, and may be discovered coincidentally on a postoperative cholangiogram. Symptomatic patients may present with abdominal pain, localized or generalized peritonitis, fever, and sometimes elevated serum liver enzymes and/or bilirubin.

Biliary leakage can occur at various sites and intervals after transplantation. The majority of postoperative leaks occur at the site of anastomosis or the T-tube insertion site, but also the resection surface of the graft in the case of living-donor of split-donor transplantation is a common site for leakage. Bile leakage early after liver transplantation most likely originates from the anastomosis or the T-tube insertion site. Anastomotic leaks are mainly related to errors in surgical technique and/or ischemic necrosis at the end of the bile duct. Insufficient blood supply or traction of the stitches causes ischemia, which can result in bile leakage. A hepatic artery thrombosis can lead to massive biliary necrosis resulting in dehiscence of the biliary anastomosis. Bile leakage at the T-tube insertion site can occur immediately after transplantation or after removal of the T-tube due to an insufficiently formed fistula around the tract of the bile drain. Occasionally, bile leakage occurs after percutaneous liver biopsy or iatrogenic duct damage.

Management

The management of bile leaks depends on the type of biliary anastomosis, clinical presentation, severity, and localization of the bile leak. If a leak presents shortly after surgery, the abdominal drains should be left in place and opened. Ultrasonography should be made to confirm arterial perfusion of the graft. The majority of bile leaks are due to leakage at the site of the biliary anastomosis.

A small anastomotic bile leak can usually be managed conservatively, especially when the patient is asymptomatic. Symptomatic or infected bile collections should be treated with a radiologically placed percutaneous drain. An anastomotic bile leak without disruption of the anastomosis can be successfully managed primarily nonsurgically. Stenting of the bile duct, nasobiliary drainage, sphincterotomy and a combination of these have all been used with a success rate of 85–100%. Since sphincterotomy may lead to specific complications (bleeding and perforation), it should not be routinely performed. The optimal timing of stent removal after resolution of symptoms is still unclear, but 8 weeks has been proven successful.[36] In the presence of a hepatico-jejunostomy, ERCP can be attempted, but is frequently not successful. Alternatively, a PTC drain can be placed, even in the presence of nondilated bile ducts.[26]

In the rare case of a complete disruption of the anastomosis, prompt surgery with conversion to a hepatico-jejunostomy is most appropriate. In selected cases a repeat choledochocholedochostomy can be considered. In the case of diffuse bilious peritonitis with hemodynamic instability or sepsis, direct laparotomy should always be considered.

Leakage after removal of a bile drain can be managed successfully in one-third of cases by conservative measures, including intravenous fluids, antibiotics, analgesics, and observation.[37] In the absence of improvement, ERCP with stent placement should be performed. A laparotomy is indicated when clinical signs of biliary peritonitis persist despite adequate drainage of the biliary system.

Other biliary complications

Pathogenesis, clinical presentation and management

Sphincter of Oddi dysfunction The sphincter of Oddi is a small, smooth muscle sphincter located at the junction of the bile duct, pancreatic duct, and duodenum. The sphincter controls flow of bile and pancreatic juices into the duodenum and prevents reflux of duodenal content into the ducts. Disorder of its motility is called sphincter of Oddi dysfunction. Clinically sphincter of Oddi dysfunction presents with cholestasis, dilatation of the distal extrahepatic bile duct, and cholangiographic absence of any anatomic cause for biliary obstruction.

Studies focusing on sphincter of Oddi dysfunction are scarce and often report only very few patients. Reported incidence of sphincter of Oddi dysfunction varies from 0–7%.[1,2] Development of sphincter of Oddi dysfunction after liver transplantation may be imputed to operative denervation of the sphincter of Oddi during recipient hepatectomy, leading to impairment of ampullary relaxation and increased intraductal biliary pressure.[1]

Sphincter of Oddi dysfunction after liver transplantation is an obscure diagnosis. Formal proof of this diagnosis will require pressure measurement in the bile duct lumen, which is difficult to perform in the absence of a biliary drain. In case of clinical suspicion and exclusion of any other possible cause of cholestasis, an endoscopic sphincterotomy or temporary stent placement can be performed.

Biliary casts, sludge and stones Casts, sludge and stones in the bile ducts are also known as bile duct filling defects. Sludge is a viscous collection of mucus, calcium bilirubinate, and cholesterol. When left untreated, biliary casts can develop. Casts consist of retained lithogenic material morphologically confined to bile duct dimensions. Biliary sludge and casts tend to occur within the first year after transplantation, and when given enough time they may progress to biliary stones. Bile duct filling defects are a relatively rare complication compared with biliary strictures and leaks. A 5.7% incidence of bile duct filling defects after transplantation was reported in the largest study so far, including 1650 transplanted livers.[38] Most patients with biliary stones and sludge present with cholangitis and only a small percentage present with abdominal pain. Despite the relative infrequency, studies have shown an increased rate of morbidity and mortality as a result of biliary sludge and casts, which have caused recurrent cholangitis, repeated need for surgery, graft loss, and death.[39]

The exact pathogenesis is yet to be discovered, but multiple factors contribute to bile duct filling defect formation, including ischemia, infection, and preservation injury.[13] Theoretically, anything that increases the viscosity of bile or reduces bile flow can predispose to bile duct filling defects. It is likely that ischemia contributes to the formation of filling defects both through stasis of bile (as a result of strictures) and through its direct injury to the biliary epithelium, resulting in the release of cell debris into the bile duct lumen as well as increasing the epithelial susceptibility to precipitation of lithogenic materials. Other pathogenic factors that are associated with filling defects are biliary cholesterol content, bacterial infection in relation to stents, the presence of a hepatico-jejunostomy, fungal infections and the use of cyclosporine.[2]

Stones and sludge of the biliary tree can almost universally be managed successfully by endoscopic removal. However, the long-term success of this treatment will depend on the underlying cause. If the formation of sludge or casts is caused by a local obstruction such as a biliary drain or an anastomotic stricture that can be treated successfully, removal of the obstruction may be curative. However, when biliary sludge and casts are a symptom of ischemic bile duct injury, the severity of the latter will determine the long-term success of cast removal and will determine the fate of the graft.

External compression of the biliary tract External compression of the biliary tract is a very rare type of biliary complication, characterized by extrahepatic cholestasis and jaundice. The main causes of external compression of the bile ducts are mucoceles of the cystic duct remnant and periductal lymphomas.

Although clinically relevant mucoceles of the cystic duct have been reported in several case reports; the exact incidence of this type of complication remains unclear. In one study, non-obstructive mucoceles of the cystic duct were reported in 4.5% of the liver transplant recipients studied.[40] A mucocele of the cystic duct can develop when both ends of the donor cystic duct are ligated, e.g. due to incorporation into the suture line of the biliary anastomosis. Continued endothelial secretion causes enlargement of the cystic duct and may subsequently cause extrinsic compression of the extrahepatic bile duct. External compression of the bile duct by a mucocele can usually be treated successfully by surgical excision of the cystic duct remnant.

A lymphoma in the hepatic (neo-)hilum can be caused by post-transplantation lymphoproliferative disorder and may result in compression of the extrahepatic bile ducts. While therapy should primarily focus on the medical treatment of the underlying lymphomas,[2] temporary endoscopic stenting of the bile duct may be indicated to restore bile drainage.

Kinking of redundant bile duct Excessive length of the donor or recipient bile duct can cause kinking of the bile duct, leading to bile flow obstruction. This is a rare technical complication that is mainly found after a choledochocholedochostomy. Patients may present with cholestatic liver function tests, fever due to cholangitis, or bile duct dilatation due to obstruction of the bile flow. The kinked bile duct can be repaired in two manners: 1) surgical resection of the redundant part and re-anastomosing of the bile ducts, or 2) by an endoscopic approach. The latter involves placement of an endoscopic stent to stretch the bile duct at the site of the choledochocholedochostomy. After the repair, scar tissue forms around the bile duct and prevents recurrence of kinking. The stent can usually be removed safely after 6 weeks. In selected cases, surgical or endoscopic correction of the choledochocholedochostomy is not possible and in these cases surgical conversion to a Roux-Y hepaticojejunostomy is indicated.

Bacterial cholangitis Bacterial cholangitis after liver transplantation usually presents with cholestatic liver function test abnormalities in combination with high fever, either with or without chills. The risk of cholangitis is increased in patients in whom a T-tube is used, in patients who underwent a hepatico-jejunostomy, and in patients complicated by anastomotic or non-anastomotic bile duct strictures. All of these conditions may facilitate ascending migration of bacteria into the biliary tree. When a biliary drain is present, positive bacterial cultures from the bile may support the diagnosis, although it should be noted that colonization of the bile is not infrequent in these patients. In other patients the diagnosis cholangitis is rarely supported by positive bile cultures and usually made after exclusion of other causes of fever. Management of acute cholangitis after transplantation is similar to that recommended to nontransplant patients and should include appropriate antibiotic therapy.

Summary

Biliary complications are a frequent cause of morbidity after liver transplantation. Advances in surgical techniques and preservation methods during the last decades have led to better results, but biliary complications still occur in 10–40% of the recipients and are associated with mortality rates of 8–15%. Partial liver grafts (e.g. split livers and livers from living donors) as well as livers from extended-criteria donors (e.g. DCD donors), are associated with a relatively high risk of biliary complications. Of all biliary complications, bile duct strictures and bile leakage are most common after liver transplantation. While bile leakage and anastomotic bile duct strictures can usually be managed successfully without long-term sequelae, non-anastomotic biliary strictures are the most troublesome type of biliary complication. NAS are often multifocal and can be difficult to treat by endoscopic techniques. When associated with recurrent cholangitis, jaundice or even secondary biliary fibrosis, retransplantation may be the only treatment option left. Future studies should focus on better defining the mechanism underlying NAS and on the development of effective preventive measures. In this respect it will be interesting to see if the development of machine preservation for liver grafts will result in better preservation of the bile ducts and a subsequent decrease in the incidence of this type of biliary complications.

Abbreviations

DBD: donation after brain death, DCD: donation after cardiac death, ERCP: endoscopic retrograde cholangio-pancreaticography, CT: computed tomography; MRC: magnetic resonance cholangiography, PTCD: percutaneous transhepatic cholangiodrainage, UW: University of Wisconsin

References

1. Wojcicki M, Milkiewicz P, Silva M. Biliary tract complications after liver transplantation: a review. Dig Surg 2008;25:245–57.
2. Verdonk RC, Buis CI, Porte RJ, Haagsma EB. Biliary complications after liver transplantation: a review. Scand J Gastroenterol 2006;243(Suppl):89–101.
3. Pine JK, Aldouri A, Young AL, et al. Liver transplantation following donation after cardiac death: an analysis using matched pairs. Liver Transpl 2009;15:1072–82.
4. Davidson BR, Rai R, Kurzawinski TR, et al. Prospective randomized trial of end-to-end versus side-to-side biliary reconstruction after orthotopic liver transplantation. Br J Surg 1999;86:447–52.
5. Bennet W, Zimmerman MA, Campsen J, et al. Choledochoduodenostomy is a safe alternative to Roux-en-Y choledochojejunostomy for biliary reconstruction in liver transplantation. World J Surg 2009;33:1022–5.
6. Sotiropoulos GC, Sgourakis G, Radtke A, et al. Orthotopic liver transplantation: T-tube or not T-tube? Systematic review and meta-analysis of results. Transplantation 2009;87:1672–80.
7. Weiss S, Schmidt SC, Ulrich F, et al. Biliary reconstruction using a side-to-side choledochocholedochostomy with or without T-tube in deceased donor liver transplantation: a prospective randomized trial. Ann Surg 2009;250:766–71.
8. Shaked A. Use of T tube in liver transplantation. Liver Transpl Surg 1997;3(Suppl 1):S22–3.
9. Porayko MK, Kondo M, Steers JL. Liver transplantation: late complications of the biliary tract and their management. Semin Liver Dis 1995;15:139–55.
10. Noack K, Bronk SF, Kato A, Gores GJ. The greater vulnerability of bile duct cells to reoxygenation injury than to anoxia. Implications for the pathogenesis of biliary strictures after liver transplantation. Transplantation 1993;56:495–500.
11. Buis CI, Verdonk RC, van der Jagt EJ, et al. Nonanastomotic biliary strictures after liver transplantation, part 1: Radiological features and risk factors for early vs. late presentation. Liver Transpl 2007;13:708–18.
12. Sanchez-Urdazpal L, Gores GJ, Ward EM, et al. Ischemic-type biliary complications after orthotopic liver transplantation. Hepatology 1992;16:49–53.
13. Buis CI, Hoekstra H, Verdonk RC, Porte RJ. Causes and consequences of ischemic-type biliary lesions after liver transplantation. J Hepatobiliary Pancreat Surg 2006;13:517–24.
14. Dubbeld J, Hoekstra H, Farid WRR, et al. Similar liver transplantation survival with selected cardiac death and brain death donors. Br J Surg 2010;97:744–53.
15. Buis CI, Geuken E, Visser DS, et al. Altered bile composition after liver transplantation is associated with the development of nonanastomotic biliary strictures. J Hepatol 2009;50:69–79.
16. Hoekstra H, Porte RJ, Tian Y, et al. Bile salt toxicity aggravates cold ischemic injury of bile ducts after liver transplantation in Mdr2+/– mice. Hepatology 2006;43:1022–31.
17. Feng L, Zhao N, Yao X, et al. Histidine–tryptophan–ketoglutarate solution vs. University of Wisconsin solution for liver transplantation: a systematic review. Liver Transpl 2007;13:1125–36.
18. Canelo R, Hakim NS, Ringe B. Experience with hystidine tryptophan ketoglutarate versus University Wisconsin preservation solutions in transplantation. Int Surg 2003;88:145–51.
19. Moench C, Moench K, Lohse AW, Thies J, Otto G. Prevention of ischemic-type biliary lesions by arterial back-table pressure perfusion. Liver Transpl 2003;9:285–9.
20. Sebagh M, Yilmaz F, Karam V, et al. The histologic pattern of "biliary tract pathology" is accurate for the diagnosis of biliary complications. Am J Surg Pathol 2005;29:318–23.
21. St Peter S, Rodriquez-Davalos MI, Rodriguez-Luna HM, Harrison EM, Moss AA, Mulligan DC. Significance of proximal biliary dilatation in patients with anastomotic strictures after liver transplantation. Dig Dis Sci 2004;49:1207–11.
22. Kok T, Van der Sluis A, Klein JP, et al. Ultrasound and cholangiography for the diagnosis of biliary complications after orthotopic liver transplantation: a comparative study. J Clin Ultrasound 1996;24:103–15.
23. Boraschi P, Donati F, Gigoni R, et al. MR cholangiography in orthotopic liver transplantation: sensitivity and specificity in detecting biliary complications. Clin Transplant 2009;24:E82–7.
24. Chahal P, Baron TH, Poterucha JJ, Rosen CB. Endoscopic retrograde cholangiography in post-orthotopic liver transplant population with Roux-en-Y biliary reconstruction. Liver Transpl 2007;13:1168–73.
25. Kawano Y, Mizuta K, Hishikawa S, et al. Rendezvous penetration method using double-balloon endoscopy for complete anastomosis obstruction of hepaticojejunostomy after pediatric living donor liver transplantation. Liver Transpl 2008;14:385–7.

26. Righi D, Franchello A, Ricchiuti A, et al. Safety and efficacy of the percutaneous treatment of bile leaks in hepaticojejunostomy or split-liver transplantation without dilatation of the biliary tree. Liver Transpl 2008;14:611–5.
27. Kurzawinski TR, Selves L, Farouk M, et al. Prospective study of hepatobiliary scintigraphy and endoscopic cholangiography for the detection of early biliary complications after orthotopic liver transplantation. Br J Surg 1997;84:620–3.
28. Verdonk RC, Buis CI, Porte RJ, et al. Anastomotic biliary strictures after liver transplantation: causes and consequences. Liver Transpl 2006;12:726–35.
29. Jagannath S, Kalloo AN. Biliary complications after liver transplantation. Curr Treat Options Gastroenterol 2002;5:101–12.
30. Bourgeois N, Deviere J, Yeaton P, et al. Diagnostic and therapeutic endoscopic retrograde cholangiography after liver transplantation. Gastrointest Endosc 1995;42:527–34.
31. Sharma S, Gurakar A, Jabbour N. Biliary strictures following liver transplantation: past, present and preventive strategies. Liver Transpl 2008;14:759–69.
32. Zoepf T, Maldonado-Lopez EJ, Hilgard P, et al. Balloon dilatation vs. balloon dilatation plus bile duct endoprostheses for treatment of anastomotic biliary strictures after liver transplantation. Liver Transpl 2006;12: 88–94.
33. Cantu P, Tenca A, Donato MF, et al. ERCP and short-term stent-trial in patients with anastomotic biliary stricture following liver transplantation. Dig Liver Dis 2009;41:516–22.
34. Gomez CM, Dumonceau JM, Marcolongo M, et al. Endoscopic management of biliary complications after adult living-donor versus deceased-donor liver transplantation. Transplantation 2009;88:1280–5.
35. Verdonk RC, Buis CI, van der Jagt EJ, et al. Nonanastomotic biliary strictures after liver transplantation, part 2: Management, outcome, and risk factors for disease progression. Liver Transpl 2007;13: 725–32.
36. Morelli J, Mulcahy HE, Willner IR, et al. Endoscopic treatment of post-liver transplantation biliary leaks with stent placement across the leak site. Gastrointest Endosc 2001;54:471–5.
37. Shuhart MC, Kowdley KV, McVicar JP, et al. Predictors of bile leaks after T-tube removal in orthotopic liver transplant recipients. Liver Transpl Surg 1998;4: 62–70.
38. Sheng R, Ramirez CB, Zajko AB, Campbell WL. Biliary stones and sludge in liver transplant patients: a 13-year experience. Radiology 1996;198:243–7.
39. Shah JN, Haigh WG, Lee SP, et al. Biliary casts after orthotopic liver transplantation: clinical factors, treatment, biochemical analysis. Am J Gastroenterol 2003;98:1861–7.
40. Caputo M, Piolanti M, Riccioli LA, et al. Nonobstructive residual mucocele of the cystic duct. Reassessment of complications in our 13 years' experience with liver transplantation. Radiol Med 2000;100:354–6.

30 Role of histopathology

Achim Weber

Swiss HPB and Transplantation Centers, Institute of Surgical Pathology, Department of Pathology, University of Zürich, Switzerland

Key learning points

- The role of histopathology in the context of liver transplantation is not restricted to biopsies of the allograft liver, but also includes examination of the prospective recipient's liver, the donor organ, and the liver explant.
- The role of histopathology in the context of liver transplantation ranges from confirming the clinical diagnosis to being the defining criterion.
- Acute cellular rejection is diagnosed and graded by histopathology.
- To get the maximum informative value from a liver biopsy, histopathologic findings have to be correlated with clinical findings, laboratory values, and results of imaging procedures.

Introduction

Histologic evaluation of liver tissue is a diagnostic means at several instances in the management of patients with liver transplantation. Different approaches can be taken to systematically depict circumstances in which histology is performed. A clinically focussed approach is oriented according to the time in relation to the transplantation. A more systematic approach is to categorize according to the aetiology of underlying liver disease. From the perspective of histopathology, a morphology-based approach, i.e. a categorization based on histopathologic patterns, is obvious. This would mean to basically depict the algorithms a histopathologist has to have in mind when reading a slide. Comprehensive overviews to the approach to liver biopsies from a histopathologic perspective were recently published.[1,2] Of course the different potential approaches mentioned are overlapping. This chapter discusses the histopathology of liver transplantation in selected topics – not at all claiming to cover the complete spectrum of disease relevant to liver transplant pathology. This chapter does not strictly follow one of the earlier mentioned systematics – it is mainly structured according to disease categories, but also partly depicted according to the timeframe in relation to transplantation. Since causes of liver graft dysfunction tend to occur at characteristic times after transplantation, knowledge of the time after transplantation in addition to the original disease and kind of liver injury is the basis for considerations in differential diagnosis. These considerations are correlated with the histologic findings needed to reach the correct diagnosis.

For histopathology to have a role in the management of patients with liver transplantation, it has to be embedded into the clinical context. The value of histopathologic examination is largely dependent on a clinicopathologic correlation. Knowledge of the original disease and the time after transplantation is crucial for the interpretation of post-transplant biopsies, since these factors influence the spectrum of pathologic differential diagnoses. The more precise and complete the information given to the histopathologist, the more precise and complete

Medical Care of the Liver Transplant Patient, Fourth Edition. Edited by Pierre-Alain Clavien, James F. Trotter.

the reading and interpretation of histology can be expected. Therefore, a meaningful interpretation requires communication between clinicians and pathologists.

Histopathology prior to transplantation and explanted organs

Notably, histopathology plays a role for liver transplantation already prior to transplantation. First of all, histologic examination of a liver biopsy taken from a transplant candidate can be helpful for the decision to proceed to transplantation. This is particularly relevant in patients with acute liver failure. Although a liver biopsy naturally comprises only a minor part of the organ parenchyma that is not necessarily representative for the whole organ, histology can provide information concerning the extent and – on repeated biopsies – the dynamics of liver cell damage as well as the potential of regeneration. These findings can accelerate or delay the decision for transplantation (Figure 30.1A).

Furthermore, in cases of acute liver failure in which the underlying etiology is not (completely) clear, examination of the liver explant can lead to an exact diagnosis, which again is helpful for post-transplant management of patients. In particular, in cases of liver transplantation due to acute liver failure, histologic examination of the liver explant also serves as a means of quality control by documenting the degree of liver damage thereby reinforcing (or questioning) the decision for liver transplant. In contrast to a liver biopsy, examination of the whole organ is not hampered by a sampling error due to heterogeneity of disease manifestation (Figure 30.1 B).

Histology is also a means of donor organ evaluation. Although still a minor fraction (10% in the Swiss Hepato-Pancreato-Biliary (HPB) Center in 2009), organs from living donors are used for transplantation.[3] A thorough medical evaluation of potential organ donors is performed, which routinely includes a liver biopsy in many centers. Donor organ evaluation is also performed on cadaveric livers. The risk of allograft failure to a large degree depends on the condition of the graft. Suspicion of damage to the potential graft can lead to biopsies prior to transplantation. The use of extended-criteria donors, e.g. donors with age >60 years, severe steatosis (>30% macrovesicular steatosis; >60% macrovesicular or microvesicular steatosis), extended cold ischemia time >12 h, and donation after cardiac death[4,5] led to increased requests for histologic evaluation of cadaveric donor organs. In this setting, fatty change of the potential graft, mostly suspected on macroscopic inspection of the organ, is by far the most frequent indication for biopsy in the Swiss HPB Center as well as in most other centers.

Apart from non-alcoholic fatty liver disease (NAFLD), other diseases like chronic hepatitis, storage diseases and fibrosis can also be discovered. NAFLD is the most common reason for donor disqualification of live or cadaveric donor organs. It is generally accepted that severe steatosis is associated with bad organ function. Evaluation is performed by frozen section (Figure 30.2). Although there is no strict threshold for the acceptability of a fatty liver, macrovesicular steatosis affecting more than 60% of hepatocytes is generally regarded as a reason to discard the graft. It increasingly becomes clear that the currently practised approach to determine fat content of the liver by histology has a lot of limitations including a highly questionable reproducibility of quantification[6] and oversimplification of fat as fat not taking into account the different biochemical compositions. However, as long as no better tools than the earlier described procedure are established for the quantitative and qualitative assessment of liver fat, simple quantification of liver fat by histology will be a means for providing information on which the transplant surgeon has to decide if to accept or reject a fatty liver. Owing to the urgent need of liver grafts, severely steatotic grafts should not generally be discarded.[7] However, the final decision is not solely dependent on the donor organ itself but also determined by the prospective recipient. A liver with a high fat content is more likely to be accepted for a prospective recipient in generally good condition who most likely does better with a fatty organ.

Histopathology of the allograft transplant liver

The time after transplantation is usually divided into the early, mid, and late post-transplant period. This is helpful since the incidence of differential diagnoses observed in allograft transplant livers varies over

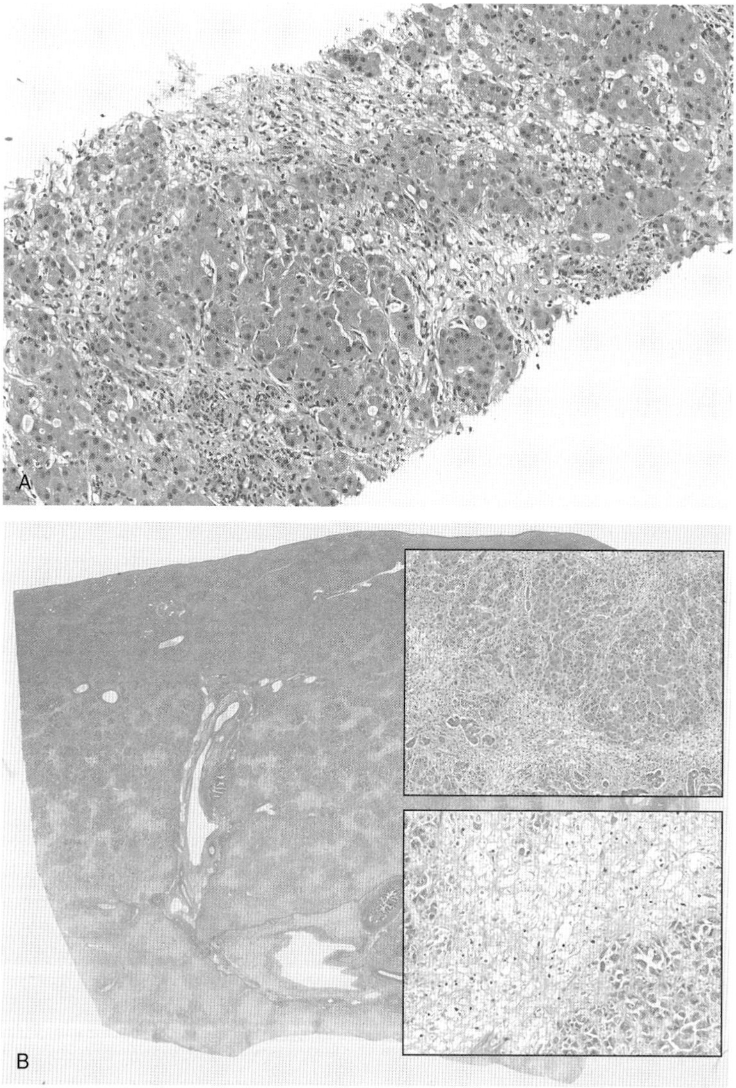

Figure 30.1 Indication for liver transplantation and quality control of liver explants. (A) Liver biopsy of a patient with acute liver failure revealing widespread fresh hepatocyte necrosis, collapse of liver plates, and inflammation. (B) Liver explant of the same patient (1 d after the biopsy was taken) with widespread liver necrosis affecting more than half of the liver cells in subcapsular areas (upper insert) to subtotal liver cells mass in other areas (lower insert), illustrating heterogeneity of changes (H&E)

time. The division is not exact, however, and time frames to categorize into early, mid, and late post-transplant periods are not consistently used in the literature.[2,8] Nevertheless, the different histopathologic findings are discussed following the time course after transplantation.

In some centers, "time-zero" biopsies are routinely performed to get a baseline histologic picture. These may be helpful in predicting development of significant preservation injury. Sinusoidal neutrophilic infiltrates and hepatocyte necrosis are signs of preservation injury and can point to initial poor graft function.[9]

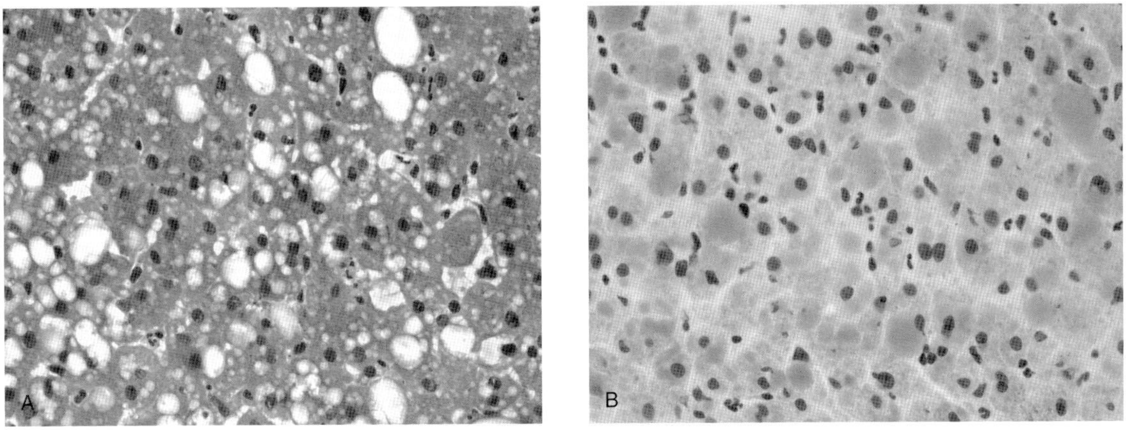

Figure 30.2 Evaluation of a potential donor organ for fat content (A) Liver biopsy of potential donor organ revealing little macrovesicular, but severe microvesicular steatosis. (Frozen section, H&E). (B) Sudan Red staining performed on frozen material to visualize fat inclusion and facilitate fat quantification in particular of microsteatosis

After this, liver biopsy is mostly performed in response to clinical signs of abnormal liver function or changes of laboratory findings indicating hepatocellular (transaminases) or biliary (alkaline phosphatase, bilirubin, γ-GT) injury. In many situations, clinical findings and liver enzyme abnormalities are not sufficient in differentiating diverse conditions potentially requiring different therapy.

The most frequent causes underlying allograft dysfunction or failure vary according to the time in relation to transplantation. The early post-transplantation period is determined mostly by post-transplant abnormalities including "cryopreservation/reperfusion injury," vascular complications, and rarely already by acute cellular rejection. The mid and late post-transplantation period is determined by acute cellular rejection, delayed vascular complications, chronic rejection, transplantation-related *de novo* diseases including infections, and recurrent disease.[10]

Hematoxylin and eosin (H&E) stain of formalin-fixed, paraffin-embedded percutaneous or transjugular liver biopsies is sufficient for most situations. Useful ancillary staining techniques include immunostaining for cytokeratin 7 (CK7) to visualize bile ducts and ductular metaplasia, immunostaining for human cytomegalovirus (CMV) and Epstein–Barr virus (EBV) proteins as well as EBV *in situ* hybridization (EBER).

Early and mid post-transplantation period

The term "cryopreservation/reperfusion injury" already indicates that this condition refers to the damage that occurs during liver storage in cold preservation solution followed by reperfusion in the recipient. Hepatocytes and sinus endothelial cells are affected, and patients frequently show prolonged elevation of transaminases and cholestatic parameters. The extent of cryopreservation/reperfusion injury can be determined by histology.[11] Mild cryopreservation/reperfusion injury is characterized by hepatocellular swelling, detachment, and rounding up of hepatocytes as well as microvesicular steatosis. Severe cryopreservation/reperfusion injury is characterized by confluent, sometimes zonal necrosis, and neutrophilic infiltrates.

Lipopeliosis, a typical lesion of the early post-transplant period, develops in fatty organs due to ischemia or cryopreservation/reperfusion injury. It occurs when fat is released from the hepatocytes and stored in the sinusoids.[12] On biopsy, empty spaces representing fat extruded from hepatocytes and stored in sinusoids are visible. Macrophages can be appreciated surrounding fat droplets (Figure 30.3A and D). Lipoeliosis is a reversible lesion, however it may cause prolonged cholestasis, thus prompting

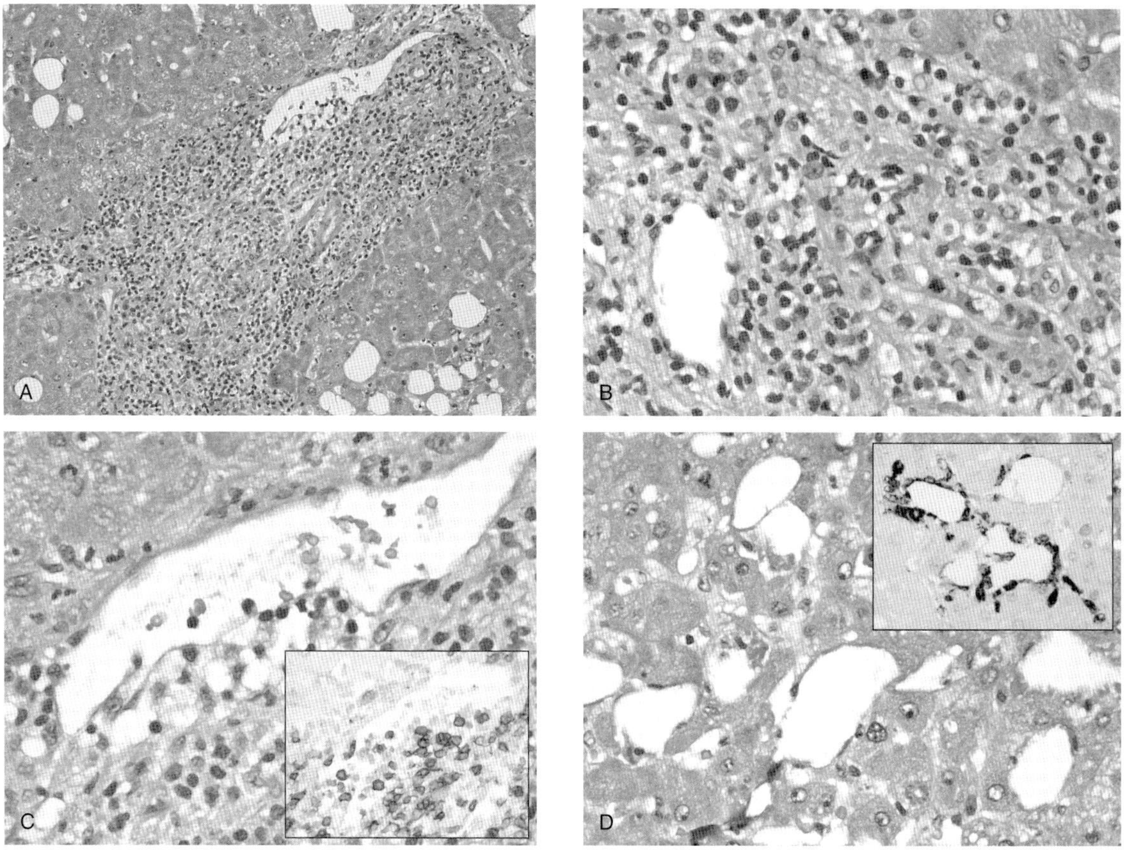

Figure 30.3 Early post-transplant liver biopsy with acute cellular rejection and lipopeliosis. (A) Low-power view of a portal field showing signs of acute rejection: portal inflammation, phlebitis of portal vein, and bile duct injury. Adjacent lobular parenchyma reveals lipopeliosis (lower right and upper left corner). (B) High-power view showing a dense mixed inflammatory infiltrate and bile duct injury. (C) Detail of phlebitis with subendothelial lymphocytes lifting the endothelium. Insert: CD3 immunostaining highlights T-cells. (D) High-power view of lobular parenchyma showing empty spaces representing fat droplets located in sinusoids (not in hepatocytes) and surrounded by macrophages. Insert: CD68 immunostaining confirms that macrophages surround the extruded fat. (H&E)

liver biopsy. It is important for this lesion to be recognized and known as a condition underlying cholestasis in the early post-transplant period.

Acute cellular rejection

In most centers, acute cellular rejection is the most frequent cause underlying graft dysfunction in the early period. Therefore it is also the most frequently asked clinical question prompting a liver biopsy. Targets of acute cellular rejection are the bile duct epithelia and vascular endothelial cells. Both are infiltrated by inflammatory cells resulting in a typical morphologic picture. Histopathology is the basis for diagnosing and grading the components of acute cellular rejection. Acute rejection histologically is characterized by:

1. A predominantly mononuclear, but mixed portal inflammatory infiltrate including lymphocytes (mostly CD8-positive T-cells), eosinophils, and also blastic cells. Lobular regions between the portal tract and

pericentral region are typically spared, which is a useful feature for discriminating acute cellular rejection from hepatitis.
2. Subendothelial inflammation of portal or central hepatic venules (phlebitis, endothelitis).
3. Bile duct damage and inflammation.[13] At least two of these findings are required for the diagnosis.
Severity of acute cellular rejection is determined by the Banff scoring system[14] comprising these three criteria: portal inflammation, bile duct damage/injury, and venous endothelitis. All three parameters are scored from 0 to 3, resulting in a total score ranging from 0 to 9, the rejection activity index (RAI). RAI scores 1–2 are categorized as indeterminate, RAI scores 3–4 as mild, RAI scores 5–6 as moderate, and >6 as severe. The total RAI score correlates with graft failure.[15] Most episodes of rejection detected by biopsy are mild to moderate. Figure 30.3 shows an example of moderate acute cellular rejection combined with lipopeliosis. Late acute rejection, occurring several months after transplantation, can differ from the early phase of acute rejection. Although mostly similar to the early phase of acute rejection, it can show minimal or no portal tract changes, less venous subendothelial infiltrates, or more necro-inflammatory lobular activity.[16] This pattern can be more difficult to discriminate from recurrent chronic viral hepatitis, and both conditions may also coexist.

Since inflammatory activity is a constituent of acute cellular rejection the most challenging histopathologic differential diagnoses comprise other inflammatory diseases, in particular viral hepatitis. These include (recurrent) hepatitis C and hepatitis B as well other viral infections like CMV and EBV (see later). Owing to its high incidence, recurrent viral hepatitis C is the most frequent differential diagnosis to acute cellular rejection and at the same time one of the most common diagnostic dilemmas due to the diametrically opposite therapeutic consequences of acute rejection and viral hepatitis. On the one hand, untreated acute cellular rejection may progress to chronic rejection and graft failure. On the other hand, immunosuppressive treatment for acute cellular rejection harbors an increased risk of allograft fibrosis and cirrhosis. Histopathologic features favoring acute cellular rejection over recurrent HCV infection are: 1) a mixed portal inflammatory infiltrate including eosinophils and blastic cells in contrast to a more monomorphic, mostly lymphocytic infiltrate in hepatitis C, 2) the lack of significant lobular inflammation apart from the portal tract and pericentral region in contrast to lobular necro-inflammatory activity in hepatitis C, and 3) significant bile duct damage that is not an integral part of hepatitis C infection (HCV). These histologic features have to be carefully taken into account to find out the dominating underlying pathology. For the discrimination between acute cellular rejection and recurrent HCV infection, it is implicitly advisable to also consider clinical and laboratory findings including liver enzymes and HCV RNA levels in addition to the histopathologic findings.

Bile duct complications

The bile duct system is frequently affected by ischemic or traumatic injury.[17] Such injury potentially leads to biliary strictures,[18] which can occur early and late, at sites of anastomosis or non-anastomotic sites. Development of jaundice or abnormal γ-GT and AP can prompt diagnostic work-up including liver biopsy. The histopathologic changes in transplanted livers are similar to findings in native livers. Obstructive/stricturing bile duct changes are characterized by portal and periductal edema, a portal inflammatory infiltrate predominantly by neutrophils, frequently neutrophils in bile duct epithelia or lumina, ductular reaction (which can be visualized by CK7 immunostaining), and frequently hepatocellular and canalicular cholestasis. In particular in the early post-transplant period, biliary tract complications are frequent among the differential diagnosis. The transplant liver – in contrast to the native liver – lacks a collateral arterial supply. Since the hepatic artery supplies the intra- and extrahepatic bile ducts, these are damaged by insufficient blood flow also potentially leading to biliary tract strictures. Helpful histopathologic features to discriminate portal tract changes due to biliary complications like strictures from portal tract changes related to acute rejection are: 1) a predominantly neutrophilic infiltrate compared to the mixed infiltrate of acute cellular rejection, 2) a relatively normal bile duct epithelium with normal nucleus-to-cytoplasma ratio in contrast to the reactive changes observable in acute cellular rejection, 3) a periductal edema, and 4) a ductular reaction, which typically is lacking in acute cellular rejection (Figure 30.4A).

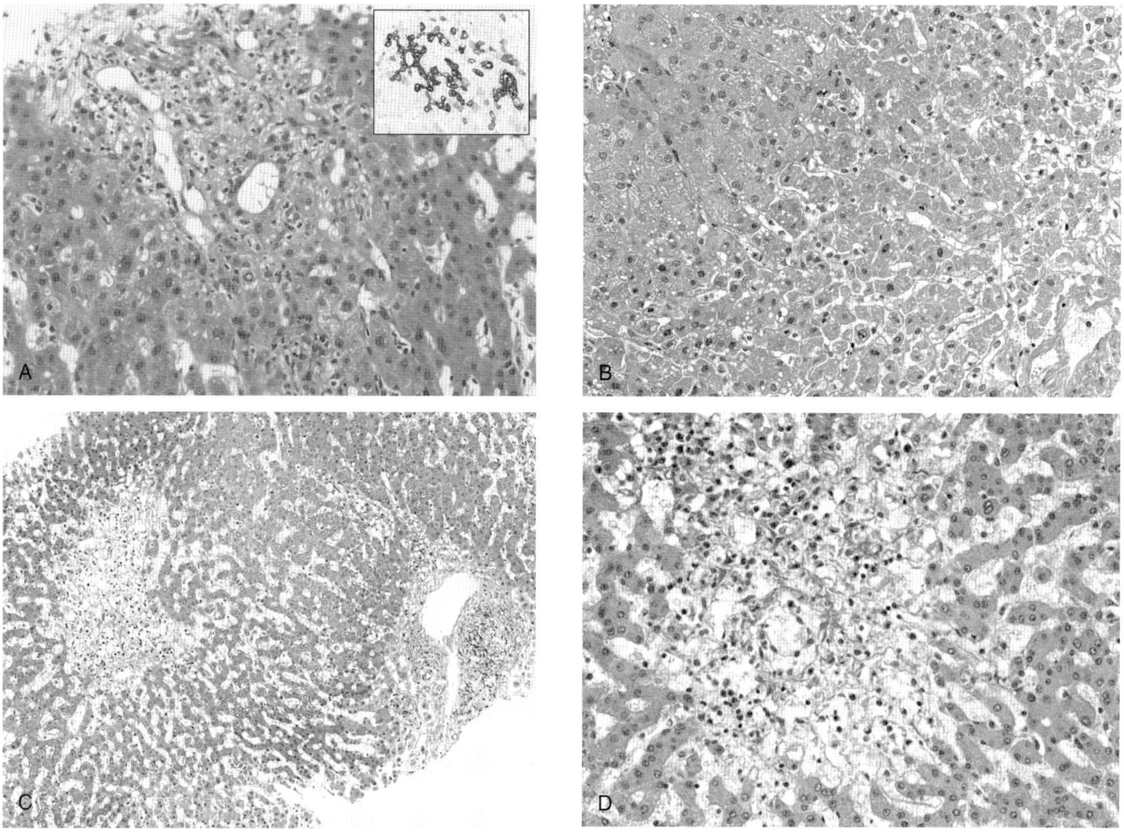

Figure 30.4 Early post-transplant liver biopsy revealing biliary or vascular complications. (A) Liver biopsy revealing portal tract edema, a mixed portal infiltrate including neutrophils and bile duct affection. Insert: CK7 immunostaining highlights ductular reaction and metaplasia. Changes were caused by bile duct obstruction due to stenosis of the anastomosis. (H&E). (B) Liver biopsy from a patient who developed thrombosis of hepatic artery on the second day post transplantation. Histology revealed ischemic damage with confluent fresh necroses in pericentral areas (right half of the picture). Note the lack of inflammatory reaction. (H&E). (C) Liver biopsy from a patient who developed abdominal pain and ascites in the early post-transplant period. Histology revealed dilatation of the portal vein (right side of the picture) and pericentral necrosis, dilatation of sinusoids and central vein obstruction (left side). (H&E). (D) EvG staining of the central vein area highlights obstruction of the central vein. Clinical work-up revealed obstruction of the vena cava

Vascular complications

Complications of vascular anastomoses, preferentially occurring during the first months after transplantation are among the most frequent technical complications that can lead to graft damage. Vascular complications primarily affect the hepatic artery and its tree. Thromboses of the hepatic artery mostly occur at or close to the anastomosis. Hepatic artery thromboses can be asymptomatic but mostly cause severe problems like hepatic infarcts, ischemic cholangiopathy, or fulminant hepatic failure. Owing to variable manifestation in different areas and sampling errors, histologic changes due to hepatic artery thrombosis cannot reliably be detected by liver biopsy. Findings can be variable and range from unremarkable changes, centrilobular hepatocyte swelling, biliary tract obstruction or cholangitis to frank ischemic necrosis (Figure 30.4B).

Portal vein thrombosis occurs less frequently than thrombosis of the hepatic artery. Complete portal vein thrombosis can result in widespread necrosis, ascites, and portal hypertension. Incomplete thrombosis can lead to smaller infarcts, hepatocyte atrophy, steatosis, or nodular regenerative hyperplasia (NRH). Morphologically, a compromised portal vein blood supply can be difficult to discriminate from impaired hepatic venous drainage. Findings that favor impaired hepatic venous drainage over portal vein problems include red blood congestion in centrilobular areas and obliterative central venopathy. In such instances, histopathology often is not sufficient in finally discriminating between these two underlying causes, and angiography and/or ultrasonography are needed.

Complications of the hepatic vein and vena cava are relatively rare, but once manifest they lead to significant clinical symptoms and histologic changes including an increased portal vein/vena cava pressure gradient. The acute situation is characterized by centrilobular congestion, central vein dilation, centrilobular necrosis, and pericentral hemorrhage. Chronic changes comprise perivenular fibrosis, central vein obstruction/occlusion (Figure 30.4C and D), and also NRH. Further potential findings include a ductular reaction that can resemble changes caused by biliary tree obstruction. The morphologic changes related to complications of the hepatic vein and vena cava reveal a broad histopathologic differential diagnosis including drug reactions and paucicellular presentations of immune reactions including acute and chronic rejection. Again, clinical work-up including examination of venous outflow by angiography and ultrasonography should point to the right direction, underlying the importance of a clinicopathologic correlation for the diagnosis of vascular complications.

Late post-transplantation period

The spectrum of disease observed in the late post-transplantation period is partly overlapping with the diseases observed earlier. However, incidences change, and whereas acute cellular rejection decreases with advanced time after transplantation, other diseases are increasingly observed including recurrence of the primary hepatic disease that led to transplantation, various infections, and chronic rejection.[8]

Chronic rejection

Chronic rejection is the third category of rejection after antibody-mediated rejection and acute cellular rejection. Whereas antibody-mediated rejection, a rare condition, occurs during the first weeks, and acute cellular rejection at any time, but mostly during the first months after transplantation, chronic rejection develops from severe or unresolved acute cellular rejection.[19] Patients with previous severe or unresolved acute cellular rejection developing progressive cholestasis on clinic presentation and a biliary pattern of blood values (γ-GT, AP) are highly suspicious of suffering from chronic rejection. The structures mainly affected by chronic rejection are the portal tract, in particular the bile ducts, and the pericentral regions. According to the Banff schema, early chronic reaction is separated from late chronic reaction.[19]

Early chronic reaction is characterized by a portal inflammation that compared to the infiltrate of acute cellular rejection is less severe and has fewer eosinophils. Furthermore, early chronic rejection targets the small bile ducts leading to biliary degenerative changes and loss of bile ducts.[20] It is important not to miss the sometimes subtle features of early chronic rejection comprising eosinophilic changes of the cytoplasm, nuclear hyperchromasia and uneven nuclear spacing.

Late chronic rejection has evolved when more than half of the bile ducts are lost. In addition, changes in the pericentral area can be found including focal obliteration of the central vein and perivenular fibrosis as well as loss of portal tract hepatic arterioles. Other characteristic changes of chronic rejection affect large perihilar hepatic arteries in the form of intimal inflammation, foam cell depositions and fibrointimal proliferation leading to luminal narrowing or occlusion as well as the large perihilar bile ducts that are damaged. In contrast to changes in portal tract, lobular and central vein regions, pathology of the perihilar region naturally cannot be detected by a percutaneous or transjugular liver biopsy. Therefore, they cannot be used for the staging of chronic rejection on liver biopsies. Nevertheless, liver biopsies are performed in cases of chronic rejection in order to get information concerning the likelihood of recovery of liver function. Early chronic rejection still has the potential for recovery whereas late chronic rejection would favor considering

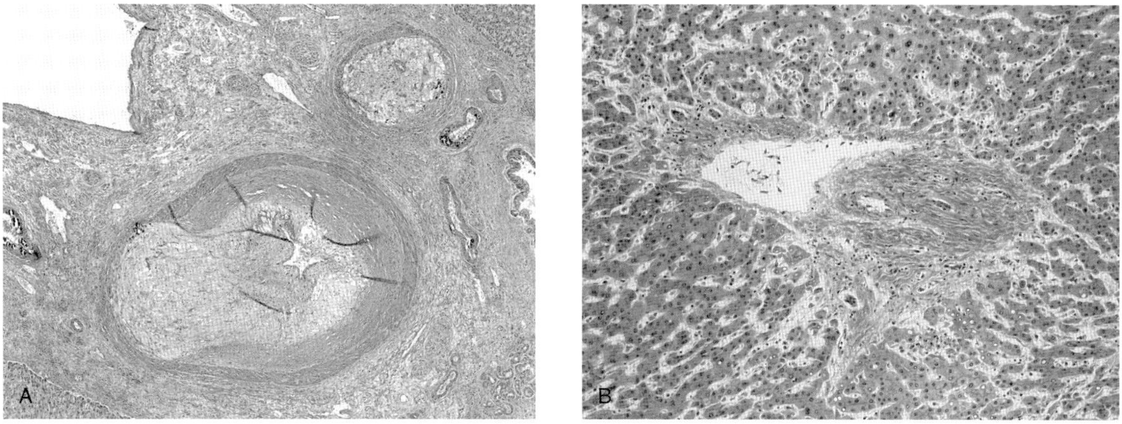

Figure 30.5 Explant of a liver transplantat with chronic (ductopenic) rejection. (**A**) Obliterative rejection arteriopathy with dense intimal foam cell aggregates resulting in subtotal stenosis of arterial lumen. Numerous calcifications of vessel walls are also seen. (H&E). (**B**) Higher magnification of a portal tract in chronic rejection shows a branch of the hepatic artery and portal vein, but no interlobular bile duct. (H&E)

retransplantation if possible. The result of a liver biopsy provides valuable information for this decision. The full spectrum of findings characterizing chronic rejection including perihilar arterial and bile duct changes can be observed in organs explanted due to liver failure and resulting from chronic rejection (Figure 30.5).

Recurrent diseases

The long-term fate of patients with liver transplantation is mainly determined by diseases induced by the transplantation and immunosuppressive therapy and/or recurrence of the original disease. The spectrum of diseases leading to liver transplantation is broad and comprises the following most important categories: 1) viral infections (mainly chronic HCV and HBV infections), 2) chronic cholestatic and autoimmune diseases like autoimmune hepatitis (AIH), primary biliary cirrhosis (PBC), and primary sclerosing cholestasis (PSC), 3) toxic damage, 4) metabolic diseases, and finally 5) tumors. Accordingly, the risk of disease recurrence in the transplant liver varies substantially, ranging from marginal as in toxic insults or hepatitis A over significant (about 20–50%) as in the chronic cholestatic and autoimmune diseases like AIH, PBC, and PSC to nearly universal like in HBV and HCV.[2,21–24]

In a patient with clinical deterioration or worsening of laboratory parameters in the post-transplant course, liver biopsy not only can be helpful to detect recurrence of the original disease but also rule out other concurrent or coexisting disorders. For example, as discussed earlier, in patients who have recurrent chronic HCV proven by detection of the virus in blood, biopsy can confirm disease activity and reveal that there is no concurrent acute cellular rejection.

Recurrence of HCV infection occurs early in nearly all patients transplanted because of chronic HCV infection. Clinical presentation is similar to HCV infection in the native liver. Although progression of the disease depends on the immune status and can vary from an indolent course to rapid progression of fibrosis leading to cirrhosis, it behaves generally more aggressively than HCV infection of the nongraft liver. Histopathologic changes are similar to those of HCV infection in the native liver. The acute infection is characterized by hepatocyte necrosis, lobular disarray, and mild portal inflammation of mononuclear cells. Even a mild bile duct injury may be observed, which in this setting is difficult to delineate from the bile duct damage of acute cellular rejection, as discussed earlier. The chronic HCV infection reveals an increase of the portal infiltrate, sometimes with lymphoid aggregates, some degree of interphase hepatitis, and necro-inflammatory activity (Figure 30.6).

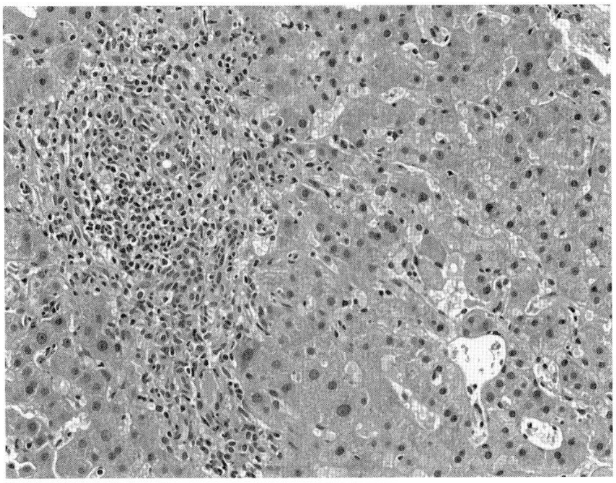

Figure 30.6 Recurrent hepatitis C infection. Characteristic histologic features include portal inflammation with lymphocytes and plasma cells forming lymphoid aggregates with interphase activity and lobular necro-inflammation with apoptotic bodies. The lack of significant diffuse bile duct damage and endothelitis are helpful for the discrimination against cellular rejection. (H&E)

Recurrent HBV infection occurs in three phases similar to HBV infection in native livers, i.e. incubation, acute, and chronic infection. However, compared to HBV infection in native livers, it generally has a more aggressive course with higher inflammatory activity and more rapid progression of fibrosis. Histopathologic findings are similar to those observed in nongraft livers including portal inflammation, lobular disarray and necro-inflammatory activity as well as Kupffer cell activation and ductular reaction. Later in the course, ground glass cells can be found. Diagnosis of HBV can be confirmed by immunostaining for HBV surface (HBsAg) and core (HBcAg) antigen.

Both, recurrent HVB and HCV can result in the aggressive course of fibrosing cholestatic hepatitis. Histopathologic findings of fibrosing cholestatic hepatitis include an inflammatory infiltrate of variable activity, widespread hepatocyte swelling and degeneration, extensive portal fibrosis with newly formed fibrous bands, bile duct involvement in the form of ductular reaction as well as severe canalicular and cellular cholestasis. It is important not to overlook or misinterpret these findings in order to prompt adequate clinical management and therapy.

Diagnosis of recurrent AIH is challenging. As for the native liver, it is based on biochemical, serologic and histopathologic findings. Owing to similar biochemical and histologic findings as in acute cellular rejection and the immunosuppressive therapy due to transplantation, however, it is difficult to use the common diagnostic criteria for AIH. Sometimes it has to rely solely on histopathologic findings. These are not specific for AIH and have to be distinguished from other inflammatory processes including acute cellular rejection. Early changes comprise a lobular inflammation and hepatocyte rosetting, changes of the chronic phase include a significant portal inflammation with plasma cells and prominent interphase hepatitis, and sometimes a pericentral inflammation resembling the pattern found in acute cellular rejection.[25]

Histopathologic findings of recurrent PBC and PSC are similar to those found in native livers. These include a portal inflammation and bile duct damage in PBC, making it difficult to distinguish from acute cellular rejection. Loss of bile ducts is a hallmark of both PSC and chronic rejection. Since both are also characterized by a cholestatic pattern of liver enzymes, differential diagnosis can be challenging.[2]

A proportion of liver transplantation is performed because of liver tumors,[23] mainly hepatocellular carcinoma,[26] but also cholangiocarcinoma,[27] and rare tumor entities like hemangioendothelioma.[28,29] Although due to the impact of imaging-based methods, primary diagnosis of HCC by liver biopsy is a bit exceptional, there is still the general rule that histologic (or cytologic) confirmation is indispensable for making a diagnosis of a neoplasm. Similarly, if a lesion is detected in a transplant liver, it is crucial to confirm tumor recurrence in order to exclude a mass lesion of non-neoplastic nature, in particular infections, or a *de novo* tumor that might result in completely different management of the patient. In rare cases, tumors can also be incidentally detected in liver biopsy taken for other indications, e.g. transplant rejection at times when they have still escaped imaging methods (Figure 30.7).

Infectious diseases in liver transplants

Apart from recurrent viral infections, other viral and nonviral infectious agents can affect the liver graft.

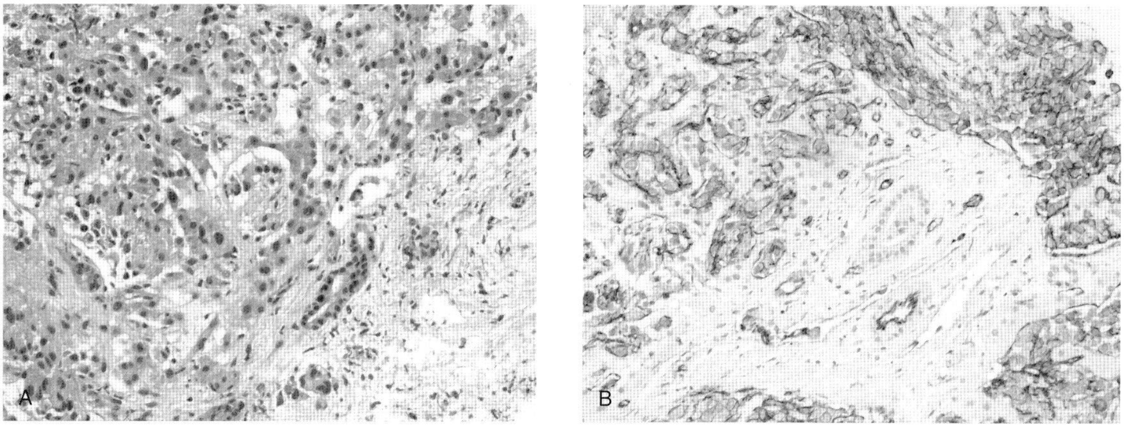

Figure 30.7 Recurrent epithelioid hemangioendothelioma. Biopsy was performed because of suspected rejection. (**A**) Tumor cells infiltrating periportal sinus and portal tract. (H&E). (**B**) CD31 immunostaining highlights tumor cells and sinusoid walls

These comprise newly acquired infections as well as re-activation of mostly opportunistic diseases fostered by immuosuppression. The spectrum includes human CMV, EBV and fungi to mention only the most important ones. Most infectious diseases in the transplant liver morphologically do not differ from those in other organs. Owing to their importance, EBV and CMV infection of the transplant liver are briefly mentioned. EBV-related diseases of the liver include EBV hepatitis and post-transplant lymphoproliferative disorders (PTLDs).

The spectrum of histopathologic changes is broad ranging from a typical EBV hepatitis characterized by a mild portal and sinusoidal infiltrate of sometimes atypical lymphocytes over a more unspecific hepatitis to a pattern with large atypical mononuclear cells to the various forms of PTLD.[2] If EBV infection is among the differential diagnoses in a transplant liver, confirmation of the diagnosis should be aimed by EBV-encoded RNA (EBER) *in situ* hybridization, and suspicion should be reported to clinicians to prompt serologic confirmation.

Liver involvement in the form of CMV hepatitis is a serious complication of post-transplant CMV infection. Clinically, it can be suspected if graft failure and rise of serum transaminases is observed, however diagnosis of CMV hepatitis should be confirmed by liver biopsy. Histopathologic features of CMV hepatitis are variable. Diagnosis is uncomplicated if the characteristic large eosinophilic intranuclear CMV inclusions can be seen. Hepatocytes with CMV inclusions may be surrounded by small clusters of neutrophils forming microabscesses. CMV hepatitis reveals mild lobular disarray and spotty necrosis as well as mononuclear or mixed portal infiltrate and sometimes mild bile duct damage. Differential diagnostic problems arise if the above mentioned characteristic findings are missing since CMV hepatitis has overlapping features with (recurrent) HBV and HCV infection, EBV infection, and especially acute cellular rejection, which also may coexist. In such instances, immunostaining for CMV antigens can point the investigator in the right direction.[30]

Conclusion

Histopathology plays a major role at several times and instances in the management of liver transplantation. Histopathology is not confined to biopsies of the liver allograft, but can also provide critical information on the potential recipient (native) liver, which can speed up or delay indication for (re)-transplantation. Furthermore, histopathology is useful for evaluating donor organ quality, i.e. mainly liver fat content, and also pathologies of the liver explant for quality control purposes. The most frequent indication for liver biopsy in the allograft is the question of acute cellular rejection. Histopathology is the basis of diagnosing and grading acute cellular rejection, and results are crucial for therapeutic decisions concerning immunosuppressive treatment. As generally in histopathology, and in particular for interpretation of allograft biopsies, accurate diagnosis and usefulness of information from pathology depends on interaction between clinicians and pathologists. Histopathologic findings in a liver allograft biopsy have to be correlated with relevant clinical information, including imaging and laboratory results as well as previous biopsies to in order obtain the maximum amount of information from a biopsy as a basis for further decision making in management of the transplant patient.

Abbreviations

AP: alkaline phosphatase, AIH: autoimmune hepatitis, CK7: cytokeratin 7, CMV: cytomegalovirus, EBV: Epstein–Barr virus, γ-GT: gamma glutamyl transpeptidase, H&E: hematoxylin and eosin staining, NAFLD: non-alcoholic fatty liver disease, NRH: nodular regenerative hyperplasia, OLT: orthotopic liver transplantation, PBC: primary biliary cirrhosis, PSC: primary sclerosing cholestasis, RAI: rejection activity index

References

1. Demetris A, Marida M, Nalesnik M, et al. Histopathology of liver transplantation. In: Ruiz P, ed. Transplantation pathology. New York: Cambridge University Press; 2009:111–84.
2. Adeyi O, Fischer SE, Guindi M. Liver allograft pathology: approach to interpretation of needle biopsies with clinicopathological correlation. J Clin Pathol 2010;63:47–74.
3. Dutkowski P, De Rougemont O, Mullhaupt B, Clavien PA. Current and future trends in liver transplantation in Europe. Gastroenterology 2010;138:802–809;e801–4.
4. Alkofer B, Samstein B, Guarrera JV, et al. Extended-donor criteria liver allografts. Semin Liver Dis 2006;26: 221–33.
5. Durand F, Renz JF, Alkofer B, et al. Report of the Paris consensus meeting on expanded criteria donors in liver transplantation. Liver Transpl 2008;14:1694–707.
6. El-Badry AM, Breitenstein S, Jochum W, et al. Assessment of hepatic steatosis by expert pathologists: the end of a gold standard. Ann Surg 2009;250: 691–7.
7. McCormack L, Petrowsky H, Jochum W, Mullhaupt B, Weber M, Clavien PA. Use of severely steatotic grafts in liver transplantation: a matched case–control study. Ann Surg 2007;246:940–6; discussion 946–8.
8. Washington K. Update on post-liver transplantation infections, malignancies, and surgical complications. Adv Anat Pathol 2005;12:221–6.
9. Busquets J, Figueras J, Serrano T, et al. Postreperfusion biopsies are useful in predicting complications after liver transplantation. Liver Transpl 2001;7:432–5.
10. Jain A, Reyes J, Kashyap R, et al. Long-term survival after liver transplantation in 4,000 consecutive patients at a single center. Ann Surg 2000;232:490–500.
11. Kakizoe S, Yanaga K, Starzl TE, Demetris AJ. Evaluation of protocol before transplantation and after reperfusion biopsies from human orthotopic liver allografts: considerations of preservation and early immunological injury. Hepatology 1990;11:932–41.
12. Ferrell L, Bass N, Roberts J, Ascher N. Lipopeliosis: fat induced sinusoidal dilatation in transplanted liver mimicking peliosis hepatis. J Clin Pathol 1992;45: 1109–10.
13. International Working Party. Terminology for hepatic allograft rejection. Hepatology 1995;22:648–54.
14. Banff schema for grading liver allograft rejection: an international consensus document. Hepatology 1997;25: 658–63.
15. Demetris AJ, Ruppert K, Dvorchik I, et al. Real-time monitoring of acute liver-allograft rejection using the Banff schema. Transplantation 2002;74:1290–6.
16. Demetris AJ, Adeyi O, Bellamy CO, et al. Liver biopsy interpretation for causes of late liver allograft dysfunction. Hepatology 2006;44:489–501.
17. Pascher A, Neuhaus P. Bile duct complications after liver transplantation. Transpl Int 2005;18:627–42.
18. Verdonk RC, Buis CI, Porte RJ, Haagsma EB. Biliary complications after liver transplantation: a review. Scand J Gastroenterol 2006;243:89–101.
19. Demetris A, Adams D, Bellamy C, et al. Update of the International Banff Schema for Liver Allograft Rejection: working recommendations for the histopathologic staging and reporting of chronic rejection. An International Panel. Hepatology 2000;31:792–9.
20. Lunz JG 3rd, Contrucci S, Ruppert K, et al. Replicative senescence of biliary epithelial cells precedes bile duct loss in chronic liver allograft rejection: increased expression of p21(WAF1/Cip1) as a disease marker and the influence of immunosuppressive drugs. Am J Pathol 2001;158:1379–90.
21. Ayata G, Gordon FD, Lewis WD, et al. Liver transplantation for autoimmune hepatitis: a long-term pathologic study. Hepatology 2000;32:185–92.

22. Gow PJ, Chapman RW. Liver transplantation for primary sclerosing cholangitis. Liver 2000;20:97–103.
23. Hoti E, Adam R. Liver transplantation for primary and metastatic liver cancers. Transpl Int 2008;21:1107–17.
24. Kotlyar DS, Campbell MS, Reddy KR. Recurrence of diseases following orthotopic liver transplantation. Am J Gastroenterol 2006;101:1370–8.
25. Hubscher SG. Recurrent autoimmune hepatitis after liver transplantation: diagnostic criteria, risk factors, and outcome. Liver Transpl 2001;7:285–91.
26. Tanwar S, Khan SA, Grover VP, Gwilt C, Smith B, Brown A. Liver transplantation for hepatocellular carcinoma. World J Gastroenterol 2009;15:5511–16.
27. Petrowsky H, Hong JC. Current surgical management of hilar and intrahepatic cholangiocarcinoma: the role of resection and orthotopic liver transplantation. Transplant Proc 2009;41:4023–35.
28. Lerut JP, Weber M, Orlando G, Dutkowski P. Vascular and rare liver tumors: a good indication for liver transplantation? J Hepatol 2007;47:466–75.
29. Rodriguez JA, Becker NS, O'Mahony CA, Goss JA, Aloia TA. Long-term outcomes following liver transplantation for hepatic hemangioendothelioma: the UNOS experience from 1987 to 2005. J Gastrointest Surg 2008;12:110–16.
30. Colina F, Juca NT, Moreno E, et al. Histological diagnosis of cytomegalovirus hepatitis in liver allografts. J Clin Pathol 1995;48:351–7.

PART THREE

Chronic Problems in the Transplant Recipient

31

Medical problems after liver transplantation

Eberhard L. Renner and Marco Puglia

Multiorgan Transplant Program, University Health Network, University of Toronto, Toronto, Canada

Key learning points

- With survival after liver transplant continuing to improve, cardiovascular diseases have become an important cause of late morbidity and mortality in liver allograft recipients.
- The use of immunosuppressive medications increases the risk of developing obesity, dyslipidemia, hypertension, diabetes, and the metabolic syndrome, thereby contributing to increased cardiovascular risk after liver transplantation.
- Early recognition and aggressive risk factor modification should translate into improved long-term outcomes. The liver allograft recipient should be considered high risk to develop cardiovascular disease and should be managed according to respective available published guidelines.
- Metabolic bone disease, hyperuricemia, skin disorders and issues regarding family planning have taken on increased importance in the care of the liver allograft recipient. Early recognition of these problems and prompt intervention should reduce or prevent the morbidity associated with these conditions.

Introduction

With long-term survival after liver transplantation having become the rule, the care for medical problems potentially arising over time in the liver transplant recipient has gained increasing importance. Medical management must aim at minimizing long-term morbidity and mortality and, thus, at optimizing long-term quality of life and survival.

Conceptually, long-term medical problems occurring in the liver transplant recipient can be divided into: 1) medical problems that are related to the liver transplant and/or immunosuppression *per se*, and 2) medical problems that are unrelated to transplant/immunsuppression, i.e. are encountered in a similar frequency in an age- and sex-matched nontransplant population. The latter will not be dealt with herein. Within the former, medical problems may arise in connection with overall too little or too much immunosuppression, i.e. rejection (Chapter 19), infections (Chapter 25), and tumors (Chapters 25, 27, and 29), or with recurrent underlying liver disease (Chapter 24). Other medical problems are associated with, and/or facilitated by, commonly used immunosuppressive agents. These include obesity, arterial hypertension, dyslipidemia, diabetes mellitus, cardiovascular risk, gout, osteoporosis, and kidney failure. With the exception of the latter (Chapter 26), these, as well as some issues regarding skin disorders and family planning are discussed in this chapter.

Obesity

Weight gain is common after liver transplantation. In a cohort of 774 adult liver transplant recipients from three centers, body mass index (BMI) (corrected for ascites) increased from 24.8 kg/m^2 pre-transplantation

Medical Care of the Liver Transplant Patient, Fourth Edition. Edited by Pierre-Alain Clavien, James F. Trotter.

to 27.0 kg/m^2 in the first post-transplant year and to 28.1 kg/m^2 in the second post-transplant year, with little change thereafter.[1] Moreover, 21.6% of non-obese liver transplant recipients became obese (BMI ≥ 30 kg/m^2) within 2 years after grafting.[1] Thus, an overall post-transplant prevalence of obesity (BMI ≥ 30 kg/m^2) of around 20%[2] and of overweight (BMI ≥ 25 kg/m^2) of more than 30% was found in some series.[3] These prevalence rates are likely to increase further in the future due to increasing numbers of obese patients being transplanted for cirrhosis related to non-alcoholic fatty liver disease and the increasing prevalence of being overweight and obese in the general population. Transplant-specific risk factors for postoperative weight gain include therapy with steroids[1] and presumably the choice of calcineurin inhibitor.[1,2] While the prevalence rates of those overweight and obese post liver transplantation were slightly – albeit not always statistically significant – higher than in the normal population,[1,4] they likely contribute to the increased incidence of diabetes mellitus, arterial hypertension, dyslipidemia and thus cardiovascular risk in these patients (see later). In addition, overweight/obesity is a risk factor for non-alcoholic fatty liver disease including its potentially progressive variant, non-alcoholic steatohepatitis, which has been reported to occur *de novo* in the graft.[5] The risk of developing health problems according to BMI and waist circumferences, as published by Health Canada,[6] is summarized in Table 31.1 A,B.

Table 31.1 Classification/terminology and relative risk to health

A.

Classification	BMI* category (kg/m^2)	Risk of developing health problems
Underweight	<18.5	Increased
Normal weight	18.5–24.9	Least
Overweight	25.0–29.9	Increased
Obese	≥30.0	
Class I	30.0–34.9	High
Class II	35.0–39.9	Very high
Class III	≥40.0	Extremely high

B.

Waist circumference (cm)	Risk of developing health problems
Men ≥102	Increased
Women ≥88	Increased

*BMI values are age and gender independent and may not be correct for all ethnic groups

Given the high rate of becoming overweight or obese post liver transplant, it seems reasonable to consider routine prophylactic counseling on diet and regular exercise for all transplant recipients (and their partners) within 3 months post transplant. Lifestyle measures should be reinforced and repeat therapeutic counseling offered once BMI increases to ≥25.0 kg/m^2. The potential benefit of other measures in the morbidly obese (BMI ≥40.0 kg/m^2), including orlistat and bariatric surgery, has not been assessed in the post-liver-transplant setting. Such measures, however, bear a risk of interfering with absorption and/or metabolism of immunosuppressive drugs.

Dyslipidemia

Dyslipidemia is common after liver transplantation, thus, hypercholesterolemia has been reported in one-third to two-thirds of liver transplant recipients and hypertryglyceridemia in some 10–50% of liver transplant recipients,[2] with many, but not all of these patients, having mixed hyperlipidemia. Compared with other solid organ transplant recipients, both prevalence and extent of dyslipidemia are generally less in patients with a liver transplant. In a comparative study, serum cholesterol levels averaged 180 mg/dl in liver transplant compared with 226 mg/dl in kidney transplant recipients.[7]

Transplant-specific risk factors for development of post-transplant dyslipidemia include anti-rejection medications, in particular steroids,[7] calcineurin inhibitors (with tacrolimus likely, but debatably, causing somewhat less hypercholesterolemia than cyclosporine),[8] and mTOR inhibitors (sirolimus and everolimus), which typically lead to more pronounced elevation of triglycerides than cholesterol.[9]

Although not formally proven beyond doubt, it seems reasonable to assume that, as in the nonliver-transplant population, cardiovascular risk increases

Table 31.2 ATP III risk categories

Risk category (10-year risk for coronary event)	Definition
High (>20%)	Coronary heart disease (CHD) (history of myocardial infarction, unstable angina, stable angina, coronary artery procedures (angioplasty or bypass surgery), or evidence of clinically significant myocardial ischemia) or CHD risk equivalents (clinical manifestations of noncoronary forms of atherosclerotic disease (peripheral arterial disease, abdominal aortic aneurysm, carotid artery disease with transient ischemic attacks or stroke of carotid artery origin) or >50% obstruction of a carotid artery, diabetes, and ≥2 risk factors with 10-year risk for hard CHD >20%)
Moderately high (10–20%)*	≥2 of the following risk factors: • Cigarette smoking
Moderate (<10%)*	• Arterial hypertension (BP ≥140/90 or on antihypertensive medication) • Low HDL cholesterol (<40 mg/dl, i.e. <1.03 mmol/L) • Family history of premature CHD (CHD in male first-degree relative <55 years of age; CHD in female first-degree relative <65 years of age) • Age (men ≥45 years, women ≥55 years)
Low†	0–1 of the above risk factors

*Calculator available at www.nhlbi.nih.gov/guidelines/cholesterol
†Almost all people with 0 or 1 risk factor have a 10-year risk <10%; a 10-year risk assessment is thus not necessary.
(Modified from reference [10])

in liver transplant recipients with increasing duration and severity of dyslipidemia (see later). Thus, for assessment of cardiovascular risk and for determining thresholds for therapeutic interventions in dyslipidemia, current guidelines and recommendations proposed for the nontransplant population by the respective experts/associations should be followed. The National Cholesterol Education Program Adult Treatment Panel III Guidelines from the USA stratify patients according to their 10-year risk of experiencing a coronary event (Table 31.2) and propose the intervention thresholds outlined in Table 31.3.[10] In 2006, the Canadian Cardiovascular Society put forward updated, more stringent evidence-based guidelines recommending a primary target LDL <2.0 mmol/L for high-risk individuals (Table 31.4).[11] The typical adult liver transplant recipient is in his/her mid-50s, hypertensive, and/or diabetic (see later); many liver transplant recipients therefore fall into at least the moderately high-risk group.

Of the currently available low-density lipid (LDL)–cholesterol-lowering drugs (i.e. HMG-CoA reductase inhibitors or statins), pravastatin and cerivastatin have been formally shown to be safe in liver transplant patients in controlled clinical trials.[12,13] Pravastatin is not prone to drug interactions with calcineurin inhibitors since it has little affinity to the cytochrome P450 system, in particular CYP3A4. Apart from myopathy and other potential side effects, statins led to dose-dependent, reversible hepatic toxicity (alanine amino transferase (ALT) elevation) in approximately 1–3% of patients; close monitoring of liver enzymes is therefore advisable when starting liver transplant recipients on statins. It remains to be determined whether HMG-CoA reductase inhibitors exert beneficial effects beyond lowering LDL cholesterol in liver transplant recipients such as immunomodulatory effects reported from heart and kidney transplant recipients[14] and the stimulation of bone formation observed in postmenopausal women.[15]

Table 31.3 ATP III LDL cholesterol goals and intervention thresholds for therapeutic lifestyle intervention (TLC) and drug therapy in different risk categories (Modified from reference [10])

Risk category	LDL cholesterol goal	Intervention threshold	
		Lifestyle	Drug therapy*
High	<100 mg/dl (<2.59 mmol/L) (optional: <70 mg/dl (<1.81 mmol/L))†	≥100 mg/dl (≥2.59 mmol/L)‡	≥100 mg/dl (≥2.59 mmol/L) (<100 mg/dl (<2.59 mmol/L): consider drug options)§
Moderately high	<130 mg/dl (<3.36 mmol/L)″	≥130 mg/dl (≥3.36 mmol/L)‡	≥130 mg/dl (≥3.36 mmol/L) (100–129 mg/dl (2.59–3.35 mmol/L): consider drug options)**
Moderate	<130 mg/dl (<3.36 mmol/L)	≥130 mg/dl (≥3.36 mmol/L)	≥160 mg/dl (≥4.14 mmol/L)
Low	<160 mg/dl (<4.14 mmol/L)	≥160 mg/dl (≥4.14 mmol/L)	≥190 mg/dl (≥4.91 mmol/L) (160–189 mg/dl) (4.14–4.90 mmol/L: LDL-lowering drug optional)

*When LDL-lowering drug therapy is employed, it is advised that intensity of therapy be sufficient to achieve at least 30–40% reduction in LDL–cholesterol levels

†Very high risk favors the optimal LDL–cholesterol goal of <70 mg/dl, and in patients with high triglyceride, non-HDL–cholesterol <100 mg/dL

‡Any person at high or moderately high risk who has a lifestyle-related risk factor (e.g. obesity, physical inactivity, elevated triglycerides, low HDL–cholesterol, or metabolic syndrome) is a candidate for therapeutic lifestyle changes to modify these risk factors regardless of LDL–cholesterol level

§If baseline LDL–cholesterol is <100 mg/dl, institution of an LDL-lowering drug is a therapeutic option on the basis of available clinical trials. If a high-risk person has high triglycerides or low HDL–cholesterol, combining a fibrate or nicotinic acid with an LDL-lowering drug can be considered

″Optional LDL goal <100 mg/dl

**For moderately high-risk persons, when LDL–cholesterol level is 100–129 mg/dl, at baseline or on lifestyle therapy, initiation of an LDL-lowering drug to achieve an LDL–cholesterol level <100 mg/dl is a therapeutic option on the basis of available trial results

Arterial hypertension

Arterial hypertension is common in liver transplant recipients. Some 40–80% of liver transplant recipients develop arterial hypertension within months to years after transplant. Compared with a normal population, age-adjusted prevalence rates of arterial hypertension have been reported to be increased to 3.07 (95% confidence interval (CI) 2.35–3.93) in long-term survivors (≥5 years) after liver transplantation.[4]

Risk factors for developing arterial hypertension are prevalent in liver transplant recipients and include immunosuppressive therapy with steroids and calcineurin inhibitors, obesity, and the metabolic syndrome.[16,17] Both glucocorticoids and cyclosporine promote sodium and water retention by the kidney, the former via a mineralocorticoid side effect and the latter via sympathetic nerve-mediated renal vasoconstriction.[18] The reversible cyclosporine-mediated renal vasoconstriction together with a more chronic calcineurin inhibitor-associated interstitial nephropathy

Table 31.4 Risk categories and treatment recommendations – Canadian Cardiovascular Society 2006

Risk level	10-year CAD risk	Recommendations
High	>20%	Treatment targets: Primary: LDL-C <2.0 mmol/L Secondary: TC/HDL-C <4.0
Moderate	10–19%	Treat when: LDL-C >3.5 mmol/L or TC/HDL-C >5.0
Low	<10%	Treat when: LDL-C >5.0 mmol/L or TC/HDL-C >6.0

adds up to calcineurin inhibitor nephrotoxicity (see Chapter 26), which predisposes further to arterial hypertension. This may lead to a vicious cycle, with increasing hypertension again aggravating further kidney dysfunction. Moreover, calcineurin inhibitors seem to have direct vasoconstrictive effects. Thus, cyclosporine has been shown to induce in human vascular smooth muscle cells *in vitro* upregulation of angiotensin II receptors and sensitization to angiotensin-mediated Ca-dependent contraction,[19] as well as upregulation of vasopressin receptors.[20]

As in the nontransplant population, arterial hypertension likely adds to the cardiovascular risk of these patients,[17] which is already elevated by the high prevalence of obesity, dyslipidemia, and diabetes. According to the Seventh Report of the Joint National Committee on Prevention, Detection, Evaluation, and Treatment of High Blood Pressure,[17] the definitions and thresholds for intervention given in Table 31.5 apply.

Lifestyle modification, including weight loss, adopting a healthy diet, and increasing physical activity, is an important aspect in the management of arterial hypertension. Table 31.6 outlines the recommended modifications and the approximate reduction in systolic blood pressure expected if these measures are implemented.[17]

Pharmacotherapy of arterial hypertension in the liver transplant recipient is in principle not different from that in the nontransplant patient and there is a multitude of drugs available (for review see Ref.[17]). The following summarizes a few issues specific to liver transplant recipients that are worth mentioning:

1. Steroid withdrawal has been shown to decrease blood pressure in liver transplant recipients.[21]
2. Many patients on calcineurin inhibitors have increased uric acid plasma levels. Concomitant use of thiazide diuretics may further increase hyperuricemia in such patients and precipitate gout attacks.
3. Many patients on calcineurin inhibitors have increased plasma potassium levels. Concomitant use of ACE inhibitors and AT-II blockers may further the risk of clinically relevant hyperkalemia.
4. Calcium channel blockers interfere with calcineurin inhibitor metabolism (inhibition of or competition for CYP3A4) and may lead to elevated cyclosporine and tacrolimus plasma levels. This is of clinical relevance for the nondihydropyridines diltiazem and verapamil, less so for the dihydropyridines, except nicardipine. Moreover, dihydropyridine calcium channel blockers have been shown to protect against calcineurin inhibitor-mediated nephrotoxicity and to lower calcineurin inhibitor-induced hyperuricemia.[22] Dihydropyridine calcium channel blockers such as amlodipine or nifedipine may therefore be considered as first-choice antihypertensive pharmacotherapy in liver transplant recipients. Their most common side effect, peripheral edema, may be counteracted and the antihypertensive effect increased by adding a low dose of a thiazide.

Table 31.5 High blood pressure – definition and threshold for intervention*

Category*	Blood pressure†		Intervention
	Systolic‡	Diastolic‡	
Normal	<120		–
Prehypertension§	120–139	80–89	Lifestyle modification″ Consider 24 h blood pressure monitoring**
Hypertension††	≥140	≥90	Lifestyle modification″ Drug therapy‡‡
If diabetic†† or Impaired kidney function†† (GFR <60 ml/min/1.72 m^2) or Albuminuria†† (>300 mg/d or >200 mg/g creatinin)	>130		Lifestyle modification″ Drug therapy‡‡

*Modified from Ref. [17]. Applies to adults aged 18 and older; the classification is based on the average of ≥2 properly measured, seated blood pressure readings on each of ≥2 office visits

†In mmHg

‡Diastolic blood pressure is a more potent cardiovascular risk factor than systolic blood pressure until the age of 50 years; thereafter, systolic blood pressure is more important.[17] Treatment of systolic hypertension warrants attention, especially in those ≥50 years old

§Pre-hypertension is not a disease category, but identifies subjects at high risk of developing hypertension

″Pre-hypertensive subjects should be advised to practice lifestyle modification in order to reduce their risk of developing hypertension; lifestyle modification is an indispensable part of therapy in hypertensive subjects. Lifestyle modification includes dietary measures in order to decrease overweight/obesity and ideally to reach/maintain a body mass index of 18.5–24.9 kg/m^2, reduction of sodium intake to 6 g NaCl/d, regular aerobic physical activity, and moderation of alcohol consumption. Each of these is able to reduce blood pressure by 2 to up to 20 mmHg[17]

**A loss of the physiologic night-time decrease in blood pressure or night-time hypertension is common in liver transplant recipients.[51,52] Office blood pressure measurements may therefore underestimate average blood pressure in these patients and 24 h ambulatory blood pressure monitoring should be liberally utilized if pre-hypertension develops

††Many liver transplant recipients fall into this category. In (nontransplant) patients with diabetes or chronic kidney disease (defined as glomerular filtration rate <60 ml/min/1.72 m^2 or albuminuria >300 mg/d or >200 mg/g creatinin), rigorous blood pressure control decreases progression of chronic kidney disease (for detail see Ref. [17]). The recommended blood pressure limits are lower than in the absence of these co-morbidities

‡‡Start pharmacotherapy, if lifestyle modification does not reduce blood pressure below 140/90 (130/80 for subjects with diabetes or chronic kidney disease); for choice of drugs see Ref. [17] and text

Diabetes mellitus

Diabetes is common in liver transplant recipients. Conceptually, diabetes already present prior to liver transplantation is distinguished from diabetes developing *de novo* only after liver transplantation, i.e. new-onset post-transplant diabetes. Prevalence rates of pretransplant diabetes mellitus of 10–15%[23–25] and new-onset post-transplant diabetes of <10% to up to 40%[8,23–26] have been reported in liver transplant recipients. The wide range of values reported, particularly with the latter, is in part due to differences in the definition of diabetes. Even the largest study reporting a prevalence rate of new-onset post-transplant diabetes of 37.7% (28.3% transient and 9.4% persistent) in 555 liver transplant recipients

Table 31.6 Lifestyle modifications to manage hypertension

Modification	Recommendation	Approximate SBP reduction
Weight reduction	Maintain healthy body weight (BMI 18.5–24.9 kg/m^2)	5–20 mmHg/10 kg weight loss
Adopt DASH eating plan	Consume a diet rich in fruits, vegetables and low fat dairy products with a reduced content of saturated and total fat	8–14 mmHg
Dietary sodium reduction	Reduce dietary sodium intake to <100 mmol/d (2.4 g sodium)	2–8 mmHg
Physical activity	Engage in regular aerobic physical activity such as brisk walking (at least 30 min/d, most days of week)	4–9 mmHg

DASH: Dietary Approaches to Stop Hypertension

followed for a median of 5 years at three American centers likely underestimated the true prevalence, since it defined diabetes as the use of antidiabetic medication.[26]

The high prevalence of diabetes in liver transplant recipients may, in part, be explained by the association of hepatitis C virus (HCV) infection with insulin resistance/type 2 diabetes[25–29] and by HCV-related end-stage liver disease (ESLD) being the single most common indication for liver transplantation in the West. Thus, the relative risk of pretransplant diabetes has been reported to be increased more than threefold (adjusted odds ratio (OR) 3.77, 95% CI 1.80–7.87)[27] and that of new-onset post-transplant diabetes 2.5- to fivefold in HCV-infected compared with nonHCV-infected patients, respectively.[25] While the exact mechanism(s) for this association of HCV infection and insulin resistance/type 2 diabetes remain(s) to be defined, HCV-induced TNF-alpha production might be involved (for review see Ref. [29]).

Moreover, an increasing number of liver transplants are performed for ESLD due to non-alcoholic steatohepatitis, the underlying insulin resistance likely persisting after transplantation.

Risk factors for developing/aggravating insulin resistance and type 2 diabetes are prevalent post liver transplant and include weight gain, as discussed earlier, but also immunosuppressive therapy with corticosteroids and calcineurin inhibitors, in particular tacrolimus. Corticosteroid dose has been linked to post-transplant diabetes,[23,25] and post-transplant diabetes was found to be around two times more frequent with tacrolimus-based than with cyclosporine-based regimens.[8,25]

As in the nontransplant population, diabetes in liver transplant recipients is associated with significant morbidity and mortality. Thus, in a case–control study, pretransplant diabetes was found to significantly increase post-transplant morbidity, in particular from cardiovascular, infectious, and renal diseases, and to decrease 5-year survival after liver transplantation from 67.7 to 34.5%.[30] Similarly, new-onset post-transplant diabetes was found to be associated with significantly increased morbidity, in particular from cardiovascular, infectious, and neurologic/neuropsychiatric diseases, and with a significantly decreased 2- to 5-year survival in most,[23] but not all studies.

Precise diagnostic criteria and terminology is a prerequisite for classification of dysglycemic disorders. Table 31.7 summarizes the respective criteria according to the American Diabetes Association.[31] These guidelines now include a HbA1c of ≥6.5% as diagnostic of diabetes mellitus. Moreover, and similar to the prognostic value of impaired glucose tolerance and impaired fasting glucose, a HbA1C of 5.7–6.4% increases the risk of developing diabetes.[31]

Impaired fasting glucose and impaired glucose tolerance are often termed "prediabetes"; they are per se not disease entities, but carry the risk of progressing to overt diabetes with time. Impaired fasting glucose and impaired glucose tolerance (insulin resistance) are associated with metabolic syndrome and through that with increased cardiovascular risk.

New-onset post-transplant diabetes has been recently reviewed by an international expert panel; the resulting consensus guidelines have been

Table 31.7 Terminology and diagnostic criteria of diabetes and dysglycemic disorders

	Fasting plasma glucose (mmol/L)		2 h plasma glucose in a 75 g oral glucose tolerance test (mmol/L)
Impaired fasting glucose	5.6–6.9		NA
Impaired fasting glucose (isolated)	5.6–6.9	and	<7.8
Impaired glucose tolerance (isolated)	<5.6	and	7.8–11.0
Impaired fasting glucose and impaired glucose tolerance	5.6–6.9	and	7.8–11.0
Diabetes	≥7.0	or	≥11.1

published.[32] New-onset post-transplant diabetes was felt to resemble type 2 diabetes and the management aspects and differences given in Table 31.8 were emphasized.

Metabolic syndrome and cardiovascular risk

Metabolic syndrome is a clustering of cardiovascular risk factors, including overweight/obesity, dyslipidemia, insulin resistance, and arterial hypertension. Table 31.9 depicts the operational diagnostic criteria for metabolic syndrome according to Ref. [33] Other panels/organizations have used similar definitions/diagnostic criteria (for review see Ref. [34]).

The diagnosis of metabolic syndrome is made if ≥3 of the earlier-mentioned risk factors are present.

Many of the aforementioned studies in liver transplant recipients focused on some component(s) of metabolic syndrome, but did not employ strict criteria for diagnosing the syndrome itself. Thus, exact prevalence rates of metabolic syndrome in liver transplant recipients are lacking. However, from all the aforementioned studies, it seems clearly conceivable that metabolic syndrome is highly prevalent among liver transplant recipients. Intuitively, it seems to also make sense that the clustering of cardiovascular risk factors within metabolic syndrome should carry an increased risk for developing cardiovascular events, i.e. for cardiovascular morbidity and mortality. This is corroborated by an, albeit nontransplant, population-based study from Finland[35] and by the fact that the Framingham equation for estimating cardiovascular risk contains with high-density lipid (HDL)–cholesterol and blood pressure two components of metabolic syndrome (for discussion see Ref. [34]).

Using the Framingham equation and comparing with an age- and sex-matched normal population, a recent study from a single center predicted an almost twofold increased 10-year risk for coronary events in 181 consecutive liver transplantation recipients at a median of 54 months after grafting.[36] While the observed cardiovascular event rate in the latter study did not differ from that in the normal population, another study clearly demonstrated a 3.07fold (95% CI 1.98–4.43) and 2.56fold (CI 1.52–4.05) increased risk for ischemic cardiac events and for cardiovascular death, respectively, in 100 consecutive liver transplant recipients followed for a median of 3.9 years after grafting.[37] With long-term survival becoming routine after liver transplantation, cardiovascular morbidity and mortality will likely also become increasingly relevant in liver transplant recipients, just as it is well known for recipients of other solid-organ transplants such as the kidney.

Therapy of metabolic syndrome consists of lifestyle modifications, i.e. reduction of overweight/obesity by dietary measures and exercise, and, if this alone is insufficient in eliminating cardiovascular risk factors, of pharmacotherapy aimed at controlling dyslipidemia, insulin resistance, and blood pressure, as outlined earlier.

Hyperuricemia and gout

Hyperuricemia is common in liver transplant recipients and was observed on average in 47 and 86% of

Table 31.8 Selected aspects of the management of new-onset post-transplant diabetes and differences/similarities to that of Type II diabetes*

Management aspect	Recommendation/frequency of testing	Comments
FPG testing	Weekly for first post-transplant month	Identify patients with dysglycemia
	At 3, 6, and 12 months	
	Annually thereafter	
OGTT	Consider in patients with normal FPG or those with impaired glucose tolerance	Utility not validated in this population
Tailoring immunosuppressive therapy	Decrease/withdraw corticosteroids as soon as possible	Consider switching to calcineurin inhibitor-free regimen in poorly controlled
	Consider switching to cyclosporine in poorly controlled tacrolimus-treated patients	cyclosporine-treated patients
Lifestyle modification	Council all patients with elevated FPG and/or abnormal OGTT regarding dietary measures, weight reduction, and exercise	
Oral agent pharmacotherapy Monotherapy		
Base choice of agent mainly on safety†	Comparative efficacy/tolerability not formally explored in this population	
	Consider potential of serious adverse events in patients with renal impairment	
Combination	Use same combinations as in nontransplant type 2 diabetics†	Efficacy/tolerability not formally explored in this population
Insulin + oral agent pharmacotherapy	Consider in patients poorly controlled on oral agent combination pharmacotherapy alone	Efficacy/tolerability not formally explored in this population
Self-monitoring of blood glucose	Essential component of management of patients receiving oral agent pharmacotherapy/insulin	Similar to recommendation for patients with type 2 diabetes‡
HbA1C	In patients with diabetes:	Interpret with care in patients with anemia/renal impairment
	Measure every 3 months	
	Intervention if HbA1C ≥6.5%	
Microalbuminuria	In patients with diabetes: consider annual screening	Not validated in this population
Diabetic complications	In patients with diabetes: screen annually	Similar to recommendation for patients with type 2 diabetes‡
Lipid levels	In patients with diabetes: evaluate annually	Similar to recommendation for patients with type II diabetes‡
Dyslipidemia	In patients with diabetes: aggressive lipid-lowering therapy according to NCEP§	All patients considered at high risk of coronary heart disease (CHD)
Hypertension	In patients with diabetes: keep blood pressure <130/80	Value of blood pressure lowering not tested in this population

*Modified for liver transplant setting from Ref. 32

†For review see Ref. 32

‡see Ref. 35

§see Ref. 10. FPG: fasting plasma glucose, OGTT: oral glucose tolerance test, NCEP: National Cholesterol Education Program

Table 31.9 Clinical identification of metabolic syndrome using NCEP ATP III criteria*

Risk factor	Defining level†
Fasting plasma glucose	≥5.6 mmol/L
Arterial blood pressure	≥130/85 mmHg
Fasting triglycerides	≥1.7 mmol/L
HDL–cholesterol	
Men	<1.0 mmol/L
Women	<1.3 mmol/L
Abdominal obesity	Waist circumference
Men	>102 cm
Women	>88 cm

*See refs 32,33

†The diagnosis of metabolic syndrome is made when ≥3 of the risk factors are present

patients 40 and 98 months after transplantation in two single-center series (n = 134 and 75, respectively).[38,39] The prevalence of hyperuricemia did not differ in cyclosporine- and tacrolimus-treated patients[38] and led to the clinical manifestation of gout in 6 and 2.6%, respectively.[38,39]

Hyperuricemia in liver transplant recipients is attributable to decreased renal uric acid clearance, rather than increased uric acid production. This seems largely due to a calcineurin inhibitor-induced decrease in glomerular filtration rate,[40] but a calcineurin inhibitor-induced decreased tubular uric acid secretion may contribute.[41] Additional factors predisposing to hyperuricemia in post-liver-transplant patients include obesity and diuretic therapy, in particular with thiazides.

Hyperuricemia may further impair already decreased renal function (glomerular filtration rate), thus leading to more uric acid retention, increased hyperuricemia, and, thus, establishing a vicious cycle for renal function in liver transplant recipients. Indeed, allopurinol treatment of hyperuricemic liver transplant recipients with increased serum creatinin has been shown to improve renal function in a retrospective analysis.[38]

Colchicin is the treatment of choice for acute gout attacks in the liver transplant recipient. Nonsteroidal anti-inflammatory drugs should be used with caution, since they bear the risk of further decreasing glomerular filtration rate, and thus uric acid clearance, by inhibiting renal prostaglandin synthesis. Allopurinol should be used as maintenance therapy to decrease uric acid blood levels and to secondarily prevent subsequent attacks in all patients with a history of gout. In addition, diuretic use should be critically re-evaluated in these patients and, in particular, thiazides discontinued, if possible. In the absence of manifest gout, allopurinol maintenance therapy may be considered in hyperuricemic patients with impaired glomerular filtration rate (elevated serum creatinin) in an attempt to improve renal function.[38] Allopurinol by inhibiting xanthine oxidase interferes with azathioprine metabolism. This may lead to cumulation of a myelotoxic azathioprine metabolite and potentially life-threatening bone marrow suppression. For safety reasons, azathioprine should therefore not be used concomitantly with allopurinol. There are no drug interactions between allopurinol and mycophenolic acid preparations (mycophenolate mofetil or mycophenolate sodium). Mycophenolic acid preparations can therefore safely replace azathioprine, if concomitant treatment with allopurinol is necessary.

Osteoporosis

Osteoporosis is a common finding in liver transplant recipients. Pooling results from cross-sectional studies and osteoporosis of the lumbar spine and hip (T-score in dual x-ray absorptiometry (DEXA) <–2.5, i.e. bone mineral density >2.5 standard deviations below the mean for young healthy adults) was found in 32 and 27% of liver transplant recipients in a recent comprehensive review.[42] An additional proportion of post-liver-transplant patients have severely reduced bone mineral density (osteopenia with Z-scores between −1 and −2.5).

Longitudinal studies demonstrate that bone mineral density decreases rapidly in the initial 3–6 months post transplant and subsequently stabilizes or improves again and reaches pretransplant levels in many patients at 1 year following grafting (for review see Ref. 42).

Factors affecting osteopenia/osteoporosis in post-liver-transplant patients include pretransplant osteopenia/osteoporosis attributable to chronic ESLD (not only the cholestatic entities; for a review see Ref

42), perioperative immobilization, and immunosuppression with corticosteroids and calcineurin inhibitors. Corticosteroids inhibit intestinal calcium absorption and have in part cytokine-mediated, direct effects on bone metabolism. The calcineurin inhibitors cyclosporine and tacrolimus have both been shown to cause bone loss (high-turnover osteoporosis) in animal models.[43] In addition, all other recognized risk factors for bone loss, including gender, hypogonadism/postmenopausal state, age, and smoking, also pertain to liver transplant recipients.

Based on the aforementioned information, it is not surprising that osteoporotic fractures, in particular of trabecular bone such as the vertebrae of the lumbar spine, occur in up to 30% of liver transplant recipients, typically within the first 3–6 months post transplant (for a review see Ref. 42). Compression fractures of the lumbar spine early post transplant impact on quality of life and mobilization, and often delay full rehabilitation with reintegration into daily life and professional activities.

It is therefore recommended that patients with chronic ESLD undergo a bone-density measurement at the lumbar spine and at the femoral neck (DEXA) at least during evaluation for liver transplantation.[40] All cirrhotic patients including liver transplant candidates should get counseling regarding lifestyle measures (exercise and smoking cessation) and vitamin D (400–800 IU/d) and calcium (1–1.5 g/d) supplements. Biphosphonates should be started in patients with bone density measurements falling into the osteoporotic range and/or with a history of osteoporotic fractures. Hormone replacement therapy should be considered in appropriate patients.[42] This is aimed at preserving as much bone mass as possible up to transplant. After liver transplantation, corticosteroids should be tapered and withdrawn as soon as possible. Liver transplant recipients may profit from continuing vitamin D and calcium supplements, which are approved for prevention of corticosteroid-induced bone loss and have been shown to inhibit post-transplant bone loss in kidney and kidney/pancreas transplant recipients.[44] Continuing hormone replacement therapy should be considered in appropriate patients. In patients with pretransplant osteoporosis/osteoporotic fractures, it also seems reasonable to continue biphosphonates post transplant. It seems reasonable to repeat bone density determination at 1 year after transplantation (or, as a baseline, if osteoporotic fractures occur) and adjust therapy accordingly.

Skin disorders

The skin of liver transplant recipients requires special attention. The mucocutaneous lesions associated with specific hepatic diseases and the dermatologic manifestations of ESLD usually improve or disappear after liver transplantation. The skin of the liver transplant patient may, however, provide crucial diagnostic clues such as maculopapular lesions of the extremities, potentially heralding graft vs host disease.[45] In addition, liver transplant recipients are at risk of developing a number of skin disorders including infections with rare organisms alone or in combination, and non-melanoma skin cancer, in particular squamous cell carcinoma.[45,46] The relative risk of developing squamous cell carcinoma has been found to be seventy- to one hundredfold higher after liver transplantation than in the general population[46,47] and to increase with the frequency and extent of lifetime sun exposure.[46]

Liver transplant recipients should therefore be advised to protect their skin from intense exposure to sunlight, the best protection being to wear dark clothes. When exposure is unavoidable, sun block should be applied 30 min before exposure and frequently reapplied. They should be counseled to periodically check their integument themselves and to have less accessible regions such as the back checked by a partner. In addition, the transplant physician or a dermatologist should annually examine the entire integument of every liver transplant recipient including the oral cavity and perianal area. A dermatologist should be consulted for evaluation of any suspicious lesion. Such systematic examination permits acting on early precancerous lesions such as actinic keratosis, oral leukoplakia, and verrucae, and prevents their progression to stages requiring extensive (plastic) surgery.

Family planning

Secondary amenorrhea is frequent in premenopausal women suffering from ESLD. Within months of successful liver transplantation menses and libido return in approximately 90% of these women.[48] Obviously, genetic counseling should be offered to patients who were transplanted for an inheritable disease. Numerous successful deliveries in liver graft recipients have been reported.[49] Any pregnancy in a liver transplant recipient should, however, be regarded as a high-risk pregnancy as hypertension, pre-eclampsia, intrauterine growth retardation, and prematurity are more frequent in these patients than in the general population.[50] Respective close monitoring is therefore mandatory. It seems advisable for women to wait at least 1 year after transplantation before planning to conceive;[49] this allows the mother to recover from transplant surgery and any potential early complication, as well as to reach stable allograft function with low-level maintenance immunosuppression. Calcineurin inhibitors and azathioprine can be maintained during the pregnancy;[50] sirolimus, mycophenolate, and other newer immunosuppressive drugs should be stopped and replaced due to the lack of sufficient safety data.[50] Contraception with intrauterine devices is generally discouraged in liver transplant recipients because of the risk of pelvic infectious complications.

References

1. Everhart JE, Lombardero M, Lake JR, et al. Weight change and obesity after liver transplantation: incidence and risk factors. Liver Transpl Surg 1998;4:285–96.
2. Guckelberger O, Bechstein WO, Neuhaus R, et al. Cardiovascular risk factors in long-term follow-up after orthotopic liver transplantation. Clin Transpl 1997;11: 60–5.
3. Aberg F, Hockerstedt JA, Isoniemi H. Cardiovascular risk profile of patients with acute liver failure after liver transplantation when compared with the general population. Transplantation 2010;89:61–8.
4. Sheiner PA, Magliocca JF, Bodian CA, et al. Long-term medical complications in patients surviving > or = 5 years after liver transplant. Transplantation 2000;15: 781–9.
5. Burke A, Lucey MR. Non-alcoholic fatty liver disease, non-alcoholic steatohepatitis and orthotopic liver transplantation. Am J Transplant 2004;4:686–93.
6. Health Canada. Canadian guidelines for body weight classification in adults. Ottawa, ON: Health Canada 2003. Publication H49-179/2003E. (http://www.hc-sc.gc.ca/hpfb-dgpsa/onpp-bppn/weight_book_tc_e.html).
7. Fernandez-Miranda C, dela Calle A, Morales JM, et al. Lipoprotein abnormalities in long-term stable liver and renal transplant patients. A comparative study. Clin Transpl 1998;12:136–41.
8. Levy G, Villamil F, Samuel D, et al. Results of lis2t, a multicenter, randomized study comparing cyclosporine microemulsion with C2 monitoring and tacrolimus with CO monitoring in de novo liver transplantation. Transplantation 2004;77:1632–9.
9. Ross H, Pflugfelder P, Haddad H, et al. Reduction of cyclosporine following the introduction of everolimus in maintenance heart transplant recipients: a pilot study. Transplant Int 2010;23:31–7.
10. Grundy SM, Cleeman JI, Merz NB, et al. for the Coordinating Committee of the National Cholesterol Education Program. Implications of recent trials for the National Cholesterol Education Program Adult Treatment Panel III Guidelines. Circulation 2004;110: 227–39.
11. McPherson R, Frohlich J, Fodor G, Genest J. Canadian Cardiovascular Society position statement – recommendations for the diagnosis and treatment of dyslipidemia and prevention of cardiovascular disease. Can J Cardiol 2006;22:913–27.
12. Imagawa DK, Dawson S 3rd, Holt CD, et al. Hyperlipidemia after liver transplantation: natural history and treatment with the hydroxy-methylglutaryl-coenzyme A reductase inhibitor pravastatin. Transplantation 1996;62:934–42.
13. Zachoval R, Gerbes AL, Schwandt P, et al. Short-term effects of statin therapy in patients with hyperlipoproteinemia after liver transplantation: results of a randomized cross-over trial. J Hepatol 2001;35: 86–91.
14. Neal DA, Alexander GJ. Can the potential benefits of statins in general medical practice be extrapolated to liver transplantation? Liver Transpl 2001;7: 1009–14.
15. Edwards CJ, Hart DJ, Spector TD. Oral statins and increased bone-mineral density in postmenopausal women. Lancet 2000;355:2218–19.
16. Hricik DE, Lautman J, Bartucci MR, et al. Variable effects of steroid withdrawal on blood pressure reduction in cyclosporine-treated renal transplant recipients. Transplantation 1992;53:1232–6.
17. Chobanian AV, Bakris GL, Black HR, et al. Seventh report of the Joint National Committee on Prevention, Detection, Evaluation, and Treatment of High Blood Pressure. Hypertension 2003;42:1206–52.
18. Moss NG, Powell SL, Falk RJ. Intravenous cyclosporine activates afferent and efferent renal nerves and causes sodium retention in innervated kidney in rat. Proc Natl Acad Sci USA 1985;822:8222–6.

19. Avdonin PV, Cottet-Maire F, Afanasjeva GV, et al. Cyclosporine A up-regulates angiotensin II receptors and calcium responses in human vascular smooth muscle cells. Kidney Int 1999;55:2407–14.
20. Krauskopf A. Vasopressin type 1A receptor up-regulation by cyclosporin A in vascular smooth muscle cells is mediated by superoxide. J Biol Chem 2003;278:41685–90.
21. Gomez R, Moreno E, Colina F, et al. Steroid withdrawal is safe and beneficial in stable cyclosporine-treated liver transplant patients. J Hepatol 1998;28:150–6.
22. Chanard J, Toupance O, Lavaud S, et al. Amlodipine reduces cyclosporin-induced hyperuricaemia in hypertensive renal transplant recipients. Nephrol Dial Transpl 2003;18:2147–53.
23. Navasa M, Bustamante J, Marroni C, et al. Diabetes mellitus after liver transplantation: prevalence and predictive factors. J Hepatol 1996;25:64–71.
24. Knobler H, Stagnaro-Green A, Wallenstein S, et al. High incidence of diabetes in liver transplant recipients with hepatitis C. J Clin Gastroenterol 1998;26: 30–3.
25. Aedosary AA, Ramji AS, Elliott TG, et al. Post-liver transplantation diabetes mellitus: an association with hepatitis C. Liver Transpl 2002;8:356–61.
26. Khalili M, Lim JW, Bass N, et al. New onset diabetes mellitus after liver transplantation: the critical role of hepatitis C infection. Liver Transpl 2004;10: 349–55.
27. Mehta SH, Brancati FL, Sulkowski MS, et al. Prevalence of type 2 diabetes mellitus among persons with hepatitis C virus infection in the United States. Ann Int Med 2000;133:592–9.
28. Bigam DL, Pennington JJ, Carpentier A, et al. Hepatitis C-related cirrhosis: a predictor of diabetes after liver transplantation. Hepatology 2000;32:87–90.
29. Knobler H, Schattner A. TNF-(alpha), chronic hepatitis C and diabetes: a novel triad. Q J Med 2005;98:1–6.
30. John RR, Thuluvath PJ. Outcome of liver transplantation in patients with diabetes mellitus: a case control study. Hepatology 2001;34:889–895.
31. American Diabetes Association. Diagnosis and classification of diabetes mellitus. Diabetes Care 2010;33(Suppl 1):S62–9.
32. Davidson JA, Wilson A on behalf of the International Expert Panel on New-Onset Diabetes after Transplantation. New-onset diabetes after transplantation 2003 International Consensus Guidelines. Diabetes Care 2004;27:805–12.
33. Grundy SM, Cleeman JI, Daniels SR, et al. American Heart Association; National Heart, Lung, and Blood Institute. Diagnosis and management of the metabolic syndrome: an American Heart Association/National Heart, Lung, and Blood Institute Scientific Statement. Circulation 2005;112:2735–52.
34. Grundy SM, Brewer B, Cleeman JI, et al. for the conference participants. Definition of the metabolic syndrome. Report of the National Heart, Lung, and Blood Institute/American Heart Association Conference on scientific issues related to definition. Circulation 2004;109: 433–8.
35. Lakka HM, Laaksonen DE, Lakka TA, et al. The metabolic syndrome and total and cardiovascular disease mortality in middle-aged men. JAMA 2002;288: 237–52.
36. Neal DA, Tom BD, Luan J, et al. Is there disparity between risk and incidence of cardiovascular disease after liver transplant? Transplantation 2004;77: 93–9.
37. Johnston SD, Morris JK, Cramb R, et al. Cardiovascular morbidity and mortality after orthotopic liver transplantation. Transplantation 2002;73:901–6.
38. Neal DAJ, Tom BDM, Gimson AES, et al. Hyperuricemia, gout, and renal function after liver transplantation. Transplantation 2001;72:1689–91.
39. Shibolet O, Elinav E, Ilan Y, et al. Reduced incidence of hyperuricemia, gout, and renal failure following liver transplantation in comparison to heart transplantation: a long-term follow-up study. Transplantation 2004;77: 1576–80.
40. Zurcher R, Bock HA, Thiel G. Hyperuricemia in cyclosporin-treated patients: GFR-related effect. Nephrol Dial Transpl 1996;11:153–8.
41. Marcen R, Gallego N, Orofino L, et al. Impairment of tubular secretion of urate in renal transplant patients on cyclosporin. Nephron 1995;70:307–13.
42. Leslie WD, Bernstein CN, Leboff MS. AGA technical review on osteoporosis in hepatic disorders. Gastroenterology 2003;125:941–6.
43. Cvetkovic M, Mann GN, Romero DF, et al. The deleterious effects of long-term cyclosporin A, cyclosporin G, and FK 506 on bone mineral metabolism in vivo. Transplantation 1994;57:1231–7.
44. Josephson MA, Schumm LP, Chiu MY, et al. Calcium and calcitriol prophylaxis attenuates posttransplant bone loss. Transplantation 2004;78:1233–6.
45. Schmied E, Dufour JF, Euvrard S. Nontumoral dermatologic problems after liver transplantation. Liver Transpl 2004;10:331–9.
46. Mithoefer AB, Supran S, Freeman RB. Risk factors associated with the development of skin cancer after liver transplantation. Liver Transpl 2002;8: 939–44.
47. Lindelof B, Sigurgeirsson B, Gabel H, et al. Incidence of skin cancer in 5356 patients following organ transplantation. Br J Dermatol 2000;143:513–19.

48. Cundy TF, O'Grady JG, Williams R. Recovery of menstruation and pregnancy after liver transplantation. Gut 1990;31:337–8.
49. Nagy S, Bush MC, Berkowitz R, et al. Pregnancy outcome in liver transplant recipients. Obstet Gynecol 2003;102:121–8.
50. Heneghan MA, Selzner M, Yoshida EM, et al. Pregnancy and sexual function in liver transplantation. J Hepatol 2008;49:507–19.
51. Van de Borne P, Gelin M, Van de Stadt J, et al. Circadian rhythms of blood pressure after liver transplantation. Hypertension 1993;21:398–405.
52. Taler SJ, Textor SC, Canzanello VJ, et al. Loss of nocturnal blood pressure fall after liver transplantation during immunosuppressive therapy. Am J Hypertens 1995;8:598–605.

32 Prevention and treatment of recurrent HBV and HCV infection

Ed Gane
New Zealand Liver Transplant Unit, Auckland City Hospital, Auckland, New Zealand

Key learning points

- Interferon (IFN)-based therapy does not increase the risk of acute rejection.
- Combination pegylated IFN plus ribavirin in patients with established recurrent hepatitis C achieves sustained virologic response (SVR) rates of 15–30%.
- Combination pegylated IFN plus ribavirin in patients early post transplant (pre-emptive therapy) has poor tolerability and efficacy and is not currently recommended.
- Combination pegylated IFN plus ribavirin in patients awaiting liver transplantation has poor tolerability and efficacy and should only be considered in well-compensated liver disease.
- The hepatitis C virus (HCV) genotype is the best predictor for SVR following antiviral therapy in the treatment of established recurrent hepatitis C.
- Hepatitis B immunoglobulin (HBIG) reduces hepatitis B virus (HBV) re-infection to <40%, with lower efficacy in those with detectable HBV DNA levels prior to transplantation.
- Combination HBIG plus lamivudine reduces recurrence rates to <5%.
- IM HBIG plus lamivudine reduces costs by 90% without loss of efficacy.
- Recurrent HBV infection can be effectively treated by combination oral antiviral therapy.

Liver transplantation for chronic hepatitis C

Almost 200 million people are currently infected with chronic HCV, with the highest rates reported in the Middle East, eastern Europe and Southeast Asia.[1] Although the incidence of HCV infections has fallen following exclusion of HCV-positive blood donors and reduction in the incidence of IV drug use (IDU)-associated HCV,[2–4] this is an aging cohort and the proportion with cirrhosis will double over the next decade.[5] The demand for liver transplantation for HCV-related hepatocellular carcinoma and liver failure is projected to treble by the year 2030.[6–8]

Recurrent hepatitis C infection is universal and occurs at the time of reperfusion. The natural history of recurrent hepatitis C is accelerated, with 20–40% progressing to cirrhosis within 5 years. Recurrent hepatitis C is associated with reduced graft and patient survival and has been compared to these losses in HCV-negative recipients.

The best predictor of rapid fibrosis progression is the grade of necroinflammation at 1 year post transplant.[9–11] In addition, multiple host, donor, and viral pretransplant predictors have been identified, including pretransplant viral load,[12] donor age[13–16] and high-dose steroid therapy for acute rejection.[17]

Prevention of recurrent HCV infection

Peritransplant prophylaxis

Initial allograft infection occurs at reperfusion, therefore prevention requires neutralization of any circulating virus following removal of the native liver.

Medical Care of the Liver Transplant Patient, Fourth Edition. Edited by Pierre-Alain Clavien, James F. Trotter.

Prior to the elimination of antiHCV-positive blood donors, it was noted that in patients transplanted for HBV/HCV co-infection, perioperative administration of very high IV doses of polyclonal immunoglobulin appeared to protect French patients from recurrent HCV infection as well as recurrent HBV.[18] These observations led to the proposal that immunoglobulin preparations that contained large amounts of polyclonal HCV anti-envelope antibodies could prevent primary HCV infection of the graft. Although single post-exposure infusion of concentrated polyclonal hepatitis C immunoglobulin HCIG may delay clinical infection in chimpanzees and repeated doses may suppress viremia,[19] no such benefit has been demonstrated in the trials to date of perioperative infusions of high-dose IV hepatitis C immunoglobulin. Neither monoclonal nor polyclonal HCIG decreased either the incidence, time of onset, or severity of recurrent hepatitis C.[20–22] The best prospects for perioperative prophylaxis now lie with the development of combinations of direct-acting antiviral therapies, of which more than 20 agents are in clinical development, from four classes (nucleoside polymerase inhibitors, non-nucleoside inhibitors, NS3/4a protease inhibitors, and cyclophyllin inhibitors). Combination direct-acting antiviral (DAA) studies have already commenced in patients with chronic hepatitis C,[23] but none are currently planned in patients either awaiting or post liver transplantation, reflecting concerns about potential toxicity in liver failure and direct drug interactions with the calcineurin inhibitors. These proof-of-concept studies must be performed, however, given the likelihood that combination DAAs without cross-resistance may provide safe and effective perioperative prophylaxis to prevent recurrent hepatitis C infection of the allograft.

Pretransplant treatment on the waiting list

The aim for treating transplant candidates whilst on the waiting list is to prevent recurrent hepatitis C infection through eradication prior to transplant. Unfortunately, the adherence of both pegylated IFN and ribavirin is decreased in patients with end-stage liver disease because of increased risks of sepsis and bleeding in patients with neutropenia and thrombocytopenia from hypersplenism and increased risk of hemolysis from functional renal impairment. IFN-induced flares may also precipitate acute decompensation and death in patients with advanced liver disease.[24] In a pilot study of 32 patients listed with decompensated cirrhosis (mean Child–Pugh score (CPS) = 12 ± 1), less than half were suitable for IFN treatment, only 33% had end-of-treatment response (ETR), and none achieved SVR. Almost 90% withdrew from the study because of serious adverse events (SAEs), namely sepsis, encephalopathy, or bleeding.[25] In a second study of 124 patients with less advanced disease (mean CPS = 7 ± 2), a low accelerating dose regimen was adopted, whereby patients were started on half-dose of both pegylated IFN and ribavirin with incremental increases as tolerated over the next 4 weeks. This was better tolerated, with 15 (12%) developing SAEs; four of these patients died.[26] A total of 30 (24%) patients achieved SVR, half of whom were delisted because of clinical improvement. A total of 12 patients were transplanted after a documented SVR and none developed recurrent HCV infection. In comparison, three patients were transplanted whilst PCR negative but whilst still on treatment and two-thirds recurred. Subsequent studies of pretransplant treatment of HCV have also reported poor tolerability and efficacy and would support a cautious approach to antiviral therapy prior to liver transplantation. The most recent Asia and Pacific Association of the Study of the Liver consensus statement suggests that patients with decompensated hepatitis C should only be considered for treatment in an experienced liver unit, preferably a transplant centre.[27]

A low ascending dose regimen should be adopted and supportive therapies to prevent variceal bleeding, infections and correct cytopenias are recommended. To avoid precipitating life-threatening encephalopathy, spontaneous bacterial peritonitis (SBP) and hepatorenal syndrome, treatment should be limited to those with a CPS ≤7 and a MELD score ≤18, without clinical ascites and with a baseline platelet count >60 000. The best candidates for treatment are those with well-compensated cirrhosis, i.e. those listed for hepatocellular carcinoma (HCC). The option of delaying transplantation until completion of 48 weeks' treatment and further 24 weeks' follow up to conform SVR is not practical in patients listed for HCC. The other group of potential candidates with well-compensated liver disease for pretransplant treatment are those awaiting live-donor liver transplantation.[28] It is likely once their safety and efficacy is demonstrated in compensated HCV infection that the combination DAA regimens will be studied in patients awaiting transplantation. The advantage of these patients is that the likely duration of therapy will be short, 8–16 weeks, thereby allowing successful eradication without unnecessarily delaying the date of transplantation. In addition, the rapid, potent viral suppression achieved by these regimens may rescue many or most patients listed for liver failure.

Management of recurrent HCV infection

Management of the recipient with recurrent hepatitis C involves strategies that may prevent HCV-related graft loss through prevention or delay in the rate of progression of fibrosis in the graft. These include lifestyle factors, such as avoidance of alcohol and prevention of hepatic steatosis through management of metabolic syndrome and post-transplant diabetes mellitus. There is now abundant evidence that optimization of immunosuppression is also important. Recent changes in immunosuppression practices may have contributed to the lack of improvement in long-term outcomes following transplantation for hepatitis C compared to those reported following transplantation for other conditions. Both overimmunosuppression in the early post-transplant period (especially pulse steroid therapy or antilymphocyte antibody therapy for management of acute rejection) and rapid weaning of maintenance immunosuppression during the first year are both associated with more rapid fibrosis progression and increased HCV-related graft loss. Avoidance of adjuvant immunosuppression and maintaining patients long term on low-dose prednisone or the addition of azathioprine may actually protect against rapid progression of recurrent hepatitis C.[29–32]

The most important management of recurrent hepatitis C is eradication of HCV infection through successful antiviral therapy; this is associated with improved graft and patient survival.[33] This has been associated with improved patient and graft survival, even in patients with established recurrent HCV cirrhosis, where SVR is associated with reduction in portal hypertension.[34]

Unfortunately, liver transplant recipients with recurrent HCV infection often have multiple baseline negative predictors for response to IFN-based therapy. Pretreatment viremia levels are increased 1–2 logs by immunosuppression following liver transplantation, often exceeding 10^7 units/ml.[35–37] A viral load >400 000 IU/ml will be present in >90% of liver transplant recipients, the cut-off associated with a low response to the current standard of care (SOC). In addition to increasing viral replication, immunosuppression also has direct effects on the efficacy of IFN, blunting the initial antiviral effect (Phase One slope).[38] Immunosuppression also blunts both innate immune responses and HCV-specific T-cell immune responses, which may contribute to the high relapse rate after cessation of therapy.[39–41]

The most important factor, however, which reduces the efficacy of current antiviral therapy, is poor adherence, due to poor tolerability of both IFN and ribavirin. Dose reduction must be undertaken in >80% and almost 30% must cease therapy because of adverse effects.

Ribavirin tolerability is affected by increased severe hemolysis because of reduced renal clearance following liver transplantation.[42] In nontransplant patients, hemolysis necessitated ribavirin dose reduction in <10% whilst in liver and kidney transplant recipients, ribavirin dose was reduced in 40–66% and stopped in 10–33%.[43–50] Strategies to improve ribavirin adherence include supportive transfusions and erythropoietin, although the latter has not been associated with improved response rates in nontransplant patients.[51] Adjusting ribavirin dose according to a renal function algorithm is possible if monitoring assay of plasma ribavirin levels is available. The dose can then be adjusted to target trough plasma ribavirin levels of 10–15 mmol/L.[52] This assay, however, is not yet widely available.

IFN tolerability is also reduced following transplantation, with increased dose-related cytopenias leading to treatment cessation in almost 20% of liver transplant recipients.[43–50] Depression may also be more common, leading to treatment cessation in almost 20% of liver transplant recipients.[53–55] Pre-emptive use of selective serotonin reuptake inhibitor (SSRI) prophylaxis may help prevent this complication and improve adherence.[56] IFN is an immunomodulator that upregulates HLA class I antigen expression and therefore could potentially increase the risk of allograft rejection.[57] Despite an early report of increased chronic rejection during IFN monotherapy, no other studies have observed an increased risk of either acute or chronic rejection in recipients who received antiviral therapy.[58–62] It would seem prudent to delay IFN-alpha therapy in any patient with either established chronic rejection or recurrent severe acute rejection.[63]

Overall SVR rates with the current SOC (48 weeks' combination pegylated IFN plus weight-based ribavirin) in liver transplant recipients with recurrent hepatitis C range from 20 to 35%, which is significantly lower than those achieved in nontransplant patients with chronic HCV infection. As in nontransplant HCV, HCV genotype 2/3 infection is associated with a higher SVR in recurrent hepatitis C. SOC achieves SVR in 40–85% of transplant recipients with recurrent HCV genotype 2/3 infection compared to only 15–34% in those with genotype 1.[33,64–66]

The most popular antiviral strategy is targeting those recipients at highest risk for recurrent cirrhosis and graft loss. The best predictor of rapid fibrosis progression is the grade of necroinflammation and stage of fibrosis in the 1-year protocol allograft biopsy.[67–70] However, early fibrosis stage is also associated with higher SVR, suggesting that treatment should not be delayed until significant allograft injury has developed.

Recently, host genotyping (SNP of rs12979860, near IL28-alpha) has been demonstrated to be the most important baseline predictor of SVR with an odds ratio of almost 7 in patients with the CC genotype compared to TC or TT. Recent studies suggest that this genotype also predicts SVR in liver transplant recipients with recurrent hepatitis C.[71]

On-treatment early virologic predictors are established as part of routine clinical practice in nontransplant HCV treatment. The most accurate predictors of SVR are the early virologic response (EVR), defined as: 1) HCV RNA after 12 weeks' therapy decreased ≥2 log reduction from baseline, 2) complete early virologic response (cEVR), defined as undetectable HCV RNA after 12 weeks, and 3) rapid virologic response (RVR) defined as undetectable HCV RNA after 4 weeks. These have also been validated in the treatment of recurrent hepatitis C, where the strongest positive predictor for SVR was RVR (positive predictive value (PPV) 90–100%), whilst PPV for cEVR was 69–100% and for EVR only 49–65%.[72–76] In contrast, the strongest negative predictor for SVR (i.e. absence was associated with subsequent failure to achieve SVR) was EVR (NPV 89–100%) whilst the NPV of RVR was only 53–82%. These studies would support the adoption of a 12-week stopping rule for patients who fail to achieve EVR. There is no data available yet to support reduced duration of therapy for those patients who achieve RVR.

Pre-emptive therapy

Although primary infection of the allograft occurs immediately following reperfusion, antiviral therapy in the immediate post-transplant period should delay the onset of acute hepatitis in the graft and subsequent fibrosis progression.[36,77] The advantages of treating early are that viral load and quasispecies diversity are still low and graft fibrosis is minimal or absent – all positive predictors for SVR. This is, however, offset by the poor tolerability of both ribavirin and pegylated IFN due to renal dysfunction and cytopenias from hypersplenism and concomitant medications. Early studies of pre-emptive IFN monotherapy randomized to no treatment reported delayed onset of acute hepatitis but no significant SVR and no improvement in graft or patient survival.[78–79] In a study of pre-emptive pegylated IFN plus ribavirin, almost two-thirds of screened patients were excluded because of anemia, renal dysfunction, rejection, or sepsis.[80] Of those who started treatment, 85% required dose reduction and 40% were discontinued, largely because of rejection and cytopenias. Only 9% achieved SVR and almost 30% developed a SAE during treatment. These results have reduced enthusiasm for pre-emptive therapy with combination pegylated IFN plus ribavirin. In the recent large, randomised multicentre PHOENIX study, 115 patients were randomized to receive either pegylated interferon-alfa 2a (135 mg/week for 4 weeks followed by 180 mg/week for 44 weeks) plus ribavirin (400 mg p.o. daily escalating to 1200 mg p.o. daily for 48 weeks) or no treatment. No differences in SVR were seen between those randomized to pre-emptive therapy (12/54) and those who switched to treatment (3/14). Rates of histologic recurrence, patient and graft survival were also similar.[81]

Liver transplantation for hepatitis B

Chronic hepatitis B (CHB) remains the leading indication for liver transplantation in the Asia–Pacific region. It is also the leading cause of liver-related mortality in the region, accounting for over 1 million deaths per annum, mostly due to HCC. The improving economies and availability of live-related liver donation have allowed a rapid expansion of liver transplantation within the Asia–Pacific region, where now more than 5000 transplants are performed annually for CHB.

Pretransplant treatment

The introduction of potent oral antiviral therapy provided new therapeutic options for patients with CHB, with particular benefits in patients with decompensated CHB, where potent viral suppression was followed by improvement in liver synthetic function and rescue from death or transplantation.[82–83] Despite more potent antiviral suppression than lamivudine, the efficacy of the more potent antivirals entecavir, tenofovir and telbivudine was similar in decompensated CHB.[84–87] The major benefit of these newer agents is the lower resistance rates. In addition, telbivudine appears to be associated with improvement in renal function.[87] Indeed, in many populations, there appears to be a decreasing need for liver transplantation due to a decline in decompensated CHB; HBV-related HCC has replaced liver failure as the chief indication for listing in patients with CHB.[88]

Peritransplant prophylaxis

Without prophylaxis, HBV recurs in more than 80% of cases and in all cases that are HBV DNA positive prior to transplant, resulting in accelerated liver disease and reduced graft and patient survival. As recently as 1983, an NIH Consensus statement recommended that CHB be considered an absolute contraindication to liver transplantation because of abysmal post-transplant outcomes (5-year patient survival rate <20%) achieved in the absence of any effective antiviral prophylaxis.

The first successful prevention strategy was passive immunoprophylaxis with hepatitis B immunoglobulin (HBIG). A large multicentre European study demonstrated that high-dose IV HBIG reduced the overall recurrence rate by 60%.[89] Best results were achieved in those patients with low or undetectable HBV DNA levels at the time of transplant, namely fulminant hepatic failure and hepatitis delta co-infection.[90] Poor results were achieved in patients with high HBV DNA levels at the time of transplant, reflecting the mechanisms of action of HBIG. HBIG protects the allograft through inhibition of initial hepatocyte infection by complexing with circulating virions and also by blocking intrahepatic spread. Patients with high HBV DNA at the time of transplant are at risk for early recurrence because of insufficient neutralizing antibody in the immediate perioperative phase, or late recurrence because of more rapid selection of surface escape mutants in the "a" determinant of the HBV pre-S/S genome.

Specific protocols with very high dose HBIG were developed to improve the efficacy of HBIG in patients with high levels of circulating HBV DNA. These include both fixed high doses (10 000 IU intraoperative, daily for 1 week, weekly, then monthly long term)[91] or on-demand high doses (targeting "protective" trough [anti-HBs] titers above 500 IU/ml).[92] These aggressive dosing protocols require 300 000–400 000 IU for the first year and 120 000–200 000 IU each subsequent year, with an associated annual cost around USD75–120 K for the first year and USD 50–100 K thereafter.

HBIG monotherapy must be maintained long term to prevent late recurrence following HBIG withdrawal. Persistent, low-level HBV replication can be detected in allografts up to 10 years post transplant, indicating a high risk of recurrence following HBIG withdrawal at any time post transplant.[93]

Unfortunately, the high cost and limited availability of IV HBIG preparations has limited the widespread adoption of such regimens in many countries. These issues have encouraged the development of less expensive, alternative strategies, including HBIG dose reduction, IM HBIG administration, late HBIG withdrawal in selected "low-risk" patients and total HBIG avoidance.

Reducing the dose of IV HBIG to 2000 IU/month, and targeting a lower trough anti-HBs level, has similar efficacy but is <50% the cost of the standard high-dose regimen (10 000 IU/month).[94]

IM HBIG achieves adequate neutralizing [anti-HBs] titres during the immediate post-transplant period and cannot be recommended as perioperative prophylaxis as monotherapy.[95–96] However, the addition of an oral nucleos(t)ide analogue will improve the efficacy of low-dose IM HBIG. Pretransplant administration of nucleos(t)ide analogues will suppress the circulating viral load prior to transplantation, thereby reducing the required perioperative neutralizing dose of anti-HBs. Post-transplant co-administration of nucleos(t)ide analogues with HBIG should help prevent or delay the emergence of surface escape mutants. Late breakthrough during combination HBIG plus lamivudine prophylaxis is rare and necessitates selection of variants conferring resistance to both HBIG and lamivudine, which is possible because of overlapping reading frames of major catalytic regions of the HBV polymerase gene and neutralization domains of the surface gene.[97–98]

Conversion from IV to low-dose IM HBIG in the late post-transplant period is safe and effective with [anti-HBs] titers maintained above 100 IU/ml long term. Therefore, conversion to IM administration after perioperative induction IV HBIG appears to be a cost-effective alternative to IV HBIG plus lamivudine.

Combination lamivudine plus IM HBIG also appears to be effective when used from the time of transplant with similar efficacy to that achieved with IV HBIG combined with oral nucleoside therapy (<5% recurrence after 5 years), but at only 10% of the cost.[99–100] Lamivudine plus low-dose IM HBIG is the most cost-effective prophylaxis regimen against recurrent HBV infection.[101]

Several small studies have reported that late withdrawal of HBIG (substituted with maintenance lamivudine monotherapy) may be possible in patients who were HBV DNA negative at the time of transplant.[102–104]

Attempts to replace HBIG with *de novo* production of anti-HBs through post-transplant vaccination have been disappointing, with no sustained protective responses achieved with standard recombinant vaccines.[105]

The replacement of HBIG by combination of lamivudine plus adefovir, two oral antivirals without cross-resistance, should prevent late recurrence even in those patients who are HBV DNA positive at the time of transplant. In a randomized, controlled study in patients maintained on lamivudine plus HBIG for at least 1 year post transplant, switching to lamivudine plus adefovir provided equivalent protection against HBV recurrence, but with better tolerability and reduced cost.[106]

In a recent study, the replacement of lamivudine plus HBIG by tenofovir plus emtricitabine (a nucleoside inhibitor similar to lamivudine) was well tolerated with no recurrence after 24 months.[107]

The ultimate prophylaxis will be a completely oral regimen, without the inconvenience and high cost associated with HBIG. In an Australasian prospective open-labelled pilot study, lamivudine plus adefovir started at the time of listing and continued lifelong was effective, safe, and well tolerated, and removed the need for maintenance post-transplant HBIG.[108] No recurrence has been reported after a median follow up of more than 3 years. Compared to lamivudine or adefovir, entecavir is a more potent antiviral agent with a very high genetic barrier to resistance. This agent has been used as monotherapy to prevent recurrent HBV in Hong Kong since 2007. No recurrence has been observed in the 90 patients transplanted on entecavir (personal communication, CM Lo). Future prophylactic strategies are likely to include entecavir plus tenofovir, with the latter also effective in patients with established lamivudine resistance prior to transplant.

Prophylaxis in patients with pretransplant lamivudine resistance

With the widespread use of lamivudine over recent years, an increasing proportion of patients being assessed for liver transplantation already have established lamivudine resistance. In this "high-risk" population, the combination of lamivudine and adefovir dipivoxil (ADV) is effective in preventing re-infection of the graft, with or without concomitant HBIG.[109–110] The commercially available combination of tenofovir plus emtricitabine (Truvada™, Gilead Pharmaceuticals, Foster City, CA, USA) is also likely to be effective in this population.

Treatment of recurrent hepatitis B

Although recurrent hepatitis B is now a rare event, when it does occur (with documented reappearance of both HBsAg and HBV DNA), HBIG should be withdrawn to avoid the risk of immune-complex disease. Appropriate rescue therapy should be started, preferably with a combination of two oral antiviral agents without cross-resistance, either lamivudine plus adefovir, lamivudine plus tenofovir, or entecavir plus tenofovir.

Transplantation with a liver from an anti-HBcore-positive donor

A liver from such a donor may result in *de* novo HBV infection in 40–80% of HBV-naïve recipients. This risk becomes negligible if the recipient receives long-term prophylaxis with either lamivudine or HBIG or if the recipient is seronegative for HBsAg but positive for anti-HBs.

Conclusion

Recurrence of HCV infection is universal and immediate following liver transplantation for HCV cirrhosis, and may be associated with rapid fibrosis progression in 20% of recipients. Successful eradication of HCV by antiviral therapy improves survival in liver transplant recipients with recurrent hepatitis C, however the efficacy and tolerability of current antiviral therapy is poor with SVR rates of <30%. There is an urgent need to develop more effective and better tolerated antiviral regimens for this area of unmet need. The introduction of direct-acting antivirals (polymerase and protease inhibitors) may provide new opportunities in the treatment of established recurrence and as pre- or peritransplant prophylaxis to prevent recurrent infection.

In contrast, excellent outcomes are now expected following liver transplantation for HBV and now associated with excellent long-term graft and patient survival. Lifelong HBIG immunoprophylaxis is costly and inconvenient. The use of potent oral nucleos(t)ide analogues have allowed HBIG minimization strategies. A combination of nucleos(t)ides without cross-resistance should provide a completely HBIG-free, oral prophylaxis regimen and should further improve the outcomes, tolerability and cost effectiveness of transplantation for chronic hepatitis B.

References

1. Shepard C, Finelli L, Alter M. Global epidemiology of hepatitis C infection. Lancet Infect Dis 2005;5:558–67.
2. NCHECR Report to the Ministry of Health Advisory Committee. Hepatitis C Virus Projections Working Group: Estimates and Projections of the Hepatitis C Virus Epidemic in Australia 2006. October 2006.
3. CDCCompressedMortalityFile.(http://wonder.cdc.gov/controller) (accessed 1 June 2008).
4. National Health and Nutrition Examination Surveys 1988–2006. (http://www.cdc.gov/nchs/about/major/nhanes) (accessed 1 June 2008).
5. Armstrong G, Wasley A, Simard E, et al. Prevalence of HCV infection in the United States. Ann Int Med 2006;144:705–14.
6. Wise M, Bialek S, Bell B, et al. Changing trends in HCV-related mortality in USA. Hepatology 2008;47:1128–35.
7. Davila J, Morgan R, Shaib Y, et al. HCV and increasing incidence of hepatocellular carcinoma: a population-based study. Gastroenterol 2004;127:1372–80.
8. Davis G, Albright J, Cook S. Projecting future complications of chronic hepatitis C in United States. Liver Transpl 2003;9:331–8.
9. Firpi R, Abdelmalek M, Soldevila-Pico C, et al. One-year protocol liver biopsy can stratify fibrosis progression in liver transplant recipients with recurrent hepatitis C infection. Liver Transplant 2004;10:1240–7.
10. Prieto M, Bereguer M, Rayon J, et al. High incidence of allograft cirrhosis in HCV genotype 1b following transplantation. Hepatology 1999;29:250–6.
11. Gane E, Portmann B, Naoumov N, et al. Long-term outcome of hepatitis C infection after liver transplantation. N Engl J Med 1996;334:821–7.
12. Charlton M, Seaberg E, Wiesner R, et al. Predictors of patient and graft survival following liver transplantation for hepatitis C. Hepatology 1998;28:823–30.
13. Thuluvath P, Krok K, Segev D, Yoo H. Trends in post-transplant survival in patients with HCV between 1991 and 2001 in the United States. Liver Transplant 2007;13:719–24.
14. Mutimer D, Gunson B, Chen J, et al. Impact of donor age and year of transplantation on graft and patient survival following liver transplantation for hepatiis C. Liver Transplant 2006;81:7–14.
15. Zekry A, Whiting P, Crawford D, et al. Liver transplant for HCV-associated liver cirrhosis: recipient predictors of outcomes in population with significant genotypes 3 and 4 distribution. Liver Transpl 2003;9:339–47.
16. Fasola C, Netto G, Onaca N, et al. A more severe HCV recurrence post-liver transplant observed in recent years may be explained by use of lower dose corticosteroid maintenance protocols. Hepatology 2003;38:226A.
17. Wiesner R, Demetris A, Seaberg E, et al. Acute hepatic allograft rejection: risk factors and impact on outcome. Hepatology 1998;28:638–45.
18. Feray C, Gigou M, Samuel D, et al. Incidence of hepatitis C in patients receiving immunoglobulins after liver transplantation. Ann Intern Med 1998;128:810–16.

19. Krawczynski K, Alter M, Tankersley D, et al. Effect of immune globulin on prevention of experimental HCV infection. JID 1996;173:822–8.
20. Willems B, Ede M, Marotta P, et al. HCV human immunoglobulins for the prevention of graft infection in HCV-related liver transplantation. J Hepatol 2002;36:32.
21. Davis G, Nelson D, Terrault N, et al. A randomised open-label study to evaluate the safety and pharmacokinetics of human hepatitis C immunoglobulin in liver transplant recipients. Liver Transpl 2005;11: 941–9.
22. Schiano T, Charlton M, Younossi Z, et al. Monoclonal HCV-AbXTL68 in patients undergoing liver transplantation for HCV. Liver Transpl 2006;12:1381–9.
23. Gane E, Roberts S, Stedman C, et al Interferon-free oral combination therapy with a nucleoside polymerase inhibitor (RG7128) and protease inhibitor (danoprevir/RG7227) for the treatment of chronic hepatitis C genotype 1 infection: Results of the INFORM-1 trial. Lancet 2010;376:1467–75.
24. Lock G, Reng C, Schölmerich J, et al. Interferon-induced hepatic failure in a patient with hepatitis C. Am J Gastroenterol 1999;94:2570–1.
25. Crippin J, McCashand T, Terrault N, et al. A pilot study of the tolerability and efficacy of antiviral therapy in hepatitis C-infected patients awaiting liver transplantation. Liver Transpl 2002;4:350–55.
26. Everson G, Trotter J, Forman L, et al. Treatment of advanced hepatitis C with a low accelerating dosage regimen of antiviral therapy. Hepatology 2005;42: 255–62.
27. McCaughan G, Omato M, Dore G, et al. APASL consensus statements on the diagnosis, management and treatment of hepatitis C infection. J Gastroenterol Hepatol 2007;22:615–33.
28. Halprin A, Trotter J, Everson G, et al. Posttransplant eradication by pretransplant treatment in living donor liver transplant recipients. Hepatology 2001;34: 244A.
29. Brillanti S, Vivarelli M, De Ruvo N, et al. Slowly tapering off steroids protects the graft against hepatitis C recurrence after liver transplantation. Liver Transpl 2002;8:884–8.
30. Vivarelli M, Burra P, La Barba G, et al. Influence of steroids on HCV recurrence after liver transplantation: A prospective study. J Hepatol 2007;47:793–8.
31. Berenguer M, Aguilera V, Prieto M, et al. Significant improvement in the outcome of HCV-infected transplant recipients by avoiding rapid steroid tapering and potent induction immunosuppression. J Hepatol 2006;44:717–22.
32. Samonakis D, Triantos C, Thalheimer U, et al. Immunosuppression and donor age with respect to severity of HCV recurrence after liver transplantation. Liver Transpl 2005;11:386–9.
33. Berenguer M, Palau A, Aguilera V, et al. Clinical benefits of antiviral therapy in patients in recurrent HCV. Am J Transpl 2008;8:679–87.
34. Carrion J, Navasa M, Garcia-Retortillo M, et al. Efficacy of antiviral therapy on HCV recurrence after liver transplantation: a randomized, controlled study. Gastroenterol 2007;132:1746–56.
35. Chazouilleres O, Kim M, Coombs C, et al. Quantitation of HCV RNA in liver transplant recipients. Gastroenterology 1994;106:994–9.
36. Gane E, Naoumov N, Qian K, et al. A longitudinal analysis of hepatitis C virus replication following liver transplantation. Gastroenterology 1996;110: 167–77.
37. Everhart J, Wei Y, Eng H, et al. Recurrent and new HCV infection after liver transplantation. Hepatology 1999;29:1220–6.
38. Reiberger T, Rasoul-Rockenschaub S, Rieger A, et al. Efficacy of interferon in immunocompromised HCV patients after liver transplantation or with HIV co-infection. Europ JCI 2008;38:421–9.
39. Rosen H, Hinrichs D, Gretch D, et al. Association of multispecific CD4+ response to HCV and severity of recurrence after liver transplantation. Gastroenterol 1999;117:926–32.
40. Gruener N, Jung M, Ulsenheimer A, et al. Analysis of a successful HCV-specific CD8+ T cell response in patients with recurrent HCV-infection after orthotopic liver transplantation. Liver Transpl 2004;10: 1487–96.
41. Schirren C, Zachoval R, Gerlach J, et al. Antiviral treatment of recurrent hepatitis C virus (HCV) infection after liver transplantation: association of a strong, multispecific, and long-lasting CD4+ T cell response with HCV-elimination. J Hepatol 2003;39:397–404.
42. Dumortier J, Ducos E, Scoazec J-Y, et al. Plasma ribavirin concentrations during treatment of recurrent hepatitis C with peginterferon alpha-2b and ribavirin combination after liver transplantation. J Viral Hepatol 2006;13:538–43.
43. Gopal D, Rabkin J, Corless C, et al. Treatment of progressive hepatitis C recurrence after liver transplantation with combination interferon plus ribavirin. Liver Transpl 2001;7:181–90.
44. De Vera M, Smallwood G, Rosado K, et al. Interferon and ribavirin for treatment of recurrent hepatitis C after liver transplantation. Transplantation 2001;71: 678–86.
45. Menon K, Poterucha J, El-Amin O, et al. Treatment of posttransplantation recurrence of hepatitis C with interferon and ribavirin: lessons in tolerability and efficacy. Liver Transpl 2002;8:623–9.

46. Alberti A, Belli L, Airoldi A, et al. Combined therapy with interferon and low dose ribavirin in posttransplantation recurent hepatitis C: a pragmatic study. Liver Transpl 2001;7:870–6.
47. Reddy R, Fried M, Dickson R, et al. Interferon alfa-2b and ribavirin vs. placebo as early treatment in patients transplanted for hepatitis C end-stage liver disease: results of multicenter, randomized trial. Gastroenterol 2002;122:A199.
48. Garnier JL, Chevallier P, Dubernard JM, Trepo C, Touraine JL, Chossegros P. Treatment of hepatitis C virus infection with ribavirin in kidney transplant patients. Transplant Proc 1997;29:783.
49. Daoud S, Garnier JL, Chossegros P, Chevallier P, Dubernard JM, Touraine JL. Hepatitis C virus infection in renal transplantation. Transplant Proc 1995;27: 1735.
50. Jain A, Eghtesad B, Venkataramanan R, et al. Ribavirin dose modification based on renal function is necessary to reduce hemolysis in liver transplant patients with hepatitis C virus infection. Liver Transpl 2002;8: 1007–13.
51. Shiffman M, Salvatore J, Hubbard S, et al. Treatment of chronic hepatitis C genotype 1 with Peginterferon, ribavirin and epoetin alpha. Hepatology 2007;46:371–9.
52. Rendina M, Schena A, Castellaneta N, et al. The treatment of chronic hepatitis C with peginterferon alfa-2a (40 kDa) plus ribavirin in haemodialysed patients awaiting renal transplant J Hepatol 2007;46: 768–74.
53. Zdilar D, Franco-Bronson K, Buchler N, et al. Hepatitis C, interferon alfa and depression. Hepatology 2000;31:1207–11.
54. De Bona M, Ponton P, Ermani M, et al. The impact of liver disease and medical complications on quality of life and psychological distress before and after liver transplantation. J Hepatol 2000;33:609–15.
55. Forton D, Allsop J, Main J, et al. Evidence for a cerebral effect of HCV. Lancet 2001;358:38–9.
56. Musselman D, Lawson D, Gumnick J, et al. Paroxetine for the prevention of depression induced by high-dose interferon. N Engl J Med 2001;34:961–6.
57. Slater A, Klein J, Sonnerfield G, et al. The effects of interferon in a model of rat heart transplantation. J Heart Lung Transpl 1992;11:975–8.
58. Wright T, Combs C, Kim M, et al. Interferon-alpha therapy for hepatitis C virus infection after liver transplantation. Hepatology 1994;20:773–9.
59. Gane E, Lo SK, Portmann BC, et al. A randomised study comparing ribavirin and interferon-alpha monotherapy for hepatitis C recurrence after liver transplantation. Hepatology 1998;27:1403–7.
60. Jain A, Demetris A, Manez R, et al. Incidence and severity of acute allograft rejection in liver transplant recipients treated with alfa interferon. Liver Transpl Surg 1998;4:197–203.
61. Vogel W. 40 kDA Peginterferon alfa-2a (Pegasys) in post-liver transplant recipients with established recurrent hepatitis C: Preliminary results of a randomized multicenter trial. 2005;128:631–5.
62. Stravitz R, Shiffman M, Sanyal A, et al. Effects of interferon on liver histology and allograft rejection in patients with recurrent hepatitis C following liver transplantation. Liver Transpl 2004;10:850–8.
63. Walter T, Dumortier J, Guillard O, et al. Rejection under alpha interferon therapy in liver transplant recipients. Am J Transplant 2007;7:177–84.
64. Roche B, Sebagh M, Canfora M, et al. HCV therapy in liver transplant recipients: response predictors effect on fibrosis progression and importance of initial stage of fibrosis. Liver Transpl 2008;14: 1766–77.
65. Calmus Y, Duvoux C, Pageaux G, et al. Multicentre randomised trial in HCV-infected patients treated with pegylated IFN and ribavirin followed by ribavirin alone after liver transplantation. Am J Transpl 2008;8: A1617.
66. Cescon M, Grazi G, Cucchetti A, et al. Predictors of SVR after antiviral treatment for HCV recurrence following liver transplantation. Liver Transpl 2009;15: 782–9.
67. Gane E, Portmann B, Naoumov N, et al. Long-term outcome of hepatitis C infection after liver transplantation. N Engl J Med 1996;334:821–7.
68. Prieto M, Bereguer M, Rayon J, et al. High incidence of allograft cirrhosis in HCV Genotype 1b following transplantation. Hepatology 1999;29:250–6.
69. Firpi R, Abdelmalek M, Soldevila-Pico C, et al. One-year protocol liver biopsy can stratify fibrosis progression in liver transplant recipients with recurrent hepatitis C infection. Liver Transpl 2004;10: 1240–7.
70. Neumann U, Berg T, Bahra M, et al. Fibrosis progression after liver transplantation in patients with recurrent hepatitis C. J Hepatol 2004;41:830–6.
71. Charlton M, Thompson A, Veldt B, et al. IL28B polymorphisms are associated with histological recurrence and treatment response following liver transplantation in patients with HCV with HCV infection. Hepatology 2010;52:S1:A1.
72. Hanouneh I, Miller C, Aucejo F, et al. Recurrent HCV after liver transplant: On treatment prediction of response to Peg/RBV. Liver Transpl 2008;14: 53–8.
73. Oton E, Barcena R, Moreno-Planas J, et al. Hepatitis C recurrence after liver transplantation: viral and histologic response to full-dose peg-interferon and ribavirin. Am J Transpl 2006;6:2345–55.

74. Carrion J, Marreo J, Fontana R, et al. Efficacy of antiviral therapy on HCV recurrence after liver transplantation. Gastroenterol 2007;132:1746–56.
75. Sharma P, Marrero J, Fontana R, et al. Sustained virologic response to therapy of recurrent hepatitis C after liver transplantation is related to early virologic response and dose adherence. Liver Transpl 2007;13: 1100–8.
76. Gane E, Strasser S, Crawford D, et al. A multicenter, randomized trial of combination pegylated interferon-alpha 2a plus ribavirin vs. pegylated interferon-alpha 2a monotherapy in liver transplant recipients with recurrent hepatitis C. Hepatology 2009;50:A.
77. Ballardini G, de raffele E, Groff P, et al. Timing of reinfection and mechanisms of hepatocellular damage in transplanted HCV-infected liver. Liver Transpl 2002;8:10–20.
78. Singh N, Gayowski T, Wannstedt C, et al. Interferon-alpha for prophylaxis of recurrent viral hepatitis C in liver transplant recipients. Transplantation 1998;65: 82–6.
79. Sheiner P, Boros P, Klion F, et al. The efficacy of prophylactic interferon-α in preventing recurrent hepatitis C after liver transplantation. Hepatology 1998;28: 831–8.
80. Shergill A, Khalili M, Straley S, et al. Applicability, tolerability and efficacy of pre-emptive antiviral therapy in HCV-infected patients undergoing liver transplantation. Am J Transplant 2005;5:118–24.
81. Bzowej N, Nelson D, Terrault N, et al. PHOENIX: a randomised controlled trial of peginterferon alpha 2a plus ribavirin as a prophylactic treatment for HCV. Liver Transpl 2011;528–538.
82. Villeneuve JP, Condreay LD, Willems B, et al. Lamivudine treatment for decompensated cirrhosis resulting from chronic hepatitis B. Hepatology 2000;31:207–10.
83. Fontana RJ, Hann HW, Perrillo RP, et al. Determinants of early mortality in patients with decompensated chronic hepatitis B treated with antiviral therapy. Gastroenterology 2002;123:719–27.
84. Liaw YF, Lee CM, Akarca US, et al. Interim results of a double-blind, randomized phase 2 study of the safety of tenofovir disoproxil fumarate, emtricitabine plus tenofovir disoproxil fumarate and entecavir in the treatment of chronic hepatitis B subjects with decompensated liver disease. Hepatology 2009;50(Suppl4): 409A.
85. Shim JH, Lee HC, Kim KM, et al. Efficacy of entecavir in treatment-naive patients with hepatitis B virus-related decompensated cirrhosis. J Hepatol 2011 doi:10.1016/j.jhep.2009.11.077
86. Liaw YF, Raptopoulou M, Cheinquer H, et al. Efficacy and safety of entecavir versus adefovir in chronic hepatitis B patients with evidence of hepatic decompensation. 60th Annual Meeting of the American Association for the Study of Liver Diseases; October 30 – November 3, 2009 Boston, MA, USA. Oral presentation #222.
87. Gane EJ, Chan HL, Choudhuri G, et al. Treatment of decompensated HBV cirrhosis: Results from 2 years' randomized trial with telbivudine or lamivudine. J Hepatol 2010;52:S4.
88. Kim WR, Terrault N, Pederson R, et al. Trends in waiting list registration for liver transplantation for viral hepatitis in the United States. Gastroenterol 2009;137:1680–6.
89. Samuel D, Muller R, Alexander G, et al. Liver transplantation in European patients with the hepatitis b surface antigen. N Engl J Med 1993;329:1842–7.
90. Marzano A, Salizzoni M, Dbernardi-Venon W, et al. Prevention of hepatitis B recurrence after liver transplantation in cirrhotic patients treated with lamivudine and passive immunoprophylaxis. J Hepatol 2001;34: 903–910.
91. Terrault N, Zhou S, Combs C, et al. Prophylaxis in liver transplant recipients using a fixed dosing schedule of hepatitis B immunoglobulin. Hepatology 1996;24: 1327–33.
92. McGory R, Ishitani M, Oliveira W, et al. Improved outcome of orthotopic liver transplantation for chronic hepatitis B cirrhosis with aggressive passive immunization. Transplantation 1996;61:1358–63.
93. Roche B, Gigou M, Roque-Afonso A, et al. HBV DNA persistence 10 years after liver transplantation despite successful anti-HBs passive immunoprophylaxis. Hepatology 2003;38:86–95.
94. Di Paulo D, Tisone G, Piccolo P, et al. Low-dose HBIG given "on demand" in combination with lamivudine. Transplantation 2004;77:1203–8.
95. Burbach G, Bienzle U, Neuhaus R, et al. Intravenous or intramuscular anti-HBs immunoglobulin for the prevention of HBV reinfection after orthotopic liver transplantation. Transplantation 1997;63:478–80.
96. Levitsky J, Doucette K. Viral hepatitis in solid organ transplant recipients. Am J Transplant 2009;9: S116–30.
97. Terrault N, Zhou S, McCory R, et al. Incidence and clinical consequences of surface and polymerase gene mutations in liver transplant recipients on hepatitis B immunoglobulin. Hepatology 1998;28: 555–61.
98. Bock C, Tillmann H, Torresi J, et al. Selection of HBV polymerase mutants with enhanced replication by lamivudine treatment after liver transplantation. Gastroenterology 2002;122:264–73.
99. Markowitz J, Martin P, Conrad JA, et al. Prophylaxis against hepatitis B recurrence following liver transplantation using combination of lamivudine plus

hepatitis B immunoglobulin. Hepatology 1998;28: 585–9.
100. Gane EJ, Angus PW, Strasser S, et al. Australasian Liver Transplant Study Group. Lamivudine plus low-dose hepatitis B immunoglobulin to prevent recurrent hepatitis B following liver transplantation. Gastroenterology 2007;132:931–7.
101. Dan Y, Wai C, Yeoh K, et al. Prophylactic strategies for HBV patients undergoing liver transplant: a cost-effectiveness analysis. Liver Transplant 2006;12: 736–46.
102. Naoumov N, Lopes A, Burra P, et al. Randomised trial of lamivudine vs. HBIG for long-term prophylaxis of HBV recurrence after liver transplantation. J Hepatol 2001;34:888–94.
103. Wong S, Chu C, Wai C, et al. Low risk of HBV recurrence after withdrawal of long-term HBIG in patients receiving maintenance nucleoside therapy. Liver Transplant 2007;13:374–81.
104. Buti M, Mas A, Prieto M, et al. Adherence to lamivudine after early withdrawal of HBIG plays important role in long-term prevention of HBV recurrence. Transplantation 2007;84:650–4.
105. Lo CM, Liu C, Chan S, et al. Failure of HBV vaccination in patients receiving lamivudine prophylaxis after liver transplantation for CHB. J Hepatol 2005;43: 283–7.
106. Angus PW, Patterson SJ, Strasser SI, McCaughan GW, Gane E. A randomized study of adefovir dipivoxil in place of HBIG in combination with lamivudine as post-liver transplantation hepatitis B prophylaxis. Hepatology 2008;48:1460–6.
107. Teperman L, Spivey J, Poordad F, et al. Emtricitabine/tenofovir combination +/– HBIG post-orthotopic liver transplantation to prevent hepatitis B recurrence in patients with normal to moderate renal impairment. J Hepatol 2010;52:S12.
108. Gane E, Strasser S, Angus P, et al. A prospective study on the safety and efficacy of lamivudine and adefovir prophylaxis in HBsAg-positive liver transplantation candidates. Hepatology 2007;46:479A.
109. Schiff E, Lai CL, Hadziyannis S, et al. Adefovir Dipivoxil Study 45 International Investigators Group. Adefovir dipivoxil for wait-listed and post-transplantation patients with lamivudine-resistant hepatitis B: final long-term results. Liver Transpl 2007;13:349–60.
110. Lo C, Lau G, Chan S, Ng I, Fan S. Liver transplantation for chronic hepatitis B with lamivudine resistant YMDD mutant using add-on adefovir dipivoxil plus lamivudine. Liver Transpl 2005;11:807–13.

33 Recurrence of the original disease

James Neuberger
Liver Unit, Queen Elizabeth Hospital, Birmingham, UK; NHS Blood and Transplant, Bristol, UK

Key learning points

- Autoimmune and metabolic diseases may recur in the liver allograft.
- Recurrence may be present in the presence of abnormal liver tests.
- Recurrence may affect patient and graft survival.
- For recurrent autoimmune hepatitis, early treatment with corticosteroids may reduce the risk and consequences of recurrence but there are few treatments that impact on recurrence of other diseases.

Introduction

Many diseases recur after liver transplantation; prompt recognition, diagnosis and, where appropriate, treatment is necessary to prevent unnecessary complications and maintain good graft function. Recurrence is a major cause of graft failure in some indications but the likelihood of recurrence does not correlate well with the likelihood of graft loss from recurrence.[1] Furthermore, graft loss from recurrence is probably the major factor accounting for differences in outcomes between indications[2] (Table 33.1). There is great variation in the reported incidence of most diseases and there are several reasons for this variation; perhaps one of the greatest reasons is the different practices relating to protocol biopsies: many diseases may recur in the presence of normal liver tests so those centers that perform biopsies only when indicated by abnormal liver tests will inevitably report lower rates of recurrence than those that do protocol biopsies. Other factors that influence the reported rates of recurrence include different diagnostic criteria.

The natural history of disease in the allograft is usually more rapid that in the native liver. Early recognition and prompt treatment may allow a slowing of the disease.

Primary biliary cirrhosis

The reported incidence of recurrent primary biliary cirrhosis (rPBC) is varied, with a recent systematic review of 16 studies suggesting a recurrence rate of 18% with a range of between 4 and 33%.[1] This wide variation of reported recurrence rates reflects largely the heterogeneity of the studies, due in part to differences in criteria used to define recurrence, variations in the use of protocol biopsies, sample sizes, and duration of follow up. In the majority of cases, the impact of recurrence of PBC on graft function and survival is minimal for the first decade after transplantation, with end-stage disease affecting <5%. After transplantation, itching rapidly resolves although lethargy is usually unaffected.

Diagnosis

The diagnostic criteria for PBC in the native liver is based on clinical history, cholestatic liver tests, elevations of the immunoglobulins (especially IgM) and the presence of anti-mitochondrial antibodies (AMA). Liver histology may be normal but usually shows the characteristic noncaseating granulomatous cholangitis. The interpretation of these tests in the post-transplant setting is more complicated as

Medical Care of the Liver Transplant Patient, Fourth Edition. Edited by Pierre-Alain Clavien, James F. Trotter.

Table 33.1 Frequency of recurrent disease and percentage of graft loss from recurrent disease (data from literature and Birmingham Liver Unit)

Indication	% graft loss from recurrence	Graft loss from all causes (relative to PBC)	Probability of recurrence
Primary biliary cirrhosis	1.3	1.0	18%
Primary sclerosing cholangitis	8.4	1.6	50%
Hepatitis C	14.3	2.0	95%
Alcohol	3.2	1.4	60%
Nondrug fulminant hepatic failure	2.7	1.3	3%
Non-alcoholic liver disease	3.2	1.3	30%
Autoimmune hepatitis	6.2	1.6	25%
Acetaminophen-induced liver failure	0	0.9	1%

features of recurrence may be modified by immunosuppression and the graft is subject to other causes of damage, including infective, immunologic, ischaemic, and toxic insults. Symptoms of PBC such as lethargy and pruritus are not specific for PBC and so are not diagnostic of disease recurrence. Similarly, liver tests are of limited value in the diagnosis of recurrent PBC because of their lack of specificity. Furthermore, histologic evidence of rPBC can be seen within the background of normal liver tests. Although AMA have a high sensitivity and specificity for the disease in the native liver, AMA persist after transplant, even in the absence of histologic evidence of recurrence and so may not be diagnostic of disease in the allograft. Titers may fall initially but thereafter may rise over time. Neither the titer nor specificity of AMA is associated with the risk of recurrence.

Hence, histology remains the primary tool for the diagnosis of recurrent PBC. The main finding is of florid duct lesions on liver biopsy, including mononuclear inflammatory infiltrates, formation of lymphoid aggregates, epithelioid granulomas, and bile duct damage. The differential diagnosis includes cytomegalovirus infection, hepatitis C infection, graft vs host disease, and acute and chronic rejection. It is important but relatively easy to exclude other causes before the diagnosis of rPBC is made.

Outcome

The effects of recurrent disease on graft function and patient survival are usually minor, with only a small number of cases reporting progression from recurrent disease to graft failure and re-transplantation. However, as more long-term data emerges, the reported incidence may increase.

Risk factors and management

The association of specific immunosuppressive agents with rPBC is controversial. Individual studies have suggested that use of tacrolimus is associated with earlier and more aggressive rPBC, compared with cyclosporine.[3] The mechanism responsible may relate to a possible protective effect of cyclosporine inhibiting viral replication and apoptosis, as is suggested (but not confirmed) in other settings. Cyclosporine has been shown to be of possible benefit in the treatment of PBC in the native liver although its use is limited by potential side effects, such as hypertension and renal damage.

Some have suggested that lack of corticosteroids in the immunosuppressive regime may increase the risk of recurrence whereas other studies have suggested that withdrawal of immunosuppression may increase the probability of recurrent disease. The heterogeneity of published studies, both in diagnostic criteria and follow up, make interpretation of these findings difficult.

Ursodeoxycholic acid (UDCA) is currently the only licenced medication for the treatment of PBC in the native liver, even though its mechanism of action remains uncertain. Many, but not all, studies have demonstrated improvement in liver function tests, delay in histologic progression, and improvement in survival in patients with PBC. The promising result seen with the use of UDCA in the native liver may translate into the post-transplant setting. Studies on the use of UDCA in recurrent PBC have so far demonstrated improvement in liver tests,[5] however as yet there is no evidence to suggest any benefit on patient and/or graft survival, but with further studies using larger sample sizes and longer follow up, any effect can be established. Many other agents have been tried, including other bile acids, in the treatment of PBC and, until a beneficial effect can be established in those with their native liver, it is unlikely that these will be of benefit in the allograft.

On the current, but limited evidence, it seems reasonable to offer UDCA to patients with evidence of rPBC at a daily dose of 10–15 mg/kg (although the drug is not licenced for use in this indication). There is no evidence, to date, that pre-emptive treatment with UDCA, switching from tacrolimus to cyclosporine or adding corticosteroids will affect either the risk of recurrence or the rate of progression.

Although there are no data, the practice of this author is to offer use of UDCA at a dose of 10–15 mg/kg/d when there is histologic evidence of rPBC and abnormal liver tests. There is no data on this at present, to recommend pre-emptive use of UDCA to prevent or delay the onset of rPBC but, given the safety profile and few side effects, this practice has been suggested by some. Ideally, prospective studies are indicated although logistics and other practical issues may preclude their success.

Primary sclerosing cholangitis

Primary sclerosing cholangitis (PSC) is a chronic progressive condition that involves inflammation and fibrosis of both intra-hepatic and extra-hepatic bile ducts, resulting in progressive chronic liver disease; it is commonly associated with inflammatory bowel disease. As with PBC, the reported prevalence of recurrent PSC differs widely between studies.

Evidence for recurrent PSC was based originally on a comparison of allograft liver histology and imaging of the biliary tree of those grafted for PSC and patients transplanted for nonPSC conditions but with biliary re-construction; non-anastomotic biliary strictures and characteristic biliary histology were significantly more common in the PSC group. Other studies have since confirmed such findings. Recurrent PSC is seen in up to 50% of patients at 5 years and may lead to graft loss in up to 25% at 5 years.

Diagnosis

As with PSC in the native liver, the diagnosis of rPSC is based on a combination of biochemical, radiologic and histologic findings and exclusion of other causes. Histologic changes suggestive of rPSC include biliary fibrosis, fibrous cholangitis and fibro-obliterative lesions but these findings are used more commonly as supportive of the diagnosis, due, in part, to patchy involvement and consequent sample variability and the relative lack of specificity of the findings. Findings that are suggestive of rPSC can also be seen in other pathologic conditions, including ischemia, recurrent biliary sepsis, and reperfusion injuries. Ductopenic rejection shares some features (clinical, serologic, and histologic), making it difficult to distinguish between the two conditions (which may rarely co-exist), but it is unusual for chronic rejection to be associated with multiple non-anastomotic strictures. Furthermore, increased deposition of copper-binding protein is not characteristic of chronic rejection but is found in other conditions, including rPSC.

The gold standard for the diagnosis of PSC, both in the native liver and in the graft (with the exception of the small duct disease variant) is demonstration of abnormal intra-hepatic and extra-hepatic ducts on imaging and exclusion of causes of secondary cholangitis. Other diseases can also give a similar picture of bile duct injury, including hepatic artery thrombosis/stenosis, drug toxicity, established ductopenia rejection, reperfusion injury, biliary sepsis, anastomotic strictures, and the consequences of donor/recipient ABO incompatibility. Hence, the diagnosis of rPSC is one of exclusion. Endoscopic retrograde cholangiopancreatography (ERCP) has largely been replaced by the use of magnetic resonance cholangiography (MRC). Percutaneous cholangiography may also be used. There are limited data on the use of MRC for the diagnosis of recurrent PSC, but early evidence suggests it offers a reliable and non-invasive test for the identification of biliary pathology seen in recurrent PSC. MRC is less specific for early changes and repeated episodes of infective cholangitis (bacterial or viral) may give irregularities to the bile duct walls and so lead to misleading conclusions.

Several groups have tried to identify risk factors for the development of recurrent PSC; retrospective studies[5] have identified: 1) male gender, 2) an intact colon before or during transplantation, 3) steroid-resistant rejection, 4) active colitis post transplantation, 5) use of OKT3 for the treatment of cellular rejection, 6) gender mismatch between donor, 7) cytomegalovirus infection, 8) recurrent acute cellular rejection, and 9) the presence of specific HLA-haplotypes (e.g. HLA-DRB1*08). There has been, however, little consistency between series, which probably relates to a great extent to the different protocols for detecting recurrent disease and different definitions of rPSC.

Early studies with relatively short follow up comparing patient survival have demonstrated no difference between patients with or without recurrent PSC, however, longer term data suggest recurrent disease can lead to graft loss.

Treatment

UDCA has been advocated for the treatment of PSC in the native liver: studies have demonstrated improvement in biochemical parameters, symptoms, disease progression, and survival at doses of 10–15 mg/kg/d, although higher doses may be toxic. Currently there are no robust data on the use of UDCA in the post-transplant setting for recurrent PSC. UDCA may be beneficial not only on possible development and/or progression of rPSC, but it may play a role in the prevention of colonic cancer in patients who have associated colitis.[6] Those with both PSC and 'ulcerative colitis', have a greater risk of such complications after liver transplantation. Current guidelines for treatment of PSC in the native liver do not recommend the use of UDCA as a chemoprotective agent for colon cancer and use of UDCA to prevent or treat rPSC should not be a substitute for careful surveillance for colonic cancer in these patients.

Although colectomy, before or during transplantation, may protect against recurrent disease, there is no indication for prophylactic colectomy merely to prevent recurrence of PSC.

IgG4-associated cholangitis

The syndrome of IgG4 cholangitis has only recently been recognised and it is likely that some cases diagnosed as PSC were actually IgG4 cholangitis. Several groups have re-analysed their series and up to one-quarter of patients may be re-classified. There have been few studies on recurrent IgG4 cholangitis, but one study suggested that this is associated with a greater risk and more rapid rate of recurrence compared with PSC. The benefit of corticosteroids in this indication in the allograft is not known but extrapolation from the native liver, suggests that concomitant use of corticosteroids in the immunosuppressive regime should be considered.[7]

Autoimmune hepatitis

As with PBC and PSC, autoimmune hepatitis (AIH) can re-occur in the post-transplant period. The reported rates of recurrence differ widely.[8] The diagnosis of AIH in the native liver incorporates a combination of clinical, biochemical, immunologic and histologic findings, a response to immunosuppression, and exclusion of other possible diagnoses. The scoring system developed by the International Autoimmune Hepatitis Group has not been validated for the use in recurrent AIH and many aspects included in this scoring system cannot and should not be simply and uncritically translated into the post-transplant setting.

Studies using protocol liver biopsies have shown that recurrent AIH can also occur in the background of normal liver function, so the use of abnormal transaminase as a marker of possible recurrent disease is limited in the diagnosis of recurrent AIH.[9] Testing for high titre auto-antibodies and hypergammaglobulinemia is useful in the diagnosis of suspected AIH in the native liver and, as with PBC, such markers can remain detectable post transplantation and in other causes of graft damage. An increase in the titre of auto-antibodies after liver transplantation may indicate recurrent disease, but evidence is limited and titres may be affected by immunosuppression. Furthermore, organ nonspecific antibodies may be associated with some infection and rejection, thus liver histology is essential to establish the diagnosis of recurrent disease and evaluate disease severity.

Histologic findings consistent with recurrent disease include mononuclear inflammatory infiltrates, abundant plasma cells and interface hepatitis (piecemeal necrosis). Such findings, however, are not unique to recurrent AIH and can be seen in viral hepatitis and cellular rejection.

Risk factors for recurrent AIH (rAIH) are uncertain: recipient HLA-DR3 positivity and donor HLA-DR3 negativity may be correlated with an increased risk of recurrent disease. Both chronic ductopenic and acute cellular rejection are more common in patients with recurrent disease, possibly reflecting an increase in autoimmune responsiveness of the recipient. While such HLA studies may help elucidate the mechanism of autoimmune disease, such data cannot, at present, be used to identify those at greater risk of recurrence.

Treatment

Prevention of rAIH

The degree of immunosuppression required to prevent allograft rejection may not be sufficient to prevent recurrent AIH. In part because of the different protocols to diagnose rAIH and for immunosuppression, it is difficult to draw a rational conclusion from the published literature as to the optimum immunosuppression for use in those transplanted for AIH. Because of the consequences of immunosuppression (nonspecific ones such as increased susceptibility to some infection and some cancers or specific ones such as corticosteroid-induced osteoporosis or CNI-associated nephrotoxicity), clinicians have tried to run immunosuppression at a minimum to prevent immune-mediated graft damage.

The reduction of immunosuppression, in particular corticosteroids, increases the risk of recurrence, so long-term and relatively low-dose corticosteroids (such as prednisolone 5–7.5 mg/d) has been suggested in patients who are transplanted for AIH. Use of long-term steroids is not without increased risks, so special care should be given to prevention of bone loss (with appropriate monitoring and lifestyle advice, calcium and vitamin D supplements and bisphosphonates, and other agents as clinically indicated). There is little evidence to base a recommendation on the use of other classes of immunosuppression: both ciclosporin and tacrolimus and mycophenolate are effective in the treatment of AIH in the native liver but recurrence occurs in all reported regimes.

In those who are not maintained on corticosteroids, regular monitoring of immunoglobulin levels, titres of auto-antibodies and use of protocol biopsies will be required to detect recurrence and allow early intervention. Small and anecdotal studies have suggested that treatment with tacrolimus and sirolimus are effective in the treatment of recurrent disease.

The reported outcome of recurrent disease varies: while the majority of patients will respond clinically, serologically and histologically to increased immunosuppression, some will progress to end-stage graft failure and may require a re-graft.[10]

Treatment of de novo rAIH

When rAIH is first recognized, the diagnosis should be confirmed with liver histology. Most centers will treat such patients with the introduction or increase in the use of corticosteroids, using regimes such as prednisolone 40–60 mg/d and reducing the dose when auto-antibodies and liver tests improve.

Non-alcoholic fatty liver disease

The extent and consequences of recurrent non-alcoholic fatty liver disease (NAFLD) in the allograft is uncertain: it is thought that many cases labelled as cryptogenic cirrhosis are "burnt out" NAFLD so distinguishing *de novo* and recurrent NAFLD in the graft may be difficult.[11] The diagnosis of NAFLD in the native liver involves the combination of clinical history and identifying component of the metabolic syndrome, abnormal liver function test, exclusions of other liver disease, and the identification of fatty liver on radiologic imaging or histology and, often, liver biopsy. Newer diagnostic tools including blood tests and imaging (such as FibroScan®), are of some value in both the diagnosis and staging of NAFLD in the native liver.

The diagnosis of recurrent NAFLD is similar to that in the native liver. Liver tests are not specific and radiologic findings of a fatty liver are suggestive of NAFLD but cannot differentiate NAFLD from other causes of fatty liver (such as diabetes mellitus, some infections, alcohol, and other toxins); liver histology may be needed to confirm the diagnosis, establish the extent of disease, and to exclude other causes. Histologic evidence of NAFLD can be seen in patients with normal liver function.

Factors associated with recurrence are related to the metabolic syndrome, and include high triglyceride level, hypertension, increased body mass index, and diabetes mellitus.[12] Immunosuppression can further exacerbate and/or trigger such risk factors: corticosteroids, calcineurin inhibitors and sirolimus can be associated with hypertension, increase in insulin resistance, obesity, and hypertension. Some reports suggest that tacrolimus may be associated more commonly with recurrent non-alcoholic steatohepatitis (NASH) than ciclosporine. As with NASH in the native liver, the number of risk factors correlates with the likelihood and severity of rNASH. The extent to which donor steatosis may be associated with recurrent NASH is uncertain but some series have shown a correlation between graft steatosis and the risk of *de novo* NASH several years after transplantation.

Treatment

Currently there is no definitive treatment for NAFLD and no study so far has looked at treatments for recurrent post-transplant NAFLD. The main focus of treatment for NAFLD is on modification of components associated with metabolic syndrome. Treatment of metabolic syndrome may not only prevent recurrent NAFLD in the liver graft, but also reduce the cardiovascular risk. Treatment includes weight reduction in the form of diet, exercise and, even in selected patients, bariatric surgery. The patient will usually need full support from the multidisciplinary team, including dieticians and physiotherapists to encourage a suitable reduction in oral intake and increase in physical activity.

Bariatric surgery is often high risk in the liver allograft recipient because of the consequences of the previous surgery and adhesions, so laparoscopic techniques are often not appropriate. Nonetheless there are isolated cases where this has been done safely and effectively after transplantation.

Newer anti-obesity drugs such as cannabinoid receptor antagonists, lipase inhibitors and serotonin and glucagon-like protein-1-receptor agonists have all provided early promising results in the treatment of NAFLD in the native liver. Thiazolidinediones and metformin have shown some benefit. Control of hypertension using agents that block the angiotensin system and treatment for dyslipidemia with lipid-lowering medications, such as statins and gemfibrozil have also been suggested to improve NAFLD. As yet, there is little evidence for the benefit of each treatment in the allograft recipient and few agents have a licence for use in this indication.

Alcoholic liver disease

The reported rate of relapse following transplantation for ALD is highly variable, in part because of lack of standardisation for the definition of recidivism. Some units will define recidivism as a return to any degree of alcohol consumption while others will accept the occasional lapse or use of modest amounts of alcohol on special occasions.[13] Although many patients return to some pattern of alcohol consumption, up to one-third will return to drinking excessively and may develop alcohol-related graft damage. Graft loss from alcohol use, however, occurs relatively infrequently (less that 4% in a European series).[2]

Many different strategies have been suggested in the detection of recidivism. Self-reporting is commonest, and the success rate may be increased if the patient is interviewed by someone outside the transplant team. The use of reporting by family members, friends, and carers may further improve the sensitivity. Biochemical tests including blood and urine alcohol level, carbohydrate-deficient transferrin (CDT) level, ratios of alanine transaminase (ALT) and aspartate aminotransferase (AST), mitochondrial AST (mAST), gamma-glutamyl transferase (GGT) and mean corpuscular volume (MCV) have all been well studied in the detection of alcohol abuse in the general population. Other tests have also been developed (such as sialic acid, sialic acid index of apolipoprotein J, beta-hexosaminidase, acetaldehyde adducts and the urinary ratio of serotonin metabolites, 5-hydroxytryptophol and 5-hydroxyindoleacetic acid, but are used less often and their role in this context is not fully tested. Measurement of blood, breath or urine alcohol concentration is a well-recognised tool in identifying patients with recent alcohol consumption, and it has been used in a number of studies in the post-transplant setting, however its value is limited by the relatively short detectable half-life of alcohol. The use of CDT measurement may overcome this shortfall, due to its longer half-life of between 14–17 d. An increase in CDT correlates with alcohol consumption exceeding 50–80 g/d for 2–3 weeks and it is said to be unaffected by liver disease, but use in the post-transplant setting has still provided mixed results.

With evidence pointing towards the different outcome between harmful drinking and slips, the main aim in the prevention and treatment of recurrent disease should be total abstinence. Limited data exist on the treatment of recidivism in the post-transplant setting. Medications that are commonly used for the treatment of alcohol dependence include acamprosate, naltrexone, and disulfiram, however the effectiveness and safety of these agents has not been fully evaluated in the post-transplant setting. There is concern as to the possible interaction between these medications and immunosuppression. Psychotherapeutic interventions such as the use of motivational enhancement therapy (MET), have been shown to be useful in the nontransplant setting in the treatment of alcohol abuse, and a few studies in the post-transplant setting have demonstrated promising results, but further research is needed.

At present, the key management of preventing the adverse consequences of a return to a damaging pattern of alcohol consumption is close follow up in a sympathetic and supportive role, the support of the patient's family and colleagues, introduction of substitute and supporting activities, and a rapid and appropriate response when the patient returns to alcohol consumption. Many centers use a pretransplant contract to ensure the patient will remain abstinent; although this contract cannot be enforced is the recipient returns to alcohol, it does provide a reminder if the original undertaking.

Budd–Chiari syndrome

In Europe and North America, the most common causes of Budd–Chiari syndrome (BCS) are haematologic or thrombotic conditions. BCS may also be the early herald of a myeloproliferative disorder. Where the thrombotic defect arises in the liver, such as in factor V Leiden mutation, protein C, protein S and anti-thrombin III deficiency, liver transplantation will correct the predisposing defect.

The incidence of recurrent disease ranges from between 0 and 10% and complications from other thrombotic events are not uncommon.[14] Because of the risk of recurrent disease relating to hypercoagulable conditions from some causes, most patients are started on anti-coagulation post liver transplantation, thus the need for anti-coagulation will depend on the indication.

Despite anti-coagulation, patients can still develop recurrent disease, leading to graft failure and death. In many such cases, subtherapeutic anti-coagulation can be identified as a factor to recurrent disease and this may reflect difficulties in the use of warfarin due to its narrow therapeutic window and the need for long-term monitoring. If recurrence does occur, management includes medical treatment of complications from portal hypertension, surgical shunt, transjugular intrahepatic portosystemic shunt (TIPS), and retransplantation.

Owing to the small number of cases, recommendation on the best treatment cannot be made and should be determined on an individual basis.

Metabolic diseases

Liver transplantation is curative for those metabolic diseases where the metabolic defect lies within the liver (such as Wilson's disease, alpha-1-antitrypsin deficiency, tyrosinemia, Crigler–Najjar syndrome) and for some urea cycle defects and glycogen storage diseases.

Haemochromatosis

It remains uncertain whether liver replacement "cures" haemochromatosis, but most evidence suggests that, at least in the medium term, significant and unexplained iron accumulation does not occur.

Lipid storage disorders

The defects in most lipid storage disorders are not confined to the liver so liver transplantation alone is not curative and these diseases persist.[15] At present, the optimum approach is to monitor recipients for evidence of pathologic iron overload and offer treatment when clinically indicated.

Porphyrias

These are a group of heterogeneous diseases that are occasionally an indication for transplantation, because of uncontrollable symptoms.[16] The likelihood that transplantation will cure the patient will depend on the nature of the metabolic defect. However, in some cases, there may be a significant improvement in symptoms even if there is no cure. In erythropoetic protoporphyria, there is excessive production of protoporphyrin by the bone marrow so although transplantation will correct the consequences of the resulting cholestasis and cirrhosis, the condition will remain and will cause graft failure in many but not all affected patients.

References

1. Gautam M, Cheruvattath R, Balan V. Recurrence of autoimmune liver disease after liver transplantation: a systematic review. Liver Transpl 2006;12:1813–24.
2. Rowe IA, Webb K, Gunson BK, et al. The impact of disease recurrence on graft survival following liver transplantation: a single centre experience. Transpl Int 2008;21:459–65.
3. Neuberger J, Gunson B, Hubscher S, et al. Immunosuppression affects the rate of recurrent primary biliary cirrhosis after liver transplantation. Liver Transpl 2004;10:488–91.
4. Angulo P, Batts KP, Therneau TM, et al. Long-term ursodeoxycholic acid delays histological progression in primary biliary cirrhosis. Hepatology 1999;29:644–7.
5. Cholongitas E, Shusang V, Papatheodoridis GV, et al. Risk factors for recurrence of primary sclerosing cholangitis after liver transplantation. Liver Transpl 2008;14: 138–43.
6. Loftus EV Jr, Aguilar HI, Sandborn WJ, et al. Risk of colorectal neoplasia in patients with primary sclerosing cholangitis and ulcerative colitis following orthotopic liver transplantation. Hepatology 1998;27:685–90.
7. Zhang L, Lewis JT, Abraham SC, et al. IgG4+ plasma cell infiltrates in liver explants with primary sclerosing cholangitis. Am J Surg Pathol 2010;34:88–94.
8. Hubscher SG. Recurrent autoimmune hepatitis after liver transplantation: diagnostic criteria, risk factors, and outcome. Liver Transpl 2001;7:285–91.
9. Duclos-Vallee JC, Sebagh M. Recurrence of autoimmune disease, primary sclerosing cholangitis, primary biliary cirrhosis and autoimmune hepatitis after liver transplantation. Liver Transpl 2009;15(Suppl 2):S25–34.
10. Guido M, Burra P. De novo autoimmune hepatitis after liver transplantation. Seminars in Liver Disease 2011;31:71–81.
11. Cauble MS, Gilroy R, Sorrell MF, et al. Lipoatrophic diabetes and end-stage liver disease secondary to non-alcoholic steatohepatitis with recurrence after liver transplantation. Transplantation 2001;71:892–5.
12. Dumortier J, Giostra E, Belbouab S, et al. Non-alcoholic fatty liver disease in liver transplant recipients: another story of "seed and soil". Am J Gastroenterol 2010;105: 613–20.
13. DiMartini A, Day N, Dew MA, et al Alcohol use following liver transplantation: a comparison of follow-up methods. Psychosomatics 2010;42:55–62.
14. Cruz E, Ascher NL, Roberts JP, et al. High incidence of recurrence and hematologic events following liver transplantation for Budd–Chiari syndrome. Clin Transplant 2005;19:501–6.
15. Crawford DH, Fletcher LM, Hubscher SG, et al. Patient and graft survival after liver transplantation for hereditary hemochromatosis: implications for pathogenesis. Hepatology 2004;39:1655–62.
16. Seth AK, Badminton MN, Mirza D, Russell S, Elias E. Liver transplantation for porphyria: who, when and how? Liver Transpl 2007;13:1219–27.

34 Infections in the liver transplant recipient

Nicolas J. Mueller[1] *and Jay A. Fishman*[2]
Swiss HPB and Transplantation Centers,[1]Division of Infectious Diseases and Hospital Epidemiology, University Hospital Zürich, Switzerland; [2]Transplant Infectious Disease and Compromised Host Program, Infectious Disease Division, Massachusetts General Hospital, Harvard Medical School, Boston, Massachusetts, USA

Key learning points

- Infections are a major contributor to morbidity and mortality after liver transplantation. Aggressive diagnosis and rapid intervention are the keys to improved outcomes.
- The traditional pattern of infection has been modified by new immunosuppressive agents and prophylaxis. The risk of infection must be considered based on individual risk factors as well as the immunosuppressive regimen and knowledge of immune function.
- The presence of infection should trigger consideration of reduction of immunosuppression as an integral part of the therapeutic prescription.
- Preventive measures should start before transplantation including completion of vaccination and screening for latent infections based on epidemiologic history.
- Ensuring that samples are properly handled for both histopathology and microbiology greatly improves the diagnostic yield.

Introduction

Despite improvements in the prevention, diagnosis and therapy of infectious diseases, the management of infection after liver transplantation remains challenging.[1] Increasingly potent immunosuppression has reduced the incidence of graft rejection but is associated with an increased risk of opportunistic infection and malignancy. Antimicrobial therapies required to treat established infection in the immunocompromised host are more complex than in the normal host with a significant incidence of drug toxicity and a propensity for drug interactions with the immunosuppressive agents used to maintain graft function. Thus, *a rapid and specific diagnosis*, whether microbiologic or not, is essential for successful therapy. The absence of effective therapies for some infections, including those due to hepatitis C virus (HCV) and Epstein–Barr virus (EBV), prevent the development of a consensus regarding the management of some common post-transplant infections. The general principles of post-transplant infectious disease care are reviewed with special attention to the risks of infection following liver transplantation.

General principles of infectious disease care

Some basic principles guide the clinical approach to the liver transplant recipient with suspected infection.

Medical Care of the Liver Transplant Patient, Fourth Edition. Edited by Pierre-Alain Clavien, James F. Trotter.

Infections are often disseminated or advanced at the time of presentation. Clinical signs of infection are attenuated by immunosuppression and, as a result, the diagnosis is often obscured. The progression of disease is often rapid even when due to organisms of relatively low native virulence. Antimicrobial resistance is increased in the immunocompromised host and increases over time under treatment. Susceptibility testing is required for all important infections. The urgency of diagnosis and therapy are increased.

To achieve a microbiologic cure, technical issues (such as fluid collections and leaks) must be addressed, often requiring surgical intervention with microbial sampling of all collections. Given the toxicities of therapy and drug interactions – including renal and hepatic dysfunction and altered metabolism of calcineurin inhibitors – specific diagnoses are needed to optimize therapy and minimize avoidable side effects.

Developing a differential diagnosis: infection after liver transplantation

As for any individual, the risk of infections in the organ transplant patient is determined by the interaction between two factors: the patient's *epidemiologic exposures* and the patient's *net state of immune suppression*. The epidemiology of infections after liver transplantation derives from a number of sources:

- Exposures of the recipient, either recent (nosocomial) or remote (travel, colonization).
- Exposures, often unknown, of the organ donor and carried with the graft, such as cytomegalovirus (CMV) or due to bacteremia.
- Technical misadventures in transplant surgery resulting in leaks (bile, blood, and bowel) and fluid collections prone to infection.
- Vascular (ischemia) or biliary (cholangitis) complications predisposing to graft injury and chronic infection.
- Post-transplant infections derived from exposures in the community or via travel.

The net state of immune suppression is a conceptual framework that measures factors contributing to the risk for infection. The most important factors include the: 1) dose, duration, and temporal sequence of immunosuppressive drugs; 2) presence of foreign bodies or injuries to mucocutaneous barriers (catheters, drains); 3) neutropenia; 4) devitalized tissues or fluid collections such as bile leaks and hematomas; and 5) co-infection with immunomodulating viruses that are common in the transplant patient population (CMV, EBV, hepatitis B virus (HBV) and HCV).

Timeline of infections

Multiple risk factors for infection are present in each host. When knowledge of epidemiologic exposures is combined with an understanding of the immune deficits of the host, a timeline of post-transplant infections is created based on the evolving risks for infection over time (Figure 34.1). An understanding of the risk factors for infection can be used to guide the selection of the diagnostic approach and initial therapy. The periods are approximate and vary with the immunosuppressive protocol. A more dynamic assessment of immune function (using gene expression or measurements of pathogen-specific immunity) has been proposed to emphasize the evolving state of immune function – and the variability of infectious risk between individuals.[2]

Early phase: first month post transplantation

Early after transplantation, the full impact of immune suppression has not yet been achieved. As a result, anatomic considerations (hematomas, bile leaks, vascular obstruction), surgical management issues (line sepsis, decubitus ulcers) and nosocomial infections (pneumonia, *Clostridium difficile* colitis) are the common sites and sources of infection.

In the liver recipient, the risk for peritoneal infection is a function of technical difficulties (bleeding, bowel perforation, biliary duct ischemia), early organ dysfunction (coagulopathy), and prior colonization. The risk for infection, notably fungal and enterococcal, increases with surgical complexity, bleeding, re-exploration, and the need for intensive care unit stays with prolonged intubation. Wound infections may be observed. In addition, the patient's pre-transplant condition (metabolic and physical) may determine post-transplant recovery.

Imaging studies are usually required for specific diagnosis, including CT scans, cholangiograms via

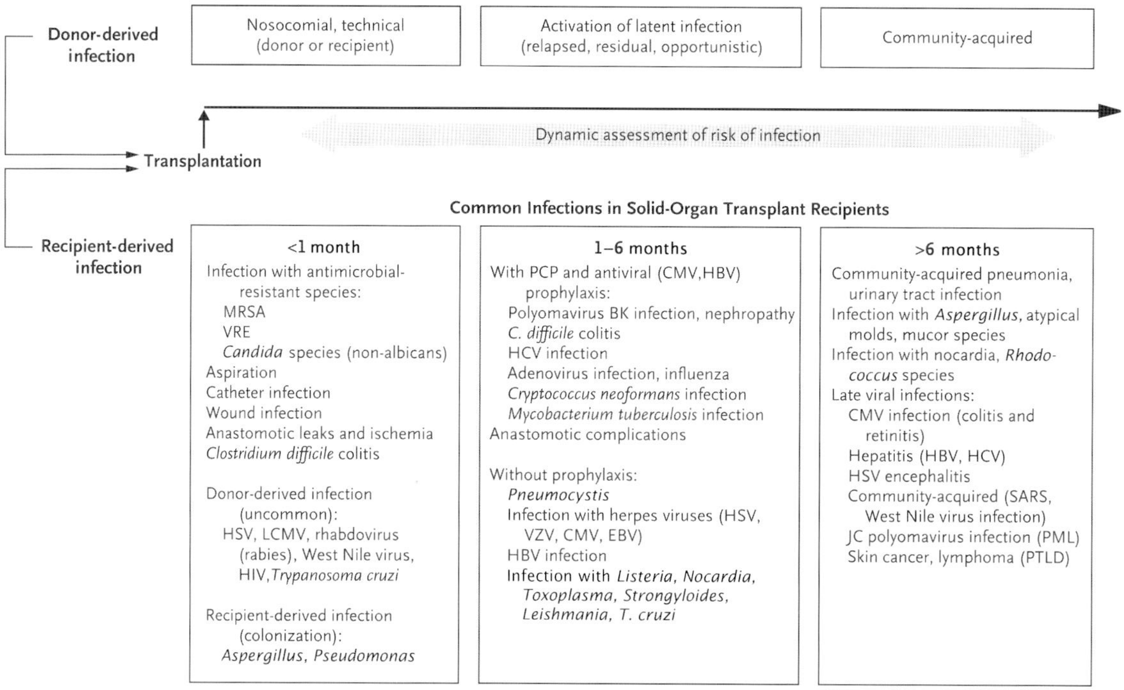

Figure 34.1 Timeline of infections after organ transplantation. The pattern of infection after solid-organ transplantation is modified by prophylaxis, intensity of immunosuppression, drug toxic effects that may cause leukopenia, or immunomodulatory viral infections. The risk of infection must be individualized by a dynamic assessment of the individual's immune function. EBV: Epstein–Barr virus, HBV: hepatitis B virus, HCV: hepatitis C virus, HIV: human immunodeficiency virus, HSV: herpes simplex virus, LCMV: lymphocytic choriomeningitis virus, MRSA: methicillin-resistant *Staphylococcus aureus*, PCP: *Pneumocystis carinii* pneumonia, PML: progressive multifocal leukoencephalopathy, PTLD: post-transplantation lymphoproliferative disorder, SARS: severe acute respiratory syndrome, VRE: vancomycin-resistant *Enterococcus faecalis*, VZV: varicella zoster virus. *N Engl J Med* 2007;357:2601–14.

ERCP or MRI for biliary tract issues, and ultrasound studies for evaluation of hepatic blood flow, notably in the portal vein and hepatic artery. Vascular ultrasound is often misleading and angiography may also be needed. Sampling of fluid collections should precede antibiotic therapy if possible, and surgical exploration should be considered early in the course of infection.

Infections were present in 64% of all liver recipients in an autopsy series.[3] Prospective series indicated a rate of severe infections of 53 to 67% in the first year post-transplant with the majority occurring during the first 2 months; the attributable mortality ranges from 8 to 26%.[4,5] Bacterial infections account for half of all infections, followed by fungal, viral, and rarely parasitic infections. Gram-negative bacteria are most common in most series (*Escherichia coli, Enterobacter, Pseudomonas*) followed by Gram-positive pathogens. Most patients with a history of infection suffered at least two episodes.

Knowledge of pretransplant colonization patterns will direct successful empirical therapy after appropriate cultures are obtained.[6] In liver recipients, the bile duct is generally colonized with colonic flora including *Candida* species and antimicrobial-resistant enterococci in addition to Enterobacteriaceae and anaerobes. Thus, in cholangitis, peritonitis, and in liver abscesses, colonic flora are generally found regardless of whether bowel perforation has occurred or bacteremia identified. Large hepatic abscesses generally require drainage for cure with prolonged antimicrobial therapy (months).

Immune deficiency due to cirrhosis, corticosteroid therapy for autoimmune hepatitis, and repetitive courses of antimicrobial therapy and prophylaxis for spontaneous bacterial peritonitis are risk factors for colonization with increasingly antimicrobial-resistant fungi and bacteria. While opportunistic infections are generally uncommon during the first month post transplant, early disseminated aspergillosis may occur related to pre-transplant colonization or to construction within the hospital environment.

Pneumonia is the most common infection not directly associated with the surgical procedure, with a spectrum of pathogens similar to that of other complex surgical patients. Empiric therapy must address nosocomial organisms, including resistance patterns for *Pseudomonas* species, Enterobacteriaceae and Gram-positive pathogens including *Stapyhlococcus aureus* (including MRSA) and enterococci. Increasingly, the Enterobacteriaceae demonstrate broad antimicrobial resistance due to extended-spectrum beta-lactamases (ESBLs) with susceptibility only to carbapenem antibiotics. The incidence of *Clostridium difficile* colitis following liver transplantation was 7% in 402 consecutive liver transplant recipients. Some studies have identified liver transplantation as a specific risk factor, while outcome was generally favorable.[7]

Disseminated viral infections are rare early after transplantation, but have been associated with fatal infection of the liver allograft early including herpes simplex virus (HSV), CMV, lymphocytic choriomeningitis (LCMV), and adenovirus infections. These may be donor- or recipient-derived infections.[8] Increased awareness of donor-derived infections has led to greater efforts at screening of organ donors.[2]

1–6 months: opportunistic infections

In the first 6 months following transplantation, the full impact of immunosuppression becomes apparent. Viral infections dominate this period, both in terms of direct viral activation and injury associated with T-cell-depleting therapies, and the so-called "indirect effects" of viral infection on the risk for other opportunistic infections, graft rejection, and malignancies.[2] Molecular assays have simplified the management of these infections.

Effective prophylaxis should prevent most cases of CMV, HSV, varicella zoster virus and *Pneumocystis* and *Toxoplasma gondii* infections. Trimethoprim-sulfamethoxazole (TMP-SMX) efficiently prevents *Pneumocystis* pneumonia, *T. gondii*, some but not all infections due to *Nocardia* and *Listeria* species, as well as many urinary, respiratory and gastrointestinal infections. Hepatitis B recurrence is well managed using an array of effective antiviral agents and passive immunization therapies. Other prophylactic strategies should be considered second line and avoided except with documented allergy to TMP-SMX.

CMV

Traditionally, CMV was the most common opportunistic infection following solid-organ transplantation. CMV disease has been associated with significant morbidity and mortality after liver transplantation.[9] Data for the immunologic effects of CMV on liver graft function are limited. CMV after solid-organ or allogeneic bone marrow transplantation is also associated with an increased incidence of bacterial (*Listeria*),[10] and fungal (*Aspergillus, Candida, Pneumocystis*),[11,12] infections. The course of hepatitis C virus infection is accelerated in patients co-infected by CMV.[13,14]

Without prophylaxis, the risk of reactivation is greatest in the seronegative recipient of a seropositive organ donor (D+R–). In the absence of effective prophylaxis, over half of all recipients will reactivate CMV and one-third will develop a febrile-neutropenic viral syndrome. Manifestations may occur in all organs, but hepatitis, enteritis, and pneumonitis are most common. With the important exception of enteritis or retinitis, CMV disease is accompanied by viremia detected by quantitative molecular assays such as the polymerase chain reaction (PCR) or the semiquantitative pp65 antigenemia assay.

Treatment should be initiated with full-dose antiviral agents (ganciclovir, foscarnet) – with lower doses risking the emergence of antiviral resistance developing during high-level viremia. Cidofovir has significant renal toxicity in patients receiving calcineurin inhibitor therapy. Generally, in severely ill patients or those with possible gastrointestinal absorption issues, initiation with IV ganciclovir is recommended. Valganciclovir has markedly improved oral bioavailability over oral ganciclovir and is a treatment option in mild to moderately ill patients with CMV disease. It should be noted that for liver transplantation, valganciclovir has no indication for treatment or prophylaxis of CMV infection. Treatment should be continued for a minimum of 14 d, generally 7–10 d minimum beyond the demonstration of viral clearance.

Other herpes viruses

The importance of the EBV virus is linked to the development of post-transplant lymphoproliferative disorder (PTLD). It is worth noting that disease is most often of B-cell origin, often extra-nodal and may present with infiltration of the graft or of the central nervous system. Prevention, diagnosis and treatment are discussed in Chapter 36. Acute infection is most commonly observed in children (recurrent B-cell lymphocytosis, fever, gastrointestinal bleeding, mass lesions of the abdomen) after transplantation. Dermatomal zoster is a common clinical presentation of varicella zoster virus (VZV) reactivation. Primary varicella is preventable by immunization before transplantation. Disseminated or CNS infection due to VZV carries a high mortality rate. Human herpesvirus 6 infection has been associated with fever, encephalopathy, pneumonitis and bone marrow suppression in the absence of CMV prophylaxis.[15]

Adenovirus and other respiratory viruses

Influenza A and B including novel (H1N1-2009) influenza A, parainfluenza 1-3, respiratory syncytial virus (RSV), and metapneumovirus may cause severe lower respiratory tract disease in transplant recipients. Unique risk factors determining the population at risk for progression to severe, lower tract disease are not defined for liver transplant recipients. Specific treatment options are limited and include drugs effective against influenza A and B (zanamavir, oseltamivir). Ribavirin has a broad *in vitro* range against many viruses including RSV and metapneumovirus, with limited proof of efficacy.[16] Prolonged replication and shedding of respiratory viruses occurs in transplant recipients, and is of uncertain clinical significance.

Adenovirus may present with pneumonitis or primary viremia with fever accompanied by end-organ manifestations such as hepatitis or enteritis. Children without pre-existing immunity are particularly vulnerable. An assessment of adenovirus viremia in 121 adult liver transplant recipients revealed an incidence of 8.3% in the first year post transplant. Most cases were asymptomatic and self-limiting.[17] Case series demonstrate a possible effect of ribavirin, cidofovir or ganciclovir, but results are ambiguous. Nucleic acid amplification assays are available for diagnosis; prolonged shedding and latency of some adenovirus serotypes should be considered when interpreting the assay data.[18]

Mycobacteria

The frequency of tuberculosis (TB) in the transplant recipient will vary according to the local endemicity. Infection may be due to reactivation in the recipient, primary infection or it may be reactivated from the donor organ. Early disease in the first year is often disseminated, with rapid diagnosis and treatment being the keys to reducing mortality. The graft is often involved in infection; infection may be difficult to distinguish from toxicities of antimicrobial therapy. Efforts to prevent disease rely on systematic screening programs and the treatment of latent TB.[19] Nontuberculous mycobacteria are increasingly identified as a cause of cryptic fever and peritonitis in transplant recipients.[20] Therapy for mycobacterial infections must be guided by susceptibility testing as each strain (both TB and nonTB) have unique characteristics *in vitro*.

Pneumocystis jiroveci

Owing to efficient prophylaxis, *Pneumocystis* pneumonia is rare during TMP-SMX prophylaxis. Alternative agents (atovaquone, dapsone, pentamidine, and others) are somewhat less effective. The clinical presentation is insidious with shortness of breath occurring early with relatively subtle findings by chest radiography. Documentation of hypoxemia and careful examination of (induced or bronchoscopic) sputum samples using immunofluorescent antibody staining will generally yield a diagnosis. Corticosteroids are useful as adjunctive therapy to both reduce pulmonary inflammation and reduce post-infection fibrosis. TMP-SMX is the agent of choice but may provoke renal toxicity. Uncommonly, clusters of infection have been observed that suggest patient-to-patient transmission.[21] Late infection may be associated with treatment of graft rejection, CMV infection, following influenza pneumonia, or with the onset of malignancy.

Pneumonia

Pneumonia in liver transplant recipients should prompt aggressive diagnostic maneuvers to obtain a specific microbiologic diagnosis. The therapies of, for example, infection due to *Aspergillus*, *Legionella* or *Nocardia* species vary widely in terms of both antimicrobial agents and toxicities, making empiric therapy inadvisable. Diagnosis of *Legionella* species requires specialized microbiologic cultivation. The urinary antigen test detects only the *Legionella pneumophila* serogroup, with moderate sensitivity. Empiric therapy (while awaiting culture data) should include therapy for atypical pathogens including *Legionella* (macrolide, flouroquinolone). *Nocardia* pneumonia is often metastatic to the central nervous system and may cause rapidly progressive, nodular or consolidative pneumonia. Radiologic evaluation of the brain is recommended and lumbar puncture should be considered, even in the absence of clinical findings. Prophylaxis with TMP-SMX will protect against many infections due to *Nocardia* species, although resistant species (e.g. among *N. nova*) have been identified. Primary therapy includes combinations of agents usually including sulfonamide, carbapenem, or third- or fourth-generation cephalosporin agents. Prolonged therapy is necessary, and some authorities recommend long-term secondary prophylaxis.[22]

Fungal infection

Fungemia or peritonitis due to *Candida albicans* and non-*albicans Candida* species (e.g. *C. glabrata, C. krusei, C. tropicalis*) are leading causes of early invasive infection after liver transplantation. Initial empiric therapy needs to consider the source and severity of disease, prior use of antifungal prophylaxis, and the local susceptibility and prevalence of specific *Candida* species. Primary therapy includes removal of indwelling IV catheters (notably those used for hyperalimentation), drainage of infected fluid collections, and correction of any surgical issues (leaks). Initial therapy should include an IV echinocandin agent until fluconazole susceptibility data are available.[23] Latter generation azole antifungals are also effective, but generally more costly with little therapeutic advantage. The polyene agents (amphotericin B and liposomal amphotericin) and flucytosine are also highly active.

Pneumonia and meningitis are common clinical presentations of infections due to *Cryptococcus neoformans*, although skin and soft tissue infections may be observed in transplant recipients. Diagnosis may be by biopsy or culture but the cryptococcal antigen assay is generally positive in cerebrospinal fluid and/or serum. Initial therapy should include amphotericin B or lipid formulations of amphotericin, generally combined with flucytosine for induction therapy in case of meningoencephalitis or disseminated disease. Fluconazole can be substituted when control is achieved or in asymptomatic individuals or for secondary prophylaxis. Inflammation associated with cryptococcal infection may cause hydrocephalus necessitating shunting and/or corticosteroid therapy. Immune reconstitution inflammatory syndrome (IRIS) may occur with symptomatic worsening if immune suppression is tapered too rapidly during therapy.[24]

Infection with *Aspergillus* species may be activated in individuals colonized pre-transplantation or as a result of new environmental or nosocomial exposures. The lungs are the primary site with dissemination commonly involving the central nervous system (CNS). Clinical signs of CNS infection necessitate radiologic and cerebrospinal fluid evaluations. The use of galactomannan and beta-glucan assays have not been proven to be useful in liver transplant recipients.[25] The positive predictive value of these assays is better in bronchoalveolar lavage fluid samples. The treatment of choice for documented infection is voriconazole; empiric therapy should utilize an amphotericin agent.

Blastomyces dermatitidis, Coccidioides immitis, Paracoccidiodes braziliensis, and *Histoplasma capsulatum* must be considered if exposure has occurred in defined geographic areas. The portal of entry of these endemic mycoses is the respiratory tract, from where dissemination can occur. Azoles are the mainstay of therapy for mild or moderate presentations (or sulfa agents for *Paracoccidioides*), while amphotericin and its lipid formulations are reserved for severe cases.[26] Increasingly, infections due to more unusual moulds including *Penicillium*, *Mucoraceae*, and *Scedosporium* species have been observed. Therapy of these fungi should be guided by susceptibility testing and surgical debridement is often needed.

T. gondii and Strongyloides stercoralis

In the absence of prophylaxis, toxoplasmosis is an important consideration in patients with systemic disease not responding promptly to empiric antimicrobial therapy or signs of central nervous system disease. Infection is generally due to reactivation of latent infection (seropositive recipient) or transmission with the graft.[27] The greatest risk for toxoplasmosis is in seronegative recipients of seropositive organs. The diagnosis is based on histology (e.g. for abnormal liver function tests, pneumonia) or seroconversion. Nuclear acid amplification testing is available for detection of disease in cerebrospinal fluid samples. Culture methods are not available routinely. Pyrimethamine and sulfadiazine induction and maintenance therapy is followed by secondary suppressive therapy by TMP-SMX.

The hyperinfection syndrome due to reactivation of *Strongyloides stercoralis* occurs with immunosuppression (and rare cases of donor-derived disease). Reactivation may occur more than 30 years after initial exposure. Presentation is generally with polymicrobial bacteremia and sepsis due to colonic organisms with dissemination of parasites and bacteria to the central nervous system. The mortality rate is high. A history of potential exposure (in Southeast Asia) in liver transplant candidates should initiate serologic screening and empiric therapy with ivermectin prior to transplantation.

Late infections

Beyond 6–12 months post transplantation, immunosuppression has generally been tapered and the impact of infection is manifest as an increased incidence of community-acquired respiratory viruses, virally mediated cancers (post-transplant lymphoproliferative syndrome, skin, and anogenital cancers), and infections associated with intensified immunosuppression for episodes of graft rejection. Relevant epidemiologic exposures occur in settings of normal activities including cooking, travel, or gardening. Common pathogens include moulds, nocardiosis, *Rhodococcus equi*, and *Legionella* species. Late viral infections may occur, notably during the treatment of graft rejection or PTLD or in patients requiring higher levels of immunosuppression.

Prevention of post-transplant infections

Vaccination

A review of vaccination status should be performed prior to transplantation, particularly for the live vaccines that are contraindicated after transplantation. Hepatitis A and B deserve special attention in liver transplant candidates. A sufficient titre demonstrating successful vaccination should be obtained for hepatitis B. Insufficient vaccine coverage and ensuing outbreaks for measles should prompt measles–mumps–rubella (MMR) vaccination in individuals without documentation of MMR vaccine born after 1957 (USA) or 1963 (Europe). Influenza vaccination is recommended on a yearly basis. Pneumoccocal vaccination is given pre transplant and at least once 5 years later. Tetanus and pertussis boosters are indicated every 10 years, or once post transplant, respectively. Varicella vaccination should be achieved pre transplant in seronegative individuals. The role of human papillomavirus (HPV) vaccination for transplant recipients is under investigation.

Special consideration should be given to travel vaccines for travel to endemic areas. Some of these vaccines (i.e. yellow fever) can only be given pre transplant. The role of appropriate vaccination of household members is also relevant.[28]

Antibacterial and *Pneumocystis* pneumonia prophylaxis

The relatively broad protection of TMP-SMX (single strength daily) is emphasized. While documented evidence is primarily available for *Pneumocystis* and *T. gondii*, infections with *Listeria*, some *Nocardia* species, intestinal pathogens such as *Isospora belli*, *Cyclospora cayetanensis* and more common respiratory, urinary, and gastrointestinal pathogens are prevented only with daily dosing regimens. The usual duration is at least 6 months to 1 year post transplantation. Discontinuation of prophylaxis should be postponed in individuals with impaired graft function, receiving higher levels of immunosuppression, and during the treatment of graft rejection or in patients with a history of CMV infection.

Antifungal prophylaxis

Antifungal prophylaxis is reserved for high-risk patients in the early phase after transplantation and for patients with latent infection due to endemic or other agents. While generally targeting *Candida* species, patients with documented exposure to endemic fungi (*Histoplasma, Coccidioides*) or *Cryptococcus* species may merit prolonged prophylaxis.[29]

Antiviral strategies

Pre-transplant screening of donors and recipients for CMV serologic status (IgG) will define the relative risk for reactivation or primary infection. Prevention of CMV will decrease the burden of disease as well as reducing overall mortality, graft loss or impaired function, and the risk for opportunistic infection ("the indirect effects"). Two strategies are employed for CMV prevention: "universal prophylaxis," where all patients at risk receive antiviral therapy for a prescribed period or "pre-emptive therapy," which relies on routine determination of CMV viremia by sensitive assay (i.e. molecular) with therapy initiated to prevent progression to clinical disease. Both approaches have advantages and pitfalls:

1. Universal prophylaxis is easier to coordinate, and some studies have suggested an impact on indirect effects (graft function/loss, opportunistic infections, and mortality).
2. Drug costs and potential for toxicity are higher with universal prophylaxis.
3. An important concern is the risk for late-onset disease after discontinuation of prophylaxis.
4. The pre-emptive strategy requires regular testing for CMV viremia, communication of results, and prompt initiation of therapy; an impact on the indirect effects of CMV has not been documented for this approach.

Most transplant centers follow a prophylactic approach at least for the patients at highest risk (donor seropositive (D+), recipient seronegative (R–)). For the intermediate risk where the recipient is seropositive, both approaches are useful. Both oral ganciclovir (3 g/d) and valganciclovir (900 mg/d) have been shown to be effective for prophylaxis, while valganciclovir (900 mg twice daily) or IV ganciclovir (5 mg/kg twice daily) should be used for pre-emptive therapy. Dosing is corrected for renal function. It is important to note that conflicting data on the efficacy of valganciclovir for prophylaxis in liver transplant recipients have resulted in a US Food and Drug Administration caution against the use of valganciclovir for this indication.[30] In D–/R– patients, antiviral prophylaxis (oral acyclovir, valacyclovir, famciclovir) targets herpes simplex and varicella zoster virus infections.

Travel

Mobility of transplant recipients has increased to include countries with limited health resources and potential exposure to transmissible diseases. Vaccinations should be completed prior to travel. Food and water precautions should be followed as for all travellers (http://wwwnc.cdc.gov/travel/content/yellowbook/home-2010.aspx). Malaria prophylaxis may interact with transplant medications. Routine prophylaxis for diarrhea is not recommended, but appropriate self-medication for self-treatment should be available.[31]

References

1. Winston DJ, Emmanouilides C, Busuttil RW. Infections in liver transplant recipients. Clin Infect Dis 1995;21: 1077–89; quiz 90–1.
2. Fishman JA. Infection in solid-organ transplant recipients. N Engl J Med 2007;357:2601–14.
3. Torbenson M, Wang J, Nichols L, Jain A, Fung J, Nalesnik MA. Causes of death in autopsied liver transplantation patients. Mod Pathol 1998;11:37–46.
4. Kusne S, Dummer JS, Singh N, et al. Infections after liver transplantation. An analysis of 101 consecutive cases. Medicine 1988;67:132–43.
5. Paya CV, Hermans PE, Washington JA 2nd, et al. Incidence, distribution, and outcome of episodes of infection in 100 orthotopic liver transplantations. Mayo Clin Proc 1989;64:555–64.

6. Russell DL, Flood A, Zaroda TE, et al. Outcomes of colonization with MRSA and VRE among liver transplant candidates and recipients. Am J Transplant 2008;8:1737–43.
7. Albright JB, Bonatti H, Mendez J, et al. Early and late onset *Clostridium difficile*-associated colitis following liver transplantation. Transpl Int 2007;20:856–66.
8. Kusne S, Schwartz M, Breinig MK, et al. Herpes simplex virus hepatitis after solid organ transplantation in adults. J Infect Dis 1991;163:1001–7.
9. Razonable RR. Cytomegalovirus infection after liver transplantation: current concepts and challenges. World J Gastroenterol 2008;14:4849–60.
10. Safdar A, Papadopoulous EB, Armstrong D. Listeriosis in recipients of allogeneic blood and marrow transplantation: thirteen year review of disease characteristics, treatment outcomes and a new association with human cytomegalovirus infection. Bone Marrow Transplant 2002;29:913–6.
11. Fortun J, Martin-Davila P, Moreno S, et al. Risk factors for invasive aspergillosis in liver transplant recipients. Liver Transpl 2002;8:1065–70.
12. Radisic M, Lattes R, Chapman JF, et al. Risk factors for *Pneumocystis carinii* pneumonia in kidney transplant recipients: a case–control study. Transpl Infect Dis 2003;5:84–93.
13. Razonable RR, Burak KW, van Cruijsen H, et al. The pathogenesis of hepatitis C virus is influenced by cytomegalovirus. Clin Infect Dis 2002;35:974–81.
14. Burak KW, Kremers WK, Batts KP, et al. Impact of cytomegalovirus infection, year of transplantation, and donor age on outcomes after liver transplantation for hepatitis C. Liver Transpl 2002;8:362–9.
15. Razonable RR, Zerr DM. HHV-6, HHV-7 and HHV-8 in solid organ transplant recipients. Am J Transplant 2009;9(Suppl 4):S97–100.
16. Ison MG. Respiratory viral infections in transplant recipients. Antivir Ther 2007;12:627–38.
17. Humar A, Kumar D, Mazzulli T, et al. A surveillance study of adenovirus infection in adult solid organ transplant recipients. Am J Transplant 2005;5:2555–9.
18. Ison MG, Green M. Adenovirus in solid organ transplant recipients. Am J Transplant 2009;9(Suppl 4: S161–5.
19. Munoz P, Rodriguez C, Bouza E. *Mycobacterium tuberculosis* infection in recipients of solid organ transplants. Clin Infect Dis 2005;40:581–7.
20. Doucette K, Fishman JA. Nontuberculous mycobacterial infection in hematopoietic stem cell and solid organ transplant recipients. Clin Infect Dis 2004;38: 1428–39.
21. Gianella S, Haeberli L, Joos B, et al. Molecular evidence of interhuman transmission in an outbreak of *Pneumocystis jirovecii* pneumonia among renal transplant recipients. Transpl Infect Dis 2010;12:1–10.
22. Clark NM. Nocardia in solid organ transplant recipients. Am J Transplant 2009;9(Suppl 4):S70–7.
23. Pappas PG, Silveira FP. *Candida* in solid organ transplant recipients. Am J Transplant 2009;9(Suppl 4): S173–9.
24. Singh N, Lortholary O, Alexander BD, et al. An immune reconstitution syndrome-like illness associated with *Cryptococcus neoformans* infection in organ transplant recipients. Clin Infect Dis 2005;40:1756–61.
25. Kwak EJ, Husain S, Obman A, et al. Efficacy of galactomannan antigen in the Platelia *Aspergillus* enzyme immunoassay for diagnosis of invasive aspergillosis in liver transplant recipients. J Clin Microbiol 2004;42:435–8.
26. Proia L, Miller R. Endemic fungal infections in solid organ transplant recipients. Am J Transplant 2009; 9(Suppl 4):S199–207.
27. Lappalainen M, Jokiranta TS, Halme L, et al. Disseminated toxoplasmosis after liver transplantation: case report and review. Clin Infect Dis 1998;27: 1327–8.
28. Danzinger-Isakov L, Kumar D. Guidelines for vaccination of solid organ transplant candidates and recipients. Am J Transplant 2009;9(Suppl 4):S258–62.
29. Winston DJ, Pakrasi A, Busuttil RW. Prophylactic fluconazole in liver transplant recipients. A randomized, double-blind, placebo-controlled trial. Ann Intern Med 1999;131:729–37.
30. Humar A, Snydman D. Cytomegalovirus in solid organ transplant recipients. Am J Transplant 2009;9(Suppl 4): S78–86.
31. Kotton CN, Hibberd PL. Travel medicine and the solid organ transplant recipient. Am J Transplant 2009; 9(Suppl 4):S273–81.

35 Cutaneous diseases in liver transplant recipients

Sylvie Euvrard and Jean Kanitakis
Department of Dermatology, Edouard Herriot Hospital Group, Hospices Civils de Lyon, Lyon, France

Key learning points

- Skin cancers represent the main long-term cutaneous complication.
- A number of skin complications (including cancers) in liver transplant recipients should be managed by optimizing immunosuppression through dose reduction and/or drug change.
- Drug-related specific cutaneous side effects may severely impact quality of life, especially in young and female patients.
- The incidence of skin cancer could be reduced by a yearly regular dermatologic examination in order to allow early detection and treatment of skin (pre)malignancies and reinforce education about sun protection.

Introduction

Few articles have so far been published on skin complications in liver transplant recipients (LTRs). Skin cancers have been briefly reported in large cohorts of LTRs,[1] but data concerning nontumoral skin manifestations have been reported only in rather short series of up to 110 patients or in isolated case reports.[2–5] LTRs present skin disorders that also develop in other solid organ transplant recipients (OTRs). The present review will focus on complications specific to LTRs. It is based on the current authors' experience on ca. 300 LTRs referred to their outpatient unit, which specializes in skin care of transplant recipients. Skin manifestations include complications linked to immunosuppression *per se*, irrespective of the medication, and specific complications due to each individual immunosuppressive drug. Skin manifestations related to rare diseases responsible for liver failure will not be considered here.

Drug-related specific side effects

These side effects are a frequent motivation for dermatologic consultation, and may have an important impact on quality of life, especially in young and female patients, potentially leading to treatment modification. They are dose dependent, but vary according to age and individual factors. Many symptoms are reversible and may improve by dosage reduction or switching to another drug. Tacrolimus (TAC) may induce alopecia within the first months after transplantation, which usually improves when the dosage is tapered. In some patients it may represent a chief complaint and prompt conversion to cyclosporine (CsA).[6] CsA-induced hypertrichosis and gingival hypertrophy are reversible but may require conversion to TAC, especially in women with hypertrichosis.[2,4] Steroid side effects have been well known for many years; they consist mainly of acne in the early post-graft period and striae distensae in

Medical Care of the Liver Transplant Patient, Fourth Edition. Edited by Pierre-Alain Clavien, James F. Trotter.

adolescents. Despite the increasing number of steroid-free regimens, other long-term side effects (such as senile purpura and skin fragility) still remain common. The use of mammalian target of rapamycin (mTOR) inhibitors is becoming more and more frequent in LTRs so that their dermatologic side effects are increasingly encountered. Cutaneous side effects of sirolimus (SRL) have been well documented, but data on everolimus (ERL) are more scarce. They include mainly mouth ulcers, edema, healing problems, folliculitis, psoriasis-like eruptions, alopecia, and hidradenitis suppurativa.[7–9] They seem to be more frequent after secondary introduction as compared with a *de novo* treatment. They are often improved by dose reduction, but may require drug discontinuation.

Skin infections

Immunodeficiency increases the risk of skin infections. While no assay is currently available to accurately measure a patient's risk of infection, this can be predicted by considering the intensity of immunosuppression and the timeline after transplantation.[10] For similar dosages of immunosuppressants, however, substantial variations in immunosuppression exist, due to differences in individual sensitivity, so that the level of immunodeficiency may be reflected better by infectious cutaneous manifestations. These can be classified into the following three groups: 1) common forms of usual infections, which should be treated as in non-immunosuppressed patients; 2) common infections presenting with unusually extensive lesions and/or progressing rapidly; and 3) a broad spectrum of uncommon infections, most of which are opportunistic ones. The second and third groups suggest excessive immunosuppression, and may develop following episodes of rejection with a resulting increase in immunosuppression. Treatment must take into account the severity of lesions. Changes in immunosuppressive regimens and routine antimicrobial prophylaxis have dramatically decreased the incidence and severity of post-transplant infections.[10]

Viral infections

Herpes group infections

The spectrum of viral infections has changed with the prophylactic use of anti-cytomegalovirus (CMV) and anti-herpes simplex virus (HSV) drugs. The clinical manifestations of herpes simplex, varicella and herpes zoster virus (HZV) infections may be modified by immunosuppression. Because of the possible visceral involvement and the association with CMV infection, it is important not to misdiagnose these infections, so as to adapt the treatment according to the course.[11]

HSV infections

A high percentage of the population at large is infected by HSV-1 and HSV-2 (50–80 and 25%, respectively). Most post-transplant HSV infections correspond to reactivations, but HSV may be transmitted by the graft to a seronegative patient and induce a severe infection. Before antiviral prophylaxis, viral shedding was detected in 60–70% of kidney transplant recipients (KTRs), and 30–45% of patients developed herpetic lesions within the first month. HSV infections are uncommon in patients receiving antiviral prophylaxis. In case of deep immunosuppression, facial or anogenital lesions manifest with large and multiple ulcers. Oral valacyclovir for 1–2 weeks may be sufficient, but IV acyclovir is needed in case of extensive lesions. Antiviral treatments prevent dissemination to internal organs. Despite the usual efficacy of anti-CMV drugs (such as gancyclovir or valgancyclovir) on HSV, resistant strains exist and these require treatment with valacyclovir.

HZV infections

As with non-immunosuppressed patients, primary varicella infection in adults may be more severe, with a higher incidence of systemic complications (such as meningoencephalitis and pneumonitis), although these were more often observed before the advent of antiviral treatments. Herpes zoster may occur at any time after transplantation and is increased by mycophenolate mofetil (MMF). HZV reactivation may manifest with recurring varicella, sparse vesicles or a typical zoster eruption affecting one or several dermatomes. The treatment depends on the clinical status. Patients with varicella and disseminated zoster should be given IV acyclovir with hospital monitoring; patients without visceral involvement may be switched to oral treatments after fever resolution. Oral valacyclovir may be sufficient for lesions with a common presentation. In children, prophylaxis relies on vaccination before transplantation, since response to varicella immunization seems poor after transplantation.

CMV infection
Deep immunosuppression after induction therapy often persists beyond the period of antimicrobial prophylaxis, and may result in late infections. Although CMV infection is common, cutaneous lesions are rare and have not been studied recently. They may manifest as a rash, vesiculobullous lesions, and oral or perineal ulcerations. The diagnosis is made by histologic examination, showing the presence of cytomegalic cells, i.e. vascular endothelial cells with intranuclear inclusions surrounded by a clear halo ("pigeon's eye" aspect), and detection of the virus *in situ* by immunohistochemistry and/or *in situ* hybridization. CMV skin infections can be treated with the usual antiviral drugs.

Poxvirus infections
Multiple spreading molluscum contagiosum lesions may be observed and are occasionally difficult to distinguish from flat warts or sebaceous hyperplasia.

Human papillomavirus infections

Human papillomavirus (HPV) infections are very common in transplant patients, however, most data of the literature should be reconsidered in the light of recent clinical and virologic studies. HPV infection of the skin is widespread and the new comprehensive polymerase chain reaction (PCR) techniques allow detection of HPV within normal-looking skin in 90% of both immunosuppressed and non-immunosuppressed populations.[12]

Common warts
The incidence of common warts in OTRs has been reported to increase with time after transplantation, reaching 50–80% of patients after 5 years. In two short series of LTRs, 13–25% of patients were reported to be HPV-infected.[2,5] A better definition of the lesions suggests that lesions described as "warts" in many publications probably correspond to keratotic lesions.[13] These present as verrucous and hyperkeratotic papules with clinical features intermediate between verrucous actinic keratoses and common warts, and correspond to premalignant or seborrheic keratoses, as well as various hyperkeratotic lesions whose clinical diagnosis is not straightforward.

External anogenital warts These are rarer than skin lesions and were found in 2% of patients in a series of 1000 OTRs[14] and 7% of 86 LTRs.[2] Owing to the frequent presence of dysplastic changes on histologic examination, biopsy is recommended.

In case of limited (cutaneous or anogenital) lesions, the usual dermatologic treatments (such as cryotherapy, laser, electrocautery or imiquimod) can be used. Extensive lesions may prompt revision of immunosuppression and necessitate additional treatments, such as oral retinoids. mTOR inhibitors have not proved to be beneficial in the absence of immunosuppression minimization.

Bacterial infections

These are a cause of concern in the immediate postgraft period, when wound infection can lead to sepsis. Nosocomial infections with resistant microorganisms (such as methicillin-resistant *Staphylococcus aureus*) may infect wounds. Folliculitis of the face and upper trunk is very common, whatever the immunosuppressive regimen. It can be treated with local antibiotics, such as erythromycin.

Fungal infections

In the long run, dermatophytoses and tinea versicolor are the commonest fungal infections. They can be treated with local treatments. In case of extensive dermatophytosis lesions, oral treatment (e.g. with terbinafin) may be required.

Opportunistic infections

The pattern of opportunistic infections has been changed due to routine prophylaxis for *Pneumocystis carinii*.[10] The risk of opportunistic infection depends on the level of immunosuppression, and is favored by specific activities such as raising pigeons or canaries (associated with *Cryptococcus neoformans* infection), marijuana abuse (associated with infection with *Aspergillus* species), gardening (increased risk of infections with black fungi) or contact with aquariums and/or swimming pools (*Mycobacterium marinum*). Cutaneous lesions may be isolated if the skin is the site of inoculation, or associated with systemic infection, and be the first clinical manifestation.

The clinical aspects are not specific. An opportunistic infection should be suspected in case of atypical suppurating lesions, abscesses, papules, nodules, or ulcers. Diagnosis requires histologic examination and cultures. Treatment of single lesions may be achieved with surgical excision. Systemic treatment may be required in the presence of multiple skin lesions and/or visceral involvement. Management should be discussed on an individual patient basis and should take into account the extension of the infection, the causal agent, and the level of immunosuppression. Minimization is recommended.

Skin malignancies

As with other OTRs, skin cancers are the most common malignancies in LTRs, however detailed studies on skin cancers in these patients are still sparse. Most data are provided in series about malignancies in general, lacking details on skin tumors. This chapter highlights the specific aspects of skin tumors in LTRs. We have recently reported that the majority of skin tumors in LTRs are accounted for by skin carcinomas (95%), followed by Kaposi's sarcoma and melanoma.[1] Other rare skin tumors (such as Merkel cell carcinoma, atypical fibroxanthomas and anogenital cancers) have been occasionally reported, as in other OTRs.

Skin carcinomas

Epidemiology

The incidence of skin carcinomas increases steadily with time after transplantation. The time-related incidence in LTR reaches 13% at 10 years, which is comparable to that in kidney transplant patients.[15] It can be expected that the long-term incidence will reach 40–60% at 20 years in Europe and the USA, as in KTRs.

The overall incidence of skin cancer in LTRs, regardless of time post transplantation, varies greatly according to the studies. The highest reported incidence (22.5%) resulted from a questionnaire sent to patients with a mean follow up of 4 years.[16] These substantial variations suggest that skin cancer is probably underreported in LTRs.

Risk factors for post-transplant skin cancer

As with immunocompetent individuals, the most important predisposing factors for skin cancer are fair color of the skin, eyes, and hair, and susceptibility to sunburn. Other intrinsic factors include older age at, and history of skin cancer prior to transplantation, male sex, and specific genetic factors such as polymorphisms in p53, gluthathione transferase, interleukin 10, folate pathway, and vitamin D receptor genes. Several of these factors are possibly related to skin type.[7,9] Among the extrinsic factors, ultraviolet (UV) radiation is the primary responsible carcinogen as suggested by the predominant location of skin carcinomas on sun-exposed areas. Although lifelong cumulative sun exposure intervenes, we have found that after the development of the first squamous cell carcinoma (SCC), strict sun protection can reduce the number of new carcinomas.[17] Several photosensitizing drugs commonly used in transplanted patients (such as diuretics and especially the association of amiloride with hydrochlorothiazide[18] or voriconazole)[19] reportedly increase the risk of skin cancer. The role of other extrinsic factors, such as smoking and alcohol, is still debated. The role of HPV in the development of SCC still remains controversial, although it is widely accepted in the development of cervical and anogenital carcinomas.[12] The new Merkel cell polyomavirus (MCPyV) could play a role.[20]

Several authors have attempted to assess the impact of the primary liver disease in LTRs on cancer development.[16,21–24] Several studies reported a higher overall incidence of cancer in patients with alcoholic cirrhosis. Furthermore, alcohol abuse is often associated with smoking, a known risk factor for several types of cancer.

A Spanish study has recently reported a twofold higher risk for skin cancer in LTRs grafted for alcoholic cirrhosis vs those grafted for a non-alcoholic disease.[24] This study found that 85% of patients with skin cancer from the alcoholic group were smokers (vs 30% in the non-alcoholic group); surprisingly, the same study reported a higher rate of BCC, even though smoking is known to increase the risk of SCC. Primary sclerosing cholangitis was found to be associated with an increased risk of skin cancer in 151 LTRs. This could be due to the immunosuppressive treatment given pre-transplantation for associated inflammatory bowel disease or autoimmune hepatitis.[15] A larger study on 8594 LTRs recorded in the Organ Procurement and Transplantation Network/United Network for Organ Sharing (OPTN/UNOS) data confirmed that patients with cholestatic liver diseases (including primary sclerosing cholangitis) and cirrhosis had an increased risk of skin cancer.[21]

The role of immunosuppressive treatments in the development of post-transplant skin carcinomas is widely recognized.[7,9] The specific clinical aspect appears to be linked to the duration, dosage, and type of immunosuppression. Skin cancers result both from the decrease of immunosurveillance and the direct oncogenic effect of specific immunosuppressants. The incidence of skin carcinomas is correlated with the load of immunosuppression. A higher rate of skin carcinomas has been observed with three- vs two-drug immunosuppressive regimens, and with normal- vs low-dose CsA ones. The decrease in new tumor development after reduction of immunosuppression has been largely documented in patients with multiple and/or aggressive skin carcinomas, and even after the first SCC.

Over the past 10 years, a number of studies have suggested that the nature of the immunosuppressant *per se* is important.[7,9] Although used for more than 40 years, azathioprine was shown recently to induce hypersensitivity to ultraviolet A (UVA) rays; the active metabolite of azathioprine is incorporated into the cellular DNA of keratinocytes and generates mutagenic reactive oxygen species when exposed to UV light. Calcineurin inhibitors reportedly have oncogenic properties linked to the production of cytokines that promote tumor growth and angiogenesis. By contrast, mTOR inhibitors (including SRL and ERL), belonging to a new class of immunosuppressants, are endowed with antitumoral properties via angiogenesis inhibition. The role of the newer-age immunosuppressants was recently assessed on ultraviolet B (UVB)-induced skin carcinogenesis. Chronically UV-exposed mice were treated with SRL, CsA, TAC and MMF in various combinations.[25,26] CsA-treated mice had the highest number of skin tumors. The reduction of large tumors was maximal with SRL alone, followed by SRL plus MMF, and MMF alone. Several clinical studies have reported a lower rate of skin cancer in KTRs treated by mTOR inhibitors as compared with those receiving calcineurin inhibitors, either in *de novo* treatment or after conversion. Conversion to SRL or ERL proved beneficial to kidney- and heart-transplant patients with skin cancer.[7–9]

Clinical features

The interval between LT and the diagnosis of skin carcinoma is similar to that observed in other OTRs, and it is shorter in patients who are older at transplantation. For patients grafted over the age of 50 years, it varies between 3 and 5 years. Skin carcinomas consist mainly in SCC and BCC (whose rates in KTRs are increased 100- and tenfold, respectively). The reversal of the SCC/BCC ratio observed in the transplant population vs control groups seems to further increase with sun exposure, immunosuppression and duration of follow up. In keeping with several studies, we have found that LTRs have a lower rate of SCC in comparison with other OTR groups[1] (unpublished data). This could be due to a shorter follow up and/or to differences in immunosuppressive regimens, which seem to be lighter in LTR *vs* kidney or heart transplant patients. Because of the field cancerization effect linked to UV radiation, LTRs show, similarly to other OTRs, a trend for simultaneous and/or sequential multiple lesions. Multiple SCCs expose to a higher risk of aggressive course, and metastatic spread has been reported. All these lesions are located on sun-exposed body zones, require repetitive destructive interventions on visible areas and severely impair quality of life. Skin cancers are often associated with multiple keratotic lesions, such as premalignant (or actinic) keratoses, Bowen's disease (*in situ* SCC), and keratoacanthoma, which seems to represent a highly differentiated SCC. Several recent works have shown that keratotic lesions, but not common warts, represent a risk factor for SCC.[12,13]

Treatment

The management of skin carcinomas in LTR depends on the type and number of lesions, as in other OTRs.[7] It consists of local treatments and additional measures to reduce the risk of subsequent tumors. Superficial BCC and premalignant keratoses may be treated without histologic examination by the usual dermatologic methods, such as cryotherapy, electocautery or CO_2 laser. Multiple lesions can be treated with topical 5-fluorouracil, imiquimod and/or diclofenac. Photodynamic therapy may be considered, although it is costly and painful. Larger, nodular lesions should be surgically excised with histologic control. Histologic examination is necessary for diagnosis, which may be clinically difficult, and for checking tumor depth and excision margins. Patients with SCC should be followed regularly every 3 months for 2 years, especially if SCCs are histologically undifferentiated, have a rapid growth, and invade the hypodermis and underlying tissues. Patients with BCC can be followed every 6–12 months according to the clinical situation. Large tumors or those on difficult anatomic sites may require multidisciplinary management. Node involvement is treated by surgery alone if there is no extracapsular spread. Radiotherapy should be avoided; it can be used as an adjuvant therapy if surgery is not feasible, and in the case of extracapsular node spread. Oral retinoids reduce the number of new lesions but frequently cause side effects. They may be used if revision of immunosuppression is not applicable or ineffective.

Immunosuppression revision is increasingly used in OTRs with skin carcinomas in order to reduce the number of new tumors. Prospective ongoing studies evaluate various immunosuppressive strategies in kidney and heart transplant recipients with skin cancer. Skin carcinomas represent a good model to assess the impact of changes of immunosuppressive treatments on carcinogenesis. Furthermore, since it appears that SCC are predictive of extracutaneous malignancies, adequate immunosuppression for skin carcinomas would prevent not only the occurrence of new skin tumors but also of extracutaneous ones. While minimization still may be considered, an increasingly used practice is conversion from calcineurin to mTOR inhibitors.

Kaposi sarcoma

Epidemiology

The incidence of Kaposi sarcoma (KS) depends on the geographic HHV8 seroprevalence; it varies from 0.14 to 0.5% in western countries and the USA to 1.5% in northern Italy and 4.1% in the Middle East. Several authors found that LTRs have a higher risk of KS and a shorter delay from transplantation to disease onset as compared with KTRs. These differences probably reflect the various immunosuppressive eras; indeed, calcineurin inhibitor-based regimens given to most LTRs increase the risk of KS (as compared with the former immunosuppressive regimen consisting of azathioprine and corticosteroids only, given in old KTRs).

Risk factors

The causative role of HHV8 for KS is now compelling and the geographic distribution of KS corresponds to the HHV8 seroprevalence (<5% in North America and Europe, 5–20% in the Mediterranean and Middle East, >50% in Central Africa). Most KS cases are due to viral reactivation after transplantation[27] but HHV8 may occasionally be transmitted via the graft, possibly leading to fulminant KS.[1] Other risk factors include male sex and older age at transplantation.

Clinical features

KS appears generally within the first year after transplantation. It manifests in 85% of patients with mucocutaneous lesions with or without visceral lesions, and in 15% of cases with purely visceral lesions. Cutaneous lesions are usually similar to those of Mediterranean KS; they consist of red–purple plaques or nodules predominating on the lower limbs, and are frequently associated with lymphedema. They may be limited to one or two lesions, or be widespread, involving any part of the body. Mucosal lesions involve mainly the mouth. Visceral lesions would be present in about 50% of patients, and concern mainly the lymph nodes, gastrointestinal tract and lungs, however the disease may be diffuse and involve any organ.

Treatment

The course of the disease depends on the depth of immunosuppression. KS usually regresses (partially or totally) after reduction of immunosuppression. Today, switch to mTOR inhibitors seems to be the first-line treatment because of its anti-angiogenic and antiproliferative effect. Additional treatment, including various chemotherapy regimens, may be necessary in case of life-threatening disease.

Other skin tumors

Melanoma

The incidence of post-transplant melanoma increases, paralleling the increase of melanoma worldwide in the population at large.[28] The risk of *de novo* melanoma would be increased 1.6- to eightfold. Melanoma occurs mainly in patients with fair skin and eyes. A large number of melanocytic nevi represent an additional risk factor. It appears that melanoma *in situ* and thin ones (of Breslow thickness <1 mm) in the transplant population have a similar course to those of the general population; however, thicker melanomas seem to have a more aggressive course in OTR. Sentinel lymph node biopsy should be considered for tumors >0.75 mm thick. The degree of immunosuppression revision should be adapted to the clinical situation. Pretransplant melanoma should be carefully screened because of the high risk of recurrence. The advised waiting time of 2 years prior to transplantation for melanoma with a Breslow thickness <1 mm has to be weighed against the vital risk to the recipient. Melanoma is the commonest tumor transmitted from the donor graft; although it remains rare, it results in metastatic spread.

Cancers of the external anogenital region

These cancers are increased 30- to 100 fold but have not been extensively studied. Risk factors include past history of genital warts, smoking, history of skin cancers and deep immunosuppression. Surgery is mandatory for invasive lesions, while *in situ* carcinomas (such as bowenoid papulosis) may be treated with imiquimod. Revision of immunosuppression is strongly recommended in all cases.

Other rare skin tumors

In addition to those mentioned earlier, other rare skin tumors (such as primary cutaneous lymphomas, Merkel cell carcinomas and atypical fibroxanthomas) are increased in OTRs. In most cases, revision of immunosuppression is advised along with local treatments.

Graft versus host disease

Acute graft vs host disease (GVH) occurs in 0.1–1% of LTRs.[3,29] Liver transplantation leads to the engraftment of a higher number of T-cells compared with transplantation of other organs. Cutaneous GVH manifests within the first two post-graft months as a generalized maculopapular rash involving the palms and soles; it is associated with fever, diarrhea and pancytopenia but no liver dysfuntion. Skin lesions may mimic toxic or infectious rashes, and the diagnosis requires histologic examination. GVH is often lethal because of uncontrollable infections. Chronic GVH may occur, and presents with lichenoid lesions and hyperpigmentation. In both cases, treatment consists in immunosuppression increase.

Conclusion

Skin disorders are frequent in LTRs and some of them should be managed by optimizing immunosuppression. Skin cancers represent the main long-term cutaneous complication in LTR. Regrettably, too many patients are not yet sufficiently screened from a dermatologic point of view (Figure 35.1). Prophylaxis

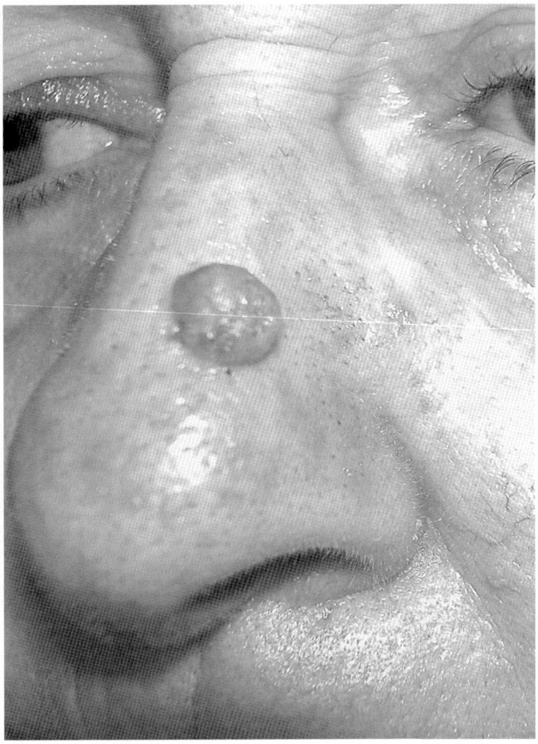

Figure 35.1 Neglected basal cell carcinoma of the nose in a 68-year-old liver transplant recipient

should be performed by regular dermatologic examination at least once a year for all patients. This allows early detection and treatment of skin (pre)malignancies and reinforces education about sun protection. The need for adequate information on sun protection has been highlighted in several publications. Recent studies have shown that better results are achieved with a reinforced education using written advice, and management by dermatologists specialized in transplant patients.[30]

References

1. Euvrard S, Kanitakis J. Skin cancers after liver transplantation: what to do? J Hepatol 2006;44:27–32.
2. Salard D, Parriaux N, Derancourt C, et al. Manifestations dermatologiques chez les transplantés hépatiques. Ann Dermatol Venéréol 2002;129:1134–8.
3. Schmied E, Dufour JF, Euvrard S. Nontumoral dermatologic problems after liver transplantation. Liver Transplantation 2004;10:331–9.
4. Hassan G, Khalaf H, Mourad W. Dermatologic complications after liver transplantation: a single-center experience. Transplant Proc 2007;39:1190–4.
5. Perera GK, Child FJ, Heaton N, O'Grady J, Higgins EM. Skin lesions in adult liver transplant recipients: a study of 100 consecutive patients. Br J Dermatol 2006;154:868–72.
6. Talbot D, Rix D, Abusin K, Mirza D, Manas D. Alopecia as a consequence of tacrolimus therapy in renal transplantation? Transplantation 1997;64:1631–3.
7. Ulrich C, Kanitakis J, Stockfleth E, Euvrard S. Skin cancer in organ transplant recipients – Where do we stand today? Am J Transplant 2008;8:2192–8.
8. Euvrard S, Boissonnat P, Roussoulières A, et al. Effect of everolimus on skin cancers in calcineurin inhibitor-treated heart transplant recipients. Transplant Int 2010;23:855–7.
9. Hofbauer G, Bouwes Bavinck JN, Euvrard S. Organ transplantation and skin cancer: basic problems and new perspectives. Exp Dermatol 2010;19:473–82.
10. Fishman JA. Infection in solid-organ transplant recipients. N Engl J Med 2007;357:2601–14.
11. Euvrard S. Pathologie cutanée infectieuse après transplantation d'organe. Ann Dermatol Venereol 1998;125:939–45.
12. Bouwes Bavinck JN, Plasmeijer EI, Feltkamp MC. Beta-papillomavirus infection and skin cancer. J Invest Dermatol 2008;128:1355–8.
13. Joly P, Bastuji-Guérin S, Francès C, et al. Squamous cell carcinomas are associated with verrucokeratotic cutaneous lesions but not with common warts in organ-transplant patients. A case–control study. Transplantation 2010;89:1224–30.
14. Euvrard S, Kanitakis J, Chardonnet Y, et al. External anogenital lesions in organ transplant recipients. Arch Dermatol 1997;133:175–8.
15. Haagsma EB, Hagens VE, Schaapveld M, et al. Increased cancer risk after liver transplantation: a population-based study. J Hepatol 2001;34:84–91.
16. Mithoefer AB, Supran S, Freeman S, Freeman RB. Risk factors associated with the development of skin cancer after liver transplantation. Liver Transplant 2002;8:939–44.
17. Euvrard S, Kanitakis J, Decullier E, et al. Subsequent skin cancers in kidney and heart transplant recipients after the first squamous cell carcinoma. Transplantation 2006;81:1093–100.
18. Jensen AO, Thomsen HF, Engebjerg MC, et al. Use of photosensitising diuretics and risk of skin cancer: a population-based case–control study. Br J Cancer 2008;99:1522–8.
19. Vanacker A, Fabré G, Van Dorpe J, et al. Aggressive cutaneous squamous cell carcinoma associated with prolonged voriconazole therapy in a renal transplant patient. Am J Transplant 2008;8:877–80.
20. Kassem A, Technau K, Kurz AK, et al. Merkel cell polyomavirus sequences are frequently detected in non-melanoma skin cancer of immunosuppressed patients. Int J Cancer 2009;125:356–61.
21. Otley C, Cherikh WS, Salsche SJ, McBride MA, Christenson LJ, Kauffman HM. Skin cancer in organ transplant recipients: effect of pretransplant end-organ disease. J Am Acad Dermatol 2005;53:783–90.
22. Euvrard S, Claudy A. Post-transplant skin cancer: The influence of organ and pre-transplant disease. Cancer Treat Res 2009;146:65–74.
23. Herrero JI, Espana A, Quiroga J, et al. Nonmelanoma skin cancer after liver transplantation. Study of risk factors. Liver Transpl 2005;11:1100–6.
24. Jimenez-Romero C, Manrique Municio A, Marques Medina E, et al. Incidence of de novo nonmelanoma skin tumors after liver transplantation for alcoholic and non-alcoholic liver diseases. Transplant Proc 2006;38:2505–7.
25. Wulff BC, Kusewitt DF, VanBuskirk AM, et al. Sirolimus reduces the incidence and progression of UVB-induced skin cancer in SKH mice even with co-administration of cyclosporione A. J Invest Dermatol 2008;128:2467–73.
26. De Gruijl F. Early and late effects of the immunosuppressants rapamycin and mycophenolate mofetil on UV carcinogenesis. Int J Cancer 2010;127:796–804.

27. Frances C, Marcelin AG, Legendre C, et al. The impact of preexisting or acquired Kaposi sarcoma herpesvirus infection in kidney transplant recipients on morbidity and survival. Am J Transplant 2009;9:2580–6.
28. Zwald FO, Christenson LJ, Billingsley EM, et al. Melanoma in solid organ transplant recipients. Am J Transplant 2010;10:1297–304.
29. Kohler S, Pasher A, Junge G, et al. Graft versus host disease after liver transplantation – a single center experience and review of literature. Transplant Int 2008;21:441–51.
30. Ismail F, Mitchell L, Casabonne D, et al. Specialist dermatology clinics for organ transplant recipients significantly improve photoprotection and levels of skin cancer awareness. Br J Dermatol 2006;155:916–25.

36 Post-transplant lymphoproliferative disorder and other malignancies after liver transplantation

Natasha Chandok[1] *and Kymberly D.S. Watt*[2]
[1]Division of Gastroenterology, Multi-Organ Transplant Program, University of Western Ontario, London, Ontario, Canada; [2]Division of Gastroenterology/Hepatology, William J. von Liebig Transplant Center, Mayo Clinic & Foundation, Rochester, MN, USA

Key learning points

- Post-transplant lymphoproliferative disorder and solid-organ malignancies are common causes of morbidity and mortality after liver transplantation.
- Liver transplant recipients are at risk for cancer development through a variety of mechanisms, including immunosuppression and susceptibility to viral infections, which play a role in carcinogenesis.
- Screening programs are important in the care of transplant recipients.
- Strategies to minimize immunosuppression may be useful in the prevention and treatment of malignancy after transplantation.

Introduction

Over the past 4 decades, the practice of liver transplantation (LT) has witnessed an incremental improvement in the short-term survival of patients receiving LT. The focus has now shifted to understand risk factors associated with long-term survival for these patients. Malignancy in recipients has emerged as a prevailing cause of late morbidity and mortality.[1–3] The cumulative incidence of any post-transplant *de novo* malignancy is depicted in Figure 36.1. Skin cancer and post-transplant lymphoproliferative disease (PTLD) comprise the most common malignancies after LT, followed by other solid-organ cancers involving the colorectal, lung, genitourinary, and oropharyngeal systems.[4] In many studies, breast and prostate cancer are not observed at significantly increased frequency among LT recipients.

LT recipients have several risk factors for the development of malignancies post transplant. Many of these risk factors such as smoking, alcohol, sun exposure and a personal history of malignancy before transplantation increase a recipient's probability of cancer after liver transplantation. In addition, post-transplant risk factors including immunosuppression and susceptibility to infections linked to carcinogenesis add an incremental risk for these patients.

PTLD

For over 30 years, PTLD has been a dreaded complication among organ transplant recipients. PTLD is a heterogeneous assortment of lymphoproliferative disorders described as a monoclonal or polyclonal expansion of lymphocytes, usually of B-cell origin

Medical Care of the Liver Transplant Patient, Fourth Edition. Edited by Pierre-Alain Clavien, James F. Trotter.

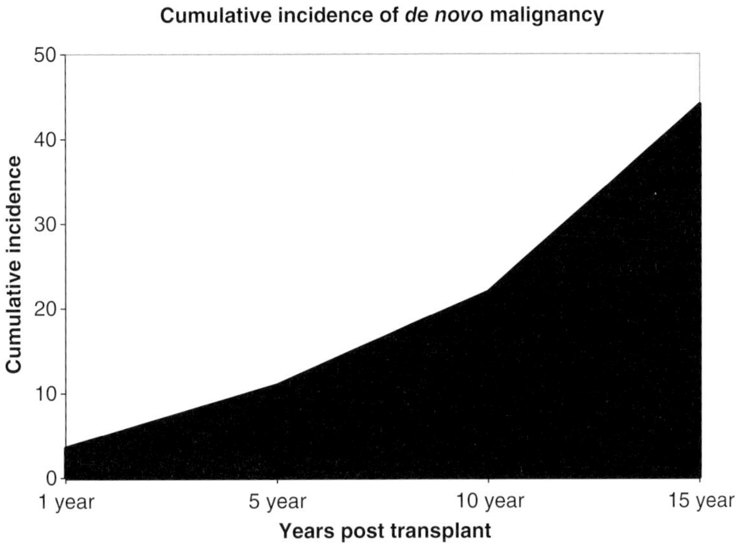

Figure 36.1 The cumulative incidence of *de novo* malignancy after liver transplantation. Based on data extracted from Haagsma et al., Finkenstadt et al., and Watt et al.[4,19,20]

(but it can be, less commonly, T-cell or rarely natural killer cell based). Unlike nonHodgkin lymphomas in immunocompetent hosts, PTLD is often extranodal and the majority are large B-cell-based lymphomas (not the low-grade B-cell variety seen more frequently in immunocompetent patients).[5,6] PTLD cells are generally of host origin, but can, on rare occasions, be of donor origin. In that circumstance the disease is usually limited to the allograft. PTLD is commonly associated with the Epstein–Barr virus (EBV), but EBV-negative disease does occur.[7,8]

Epidemiology and risk factors

The incidence of PTLD following LT ranges from 1 to 5% in most studies.[4,5,9] The risk of PTLD depends on the length of time since transplantation (or length of clinical follow up), EBV infection, recipient age, possibly sex of the recipient, and the degree of immunosuppression.[3,5,10] In a retrospective, single-center analysis of 1206 LT recipients at the Mayo Clinic, Kremers et al. found 37 cases of PTLD. The cumulative incidence was 4.7% at 15 years, with the highest incidence (1.1%) noted in the first 18 months.[5] Similarly, a large database study reported a cumulative incidence of hematologic malignancy (83% of which were PTLD) of 1.5, 1.9 and 3.2% at 1, 5 and 10 years post transplant.[4]

Several risk factors for the development of PTLD after LT have been identified. Within the first 4 years following LT, the majority of PTLD cases are related to EBV infection; thereafter the majority of PTLD cases occur in EBV-negative subjects.[5] There is conflicting data in the literature as to whether male gender and young age in the adult LT recipient increase the risk of PTLD, but certainly PTLD is more frequently seen in the pediatric population than the adult population.[3,11] There appears to be no difference in PTLD incidence with viral etiology of liver disease (hepatitis B or C virus), calcineurin inhibitor agent (tacrolimus or cyclosporine), re-transplantation, cytomegalovirus (CMV) mismatch, or length of steroid maintenance period.[5,11] Interestingly, transplantation for fulminant hepatitis has been associated with a significantly higher risk of PTLD within 18 months of LT, with a reported hazard ratio (HR) of 2.6 ($P < 0.01$).[5] This may be a reflection of increased immunosuppression in these individuals, as high-dose steroids and muromonab-CD3 (OKT3) have also been associated with PTLD (HR 4.5 and

3.9, respectively, $P < 0.01$).[5] Overall, these findings suggest that greater immunosuppression increases a recipient's likelihood of PTLD.

Pathogenesis

Immunosuppressed states predispose to lymphoid neoplasms due to a complex interplay of immunologic mechanisms and environmental exposures. EBV plays an especially important role in the pathophysiology of most cases of PTLD.

EBV is a ubiquitous DNA herpesvirus that infects the majority of the global population in childhood. Infection in childhood is usually asymptomatic or mild and self-limiting, whereas primary infection in adulthood may manifest as the syndrome of infectious mononucleosis. After primary infection, individuals are lifelong carriers as EBV persists in a latent state in B-cell lymphocytes. Infection of B cells with EBV results in either viral replication and B-cell destruction, or propagation of the B-cell with only partial EBV genome expression, leading to latent EBV infection. Cytotoxic T-cells repress the production of transformed B-cells in immunocompetent hosts, but in immunosuppressed subjects, T-cells lose their surveillance abilities, enabling replication of infected lymphocytes. The risk of PTLD is amplified in subjects who are seronegative for EBV at the time of transplantation. It is speculated that EBV-negative recipients who receive a seropositive organ and/or develop primary EBV infection have a much higher probability of developing PTLD.[6,8,10] This may explain why children are more susceptible to PTLD, as they may be more likely to be EBV negative at the time of their transplant.

Immunosuppression with calcineurin inhibitors, purine analogs and steroids to prevent hepatic allograft rejection causes T-cell dysregulation, thereby enabling proliferation of EBV-infected B-cells. Eventually, this proliferation can culminate in lymphoma. Lymphocytic proliferation is polyclonal, but with mutation and growth selection, monoclonal growth ensues.

The pathogenesis of EBV-negative PTLD is less understood. There is, however, an increasing frequency of reported EBV-negative cases of PTLD.[7] This form of PTLD tends to occur later after transplantation and is associated with a worse prognosis.[7] Evidence of immune-mediated injury, which predisposes to PTLD includes a significant association of PTLD with high-dose steroid therapy and OKT3.[5] Supporting this notion is the higher rates of PTLD observed following small bowel, heart, lung, or kidney transplantation, where recipients receive more aggressive immunosuppression than LT recipients.

Clinical manifestations

PTLD can be localized or disseminated. The spectrum of clinical presentation is broad and initially nonspecific. Manifestations may include fever, night sweats, malaise, lymphadenopathy, unintentional weight loss, gastrointestinal symptoms such as nausea or diarrhea, or respiratory or neurologic symptoms. Often these patients can present with subtle signs and symptoms, so a high index of suspicion is required to diagnosis PTLD. The three most frequent sites of involvement of PTLD are the lymphatic system, the gastrointestinal system (including the liver), and the renal systems.[10] T-cell PTLD not associated with EBV generally occurs at extranodal sites, including the central nervous system (CNS). Unfortunately, patients with PTLD can deteriorate precipitously, thus rapid diagnosis and treatment are needed.

In addition to the clinical exam, cross-sectional imaging including CT scan, MRI and/or PET scanning is required. Serologic support with LDH levels and EBV serology are helpful. A tissue biopsy is mandatory for diagnosis and staging of the malignancy, with excisional biopsy preferred over needle biopsies.

Treatment and prognosis

More research is needed to guide the optimal timing and treatment approach to malignant PTLD. Generally, a stepwise approach is employed, with the best tolerated strategies employed first. As PTLD is relatively uncommon, prospective trials are unlikely to occur.

Most patients with mild PTLD respond well to a reduction or withdrawal of immunosuppression; this intervention enables a patient's immune system to control propagating lymphocytes. The short-term success of immunosuppression reduction is 40 to 70%.[12] Predictors of poor response to immunosuppressant reduction include: polyclonal, as opposed to monoclonal, PTLD; CNS involvement; EBV-negative disease; and T-cell PTLD.[8] PTLD that responds inadequately to such conservative measures, requires consideration for other treatment modalities, including surgery, radiation, and chemotherapy.

Acyclovir and ganciclovir, which inhibit EBV DNA replication, have not been definitively shown to be effective in preventing or treating PTLD.[13] There are also anecdotal reports that interferon alfa, which has antiviral properties, is effective in the treatment of B-cell PTLD in some, but this agent has also not been studied prospectively.[14] IV immunoglobulin has similarly been used as an ancillary treatment for PTLD, alone or in combination with interferon alfa, but its impact on PTLD is questionable.

Rituximab is an anti-CD20 antibody that can be used as a second-line agent when immunosuppression reduction is inadequate. It has been associated with a 44% remission rate when used as a single agent along with immunosuppression reduction,[15] and appears to be well tolerated in these patients.

Cyclophosphamide, adriamycin, oncovin, and prednisone (CHOP) therapy, combined with immunosuppression reduction, has been used in patients with aggressive PTLD with limited success, in large part due to significant relapse rates. In a series of 26 patients with PTLD, Choquet et al. reported an overall response rate of 65%, with median overall and progression-free survival rates of 13.9 and 42 months.[16] Such regimens have significant toxicities and are associated with a high mortality rate. Frequently, CHOP is combined with rituximab, to permit reduction in doses of toxic alkylating agents and anthracyclines, thereby minimizing serious adverse events.

There is no standard approach to patients who relapsed, or were refractory, to standard chemotherapy and immunosuppression reduction. Rituximab may be a reasonable salvage agent to explore in this setting, if not used previously. Trappe et al., reported on a small series of patients in which rituximab was used after chemotherapy; they reported a 43% rate of complete remission and 14% rate of partial remission, with no therapy-associated toxicity.[17]

Surgical resection or localized radiation may be of benefit in some patients with PTLD. Such an approach may be curative in patients with focal disease. Surgical resection may also be of benefit to debulk a large burden of disease, but this is largely only performed if the lesion has clinical consequences (e.g. bowel obstruction). Radiation is also an option in patients with PTLD, particularly those with CNS involvement.

PTLD in LT recipients portends a poor survival, with only 50% of patients alive 2 years after diagnosis.[5] In a multi-center prospective analysis, Watt et al. found a 44% and 58% mortality rate at 1 and 5 years, respectively, following the diagnosis of PTLD.[4] Late-onset PTLD responds less favorably to treatment and has an even worse prognosis.[6] The strongest predictors of poor outcomes from PTLD are suboptimal performance status, clinical stage III or IV disease, CHOP as first-line therapy, and numerous extra-nodal site involvement.[12]

Solid-organ malignancies in liver transplant recipients

Solid-organ malignancies following LT are among the most frequent causes of late morbidity and mortality among recipients.[1,2] Like PTLD, the possibility of developing a solid organ malignancy is increased in LT recipients because immunosuppression decreases immune surveillance mechanisms against malignant cells and renders the host vulnerable to viruses with oncogenic properties.

Epidemiology

The overall risk for solid-organ malignancy among LT recipients is 2–4 times higher than in the general population matched for sex and age.[2–4,18] Analysis of the National Institute of Diabetes and Digestive and Kidney Diseases' (NIDDK) liver transplantation prospective database found that 171 of 798 adult LT recipients from 1990 to 1994 developed *de novo* malignancies over 12 years of follow up. In this study of 147 skin cancers, 29 hematologic cancers and 95 solid-organ malignancies, the probability of developing any *de novo* malignancy was 28%, and of a solid-organ malignancy was 13.6% at 10 years.[4] Furthermore, a retrospective Austrian study found that of 779 consecutive LT recipients, 12.3% developed 105 malignancies.[19] In this study, Finkenstadt et al. determined that the cumulative risk for *de novo* cancer was 10, 24, 32 and 42% at 5, 10, 15 and 20 years after LT; the most frequent tumors in this Austrian cohort were skin cancer (17%), lung cancer

Table 36.1 10-year probability of developing specific malignancies

Source	Any malignancy	Gastrointestinal malignancy	Lung malignancy	Genito-urinary malignancy	Oropharyngeal malignancy
Watt et al[4]	13.6%	3.6%	2.2%	1.8%	1.1%
CDC	6.5%	0.62%	0.7%	0.13–0.54*	0.07–0.21*

Based on data extracted from Watt et al.[4] and historic data available on the Centers for Disease Control (CDC): National Cancer Institute (NCI) website http://seercancergov/csr/1975_2005/ 2005 for the 10-year probability of malignancy estimates for individuals (mean age 50) from 1990–1994 (to match the study by Watt et al.)
*Probability range reflects different sites within the genitourinary tract or oropharyngeal region

(16%), and oropharyngeal carcinoma (11%).[19] Lung cancer, gastrointestinal cancer, oropharyngeal, and genitourinary cancers are the most prevalent cancers found in most series.[4,19–21] The probability of developing any of these more common malignancies is outlined in Table 36.1. A Finnish study comparing LT recipients with the general population found an overall standardized incidence ratio (SIR) calculated as observed to expected) for the development of malignancy to be 2.59; this rate was higher among men (4.16) than women (1.74), higher among children vs adults (18.1), and higher within 2 years following transplantation (3.17).[3]

Risk factors and pathogenesis

Age is a risk factor for most cancers. Unlike PTLD, where children and young adults have high rates of lymphoma, the prospective analysis of the NIDDK multicenter database indicates that the risk of solid-organ cancer increased in a unidirectional fashion with age by decade after LT.[4,19]

While carcinogenesis is clearly multifactorial, immunosuppression is thought to be a principal component in the development of cancer after transplantation. It is believed to be related to the overall state of immunosuppression and not a direct association between specific immunosuppressive agents. Although initial evidence suggested an increased risk of malignancy in patients treated with azathioprine and/or cyclosporine, it was hard to determine the direct effect, as these patients had a higher incidence of rejection and likely overall immunosuppression.[22] Indeed, Watt et al. were unable to find specific immunosuppressive medications (e.g. cyclosporine vs tacrolimus), nor the specific use of anti-lymphocyte agents to be associated with higher risk of *de novo* nonPTLD, malignancy.[4] Studies have also failed to show a direct association between rejection episodes and the development of malignancy.[4,18]

A variety of well-known environmental exposures that contribute to carcinogenesis may impose an additive or synergistic risk for cancer development, in conjunction with immunosuppression, among transplant recipients. Primary examples of these environmental exposures include sunlight, alcohol, and smoking. A quantity of sun exposure in fair-skinned transplant recipients is a proven risk factor for skin malignancy, and counseling on sun protection and regular dermatologic examinations is imperative.[23] Routine application of broad-spectrum sunscreens has been prospectively validated as an effective method to prevent actinic keratoses and invasive squamous cell carcinomas in particular.[24]

Alcohol and smoking have well-established associations with a variety of malignancies. Alcohol and tobacco exposures have been shown to increase cancer risk in the cirrhotic patient prior to transplantation and immunosuppression.[25] The magnitude of the risk of ongoing alcohol and/or smoking on the development of cancers after LT is unknown. A number of studies have shown that patients who were transplanted for alcoholic liver disease have higher rates (9–18%) of malignancy post-transplantation as compared to patients with no prior history of excessive alcohol exposure.[4,19,22,26] Patients with alcoholic liver disease are in the highest risk group for lung, oropharyngeal, and GI malignancies.

In a case–control study of recipients transplanted for alcoholic liver disease vs non-alcoholic liver diseases, the incidence of lung cancer was significantly greater at 4.3% in the alcohol-exposed group vs 0.7% in the control group.[27] These findings are similar to the rates found in the NIDDK study (4.8 vs 1.3% 10-year cumulative incidence).[4] The mean time to lung cancer diagnosis was significantly reduced in patients who also smoked.[27,28] LT recipients exposed to smoking and/or excess alcohol are also at higher risk for oropharyngeal carcinoma, which represents 11% of post-transplant malignancies and in a large Austrian series.[19] The 10-year cumulative incidence of 4.6% is over 10× that of the rest of the transplant population.[4,22] The 10-year cumulative risk for a GI malignancy is also twice as much as the nonprimary sclerosing cholangitis (PSC) transplant population (5 vs 2.4%). This data suggests a need for continued counseling against these exposures.

Alcoholic liver disease is not the only example where underlying liver disease appears to correlate with the likelihood of cancer development after LT. Patients with underlying PSC were also found to be at highest risk (22%) for *de novo* malignancy within a decade of transplantation.[4] For unclear reasons PSC patients were found to have more risk for skin as well as hematologic malignancies than the rest of the transplant population. This may be related to the longer duration of immunosuppression relating to management of coincident inflammatory bowel disease (IBD), or to relative vitamin D (and its anti-proliferative property) deficiency secondary to chronic cholestasis. These theories would also suggest a higher risk for autoimmune hepatitis patients or even primary biliary cirrhosis patients, but this was not the case. This suggests other factors are involved in the increased risk.

Patients with PSC may be at higher risk for colorectal cancer (CRC), in particular because of concomitant IBD. Approximately 5% of patients transplanted for PSC will develop colorectal carcinoma.[29] Patients with PSC and IBD were more likely to develop CRC than patients with either PSC alone or IBD alone. This risk is difficult to accurately determine since this patient population is usually more stringently screened than the rest of the transplant population and several patients with IBD may have had a colectomy, thereby eliminating their risk for CRC. Vera et al. determined a cumulative risk of CRC in PSC/IBD patients with intact colons to be 14% at 5 years and 17% at 10 years.[29]

The bulk of the evidence suggests that liver transplant recipients, particularly with a history of IBD, PSC or alcohol, are at higher risk for CRC and thus require more aggressive screening in these populations to enable earlier detection than is currently published in multi-society guidelines. Albright et al. found that post-LT adenomatous polyps were detected in 47.3% of patients with pre-LT polyps vs 6.7% of patients without pre-LT polyps ($P < 0.001$). Patients with alcoholic liver disease had a significantly higher rate of adenoma formation (50 vs 11.1%, $P < 0.001$).[30] The risk of CRC, as well as most other malignancies, appears to be cumulative, and increases with time after transplantation.

As in the case of PTLD, viruses with oncogenic potential are an important theoretical risk factor for cancer development in transplant recipients. Malignancies such as Kaposi sarcoma (KS) and cervical cancer, related to human-herpes-virus 8 infections and human papillomavirus, respectively, are observed at higher frequencies. Di Benedetto et al. reported an incidence of KS of 2.1% among 285 consecutive recipients of LTs from 2000 to 2006.[31] In a German study assessing 98 women before and after LT, female liver transplant recipients were observed to have a higher risk of developing cervical dysplasias and neoplasias regardless of calcineurin inhibitor used (cyclosporine or tacrolimus); this confirms the need for regular internal examinations and Pap smears after LT.[32] The human papillomavirus virus increases the risk of other squamous cell cancers such skin cancer, anal cancer, and oropharyngeal/head and neck cancer.[30,33]

Another potential risk factor, unique to transplant recipients, is the possibility of donor-transmitted malignancy. With careful consideration of the donor before and at the time of procurement, this phenomenon is generally uncommon and the subject of case reports.

Diagnostic strategies, prognosis and treatment

Given that LT recipients have higher rates of numerous malignancies than the general population, systematic screening programs are of great importance. Finkelstedt et al. found than an intensified surveillance protocol drastically increased the detection of *de novo* cancers from 4.9 to 13%.[19] Moreover, the screening program led to the malignancies being diagnosed at earlier stages, and the median survival of nonskin cancers increased from 1.2 to 3.3 years.[19] Such impressive outcomes were replicated in another study by Herrero et al., suggesting that a surveillance protocol can be life saving for LT recipients.[21] The need for structured screening for prevention and earlier diagnosis of malignancies cannot be overstated, especially in light of studies that show that outcomes after malignancies are significantly worse in LT recipients than in the general population.[4,22,34]

The approach to treatment of malignancies in LT recipients is generally similar to that in the untransplanted population. Transplant physicians, however, may consider reduced immunosuppression and/or switching the calcineurin inhibitor to the mTOR inhibitor, rapamycin. Rapamycin has multiple antitumor effects, including suppression of angiogenesis, cell proliferation, and cell survival. Emerging evidence, largely from renal transplant recipients, reveals that rapamycin reduces nonmelanoma skin cancer and is associated with improved survival.[35,36] The use of rapamycin to reduce recurrence of disease in the transplant recipient with hepatocellular carcinoma has shown conflicting results. Further prospective studies on post-transplant malignancies are needed in LT recipients to better characterize their prognosis and optimal management.

Figure 36.1 illustrates the cumulative incidence of *de novo* malignancy after liver transplantation. Based on data extracted from Haagsma et al., Finkenstadt et al., and Watt et al.[4,19,20]

References

1. Watt K, Pedersen R, Kremers W, Heimbach J, Charlton M. Evolution of causes and risk factors for mortality post liver transplantation: Results of the NIDDK long-term follow-up study 2010;10:1420–7.
2. Baccarani U, Adani GL, Serraino D, et al. De novo tumors are a major cause of late mortality after orthotopic liver transplantation. Transplant Proc 2009;41: 1303–5.
3. Aberg F, Pukkala E, Hockerstedt K, Sankila R, Isoniemi H. Risk of malignant neoplasms after liver transplantation: a population-based study. Liver Transpl 2008;14: 1428–36.
4. Watt KD, Pedersen RA, Kremers WK, Heimbach JK, Sanchez W, Gores GJ. Long-term probability of and mortality from de novo malignancy after liver transplantation. Gastroenterology 2009;137:2010–7.
5. Kremers WK, Devarbhavi HC, Wiesner RH, Krom RA, Macon WR, Habermann TM. Post-transplant lymphoproliferative disorders following liver transplantation: incidence, risk factors and survival. Am J Transplant 2006;6(Pt1):1017–24.
6. Khedmat H, Taheri S. Early onset post transplantation lymphoproliferative disorders: analysis of international data from 5 studies. Ann Transplant 2009;14:74–7.
7. Nelson BP, Nalesnik MA, Bahler DW, Locker J, Fung JJ, Swerdlow SH. Epstein–Barr virus-negative post-transplant lymphoproliferative disorders: a distinct entity? Am J Surg Pathol 2000;24:375–85.
8. Dotti G, Fiocchi R, Motta T, et al. Epstein–Barr virus-negative lymphoproliferate disorders in long-term survivors after heart, kidney, and liver transplant. Transplantation 2000;69:827–33.
9. Dhillon MS, Rai JK, Gunson BK, Olliff S, Olliff J. Post-transplant lymphoproliferative disease in liver transplantation. Br J Radiol 2007;80:337–46.
10. Khedmat H, Taheri S. Late onset post transplantation lymphoproliferative disorders: analysis of international data from 5 studies. Ann Transplant 2009;14:80–5.
11. Marques E, Jimenez C, Manrique A, et al. Development of lymphoproliferative disease after liver transplantation. Transplant Proc 2008;40:2988–9.
12. Richendollar BG, Tsao RE, Elson P, et al. Predictors of outcome in post-transplant lymphoproliferative disorder: an evaluation of tumor infiltrating lymphocytes in the context of clinical factors. Leuk Lymphoma 2009;50:2005–12.
13. Trigg ME, Finlay JL, Sondel PM. Prophylactic acyclovir in patients receiving bone marrow transplants. N Engl J Med 1985;312:1708–9.
14. Davis C, Wood B, Sabath D, Joseph J, Stehman-Breen C, Broudy V. Interferon-alpha treatment of posttransplant lymphoproliferative disorder in recipients of solid organ transplants. Transplantation 1998;66: 1770–9.
15. Choquet S, Leblond V, Herbrecht R, et al. Efficacy and safety of rituximab in B-cell post-transplantation lymphoproliferative disorders: results of a prospective multicenter phase 2 study. Blood 2006;107:3053–7.
16. Choquet S, Trappe R, Leblond V, Jager U, Davi F, Oertel S. CHOP-21 for the treatment of post-transplant lymphoproliferative disorders (PTLD) following solid organ transplantation. Haematologica 2007;92:273–4.
17. Trappe RU, Choquet S, Reinke P, et al. Salvage therapy for relapsed posttransplant lymphoproliferative disorders (PTLD) with a second progression of PTLD after

Upfront chemotherapy: the role of single-agent rituximab. Transplantation 2007;84:1708–12.
18. Yao FY, Gautam M, Palese C, et al. De novo malignancies following liver transplantation: a case–control study with long-term follow-up. Clin Transplant 2006;20:617–23.
19. Finkenstadt A, Graziadei IW, Oberaigner W, et al. Extensive surveillance promotes early diagnosis and improved survival of de novo malignancies in liver transplant recipients. Am J Transplant 2009;9: 2355–61.
20. Haagsma EB, Hagens VE, Schaapveld M, et al. Increased cancer risk after liver transplantation: a population-based study. J Hepatol 2001;34:84–91.
21. Herrero JI, Alegre F, Quiroga J, et al. Usefulness of a program of neoplasia surveillance in liver transplantation. A preliminary report. Clin Transplant 2009;23: 532–6.
22. Benlloch S, Berenguer M, Prieto M, et al. De novo internal neoplasms after liver transplantation: increased risk and aggressive behavior in recent years? Am J Transplant 2004;4:596–604.
23. Terhorst D, Drecoll U, Stockfleth E, Ulrich C. Organ transplant recipients and skin cancer: assessment of risk factors with focus on sun exposure. Br J Dermatol 2009;161(Suppl 3):85–9.
24. Ulrich C, Jurgensen JS, Degen A, et al. Prevention of non-melanoma skin cancer in organ transplant patients by regular use of a sunscreen: a 24 months, prospective, case–control study. Br J Dermatol 2009;161(Suppl 3): 78–84.
25. Sorensen HT, Friis S, Olsen JH, et al. Risk of liver and other types of cancer in patients with cirrhosis: a nationwide cohort study in Denmark. Hepatology 1998;28: 921–5.
26. Jimenez-Romero C, Manrique Municio A, Marques Medina E, et al. Incidence of de novo nonmelanoma skin tumors after liver transplantation for alcoholic and nonalcoholic liver diseases. Transplant Proc 2006;38: 2505–7.
27. Jimenez C, Manrique A, Marques E, et al. Incidence and risk factors for the development of lung tumors after liver transplantation. Transpl Int 2007;20:57–63.
28. VanderHeide F, Dijkstra G, Porte R, Kleibeuker J, Haagsma E. Smoking behavior in liver transplant recipients. Liver Transpl 2009;15:648–55.
29. Vera A, Gunson BK, Ussatoff V, et al. Colorectal cancer in patients with inflammatory bowel disease after liver transplantation for primary sclerosing cholangitis. Transplantation 2003;75:1983–8.
30. Albright JB, Bonatti H, Stauffer J, et al. Colorectal and anal neoplasms following liver transplantation. Colorectal Dis 2010:12:657–666.
31. Di Benedetto F, Di Sandro S, De Ruvo N, et al. Kaposi's sarcoma after liver transplantation. J Cancer Res Clin Oncol 2008;134:653–8.
32. David M, Olbrich C, Neuhaus R, Lichtenegger W. Occurrence of suspicious changes in cervix cytology in women after liver transplantation. Geburtshilfe Frauenheilkd 1995;55:431–4.
33. Tedeschi SK, Savani BN, Jagasia M, et al. Time to consider HPV vaccination after allogeneic stem cell transplantation. Biol Blood Marrow Transplant 2010;16:1033–6.
34. Rubio E, Moreno JM, Turrion VS, Jimenez M, Lucena JL, Cuervas-Mons V. De novo malignancies and liver transplantation. Transplant Proc 2003;35:1896–7.
35. Toso C, Merani S, Bigam DL, Shapiro AM, Kneteman NM. Sirolimus-based immunosuppression is associated with increased survival after liver transplantation for hepatocellular carcinoma. Hepatology 2009;51: 1237–43.
36. Salgo R, Gossmann J, Schofer H, et al. Switch to a sirolimus-based immunosuppression in long-term renal transplant recipients: Reduced rate of (pre)malignancies and nonmelanoma skin cancer in a prospective, randomized, assessor-blinded, controlled clinical trial. Am J Transplant 2010;10:1385.

37 Sexual function and fertility after liver transplantation

Andreas Geier and Beat Müllhaupt
Swiss HPB and Transplantation Centers, Section of Hepatology, University Hospital Zürich, Zürich, Switzerland

Key learning points

- Patients with chronic liver disease often have alterations in the normal physiology of the hypothalamic–pituitary–gonadal axis, which can affect sexual function.
- After liver transplantation, sexual function can return to normal and regular menstrual bleeding will reappear in the vast majority of women of child-bearing age within 1 year post transplant.
- After liver transplantation female patients need an effective, safe, and reversible contraceptive method to avoid an unwanted pregnancy.
- The most common maternal risks during pregnancy are: systemic hypertension and/or pre-eclampsia, both of which occur at far higher frequency than in the general population.
- The most common fetal complications in the liver transplant recipient are: prematurity, fetal distress and growth restrictions.
- It is important to know the impact of immunosuppressive drugs on pregnancy and fetal outcome.

Sexual health in patients with chronic liver disease

End-stage liver disease is a well-recognized disease that alters the normal physiology of the hypothalamic–pituitary–gonadal axis and thereby affects sexual function. In men, cirrhosis is associated with decreased levels of serum testosterone, inappropriately low levels of pituitary–gonadal stimulating hormones, luteinizing hormone and follicular-stimulating hormone, resulting in a hypogonadal state.[1–4] The elevated serum levels of estrogens and prolactin might further affect sexual function.[1,2] Although these endocrinologic effects affect patients with cirrhosis of any etiology, it has been suggested that ongoing alcohol consumption associated with end-stage alcoholic liver disease might further impact on the hypothalamic–pituitary–gonadal axis in men and women.[4]

In a survey of 53 women with chronic liver disease it was shown that >60% of these patients were suffering menstrual irregularities pre transplant, 30% had irregular menses, and 34% were amenorrhoic. This was significantly more frequent compared to women with acute liver failure, who had 18 and 9%, respectively.[5] A recent report suggested that amenorrhea occurs more often in women with hepatocellular liver disease (60%) compared to women with cholestatic liver disease (19%) ($P = 0.0009$).[6] In men, it was reported that the volume of ejaculatory fluid as well as libido/interest in sex are decreased.[2,7] The frequency of erectile dysfunction including frank impotence, has been reported to some degree in anywhere from 50 to 90% of patients with cirrhosis.[2,7] Although suspected for a long time, it was until recently unclear whether a correlation exists between the degree of sexual dysfunction and the severity of liver insufficiency. Sorrell et al. showed that sexual activity pre-transplant correlated with the MELD score.[7] They found that in patients who reported no sexual activity the Model for End-stage Liver Disease

Medical Care of the Liver Transplant Patient, Fourth Edition. Edited by Pierre-Alain Clavien, James F. Trotter.

(MELD) score (15.18) was clearly higher compared to patients with no change in sexual activity (MELD score 10.74). In addition, a similar correlation between MELD score and erectile dysfunction was also observed.

Additionally, sexual function might be further affected by underlying liver disease such as alcohol,[4] hemochromatosis,[8] other disease such as diabetes mellitus,[9] autonomic neuropathy,[10] or medications frequently used in the treatment of patients with chronic liver disease such as beta-blockers (propranolol, nadolol) or diuretics (spironolactone, furosemide).[11]

Sexual health after liver transplantation

Physiologically, the marked hypothalamic–pituitary–gonadal abnormalities of end-stage liver disease should be reversed by liver transplantation,[1,2,4] however it has been reported that some transplant recipients, especially patients with alcoholic liver disease, might have persisting abnormalities.[4,12] Regular menstrual bleeding will reappear in the vast majority of women of child-bearing age within 1 year post transplant and in some menses will resume within the first few months.[5,6,13,14] Sexual health, however, which encompasses not only sexual function but also satisfaction, is affected by more than just hormonal and endocrinologic physiology. Concomitant health issues, aging, medications as well as psychologic and social issues may also affect post-transplant sexual health. The post-transplant literature on sexual health is mixed, depending on the study population(s) and the specific questions asked. Post-transplant quality of life studies using standard but generic instruments tend to report improvements in sexual function.[15] In another study, older recipients and women reported worse sexual functioning compared to men and young patients.[16]

Regarding sexual activity, a Brazilian study of relatively young post-transplant women (mean age 44 years) found that 75% reported weekly sexual intercourse, with 70% experiencing orgasm and 70% experiencing satisfaction with their sexual health.[13] The North American experience, however, is markedly less favorable. A survey of post-liver transplant recipients (150 respondents, median age 54 years) in Canada reported that 32% experienced *de novo* post-transplant sexual dysfunction, 20% of men and 26% of women, respectively, reported decreased libido and 33% of men and 26% of women reported difficulty with orgasm.[17] Immunosuppressive drugs (approximately 60% were on tacrolimus (TAC) and 30% on cyclosporine) were blamed by 36% for sexual dysfunction followed by their liver disease (33%), other causes (18%), and depression (10%). Overall, approximately 60% reported that, despite their problems, they were "moderately" to "very satisfied" with their sexual relationships, suggesting that sexual function/performance itself is only a component of overall post-transplant sexual health. Even less favorable was an American study, where 39 post-transplant recipients were surveyed by a telephone interviewer. Overall, 44% reported decreased satisfaction with sex, and only 24% of men reported "no problems" with erectile dysfunction, although 35% did report an increased "interest in sex" and 28% reported an increased frequency of intercourse.[7]

The study by Ho et al. reported that, unknown to the transplant team, 19% of transplant respondents were using the phosphodiesterase-5 inhibitor sildenafil.[17] Experience with sildenafil has so far not been reported in liver transplant recipients, however it has been successfully used in renal transplant recipients with erectile dysfunction without adverse effects or interactions with calcineurin inhibitors.[18]

Contraception after liver transplantation

Menstrual cycles and sexual function will return in most women (>90%) of reproductive age within the first year after transplantation[13,14] and consequently women who have undergone successful OLT may conceive as early as 1 month following OLT.[19] There is therefore a clear need for contraception in fertile women after OLT, but only a few studies have investigated the different contraceptive methods in this special population. Because the data on which to base these recommendations in liver transplant patients is very limited, the experience is largely derived from the kidney transplant population.

There are no differences to the general population regarding the contraceptive methods that are available for women after liver transplantation. Some peculiarities, however, deserve special attention in this population, including an increased prevalence of chronic renal insufficiency, an increased risk of infections and (some) cancer(s), as well as systemic hypertension and an increased cardiovascular risk, a greater potential for hepatotoxicity, and drug interactions by virtue of the lifelong requirement of immunosuppressive therapy.

Interrupted intercourse and barrier methods

Periodic abstinence and coitus interruptus are ineffective methods of contraception, but are not associated with side effects or drug interactions. A total of 15 out of 16 female kidney transplant recipients from Iran with unintended pregnancies used coitus interruptus as their only form of contraception,[20] therefore this method cannot be recommended. Nevertheless, in a survey on contraceptive practices, one-quarter of US female kidney transplant recipients reported to use no contraception at all.[21]

Barrier methods, such as diaphragms and condoms are widely used in the general population, are of low cost and drug interactions are avoided. Compared to women on oral contraceptives the use of diaphragms increases the risk of urinary tract infections by a factor of two. In the transplant population this increased risk of infection can be especially problematic.[22] Condoms represent the only form of contraception that prevents transmission of (most) sexually transmitted disease(s), and should therefore be recommended for all patients without a stable sexual partner.[23] A spermicide should be added to most barrier methods to increase their efficacy. Failure rates are reported to range between 15 and 32%,[24] nevertheless, all barrier methods can be recommended for birth control in female transplant recipients.[23]

Intrauterine contraceptive devices

Currently two types of intrauterine devices (IUDs) are available: The levonorgestrel-releasing Mirena and the copper-containing ParaGard.[24] They are effective over a period of 5 (Mirena) to 10 years (ParaGard) and both are very effective with failure rates below 1% during the first year of use. In transplant patients two factors limit the use of an IUD: 1) fear of infectious complications upon insertion of a foreign body into the uterine cavity,[25] and 2) reduced effectiveness in immunosuppressed patients.[26] The fear of infectious complication, however, appears to be more theoretical than real. In cohorts of transplant patients there are so far no studies that can confirm or refute this increased risk.[25] In a prospective cohort of 156 HIV-positive women, the rate of infectious complications was not increased compared to 493 HIV-negative women.[27]

IUDs are, based on such data, classified as category 2 contraceptive devices for HIV-positive women receiving antiviral therapy. This indicates that the benefit exceeds the risk associated with use of IUDs.[24] The reduced effectiveness of the IUD among transplant patients is based on failures in two kidney transplant patients and on the theoretical basis that immunosuppression reduces the local inflammatory response.[26] This local inflammatory reaction determines the effectiveness of an IUD. The most important inflammatory cells responsible for the action of IUDs are presumably macrophages.[28] Most immunosuppressive drugs inhibit T-cell activation and their effect on macrophages is limited. On the other hand, drug interactions are obviously only of minor importance, and therefore it has recently been suggested that IUDs maybe the "perfect" option for transplant recipients.[23]

Hormonal contraception

A variety of hormonal contraceptives administered in different ways are currently available to OLT recipients with a 1-year failure rate of between 3 and 8%.[24]

Combined oral or transdermal contraceptives

The most commonly prescribed type of contraceptives are the combined oral contraceptives (COCs). The same contraindications as in the general population have to be respected in patients who underwent a solid-organ transplantation such as those with a personal history of myocardial infarction, stroke or deep vein thrombosis, smokers over the age of 35 (smoking >15 cigarettes/d), and who have migraine with focal aura, uncontrolled systemic hypertension, marked unexplained liver test abnormalities, and hepatic adenoma.[24] In addition, drug interactions are at least a theoretical concern, since COCs are metabolized by the hepatic cytochrome P450 3A4 (Cyp3A4) system.

Because cyclosporine and TAC are also metabolized by Cyp34, their serum concentration could be increased by the concurrent administration of COCs. Although of theoretical interest, these interactions are in clinical practice of minor importance. Surprisingly, the efficacy and safety of COCs has been investigated in only a few female liver transplant recipients. In one study of 15 female liver graft recipients who used hormonal contraceptives after transplantation for at least 12 months, it could be shown that COCs were effective, well tolerated, and had no impact on graft function.[29] Finally, COCs might increase the risk for cervical cancer, while at the same time they reduce the risk for endometrial and ovarian cancer.[25]

It has recently been recommended that COCs should only be used in recipients with stable graft function for at least 6–8 months and without any other contraindications for starting therapy.[30] It addition, liver value should be carefully monitored. Even less data are available for the vaginal ring and the transdermal contraceptive patch. One potential advantage of the vaginal ring could be the lack of a first-pass effect.

Progesterone-only contraceptives

For women with contraindications to estrogens the progestin-only method of contraception is a reasonable alternative. These agents can be delivered as an intramuscular injection, as an implantable device, or orally. The effect on the liver and drug interactions are minimal with progestins. As a synthetic progestin, depot medroxyprogesterone acetate (DMPA) is delivered as an injection every 3 months. Its effectiveness is high with failure rates of around 2%.[24] The most common side effects are irregular menstrual bleeding, weight gain, and decreased bone mineral density. These latter two are especially important for OLT patients, who already have to deal with weight gain post transplant and in addition they also have a high likelihood for pre-existing osteoporosis in the context of cirrhosis and end-stage chronic liver disease. An alternative to DMPA is a subcutaneous etonogestrel implant. It provides protection for up to 3 years. The side-effect profile is similar to DMPA except that the risk for reduced bone mineral density is significantly less.

Surgical sterilization

Surgical sterilization was the contraceptive method of choice in 60% of adult renal and 24% of liver transplant recipients.[14,31] Drug interactions can be avoided with surgical sterilization and in addition it is very effective in preventing unwanted conception. This method, although very effective, may not be a viable option for women who might wish to consider pregnancy in the future.

After liver transplantation, female patients need an effective, safe, and reversible contraceptive method to avoid unwanted pregnancy. Efficacy and limitations of the current contraceptive methods are summarized in Table 37.1. Today, the method of choice appears to be the IUD, however this consensus opinion is mostly derived from the nontransplant literature rather than firm data obtained in transplant patients.[23]

Table 37.1 Contraceptive methods available after liver transplantation

Method	Effectiveness	Drug interactions	Reversibility
IUD	++	–	++
COC	++	+	++
Progestin-only pill	++	(–)	++
DMPA	++	(–)	++
Barrier method	+	–	++
Surgical sterilization	+++	–	–

COC: combined oral contraceptive, DMPA: depot medroxyprogesterone acetate, IUD: intrauterine device

Pregnancy after liver transplantation

In 1978 the first successful pregnancy after OLT was reported, which led to an excellent fetal outcome despite low birth weight.[32] The fetal problems most commonly observed are fetal loss, prematurity (defined as birth occurring prior to 37 weeks' gestation) and low birth weight (<2500 g), while the risk for the mother includes systemic hypertension/pre-eclampsia, gestational diabetes, graft dysfunction and, in rare instances, maternal death. The best source of information regarding pregnancy outcomes is obtained from national registries, which have been established to record fetal and maternal outcomes following organ transplantation of any type. One of the largest reports on pregnancy outcome in patients after liver transplantation was reported by the National Transplantation Pregnancy Register (NTPR)[32] (see Table 37.2).

Maternal risks

A recent case–control study showed maternal risks to be systemic hypertension (30%) and/or pre-eclampsia (17%), both of which occur at far higher frequency than in the general population (9% and 4%, respectively).[33] Potential factors contributing to these complications are calcineurin inhibitor therapy, chronic corticosteroid use and underlying renal dysfunction. The risk of systemic hypertension, renal dysfunction and pre-eclampsia seems to be highest in patients treated with cyclosporine, followed by TAC and corticosteroids.[34] In the most recent NTPR report, rejection was reported in 2–8% of recipients and graft loss within 2 years of delivery between 6 and 10% (Table 37.2).[32] Graft dysfunction responds either to an increase of the baseline immunosuppression and rarely requires additional therapy with pulse dose methylprednisolone. On the other hand graft

Table 37.2 National Transplantation Pregnancy Registry (NTPR) Report 2009: Fetal and maternal outcomes in liver transplant recipients according to main immunosuppression[32]

Maternal factors	Cyclosporine	Cyclosporine neural	Tacrolimus
n	96	44	98
Mean transplant to conception interval	3.7 ± 2.96	8.5 ± 4.2	5.2 ± 4.5
Hypertension during pregnancy (%)	39	44	25
Diabetes during pregnancy (%)	2	0	14
Pre-eclampsia (%)	25	29	23
Rejection (%)	8	2	5
Graft loss within 2 years of delivery (%)	10	8	6
Outcome			
n	97	44	99
Therapeutic abortions (%)	10	0	0
Spontaneous abortions (%)	13	16	27
Stillborn (%)	3	0	2
Livebirths (%)	73	82	71
Livebirths			
n	71	36	70
Mean gestational age (weeks)	36.5 ± 3.8	37.4 ± 2.6	36 ± 3.6
Premature (<37 weeks) (%)	37	28	49
Low birth weight (%)	34	41	33
Cesarean section (%)	43	25	47

dysfunction is associated with increased rates of miscarriage and lower birth weights. Available evidence suggests that, overall, episodes of rejection do not occur with any greater frequency than in nonpregnant women and that liver biopsy is safe in pregnancy.[34,35]

Fetal risk

In the most recent NTPR registry report, the time interval between liver transplantation and conception varied between 3.7 and 8.5 years and the mean gestation age was around 37 weeks. Low birth weight (<2500 g) was a factor in 33–41% of newborns, which is considerably higher than in the general population. The risk of spontaneous abortion and stillbirth were between 13 and 27% and 2 and 3%, respectively.[32] In a case–control study, it was reported that the specific fetal complications that occurred significantly more frequently in liver transplant recipients were prematurity (27 vs 11%; $P < 0.0001$), fetal distress (10 vs 5%; $P = 0.0005$) and growth restrictions (4.8 vs 2.2%, $P = 0.05$).[33]

It was suggested that the interval between transplantation and conception was shorter in those who suffered abortions or miscarriages (mean 24.4 ± 24.3 months vs 47.8 ± 28.7 months; $P = 0.02$).[35] These data were supported by a recent analysis from the NTPR, which also suggested better outcomes for mothers and newborns with a transplant-to-conception interval greater than 2 years.[32] Based on these data it was concluded that pregnancy should be delayed for up to 2 years post OLT.

Mode of delivery

In a recently published population-based study, the rate of cesarean section (CS) in liver transplant recipients was significantly higher (38 vs 24%; $P = 0.0001$) compared to that in the normal population.[33] Case series and registries report a similar CS rate ranging from 32 to 63% (see Ref. [33]). Many authors report that the majority of CSs are performed for standard obstetric indications.

As shown earlier, the rate of CS is variable and may relate to differing experience in OLT and subsequent experience in managing pregnancy post OLT. A learning curve may therefore exist as evidenced by a reduction of CS rates over time in one series,[34] however this was not confirmed in the recent population-based study.[33] In addition, there is no evidence that this form of delivery reduces the risk of disease transmission to the fetus.

Effect of immunosuppression on fetal outcomes

In utero effects of immunosuppression

The necessity of continued immunosuppressive drug therapy during pregnancy and the teratogenic potential of these drugs has been a major concern, however the commonly used immunosuppressive agents seem to have a low risk of teratogenicity and fetal loss. Evidence has largely been gathered from experimental studies in animals or relatively small case series, therefore these data have significant limitations in their ability to accurately predict outcomes. In both Europe and the USA, the most commonly used immunosuppressive drugs used post OLT are TAC, cyclosporine A (CyA), prednisolone and mycophenolate mofetil (MMF). The safety of these drugs in pregnant women has been rated by the US Food and Drug Administration (FDA) based on the available evidence and are presented in Table 37.3 and Box 37.1.

CyA

It is still controversial how efficiently CyA is transferred through the placenta. Some reports find no significant placental levels whereas others demonstrate levels equivalent to those observed in maternal blood.[36,37] Its teratogenic potential however seems to be low. Premature labor, low birth weight, transient

Table 37.3 Pregnancy categories of commonly used immunosuppressive drugs (according to Ref. [32])

Drug	Pregnancy category
Corticosteroids	B
Azathioprine	D
Cyclosporine	C
Tacrolimus	C
Mycophenolate mofetil	D
Enteric coated mycophenolate sodium	D
Sirolimus	C

Box 37.1 United States of America Food and Drug Administration categories of the safety of drugs in pregnancy

A. Controlled studies show no risk:
Adequate and well-controlled studies have failed to demonstrate a risk to the fetus in the first trimester of pregnancy (and there is no evidence of risk in later trimesters)

B. No evidence of risk in humans:
Animal reproduction studies have failed to demonstrate a risk to the fetus and there are no adequate and well-controlled studies in pregnant women

C. Risk cannot be ruled out:
Animal reproduction studies have shown an adverse effect on the fetus and there are no adequate and well-controlled studies in humans, but potential benefits may warrant use of the drug in pregnant women despite potential risks

D. Positive evidence of risk:
Investigational or post-marketing data show risk to fetus. Nevertheless, potential benefits may outweigh the risk

X. Contraindicated in pregnancy:
Studies in animals or humans have demonstrated fetal abnormalities and/or there is positive evidence of human fetal risk based on adverse reaction data from investigational or marketing experience, and the risks involved in use of the drug in pregnant women clearly outweigh potential benefits

neonatal hyperkalemia and elevated serum creatinine concentrations have been reported.[38–41]

CyA is considered a class C drug in terms of its risk to pregnancy by the US FDA. According to a meta-analysis of 15 studies of women who received CyA during pregnancy, major malformations were reported in 4.1% of live births, a rate not significantly different compared to the general population.[38] Compared to immunosuppression with azathioprine and prednisone, CyA-treated kidney transplant recipients experienced fewer complications with no congenital malformations noted, although CyA-treated patients were more likely to have diabetes and systemic hypertension, and the child was more likely to have a low birth weight.[42]

Azathioprine
Azathioprine is considered relatively safe during pregnancy in both nontransplant and transplant populations,[14,38,42] although it is considered a class D drug by the FDA based on reports of congenital malformation present in some exposed infants.

TAC
As for CyA, TAC is considered a class C drug in terms of its risk in pregnancy by the FDA. After TAC became the mainstay of immunosuppression post OLT, more and more data on its safety in pregnancy emerged. In 37 pregnant women on TAC after liver transplantation, preterm delivery and low birth weight rates were found to be comparable to those of patients on other immunosuppressive drugs.[43] Among 100 pregnancies in 84 women treated with TAC, 68 pregnancies progressed to live birth and 60% of these live births were premature.[44] The neonatal malformation rate was 4% – similar to the rate associated with CyA.[38]

Corticosteroids
Prednisone is considered a class B drug in terms of its risk to pregnancy by the FDA. Only small quantities of prednisone and prednisolone appear in fetal cord blood, although both cross the placenta.[45] A systematic review of studies of women who took corticosteroids during pregnancy for nontransplant-related conditions demonstrated a 3.4fold increased risk of cleft palate.[46] Other fetal risks associated with its use are premature rupture of the membranes and intrauterine growth retardation.[47]

MMF
Two newer immunosuppressive agents have gained increasing popularity either as replacement of azathioprine or as alternatives for calcineurin inhibitors: MMF is classified by the FDA as a class D drug and sirolimus (SRL) as a class C drug in terms of risk in pregnancy. Pregnant rats and rabbits treated with MMF exhibit intrauterine death and malformations such as anophthalmia, agnathia, hydroencephaly, and diaphragmatic hernia.[48] In a large report of the NTPR, 18 kidney recipients reported 26 pregnancies with exposure to MMF.[49] There were 15 live births, and 11 spontaneous abortions. In four of the 15 children (26.7%) structural malformations were reported including hypoplastic nails and shortened fifth fingers,

microtia with cleft lip and palate, microtia alone, and in one case neonatal death with multiple malformations.[49] In another report of 119 human pregnancies with maternal exposure to MMF, outcome data was available for 65 women. The live birth rate was only 34% with a miscarriage rate of 31% and elective abortion rate of 20%.[40] In the earlier mentioned registry analysis, the reported malformation rate was 26.7%, which is considerably higher than that previously reported with a structural malformation rate of 4–5%.[49]

SRL

SRL exposure during pregnancy was reported in seven recipients (four kidney, one kidney/pancreas and two liver) reporting four live births (one infant whose mother was switched from MMF to SRL during late pregnancy had a cleft lip and palate and microtia) and three spontaneous abortions.[49] In addition, in a recent publication it was shown that immunosuppression with SRL is associated with impaired spermatogensis and reduced male fertility.[50]

In summary, it is considered safe in pregnant women to continue immunosuppression with calcineurin inhibitors (TAC or cyclosporine neoral), azathioprine and prednisone, whereas it is recommended to discontinue MMF and SRL.

Breast feeding

Most transplant physicians advise against breastfeeding due to concerns over the safety of neonatal exposure to immunosuppressants, although this is still an area of much uncertainty. Whereas corticosteroids, CyA and TAC are all known to be excreted in breast milk, no data exists for SRL and MMF.[43,51] Corticosteroids, however, are excreted in extremely low concentrations and are felt to be safe during breast feeding.[52] A wide variation of cyclosporine concentration in the breast milk has been reported, ranging from 16 μg/L to over 1000 μg/L breast milk. Even with these high concentrations in breast milk, however, they seem to be clinically unimportant, because they must exceed 2000 μg/L to reach even 10 percent of the therapeutic dose in infants, unless the clearance rate is substantially lower in infants.[51,52] On the basis of such findings some authors suggest that women who are taking cyclosporine may be allowed to breast feed their infants.[53] Less data are available regarding TAC and breastfeeding. In some studies the concentration of TAC in the breast milk was reported to range between 0.6 and 1.8 μg/L[43,54] and it was suggested that only 0.5% of the maternal dose was ingested by the newborn.[54]

In the latest publication of the NTPR database, there were no specific problems reported related to breast feeding of the children and it was concluded that due to the relatively small amount of drug reaching the breast-fed child and due to the lack of reported adverse effects, the documented benefits of breastfeeding might actually outweigh the theoretical risk of this exposure.[32]

Male recipient

According to the latest NTPR report, there are 61 recipients of a liver graft, who fathered 90 pregnancies.[32] The outcome of these pregnancies regarding percentages of live births, mean gestational age and mean birth weight is not different from that of the general population.

References

1. Guechot J, Chazouilleres O, Loria A, et al. Effect of liver transplantation on sex-hormone disorders in male patients with alcohol-induced or post-viral hepatitis advanced liver disease. J Hepatol 1994;20:426–30.
2. Madersbacher S, Ludvik G, Stulnig T, Grunberger T, Maier U. The impact of liver transplantation on endocrine status in men. Clin Endocrinol (Oxf) 1996;44:461–6.
3. van Thiel DH, Gavaler JS, Spero JA, et al. Patterns of hypothalamic–pituitary–gonadal dysfunction in men with liver disease due to differing etiologies. Hepatology 1981;1:39–46.
4. Van Thiel DH, Kumar S, Gavaler JS, Tarter RE. Effect of liver transplantation on the hypothalamic–pituitary–gonadal axis of chronic alcoholic men with advanced liver Disease. Alcoholism: Clinical and Experimental Research 1990;14:478–81.
5. Mass K, Quint EH, Punch MR, Merion RM. Gynecological and reproductive function after liver transplantation. Transplantation 1996;62:476–9.
6. Gomez-Lobo V, Burgansky A, Kim-Schluger L, Berkowitz R. Gynecologic symptoms and sexual

function before and after liver transplantation. J Reprod Med 2006;51:457–62.
7. Sorrell JH, Brown JR. Sexual functioning in patients with end-stage liver disease before and after transplantation. Liver Transplantation 2006;12:1473–7.
8. Stremmel W, Niederau C, Berger M, Kley HK, Krüuskemper HL, Strohmeyer G. Abnormalities in estrogen, androgen, and insulin metabolism in idiopathic hemochromatosisa. Ann NY Acad Sci 1988;526:209–23.
9. Adeniyi AF, Adeleye JO, Adeniyi CY. Diabetes, sexual dysfunction and therapeutic exercise: a 20 year review. Curr Diabetes Rev 2010;6:201–6.
10. McDougall AJ, Davies L, McCaughan GW. Autonomic and peripheral neuropathy in endstage liver disease and following liver transplantation. Muscle Nerve 2003;28:595–600.
11. Manolis A, Doumas M. Sexual dysfunction: the "prima ballerina" of hypertension-related quality-of-life complications. J Hypertens 2008;26:2074–84.
12. Burra P, Germani G, Masier A, et al. Sexual dysfunction in chronic liver disease: is liver transplantation an effective cure? Transplantation 2010;89:1425–9.
13. Parolin MB, Rabinovitch I, Urbanetz AA, Scheidemantel C, Cat ML, Coelho JC. Impact of successful liver transplantation on reproductive function and sexuality in women with advanced liver disease. Transplant Proc 2004;36:943–4.
14. Cundy TF, O'Grady JG, Williams R. Recovery of menstruation and pregnancy after liver transplantation. Gut 1990;31:337–8.
15. Bravata DM, Olkin I, Barnato AE, Keeffe EB, Owens DK. Health-related quality of life after liver transplantation: A meta-analysis. Liver Transpl 1999;5: 318–31.
16. Blanch J, Sureda B, Flaviá M, et al. Psychosocial adjustment to orthotopic liver transplantation in 266 recipients. Liver Transpl 2004;10:228–34.
17. Ho JK, Ko HH, Schaeffer DF, et al. Sexual health after orthotopic liver transplantation. Liver Transpl 2006;12:1478–84.
18. Barry JM. Treating erectile dysfunction in renal transplant recipients. Drugs 2007;67:975–83.
19. Jabiry-Zieniewicz Z, Bobrowska K, Pietrzak B, et al. Mode of delivery in women after liver transplantation. Transplantation Proc [doi: DOI: 10.1016/j.transproceed.2007.09.011]. 2007;39:2796–9.
20. Lessan-Pezeshki M, Ghazizadeh S, Khatami MR, et al. Fertility and contraceptive issues after kidney transplantation in women. Transplantation Proc [doi: DOI: 10.1016/j.transproceed.2004.04.090].2004;36:1405–6.
21. Mattix Kramer H. Reproductive and contraceptive characteristics of premenopausal kidney transplant reipients. Prog Transplant 2003;13:193–6.
22. Fihn SD, Latham RH, Roberts P, Running K, Stamm WE. Association between diaphragm use and urinary tract infection. JAMA 1985;254:240–5.
23. Estes CM, Westhoff C. Contraception for the transplant patient. Semin Perinatol 2007;31:372–7.
24. WHO medical eligibility for contraceptive use. 3rd edn. Geneva, Switzerland 2004.
25. Watnick S, Rueda J. Reproduction and contraception after kidney transplantation. Curr Opin Obstet Gynecol 2008;20:308–12.
26. Zerner J, Doil KL, Drewry J, Leeber DA. Intrauterine contraceptive device failures in renal transplant patients. J Reprod Med 1981;26:99–102.
27. Morrison CS, Sekadde-Kigondu C, Sinei SK, Weiner DH, Kwok C, Kokonya D. Is the intrauterine device appropriate contraception for HIV-1-infected women? Br J Obstet Gynaecol 2001;108:784–90.
28. Ortiz ME, Croxatto HB. Copper-T intrauterine device and levonorgestrel intrauterine system: biological bases of their mechanism of action. Contraception 2007;75(Suppl 6):S16–30.
29. Jabiry-Zieniewicz Z, Bobrowska K, Kaminski P, Wielgos M, Zieniewicz K, Krawczyk M. Low-dose hormonal contraception after liver transplantation. Transplant Proc 2007;39:1530–2.
30. Sucato GS, Murray PJ. Gynecologic health care for the adolescent solid organ transplant recipient. Pediatric Transplantation 2005;9:346–56.
31. O'Donnell D. Contraception in the female transplant recipient. Dial Transplant 1986;15:610–12.
32. Coscia LA, Constantinescu S, Moritz MJ, et al. Report from the National Transplantation Pregnancy Registry (NTPR): outcomes of pregnancy after transplantation. Clin Transpl 2009:103–22.
33. Coffin CS, Shaheen AAM, Burak KW, Myers RP. Pregnancy outcomes among liver transplant recipients in the United States: A nationwide case–control analysis. Liver Transplantation 2010;16:56–63.
34. Christopher V, Al-Chalabi T, Richardson PD, et al. Pregnancy outcome after liver transplantation: A single-center experience of 71 pregnancies in 45 recipients. Liver Transplantation 2006;12:1138–43.
35. Nagy S, Bush MC, Berkowitz R, Fishbein TM, Gomez-Lobo V. Pregnancy outcome in liver transplant recipients. Obstet Gynecol 2003;102:121–8.
36. Nandakumaran M, Eldeen AS. Transfer of cyclosporine in the perfused human placenta. Dev Pharmacol Ther 1990;15:101–5.
37. Walcott WO, Derick DE, Jolley JJ, Snyder DL. Successful pregnancy in a liver transplant patient. Am J Obstet Gynecol 1978;132:340–1.
38. Bar Oz B, Hackman R, Einarson T, Koren G. Pregnancy outcome after cyclosporine therapy during pregnancy: a meta-analysis. Transplantation 2001;71:1051–5.

39. Cockburn I, Krupp P, Monka C. Present experience of Sandimmun in pregnancy. Transplant Proc 1989;21: 3730–2.
40. Ostensen M, Khamashta M, Lockshin M, et al. Anti-inflammatory and immunosuppressive drugs and reproduction. Arth Res Ther 2006;8:209.
41. Venkataramanan R, Koneru B, Wang CC, Burckart GJ, Caritis SN, Starzl TE. Cyclosporine and its metabolites in mother and baby. Transplantation 1988;46:468–9.
42. Armenti VT, Ahlswede KM, Ahlswede BA, Jarrell BE, Moritz MJ, Burke JF. National Transplantation Pregnancy Registry – outcomes of 154 pregnancies in cyclosporine-treated female kidney transplant recipients. Transplantation 1994;57:502–6.
43. Jain AB, Reyes J, Marcos A, et al. Pregnancy after liver transplantation with tacrolimus immunosuppression: a single center's experience update at 13 years. Transplantation 2003;76:827–32.
44. Kainz A, Harabacz I, Cowlrick IS, Gadgil SD, Hagiwara D. Review of the course and outcome of 100 pregnancies in 84 women treated with tacrolimus. Transplantation 2000;70:1718–21.
45. Beitins IZ, Bayard F, Ances IG, Kowarski A, Migeon CJ. The transplacental passage of prednisone and prednisolone in pregnancy near term. J Pediatr 1972;81:936–45.
46. Park-Wyllie L, Mazzotta P, Pastuszak A, et al. Birth defects after maternal exposure to corticosteroids: Prospective cohort study and meta-analysis of epidemiological studies. Teratology 2000;62:385–92.
47. Lockshin MD, Sammaritano LR. Corticosteroids during pregnancy. Scand J Rheumatol Suppl 1998;107:136–8.
48. Mastrobattista JM, Katz AR. Pregnancy after organ transplant. Obstetrics and Gynecology Clinics of North America. [doi: DOI: 10.1016/j.ogc.2004.03.005]. 2004;31:415–28.
49. Sifontis NM, Coscia LA, Constantinescu S, Lavelanet AF, Moritz MJ, Armenti VT. Pregnancy outcomes in solid organ transplant recipients with exposure to mycophenolate mofetil or sirolimus. Transplantation 2006;82:1698–702.
50. Zuber J, Anglicheau D, Elie C, et al. Sirolimus may reduce fertility in male renal transplant recipients. Am J Transplant 2008;8:1471–9.
51. Moretti ME, Sgro M, Johnson DW, et al. Cyclosporine excretion into breast milk. Transplantation 2003;75: 2144–6.
52. Ito S. Drug therapy for breast-feeding women. N Engl J Med 2000;343:118–26.
53. Nyberg G, Haljamae U, Frisenette-Fich C, Wennergren M, Kjellmer I. Breast-feeding during treatment with cyclosporine. Transplantation 1998;65:253–5.
54. Gardiner SJ, Begg EJ. Breastfeeding during tacrolimus therapy. Obstet Gynecol 2006;107(Pt2):453–5.

PART FOUR

Pediatric Liver Transplantation

38 Special considerations in pediatric liver transplantation

Brandy Ries Lu[1] *and Ronald J. Sokol*[2]

[1]Sutter Pacific Medical Foundation, California Pacific Medical Center, Pediatric Gastroenterology and Hepatology, San Francisco, CA, USA; and [2]Colorado Clinical and Translational Sciences Institute, University of Colorado School of Medicine and The Children's Hospital, Aurora, CO, USA

Key learning points

- Biliary atresia is a neonatal inflammatory condition affecting intra- and extrahepatic ducts and is the most common indication for pediatric liver transplantation. It has excellent outcomes after liver transplantation, and does not recur following transplantation.
- Pediatric acute liver failure is defined based on degree of coagulopathy and hepatic encephalopathy is not required. A thorough investigation for etiology of liver failure should be undertaken.
- It is important to be aware of the technical variant grafts (reduced, split, left lateral segment) and challenging biliary and vascular anastomoses used in pediatric liver transplantation.
- Careful monitoring for Epstein–Barr virus (EBV) infection or reactivation is important after liver transplantation in order to anticipate and prevent the development of post-transplant lymphoproliferative disorder (PTLD).
- Minimizing immunosuppression in order to avoid infection, toxicity of calcineurin inhibitors, and risk for PTLD is an important concept for long-term management of pediatric liver transplant recipients.

Disease indications for liver transplantation in pediatrics

Table 38.1 shows the indications for liver transplantation in pediatrics.[1] Biliary atresia, the most common indication, is a fibro-inflammatory condition affecting neonates, in which both the intra- and extrahepatic bile ducts are injured, leading to obstruction of part of the entire extrahepatic biliary tree. The incidence varies based on geography, from approximately 1:8–10 000 in Asia[2] to 1:18 000 in Europe. There are two major forms of biliary atresia: a fetal–embryonal or congenital form (approximately 20% of cases) and an acquired or perinatal form (80% of cases). Infants with the embryonal form are often jaundiced at birth and have other congenital malformations, such as cardiovascular defects, polysplenia or asplenia, abdominal situs inversus, and intestinal malrotation. Infants with the perinatal form are often thriving term babies who develop acholic stools by 2–4 weeks of age along with direct hyperbilirubinemia and hepatosplenomegaly. Diagnosis is suggested by liver biopsy, which demonstrates bile duct proliferation (bile ductular reaction), portal tract bile duct plugging, cholestasis, and portal tract inflammation and fibrosis. Diagnosis is confirmed by exploratory laparotomy and intraoperative cholangiogram, which will show complete obstruction in the extrahepatic bile duct. The pathogenesis of the two types of biliary atresia is under investigation, but given the diversity of the two presentations, likely involves different mechanisms. The natural history of biliary atresia in the absence

Medical Care of the Liver Transplant Patient, Fourth Edition. Edited by Pierre-Alain Clavien, James F. Trotter.

Table 38.1 Indications for pediatric liver transplantation from 1995 to 2005

Primary diagnosis	No. (n = 3161)	Percentage
Cholestatic	**1685**	**53.3**
Biliary atresia	1245	39.4
Primary sclerosing cholangitis	104	3.3
Alagille syndrome	84	2.7
TPN-induced cholestasis	65	2.1
Idiopathic	44	1.4
Progressive familial intrahepatic cholestasis	42	1.3
Neonatal hepatitis	39	1.2
Other	62	1.9
Metabolic	**458**	**14.5**
Alpha-1-antitrypsin deficiency	93	2.9
Urea cycle defects	68	2.2
Cystic fibrosis	59	1.9
Wilson disease	34	1.1
Tyrosinemia	32	1.0
Primary hyperoxaluria	24	0.8
Neonatal hemochromatosis	23	0.7
Other	125	3.9
Cirrhosis	**256**	**8.1**
Autoimmune hepatitis	111	3.5
Unknown cause	80	2.5
Hepatitis C	20	0.6
Other	45	1.5
Acute liver failure	**423**	**13.4**
Unknown cause/indeterminate	307	9.7
Autoimmune hepatitis	58	1.8
Acute on chronic liver disease	18	0.6
Acute hepatitis A/B/C	13	0.4
Other	27	0.9
Tumor	**172**	**5.4**
Hepatoblastoma	115	3.6
Hemangioendothelioma	24	0.8
Hepatocellular carcinoma	20	0.6
Other	13	0.4
Drug effect	**29**	**0.9**
Other	**138**	**4.4**

Derived from the Studies of Pediatric Liver Transplantation 2006 Annual Report[1] and reproduced with permission

of surgical treatment is the development of biliary cirrhosis within months and death from liver failure by 2 years of age.

A Kasai hepatoportoenterostomy is the surgical treatment that attempts to establish bile flow by anastomosing a Roux-en-Y loop of small bowel to the dissected porta hepatis. The results of the procedure are best if performed before 45 d of life and even if drainage is achieved, progression to cirrhosis may still occur. Half of these patients undergo liver transplantation within the first 1–2 years of life and 80% during childhood.[3] Close attention to nutritional status, fat-soluble vitamin supplementation and monitoring for complications of portal hypertension are also important components of medical management. Despite the lack of a cure in the majority of patients, a successful Kasai hepatoportoenterostomy will generally allow a young child to grow and develop normally and be better prepared for liver transplantation when needed.

Other cholestatic pediatric diseases that are indications for transplantation include Alagille syndrome (AGS), primary sclerosing cholangitis, total parenteral nutrition associated cholestasis, and progressive familial intrahepatic cholestasis (PFIC). AGS is an autosomal dominant disorder caused by a variety of mutations in the *JAGGED1* gene, which is a ligand in the Notch signaling pathway that controls the development of many organs. Clinical features include chronic cholestasis due to the paucity of interlobular bile ducts, peripheral pulmonary branch artery stenosis, butterfly vertebrae, posterior embryotoxon in the eyes, characteristic facies, and renal lesions. In infancy, AGS can mimic the clinical presentation of biliary atresia, so a careful clinical examination for extrahepatic features of AGS is important, particularly before initiating invasive procedures such as exploratory laparotomy. Severity of liver disease can be variable, with most patients not developing significant portal fibrosis or portal hypertension.

Approximately 50% of patients who present in infancy will not survive into adulthood without liver transplantation or because of complications of cardiovascular lesions or intracranial vascular abnormalities.[4] Often serum cholesterol is very elevated and leads to the development of xanthomas. Pruritus can be debilitating and can be an indication for liver transplantation, as can metabolic bone disease. Primary sclerosing cholangitis is a chronic inflammatory disorder that leads to strictures and obliteration of the intra- and extrahepatic bile ducts, progressing to biliary cirrhosis with repeated episodes of bacterial cholangitis. Half of pediatric cases of primary sclerosing cholangitis are associated with inflammatory bowel disease, 27% with another disease, and 24% are idiopathic.[5] Diagnosis is confirmed with a combination of liver biopsy and cholangiography (either endoscopic or magnetic resonance). Treatment is supportive and progression to liver transplantation occurs approximately 40% of the time.[5] Total parenteral nutrition has been life saving in small children with intestinal failure. A known complication is the development of liver disease, manifested by progressive cholestasis, hepatomegaly and eventually cirrhosis, which is unique to the pediatric population. If total parenteral nutrition cannot be stopped and liver disease progresses to cirrhosis, liver transplantation (and frequently intestinal transplantation) will be required.

PFIC is in the umbrella group of autosomal recessive inherited disorders of transport proteins that share clinical features, three of which have the genetic etiology identified: PFIC1 (FIC1 disease) and PFIC 2 (BSEP disease) have low gamma-glutamyl transpeptidase (GGTP) and PFIC3 has high GGTP (MDR3 disease). Response to ursodeoxycholic acid is variable and some patients respond to partial biliary diversion. Progression of liver disease to cirrhosis, intractable pruritus or the development of hepatocellular carcinoma may require liver transplantation.

Many pediatric patients undergo liver transplantation as treatment for genetic metabolic liver diseases, including alpha-1-antitrypsin deficiency, urea cycle defects, tyrosinemia, cystic fibrosis, Wilson disease and neonatal hemochromatosis. Alpha-1-antitrypsin deficiency results from homozygous mutations in the alpha-1-antitrypsin gene and has variable presentation in children. It is one of the most common inherited diseases (one in 2500 Europeans), with only 10–20% of affected children developing liver disease, of which 20–30% will require liver transplantation.[6]

Screening is based on the PI phenotype, with the MM phenotype considered normal. Variable enzyme activity, from 40–80%, exists with phenotypes SZ, MZ, SS, and MS, while the ZZ phenotype is considered the most severe. Liver disease develops only in the PISZ and PIZZ individuals. Urea cycle defects usually present in the neonatal period with episodes of lethargy and severe hyperammonemia. Ammonia is normally detoxified to urea in the liver and enzyme defects in carbamoyl phosphate synthase I (CPS1), N-acetylglutamate synthase (NAGS), ornithine transcarbamylase (OTC), argininosuccinate synthase (ASS), or argininosuccinate lyase (ASL) cause urea cycle defects. All urea cycle defects are autosomal recessive, except for OTC deficiency, which is X-linked and explains OTC's severe presentation in males but variable presentation in females. Infants can become neurologically devastated after just one episode of prolonged hyperammonemia.

Treatment of acute episodes includes dialysis, reducing protein intake, and IV or enteral ammonia scavengers. Liver transplantation is the only effective therapy to prevent life-threatening episodes of hyperammonemia in severely affected OTC-, CPS- and NAGS-deficient patients. Hereditary tyrosinemia type I is an autosomal recessive disease, common in northern Europe and Quebec, Canada, in which an enzyme (fumarylacetoacetate hydrolase) in the degradation of tyrosine is genetically defective. Accumulation of toxic metabolites of tyrosine leads to cirrhosis and death by a few years of age. Newborn screening for urine succinylacetone, which is not performed routinely, allows for appropriate treatment of a low phenylalanine/tyrosine diet and a medication that prevents build-up of toxic metabolites (nitisinone (NTBC)) to be started. NTBC is also started when the diagnosis is established in infancy and can prevent the need for liver transplantation. When indicated, liver transplantation will cure the underlying liver disease and genetic defect.

Approximately 10–15% of children with cystic fibrosis will develop significant liver disease. The spectrum varies from cholestasis to steatosis to focal biliary cirrhosis to multilobular cirrhosis.[7] When complications of portal hypertension are significant, liver transplantation prior to deterioration of lung function is advocated. Wilson disease is the most common metabolic cause of acute liver failure in older children and adolescents and is caused by copper deposition and toxicity to the liver. Autosomal recessive mutations in *ATP7B* cause defective biliary secretion of copper and ceruloplasmin synthesis. Clinical presentation of acute liver failure includes very prominent mixed direct/indirect hyperbilirubinemia due to a combination of liver injury and non-immune hemolysis, low alkaline phosphatase, and renal failure. Diagnosis can be confirmed by the presence of Kaiser–Fleisher rings in the eyes, low ceruloplasmin level, high 24-hour urine copper excretion, and high quantitative liver copper on biopsy. Genetic testing is available when necessary. Liver transplantation is indicated for acute liver failure or chronic liver disease with decompensation unresponsive to copper chelation or zinc therapy. Neonatal hemochromatosis presents with neonatal liver failure (hypoglycemia and coagulopathy) in the first days or weeks of life. Diagnosis is confirmed by elevated ferritin levels and demonstration of excess iron deposition in extrahepatic organs, such as pancreas or heart on MRI or salivary glands on buccal biopsy. It is now believed that the disease is caused by transplacental passage of maternal IgG that activates complement on the surface of hepatocytes. The current treatment includes exchange transfusion and IV immunoglobulin, however if this fails, liver transplantation can be life saving. Neonatal hemochromatosis does not recur after transplantation.[8]

Diseases, such as autoimmune hepatitis, primary sclerosing cholangitis, and viral hepatitis, which are common in the adult population, also affect children. Autoimmune hepatitis is diagnosed based on the presence of either anti-smooth muscle antibody (type 1) or anti-liver–kidney microsomal antibody (type 2). Children with type 2 autoimmune hepatitis often tend to be younger, male, and more likely to present with acute liver failure. Of children with autoimmune hepatitis, 10–20% eventually will need liver transplantation.[9] Hepatitis B is a rare indication for pediatric liver transplantation, but adolescents with vertically acquired hepatitis C can develop cirrhosis and require liver transplantation. As in adults, hepatitis C disease recurrence after transplantation is common and poses a major clinical challenge. Hepatoblastoma is the most common pediatric liver tumor that is amenable to liver transplantation. Chemotherapy is first used to shrink the tumor and if the tumor is still not resectable and there are no metastases that cannot be resected, liver transplantation should be offered. Hepatocellular carcinoma (HCC) has a less favorable response to chemotherapy in children. The criteria used in adults for transplantation listing for HCC are generally used in children due to a high rate of reoccurrence.

Finally many pediatric patients are transplanted for acute (previously called "fulminant") liver failure, but it is important to note that different diagnostic criteria are used for pediatric acute liver failure (PALF) when compared to adults. PALF is defined as: (1) no known evidence of chronic liver disease, (2) biochemical evidence of acute liver injury, and (3) hepatic-based coagulopathy defined as INR $\geq$1.5 not corrected by vitamin K in the presence of hepatic encephalopathy or INR ≥2.0 regardless of the presence or absence of clinical hepatic encephalopathy. The pediatric criteria do not require the presence of hepatic encephalopathy because of the difficulty in assessing this finding in young children and its inconsistent presence in infants. The etiology for 49% of PALF cases is categorized as "indeterminate", followed by acetaminophen toxicity (14%), metabolic disease (10%), autoimmune (6%), infectious (6%), drug toxicity (5%), and other (11%).[10] The diagnostic evaluation for PALF is often incomplete but should include drug history (acetaminophen level, urine toxicology screen), common metabolic diseases (older children: ceruloplasmin for Wilson disease, alpha-1-antitrypsin phenotype; younger children: urine succinylacetone for tyrosinemia, ferritin for neonatal hemochromatosis, serum amino acids, urine-reducing substances for galactosemia, acylcarnitine profile for fatty acid oxidation defects, lactate/pyruvate ratio for mitochondrial hepatopathies), infection (hepatitis A/B/C, EBV, cytomegalovirus (CMV), herpes virus in infants), and autoimmune (anti-nuclear antibody, anti-smooth muscle antibody, anti-liver kidney microsomal antibody).[11] More than 50% of PALF patients will not require liver transplantation or are not candidates.

Indications for liver transplantation

The Studies of Pediatric Liver Transplantation (SPLIT) registry was initiated in 1995 as an international, multi-center registry for children undergoing liver transplantation and has prospectively followed over 3000 children. Primary indications for liver transplantation in SPLIT are shown in Table 38.1 and include: biliary atresia (39.4%); other cholestatic diseases, such as Alagille syndrome, primary sclerosing cholangitis, total parenteral nutrition induced cholestasis, and progressive familial intrahepatic cholestasis (14%); metabolic disease, such as alpha-1-antitrypsin deficiency, urea cycle defects, tyrosinemia, cystic fibrosis, Wilson disease, and neonatal hemochromatosis (14.5%); fulminant hepatic failure (13.4%); cirrhosis (8.1%), caused by autoimmune hepatitis, idiopathic, and hepatitis C; tumor (5.4%); and other (5.2%).[1]

Evaluation and preparation for liver transplantation

Evaluation of a child for liver transplantation candidacy is a multidisciplinary process that involves pediatricians, pediatric hepatologists, transplant surgeons, anesthesiologists, nutritionists, social workers, transplant coordinators, psychologists, and hospital financial officers. Staging of liver disease involves assessing liver synthetic function (serum albumin and INR), degree of cholestasis based on direct and total bilirubin, and complications of end-stage liver disease. Liver biopsy is helpful in confirming the underlying diagnosis and assessing for cirrhosis. Complications of chronic liver disease include portal hypertension, which can manifest as splenomegaly and hypersplenism, esophageal or gastric varices, spontaneous bacterial peritonitis, hepatopulmonary syndrome, portopulmonary hypertension, and ascites. Hepatorenal syndrome rarely develops in children with cirrhosis and hepatic encephalopathy is difficult to identify in infants and young children. The child's quality of life needs to be assessed and considered in the decision about whether to proceed to liver transplantation. It is important to maximize nutrition for children awaiting transplantation and to monitor for fat-soluble vitamin deficiency in cholestatic children. Immunization schedules should be followed closely and because live-virus vaccines, such as measles, mumps, rubella (MMR) and varicella, are contraindicated after transplantation, all attempts should be made to administer live-virus vaccines pre transplantation. Owing to high levels of immunosuppression after liver transplantation and less likelihood of vaccine response, routine killed-virus vaccines are deferred for at least 3 months after transplantation. Occasionally due to surgical issues, the spleen is removed during transplantation and penicillin prophylaxis against encapsulated organisms is instituted until the child is 5 years of age. EBV and CMV serologies are checked pre-transplantation and are helpful in distinguishing between the development of primary vs reactivation of disease after transplantation, and the need for post-transplant viral prophylaxis. Hepatitis A, B, and C and HIV are also routinely screened for pre transplantation. There are few absolute contraindications to liver transplantation: 1) issues with other organ systems, such as systemic sepsis that is not adequately treated, 2) severe disease involvement of the brain, heart, and/or lungs that will not be significantly improved by liver transplantation, or that will pose risks during the transplant, and 3) metastatic liver tumors that are not responsive to chemotherapy. HIV infection in a child would be handled as it would in an adult being listed for transplantation.

Allocation of organs

Two scoring systems – the Pediatric End-stage Liver Disease (PELD) and Model for End-stage Liver Disease (MELD) – are used to prioritize patients awaiting liver transplantation in the USA. The PELD scoring system is used for children up to 12 years of age, and the MELD scoring system is used for children 12 years of age and older, and adults. The separate MELD and PELD systems were developed in 2002, when it was recognized that chronic liver disease affected children much differently than adults.[12] Often renal function, and thus creatinine is preserved in children, while growth is much more affected. The PELD score incorporates age, total bilirubin, INR, albumin, and growth parameters to calculate a score that has a similar severity range when compared to the MELD. There is no maximum PELD value and negative values are possible if liver synthetic function and growth are preserved. United Network for Organ Sharing (UNOS) oversees the distribution of donated organs in the USA and donor livers are allocated based on MELD/PELD score, and the patient's size, age, and blood type. Young children can be listed for donor size up to 10 times their weight and often the age ranges are capped at 40–50 years. Blood type ABO compatibility is a priority, however infants who are very sick (e.g. with acute liver failure) may receive ABO-incompatible organs if they have not yet developed antibodies to different blood types.[13] With ABO-incompatible transplantation in older children, ABO antibody titers are checked pre-transplantation and if positive, plasmapheresis is performed both pre and post transplantation to maintain antibody titers below 1:8. Splenectomy is also performed during transplantation at most centers. Treatment also includes high-dose IV immunoglobulin.[14] Children can be listed for Status 1A, which is the highest priority: for pediatric acute liver failure, primary graft nonfunction after liver transplantation, hepatic artery thrombosis within 7 d of liver transplantation, anhepatic, or acute liver failure from Wilson disease. Status 1B is the next priority and is reserved for children who have a MELD/PELD score of at least 25 and have one of the following: mechanical ventilation, GI bleeding requiring transfusion of at least 30 ml/kg of red blood cells in a 24-hour period, renal failure requiring dialysis, or Glasgow score <10 within 48 h of listing. Metabolic diseases, such as urea cycle defects or organic acidemias, have a special listing in that children will often have preserved liver synthetic function. In view of the high risk of neurologic complications related to their metabolic disease, children are listed with an initial PELD/MELD of 30 and upgraded to status 1B after 30 d. Special listing criteria also exist for hepatocellular carcinoma, hepatoblastoma, hepatopulmonary syndrome, portopulmonary syndrome, primary hyperoxaluria, and cystic fibrosis. Pediatric donor organs will be offered to suitable pediatric candidates in each category (Status 1A, 1B, and PELD) before being offered to the adult candidates in each category.

Surgical grafts

Owing to the wide range of ages and sizes, children may receive a variety of different liver transplant grafts. Knowledge of the type of graft received is important in order to anticipate complications that can arise with each type. Whole-organ transplantation is ideal because it preserves anatomy, however it is not always possible because of the shortage of donor organs for small children. Other variations include a reduced size liver allograft, where a liver is cut to the size needed and the rest discarded; split-liver allografts, where a liver is carefully divided and placed into two patients; and living related allografts, where a live donor will provide either their left lateral segment or rarely in pediatrics the right or left lobe of the liver, see Figure 38.1.

Vascular and bile duct anastomoses of the liver graft can differ in children compared to adults due to their small size, more use of reduced or segmental grafts, and underlying etiology of liver disease. With biliary atresia, being the most common indication for liver transplantation in children, the native recipient bile duct cannot be used; thus the bile duct

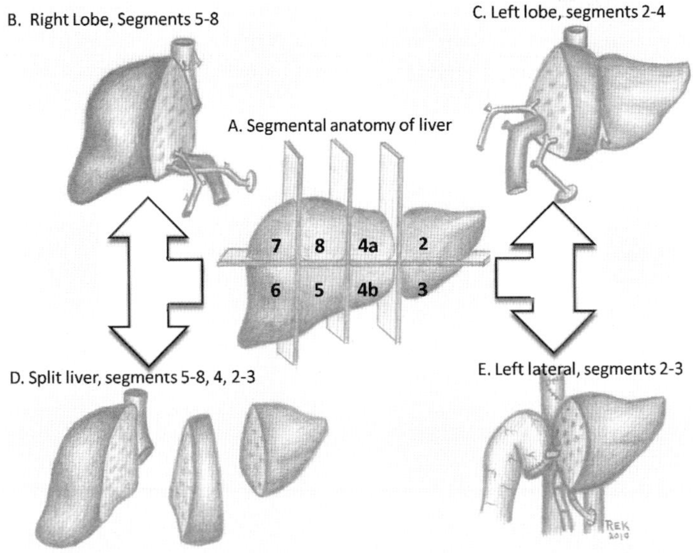

Figure 38.1 Illustrations of the different types of liver allografts used in pediatric liver transplantation. (**A**) Segmental anatomy of a whole liver. (**B**) Right hepatic lobe with segments 5–8. (**C**) Left hepatic lobe with segments 2–4. (**D**) Split liver where segments 5–8 go to one donor, segments 2–3 go to another donor, and segment 4 is discarded. (**E**) Left lateral segment with end-to-side choledochojejunostomy into a Roux-en-Y jejunal limb. Illustrations provided courtesy of Robert Kramer, MD.

reconstruction involves an end-to-side choledochojejunostomy into a Roux-en-Y jejunal limb. A bile duct anastomotic stent is often left in place for 3 months after transplantation. In infants, the hepatic artery can be very small and instead of a direct artery-to-artery anastomosis, the celiac axis of the donor liver may be implanted to the aorta. Portal vein anastomosis is usually direct between donor and recipient, however hepatic vein outflow anastomosis can vary. The most common anastomosis involves removing the recipient's retrohepatic inferior vena cava (IVC) and placing the donor's liver with intact IVC (with hepatic vein connection preserved) and sewing a suprahepatic and infrahepatic IVC anastomosis. The "piggyback" technique is often used, especially with living related or reduced-size transplantation, where it is not feasible to remove part of the donor's IVC. The recipients diseased liver is removed while preserving the native inferior vena cava. The left hepatic vein from the donor is anastomosed to the vena cava end to side. Distribution of the types of grafts used in children include: deceased whole liver (51%), reduced liver (21%), live donor liver (20%), and split liver (8%).[15]

Immunosuppression

Immunosuppression generally includes initial induction therapy on the day of transplant with high-dose (10 mg/kg/d up to 1 g) methylprednisolone intravenously for several days, dropping to 1 mg/kg/d in 3–5 d. The goal is to wean prednisone dose down quickly, with patients off of corticosteroids within 1–6 months following liver transplantation. Calcineurin inhibitors, such as cyclosporine and tacrolimus, are used in most centers for long-term suppression of allograft rejection. Most centers use tacrolimus for primary maintenance therapy (initial dose 0.1–0.15 mg/kg given every 12 h orally) because of better graft outcomes, but occasionally patients will be switched to cyclosporine because of side effects from tacrolimus.[16] Acute toxic side effects to monitor during tacrolimus therapy include hemolytic anemia, hyperkalemia, hypomagnesemia, tremors, hypertension, and headaches. Long-term side effects include nephrotoxicity, hyperglycemia, hyperlipidemia, infection, PTLD risk, and hypertension. Therapeutic levels should be followed closely, aiming for trough levels the first month after transplantation of 10–15 ng/ml, with weaning of tacrolimus to levels as low as 3–5 ng/ml 1 year post transplantation if liver function is stable and lower thereafter. If calcineurin inhibitors cannot be used immediately post transplantation, often due to underlying renal dysfunction, anti-thymocyte globulin or IL-2 receptor antagonists have been used for induction. Rapamycin (sirolimus) acts slightly differently than the calcineurin inhibitors and is considered more "renal sparing" than tacrolimus. Noted side effects include hypercholesterolemia, hypertension, and mouth sores. It is often added as a second agent after an episode of acute rejection or if there is persistent elevated EBV viremia, based on its *in vitro* suppression of EBV.[17] Mycophenolate mofetil is used as a second agent to augment immunosuppression following rejection or as a tacrolimus-sparing agent. Side effects include leucopenia, diarrhea, and abdominal pain. Careful attention should be paid to prescribing additional medicines due to interactions with the immunosuppressive medications. Cyclosporine and tacrolimus are metabolized by cytochrome P450s (CYPs). Medications that increase blood levels of immunosuppressives by inhibiting CYPs include: erythromycin/clarithromycin, amphotericin B, clotrimazole/voriconazole/fluconazole, diltiazem, verapamil, nicardipine, amlodipine, amiodarone, isoniazid, fluoxetine, oral contraceptives, cimetidine, and grapefruit. Medications that decrease immunosuppressive blood levels by inducing CYPs include: carbamazepine, phenobarbital, phenytoin, rifampin, nafcillin, and St John's wort. Frequent monitoring of tacrolimus or cyclosporine blood levels and dose adjustments are mandatory if any of these medications are begun during immunosuppression.

Complications

Complications after liver transplantation can be divided into early, often seen during the initial hospitalization after transplantation, and late, generally after patients have been discharged home. Early complications include primary nonfunction of the liver, hepatic artery or portal vein thrombosis, infection, surgical complications (such as intra-abdominal bleeding, infection, or bowel perforation), and acute cellular rejection. Primary nonfunction of the liver, with an incidence in pediatrics of 1%, manifests 12–48 h after transplantation and includes rising INR (>3), AST or ALT (>5000 IU/L), and bilirubin.[15] The only effective treatment is emergent re-transplantation. Hepatic artery thrombosis, with an incidence of 3–4%, often occurs within 7 d of transplantation and may require emergent retransplantation or may result in bile duct strictures.[15] Portal vein thrombosis does not often cause significant changes in hepatic function. A hypercoagulation work-up should be initiated, keeping in mind that the newly transplanted liver produces clotting factors, negating the usefulness of genetic tests in the evaluation. Screening with abdominal Doppler ultrasonography during the first days after transplantation is routine to detect vascular thrombosis at a time when intervention is possible. An abrupt increase in aminotransferases, bilirubin, alkaline phosphatase, GGTP, or an episode of sepsis, should trigger high suspicion for vascular compromise in the first week following transplantation. Some centers attempt to prevent hepatic artery thrombosis by maintaining hemoglobin between 8 and 10 g/L and administering dextran when the INR is <2. Prophylaxis against vascular thrombosis with oral aspirin or dipyridamole is standard for the first month after transplantation at most centers.

Serious bacterial/fungal or viral infection occurs in over half of pediatric liver transplant patients, with younger age and use of surgical variant graft associated with increased risk of developing serious infection.[18] Surgical complications include hemorrhage, particularly from the cut surface of the liver if a reduced or split graft is used, and bowel perforation due to the creation of Roux-en-Y jejunal limb with biliary reconstruction. Reduced or split-liver grafts may also have bile leaks from the cut surface, requiring drainage or surgical repair. Hyperacute rejection is rare in liver transplantation, but acute cellular rejection can occur in as soon as 7–10 d. At least one episode of cellular rejection will occur in 60% of children, which is suspected with increased AST/ALT, bilirubin, alkaline phosphatase and GGTP, and must be confirmed with liver biopsy.[15] Findings on liver biopsy include mixed portal inflammation, with occasional eosinophils, bile duct injury and endothelialitis (lymphocyte invasion under the endothelium of portal or central venules). Treatment includes IV corticosteroids and increasing immunosuppression. Early rejection, defined as within 6 months of transplantation, does not increase risk of mortality or graft failure.[18] Infants have a lower risk of rejection compared to older children, likely due to a more tolerant immune system.[18]

Late complications after liver transplantation include biliary strictures, portal vein thrombosis, chronic allograft rejection, EBV or CMV infection and PTLD. Children who undergo primary bile duct to bile duct anastomosis can develop anastomotic strictures, which may be amenable to dilation and stent placement with endoscopic retrograde cholangiopancreatography or percutaneous transhepatic cholangiography. If the problem persists or the child is too small for these interventions, conversion to choledochojejunostomy via a Roux-en-Y jejunal limb may be necessary. The hepatic artery is the sole supply of oxygen to the bile ducts and reduced flow will lead to bile duct injury, manifested by increased GGTP. Abdominal ultrasound with Doppler evaluation should always be obtained with an unexplained rise in GGTP. Acute cellular rejection can occur any time after transplant and may be clinically silent. In stable patients at least 1 year following transplant, routine laboratory evaluation (complete blood count, comprehensive metabolic panel, GGTP, immunosuppression drug levels) should be obtained every 2–3 months to monitor for biochemical signs of rejection. Chronic rejection, with an incidence of about 5%, develops after episodes of acute rejection that are not responsive to increased immunosuppression and often leads to graft loss.[15] Clinically, patients have progressive jaundice and findings on biopsy include loss of small bile ducts and a vasculopathy affecting medium and large arteries.

Up to 60% of infants and children have not been exposed to either EBV or CMV infection prior to transplantation, thus they are evaluated for EBV and CMV infection routinely post transplantation, particularly in the setting of increasing liver enzymes.[15] Most transplant centers use EBV DNA levels quantified by polymerase chain reaction (PCR) to monitor for acquisition or reactivation of infection. EBV and CMV status of the donor and recipient should be obtained to understand the risk for disease following immunosuppression. Depending on donor and recipient status, either IV ganciclovir or oral valganciclovir is used as prophylaxis for up to 6 months to 1 year post transplant. Within the first year after transplantation, 56% of EBV-negative transplant patients will convert. EBV infection is strongly associated with the development of PTLD. PTLD is a spectrum from a mononucleosis-like picture to frank lymphoma that is caused by abnormal proliferation of EBV-infected B-cells and can present in lymphoid tissue in any organ, although most commonly in the transplanted organ, lymph nodes, gastrointestinal (GI) tract, or lungs. Presentation of PTLD is variable and can include general symptoms, such as fever, weight loss, and fatigue with physical examination findings of enlarged tonsils and lymphadenopathy or it can present with a mass lesion, bowel obstruction, GI bleeding, diarrhea, respiratory symptoms or central nervous system involvement. Diagnosis is made by the histologic evidence of PTLD and EBV infection in biopsies of affected organs, such as liver, lymph nodes, or intestine. Primary EBV infection after transplantation is associated with a higher likelihood of the development of PTLD; approximately 4–6% of pediatric patients will develop PTLD within 5 years following liver transplantation.[15] Treatment entails reducing or stopping immunosuppression, addition of antivirals, and use of anti-CD20 antibody treatment or chemotherapy for nonresponders. Approximately 75% of children with PTLD will recover with appropriate therapy.

Outcomes

Children have excellent clinical outcomes after liver transplantation, likely related to the lack of recurrence of their underlying liver disease and lack of co-morbid conditions as seen in the adult population. Figure 38.2 shows that 1-year and 4-year patient survival rates are 89.8 and 85.5%, and among survivors, 1-year and 4-year graft survival rates are 84.0 and 77.3%.[1] Primary causes of death include multi-organ failure (31% of deaths), infection (28%), central nervous system complications (11%), and liver failure (11%).[19] Loss of liver allografts from rejection episodes is rare. Indications for retransplantation include hepatic artery thrombosis (32% of retransplants), chronic rejection and cholestatic

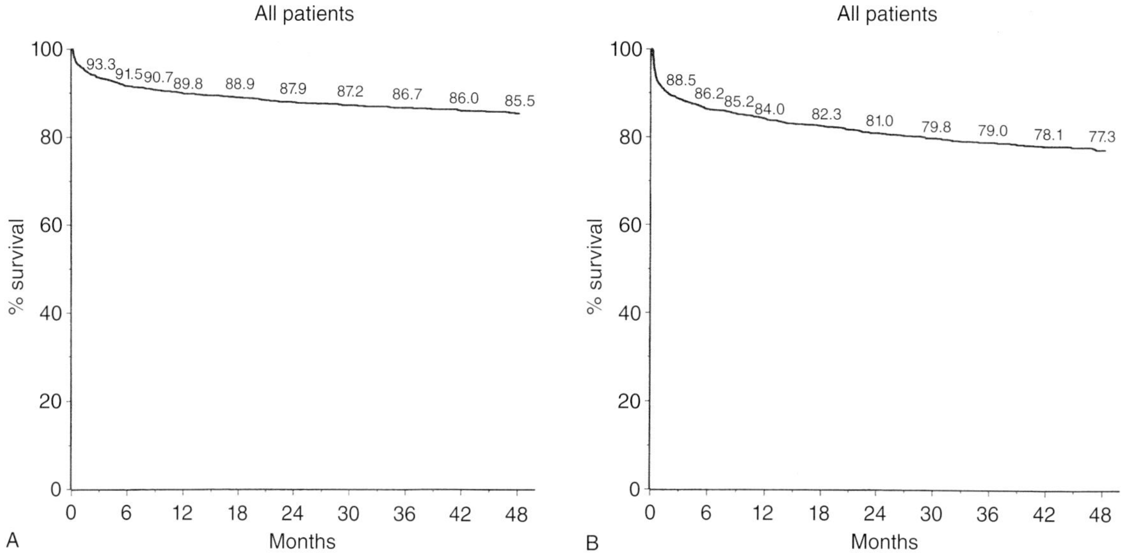

Figure 38.2 Kaplan–Meier probability of patient (**A**) and graft (**B**) survival over 4 years for pediatric liver transplantation. Derived from the Studies of Pediatric Liver Transplantation 2006 Annual Report.[1] Reproduced by permission

fibrosis (16%), primary graft nonfunction (14%), biliary complications (12%), and other indications (26%).[15] As surgical techniques advance, infants younger than 90 d are more frequently undergoing liver transplantation, with weights as low as 2.4 kg, but averaging 3.9 kg.[20] When compared to older children, the infants experienced longer hospitalizations and more frequent need for reoperation; however, there was no difference in the rates of vascular or biliary tract complications. The 1-year patient and graft survival rate for infants was 87.8 and 76.1%, which when compared to older children from the same era, was slightly lower but not significantly different.[20] Diagnosis plays a role in outcome, as children transplanted for acute liver failure have a lower 6-month survival rate compared to children transplanted for other causes (75.9 vs 90.8%).[10] Transplant-free survival in PALF is 54%; approximately 32% of PALF patients require liver transplantation and 14% die without liver transplantation.[10] Survival after transplantation for PALF is from 50 to 70%. Early recognition of PALF and referral to a pediatric liver transplant center for evaluation is important for optimal patient outcomes. Biliary atresia patients have outstanding patient and graft survival rates at 6 months of 92.4 and 86.2%, respectively.[21]

Late graft loss, after 1 year post transplantation, is rare in children and is mainly caused by chronic rejection (48.5%) and biliary strictures (20%).[22] Recurrent disease was only responsible for 3% of cases of late graft loss.[22] With the exception of autoimmune hepatitis, primary sclerosing cholangitis, and viral hepatitis, liver transplant "cures" the underlying liver disease. Though there may be ongoing systemic involvement, such as with Alagille syndrome, tyrosinemia, and alpha-1-antitrypsin deficiency, recurrent disease within the liver does not occur. Close monitoring for reoccurrence of autoimmune disease and reactivation of hepatitis B and C are key for graft survival.

Children who receive a technical variant graft (live donor, reduced, or split liver) have been shown to have an increased 30-day post-transplant morbidity compared to whole organ, but when followed for 5 years, graft survival was found to be the same.[23] There was no difference in 30-day post-transplant morbidity among the types of surgical variant grafts. When complications were compared to whole-organ grafts, variant grafts had higher frequencies of bile duct leaks (13.9 vs 3.7%), portal vein thrombosis (7.8 vs 3.6%), and other GI complications (13.2 vs 7.0%). Patients who received technical variant grafts were younger, more likely to be transplanted for acute liver failure, and spent an average of 2–3 months less on the waiting list.[23] Most children with chronic liver disease have poor growth prior to liver transplantation (height z score −1.55 at transplantation) and although growth improves after transplantation (height z score −0.68 at 2 years post transplantation), growth still does not return to baseline, particularly in patients with biliary atresia.[24] This lack of catch up growth is likely due to continued steroid exposure post transplantation, underlying liver disease, such as metabolic disease,[24] and stunting that may have occurred prior to transplantation. As a group, quality of life improves after transplantation, but does not return to baseline and families and patients report similar social and school function as cancer patients receiving chemotherapy.[25]

Transitioning to adult centers

With better graft and patient survival, many pediatric liver transplant patients will eventually need transitioning to adult practices. It is important for the adult practitioner not only to be familiar with the pediatric diseases that required liver transplantation, but also to be aware of the unique challenges posed by this young population. For many young adults transplanted as a child, medical care has been dictated by their caregivers and the young adults are unfamiliar with the responsibilities needed to manage their liver transplant.[26] Non-adherence to medications, follow-up clinic visits and laboratory tests; risk of under- or overdosing of medications; and under-recognition of ongoing liver injury or rejection becomes more prevalent as children get older. Risk factors for non-adherence include family dysfunction and poor behavior functioning in the child.[27] The transition to adult practice is often a vulnerable time and small studies have shown a decrease in medication adherence during this period.[28] Novel interventions should be considered, such as text messaging reminders about medications and specialty clinics focused on educating adolescents about their diagnosis and medications.[29,30]

Acknowledgments

Grant support: Supported in part by NIH grants U01 DK 062453, U54 RR019455, MO1 RR00069 and UL1 RR025780.

References

1. EMMES Corporation. Studies of Pediatric Liver Transplantation (SPLIT) 2006 Annual Report. 2006:1–6, 6–7, 6–12.
2. Mieli-Vergani G, Vergani D. Biliary atresia. Semin Immunopathol 2009;31:371–81.
3. Ohhama Y, Shinkai M, Fujita S, et al. Early prediction of long-term survival and the timing of liver transplantation after the Kasai operation. J Pediatr Surg 2000;35: 1031–4.
4. Hoffenberg EJ, Narkewicz MR, Sondheimer JM, et al. Outcome of syndromic paucity of interlobular bile ducts (Alagille syndrome) with onset of cholestasis in infancy. J Pediatr 1995;127:220–4.
5. Erickson NI, Balistreri WF. Sclerosing cholangitis. In: Suchy FJ, Sokol RJ, Balistreri WF, editors. Liver disease in children. 3rd ed. New York: Cambridge University Press; 2007:459–77.
6. Filipponi F, Soubrane O, Labrousse F. Liver transplantation for end-stage liver disease associated with alpha-1-antitrypsin deficiency in children: pre-transplant natural history, timing and results of transplantation. J Hepatol 1994;20:72–8.
7. Moyer K, Balistreri W. Hepatobilary disease in patients with cystic fibrosis. Curr Opin Gastroenterol 2009;25: 272–8.
8. Rand EB, Karpen SJ, Kelly S, et al. Treatment of neonatal hemochromatosis with exchange transfusion and intravenous immunoglobulin. J Pediatr 2009;155: 566–71.
9. Mieli-Vergani G, Heller S, Jara P, et al. Autoimmune hepatitis. J Pediatr Gastroenterol Nutr 2009;49: 158–64.
10. Squires RH, Shneider BL, Bucuvalas J, et al. Acute liver failure in children: The first 348 patients in the pediatric acute liver failure study group. J Pediatr 2006;148: 652–8.
11. Narkewicz MR, Dell Olio D, Karpen SJ, et al. Pattern of diagnostic evaluation for the causes of pediatric acute liver failure: an opportunity for quality improvement. J Pediatr 2009;155:801–6.
12. McDiarmid SV, Anand R, Lindbald AS, and the Principal Investigators and Institutions of the Studies of Pediatric Liver Transplantation (SPLIT) Research Group. Development of a pediatric end-stage liver disease score to predict poor outcome in children awaiting liver transplantation. Transplantation 2002;74: 173–81.
13. Stewart ZA, Locke JE, Montgomery RA, et al. ABO-incompatible decreased donor liver transplantation in the United States: a national registry analysis. Liver Transpl 2009;15:883–93.

14. Bucuvalas JC, Anand R, Studies of Pediatric Liver Transplantation Research Group. Treatment with immunoglobulin improves outcome for pediatric liver transplant recipients. Liver Transpl 2009;15:1564–9.
15. Ng VL, Fecteau A, Shepherd R, et al. Outcomes of 5-year survivors of pediatric liver transplantation: Report of 461 children from a North American multicenter registry. Pediatrics 2008;122:e1128–35.
16. Kelly D, Jara P, Rodeck B, et al. Tacrolimus and steroids versus ciclosporin microemulsion, steroids, and azathioprine in children undergoing liver transplantation: randomised European multicentre trial. Lancet 2004;364:1054–61.
17. Krams SM, Martinez OM. Epstein–Barr virus, rapamycin, and host immune responses. Curr Opin Organ Transplant 2008;13:563–8.
18. Shepherd RW, Turmelle Y, Nadler M, et al. Risk factors for rejection and infection in pediatric liver transplantation. Am J Transplant 2008;8:396–403.
19. Martin SR, Atkison P, Anand R, et al. Studies of pediatric liver transplantation 2002: Patient and graft survival and rejection in pediatric recipients of a first liver transplant in the United States and Canada. Pediatr Transplant 2004;8:273–83.
20. Sundaram SS, Alonso EM, Anand R, for the Study of Pediatric Liver Transplantation Research Group. Outcomes after liver transplantation in young infants. J Pediatr Gastroenterol Nutr 2008;47:486–92.
21. Utterson EC, Shepherd RW, Sokol RJ, et al. Biliary atresia: Clinical profiles, risk factors, and outcomes of 755 patients listed for liver transplantation. J Pediatr 2005;147:180–5.
22. Soltys KA, Mazariegos GV, Squires RH, et al. Late graft loss of death in pediatric liver transplantation: An analysis of the SPLIT database. Am J Transplant 2007;7:2165–71.
23. Diamond IR, Fecteau A, Millis JM, et al. Impact of graft type on outcome in pediatric liver transplantation. Ann Surg 2007;246:301–10.
24. Alonso EM, Shepherd R, Martz KL, et al. Linear growth patterns in prepubertal children following liver transplantation. Am J Transplant 2009;9:1389–97.
25. Alonso EM, Limbers CA, Neighbors K, et al. Cross-sectional analysis of health-related quality of life in pediatric liver transplant recipients. J Pediatr 2010;156:270–6.
26. Annunziato RA, Parkar S, Dugan CA, et al. Brief report: Deficits in health care management skills among adolescent and young adult liver transplant recipients transitioning to adult care settings. J Pediatr Psychol 2009 [cited 2010 April 1st]. Available from Oxford University Press. http://jpepsy.oxfordjournals.org.
27. Dew MA, Dabbs AD, Myaskovsky L, et al. Meta-analysis of medical regimen adherence outcomes in pediatric solid organ transplantation. Transplantation 2009;88:736–46.
28. Shemesh E, Annunziato RA, Shneider BL, et al. Improving adherence to medications in pediatric liver transplant recipients. Pediatr Transplant 2008;12: 316–23.
29. Annunziato RA, Emre S, Shneider BL, et al. Adherence and medical outcomes in pediatric liver transplant recipients who transition to adult services. Pediatr Transplant 2007;11:608–14.
30. Miloh T, Annunziato R, Arnon R, et al. Improved adherence and outcomes for pediatric liver transplant recipients by using text messaging. Pediatrics 2009;124:e844–50.

Multiple choice questions

Chapter 1

1. Which is an absolute contraindication for liver transplantation?

A. Previous breast cancer
B. Active tuberculosis
C. Cystic fibrosis
D. Portal thrombosis
E. Active substance abuse

2. What are possible indications of liver transplantation for primary biliary cirrhosis?

A. Uncontrolled pruritus
B. Bilirubin level over 50 mmol/L
C. One episode of variceal bleeding
D. Uncontrolled recurrent ascites
E. Chronic encephalopathy

3. Is this sentence correct?: "Hepatic artery thrombosis is an indication of retransplantation because it could be due to allograft rejection"

A. First part is wrong, second part is wrong
B. First part is correct, second part is wrong
C. First part is wrong, second part is correct
D. First part is correct, second part is correct, "because" is incorrect
E. First part is correct, second part is correct, "because" is correct

Chapter 2

1. Which antibiotic is indicated to prevent infections in a Child A patient with variceal hemorrhage?

A. Ciprofloxacin
B. Amoxicillin
C. First-generation cephalosporin
D. Trimethoprim-sulfamethoxazole
E. Third-generation cephalosporin

2. Which of the following statements are true?

A. Propranolol is indicated for the primary prophylaxis in patients with large varices and no previous bleeding episode.
B. Transarterial chemoembolization is mandatory to prevent tumor progression in patients with hepatocellular cancer.
C. There is no need for antibiotic prophylaxis in patients with a previous spontaneous bacterial peritonitis.
D. Hepato-renal syndrome Type 1 can be treated with terlipressin and albumin.
E. Follow-up echocardiography is not indicated in patients with a normal RVsys at baseline.

3. Is this sentence correct?: "Antibiotic prophylaxis is indicated in patients with a variceal hemorrhage because it has been shown that this improves survival"

A. First part is wrong, second part is wrong
B. First part is correct, second part is wrong
C. First part is wrong, second part is correct
D. First part is correct, second part is correct, "because" is incorrect
E. First part is correct, second part is correct, "because" is correct

Chapter 3

1. What is true about primary prophylaxis of variceal bleeding? (Choose one correct answer)

A. Patients without varices should be screened endoscopically for the appearance of varices every year.
B. Patients with large varices and those with small varices and red signs or severe liver disfunction are candidates for primary prophylaxis.
C. Endoscopic band ligation is always the treatment of choice for primary prophylaxis.
D. Propranol is better than nadolol.
E. TIPS is preferable to derivative surgery in primary prophylaxis.

Medical Care of the Liver Transplant Patient, Fourth Edition. Edited by Pierre-Alain Clavien, James F. Trotter.

2. What is true in the treatment of acute variceal bleeding? (More than one answer is possible)

A. Prophylaxis of infection with broad-spectrum antibiotics should only be given to patients with a history of previous infections.
B. In acute variceal hemorrhage, the best approach is the combined use of a pharmacologic agent, started from admission and an endoscopic procedure.
C. Patients surviving an episode of variceal bleeding are at a high risk of rebleeding; medical therapies, using beta-blockers +/– nitrates, endoscopic band ligation or both, are the recommended first-line treatments.
D. Sclerotherapy is the best endoscopic approach in the management of variceal bleeding.
E. Volemia must be carefully replaced.

3. Is this sentence correct?: "PTFE-covered stents are the treatment of choice in patients with high risk of treatment failure *because* in these patients mortality and treatment failure applying the combination of endoscopic and drug therapy is very high" (Sentences compounded with "because")

A. First part is wrong, second part is wrong
B. First part is correct, second part is wrong
C. First part is wrong, second part is correct
D. First part is correct, second part is correct, "because" is incorrect
E. First part is correct, second part is correct, "because" is correct

Chapter 4

1. Is this sentence correct?: "Because the Modification of Diet in Renal Disease (MDRD) equations are based on serum creatinine and specific patient demographics, they accurately estimate glomerular filtration rate in cirrhotics"

A. First part is right, second part is wrong
B. First part is right, second part is right
C. First part is wrong, second part is right
D. First part is wrong, second part is wrong

2. True or False? The gold standard for measuring glomerular filtration rate in cirrhosis is clearance measurement based on exogenous markers such as inulin and radiolabeled compounds

3. Which of the following is *not* a primary cause of renal failure in cirrhosis?

A. Infections
B. Hypovolemia
C. Encephalopathy
D. Hepatorenal syndrome

4. Which of the following is an established effective therapy for hepatorenal syndrome? (More than one may be correct)

A. Transjugular intrahepatic portosystemic shunt (TIPS)
B. Terlipressin with albumin
C. Molecular readsorbent recirculating system (MARS)
D. Extracorporeal liver support device

5. According to established selection criteria, liver transplant candidates need a simultaneous kidney transplant if dialysis is required for more than how many days?

A. 3 days
B. 7 days
C. 42 days
D. 180 days

Chapter 5

1. What is the best screening strategy for the diagnosis of hepatopulmonary syndrome in patients undergoing evaluation for liver transplantation?

A. Pulse oximetry
B. Arterial blood gas
C. Contrast echocardiography
D. Pulse oximetry and contrast echocardiography
E. 99mTc-macroaggregated albumin lung perfusion scan

2. Which of the following statements is/are true regarding the evaluation and treatment of liver transplant candidates?

A. The presence of right ventricular hypertrophy on echocardiography warrants right-heart catheterization
B. Beta-blockers are the preferred treatment for variceal bleeding prophylaxis in patients with POPH
C. Oral anticoagulation is mandatory in patients with documented POPH
D. Patients with portopulmonary hypertension may have normal pulmonary vascular resistance
E. Almost 20% of transplant candidates have elevated RVSP on Doppler echocardiography

3. Is this sentence correct?: "A patient with sustained response after medical treatment for portopulmonary hypertension achieving a mean pulmonary arterial pressure (mPAP) below 35 is not a candidate for liver transplantation, because his baseline mPAP was above 45"

A. First part is wrong, second part is wrong
B. First part is correct, second part is wrong
C. First part is wrong, second part is correct
D. First part is correct, second part is correct, "because" is incorrect
E. First part is correct, second part is correct, "because" is correct

Chapter 6

1. Which alcohol use diagnosis offers the best prognosis for post-transplant abstinence?

A. Alcohol dependence
B. Polydrug dependence including alcohol
C. Alcohol abuse
D. Type 1 alcohol dependence
E. Type 2 alcohol dependence

2. Useful prognostic factors in predicting post-transplant alcohol abstinence include:

A. Social stability
B. Alcohol use diagnosis
C. >6 months pre-transplant abstinence
D. Polysubstance use diagnosis
E. Vaillant's factors

3. Is this sentence correct?: "Alcoholic liver disease and alcoholic hepatitis are clear indicators of alcoholism because they occur only in the presence of alcohol dependence" (Sentences compounded with "because")

A. First part is wrong, second part is wrong
B. First part is correct, second part is wrong
C. First part is wrong, second part is correct
D. First part is correct, second part is correct, "because" is incorrect
E. First part is correct, second part is correct, "because" is correct

Chapter 7

1. What is liver transplant survival benefit?

A. The amount of time a recipient lives after liver transplant
B. The improvement in quality of life after liver transplant
C. An insurance policy for patients who survive liver transplantation
D. The difference between survival with and survival without a liver transplant
E. The difference in liver transplant survival between receiving a good graft with or a marginal graft

2. The MELD score's accuracy is limited by:

A. Gender differences in serum creatinine values relative to actual kidney function
B. Different laboratory reagents for measuring pro-thrombin time
C. Height of liver transplant candidates
D. Use of vitamin K antagonists
E. Serum sodium values

3. Is this sentence correct?: "Liver donor allocation and distribution is based on mortality risk because mortality risk is the only definition of liver transplant need"

A. First part is wrong, second part is wrong
B. First part is correct, second part is wrong
C. First part is wrong, second part is correct
D. First part is correct, second part is correct, "because" is incorrect
E. First part is correct, second part is correct, "because" is correct

Chapter 8

1. Which of the following is the best prediction of HBV recurrence post transplant?

A. Non-use of high-dose IVI HBIG
B. HBeAg positivity at the time of transplantation
C. The presence of HBV DNA in serum at the time of transplantation
D. The presence of HCC at the time of transplantation
E. The use of antiviral therapy before transplantation

2. Which of the following characterize chronic HCV infection and worse natural history post transplantation?

A. Recipient age
B. Donor age
C. Highest viral load at 3 months post transplantation
D. High levels of hepatic inflammation at 3 months post transplantation
E. Presence of F1 fibrosis in the year biopsy

3. Which of the following statements is correct?

A. Lamivudine therapy is the agent of choice to control HBV infection in the transplant setting because of low levels of drug resistance
B. Chronic HCV infection is associated with worse outcomes post transplantation because of the high prevalence of cryoglobulinemia post transplant
C. Chronic HCV is a major contraindication for liver transplantation because of the universal recurrence of infection post transplantation
D. Tenofovir is a powerful anti-HBV agent because it decreases anti-HBV B-cell responses
E. Entecavir should not be used as an antiviral agent in the setting of lamivudine resistance because of the high rate of entecavir resistance in this setting

Chapter 9

1. Key in the pathogenesis of NASH is / are

A. Insulin resistance
B. Hyperinsulinemia
C. Abnormal adipocytokine production
D. Mitochondrial dysfunction
E. All of the above

2. Recurrence of NASH after OLT can be adequately diagnosed by

A. Regular biochemical assessments
B. Protocol liver biopsies
C. Hepatic ultrasound
D. MRI-scan
E. Combination of biochemical assessments and MRI-scan

3. The most common indication for OLT in patients with Wilson's disease is

A. Acute liver failure
B. Chronic liver failure
C. Extrahepatic complications
D. Progression of the liver disease despite treatment
E. OLT for Wilson's disease is not seen, since chronic disease can be prevented

4. Iron overloading with hereditary hemochromatosis is most often seen when diagnostics testing shows

A. Increased transferrin saturation >45%, ferritin >1000 ng/mL, and Hepatic iron index >1.9
B. Increased transferrin saturation <45%, ferritin >1000 ng/mL, and Hepatic iron index <1.9
C. Increased transferrin saturation >45%, ferritin >1000 ng/mL, and Hepatic iron index <1.9
D. Increased transferrin saturation >45%, ferritin <1000 ng/mL, and Hepatic iron index <1.9
E. Increased transferrin saturation >45%, ferritin <1000 ng/mL, and Hepatic iron index >1.9

Chapter 10

1. Which is the standard medical treatment of primary biliary cirrhosis (PBC), which may prevent the need of liver transplantation in "responders" (>60% of patients treated over up to 20 years)?

A. Cholestyramine, 4 g before and after breakfast
B. Ursodeoxycholic acid, 13–15 mg/kg/d
C. Chenodeoxycholic acid, 10 mg/kg/d
D. Ursodeoxycholic acid, 28–30 mg/kg/d
E. Obeticholic acid, 10 mg/kg/d

2. Patients with primary sclerosing cholangitis have an increased risk to develop malignancies. Which malignomas have been shown to be more prevalent in PSC than in the normal population?

A. Colon carcinoma
B. Cholangiocarcinoma
C. Oesophageal carcinoma
D. Gallbladder carcinoma
E. Pancreatic carcinoma
F. Hepatocellular carcinoma

3. Is this sentence correct?: "Autoimmune hepatitis (AIH) is diagnosed on the basis of biochemical and histologic features because both a markedly elevated IgA and a typical florid, nonsuppurative cholangitis predict good response to immunosuppressive treatment of AIH"

A. First part is wrong, second part is wrong
B. First part is correct, second part is wrong
C. First part is wrong, second part is correct
D. First part is correct, second part is correct, "because" is incorrect
E. First part is correct, second part is correct, "because" is correct

Chapter 11

1. Which is an indication for cadaveric liver transplantation in patients with hepatocellular carcinoma (HCC)? (One correct answer out of five)

A. Patients with one nodule ≥5 cm
B. Only patients with HCC with portal vein thrombosis
C. Patients within Milan criteria
D. Patients without Milan criteria
E. Patients with extrahepatic disease

2. Recurrence is one of the most frequent post-surgical problems. Which patients are optimal candidates for liver transplantation after initial surgical resection? (One correct answer out of five)

A. Patients with microvascular invasion and satelitosis in surgical sample
B. Patients with more than two nodules in surgical sample
C. Patients developing several nodules beyond Milan criteria
D. Patients with a single encapsulated nodule without microvascular invasion
E. Patients with a resected nodule without microvascular invasion and without satelitosis

3. One of the major problems in LT is the shortage of donors. What strategy tries to improve this problem?

A. Use of so-called marginal livers (advanced age, steatosis)
B. Use of livers with metabolic disorders or with viral infection without significant liver injury
C. Use of the split-liver technique
D. Living donor liver transplantation
E. All of them are correct.

Chapter 12

1. A 34-year-old woman presents with jaundice and pruritus that have been progressively worsening during the past month. She was incidentally diagnosed with primary sclerosing cholangitis 2 years ago during an elective cholecystectomy. An MRI/MRCP demonstrates a dominant stricture at the hilum with a hepatic mass adjacent to the stricture. What is the most appropriate next step in the evaluation?

A. Diagnostic paracentesis
B. Alphafetoprotein level
C. Resection of the involved hepatic lobe
D. ERCP with brushings of the bile ducts for cytology
E. Ultrasound-guided percutaneous biopsy of the mass

2. In which of the following patients with CCA is liver transplantation possibly indicated?
   A. Intrahepatic CCA involving a single hepatic lobe
   B. Extrahepatic CCA with bilateral involvement to the second-degree biliary radicals with no metastases
   C. Extrahepatic CCA with metastases confined to regional lymph nodes
   D. Extrahepatic CCA with unilateral involvement in a patient with PSC with no metastases
   E. Extrahepatic CCA with a single intrahepatic metastasis

3. Is this sentence correct?: "Early placement of metallic biliary stents is recommended in CCA patients because it is critical to maintain drainage from both the right and left biliary systems"
   A. First part is wrong, second part is wrong
   B. First part is correct, second part is wrong
   C. First part is wrong, second part is correct
   D. First part is correct, second part is correct, "because" is incorrect
   E. First part is correct, second part is correct, "because" is correct

Chapter 13

1. The most common underlying prothrombotic condition associated with primary Budd–Chiari syndrome is: (One correct answer out of five)
   A. Antiphospholipid syndrome
   B. Factor V Leiden
   C. Myeloproliferative disease
   D. Paroxysmal nocturnal hemoglobinuria
   E. Antithrombin deficiency

2. Is this sentence correct?: "Somatostatin receptor scintigraphy is the most sensitive imaging modality for detection of neuroendocrine tumor metastases because chromogranin A is produced by all tumors, including those that are non-functioning" (Sentences compounded with "because")
   A. First part is wrong, second part is wrong
   B. First part is correct, second part is wrong
   C. First part is wrong, second part is correct
   D. First part is correct, second part is correct, "because" is incorrect
   E. First part is correct, second part is correct, "because" is correct

3. Caroli syndrome may be associated with hepatobiliary complications including: (More than one answer is possible)
   A. Cholangitis
   B. Intraductal biliary stones (hepatolithiasis)
   C. Ascites
   D. Cholangiocarcinoma
   E. Gastroesophageal varices

Chapter 14

1. Which of the following immunosuppressive agents commonly used as immunosuppressive therapy have anti-retroviral effects?
   A. Cyclosporine A
   B. Mycophenolate mofetil
   C. Sirolimus
   D. All the above

2. Which of the following are relative contraindications to liver transplantation in the HIV/HCV co-infected patient?
   A. CD4+ T-cell count of 110
   B. Detectable HIV RNA
   C. History of CMV retinitis
   D. Chronic cryptosporidiosis

3. Which of the following classes of anti-retroviral agents necessitate significant reduction of concurrently administered tacrolimus?
   A. Non-nucleoside reverse transcriptase inhibitors
   B. Nucleoside/nucleotide reverse transcriptase inhibitors
   C. Protease inhibitors
   D. Fusion inhibitors

Chapter 15

1. **Living-donor liver transplantation**
   A. Can be done with a left lobe graft in most adult patients
   B. Is associated with significantly higher rates of biliary complications than deceased donor transplantation
   C. Should be used for transplantation when a deceased donor graft is contraindicated (e.g. acute alcoholic hepatitis)
   D. Is associated with a mortality rate in the donor of 3–5%

2. **Living-donor liver transplantation:**
   A. Allows earlier transplant at a lower MELD score
   B. Has superior outcomes to deceased donor liver transplants
   C. Does not work for genetic diseases
   D. Is currently viewed as experimental
   E. Can be performed with a right or left lobe graft

3. **Living-donor liver transplantation should not be carried out in cases with hepatitis C because HCV recurrence is always more severe**
   A. First part is wrong, second part is wrong
   B. First part is correct, second part is wrong
   C. First part is wrong, second part is correct
   D. First part is correct, second part is correct, "because" is incorrect
   E. First part is correct, second part is correct, "because" is correct

Chapter 16

1. **Which of the following is necessary for the diagnosis of fulminant hepatic failure (FHF), i.e. the *sine qua non*?**
   A. Coagulopathy
   B. Jaundice
   C. Encephalopathy
   D. Hepatitis

2. **Which of the following are possible etiologies of FHF?** (More than one may be correct)
   A. Pregnancy
   B. Liver rupture
   C. Metastatic cancer
   D. Diabetes

3. **True or False?: According to the US Acute Liver Failure Study Group more patients with FHF spontaneously survive without a transplant than receive a transplant**

4. **Is this sentence correct?: "Because extracorporeal liver-assist devices are novel therapies for FHF, they are rapidly evolving as the standard of care in this setting"**
   A. First part is true, second part is false
   B. First part is false, second part is false
   C. First part is false, second part is true
   D. First part is true, second part is true

Chapter 17

1. **Is this sentence correct?: Clinical studies on the influence of graft steatosis on morbidity and mortality after OLT report consistent results because steatosis can be accurately quantified microscopically by pathologists:**
   A. First part is wrong, second part is wrong
   B. First part is correct, second part is wrong
   C. First part is wrong, second part is correct
   D. First part is correct, second part is correct, "because" is incorrect
   E. First part is correct, second part is correct, "because" is correct

2. **Which criteria are considered as extended criteria for the liver allograft?**
   A. Cold ischemia time >12 h
   B. Donor age over 40 years
   C. Liver steatosis >20%
   D. Split graft
   E. Nonwhite race

3. **The donor risk index is directly related to:**
   A. Post-transplant complication rates
   B. Graft survival
   C. Rejection rate
   D. MELD score
   E. Post-transplant disease transmission

Chapter 18

1. Which is the definition of a Maastricht category III DCD?

A. Dead at arrival in hospital
B. DBD but the family wishes to wait for cardiac arrest prior to organ retrieval
C. Cardiac arrest and unsuccessful resuscitation within hospital premises
D. Planned withdrawal of treatment and awaiting cardiac arrest
E. DBD but the donor unexpectedly suffers a cardiac arrest

2. Which are commonly accepted definitions of donor warm ischemia time?

A. Time from withdrawal of treatment to cardiac arrest
B. Time from post withdrawal hypotension/hypoxia to initiation of aortic perfusion
C. Time from withdrawal of treatment to skin incision
D. Time from withdrawal of treatment to initiation of aortic perfusion
E. Time from withdrawal of treatment to initiation of portal vein perfusion

3. DCD liver graft survival is inferior to DBD liver grafts because of primary nonfunction and ischemic biliary strictures?

A. First part is wrong, second part is wrong
B. First part is correct, second part is wrong
C. First part is wrong, second part is correct
D. First part is correct, second part is correct, "because" is incorrect
E. First part is correct, second part is correct, "because" is correct

Chapter 19

1. The typical West Nile virus host is a:

A. Rabbit
B. Snake
C. Fish
D. Turtle
E. Crow

2. Which of the following factors may influence transmission of a CNS tumor?

A. Prior surgery
B. Prior chemotherapy
C. Prior radiation therapy
D. Sex of the donor
E. Ventriculoperitoneal shunt

3. An HTLV-2-positive donor should never be used for organ transplantation because it is associated with a high rate of disease transmission

A. First part is wrong, second part is wrong
B. First part is correct, second part is wrong
C. First part is wrong, second part is correct
D. First part is correct, second part is correct, "because" is incorrect
E. First part is correct, second part is correct, "because" is correct

Chapter 20

1. Current preservation solutions for liver transplantation include:

A. UW solution
B. Euro-Collins solution
C. IGL solution
D. Celsior solution
E. HTK solution

2. Arterial reconstruction during liver transplantation: (There will be more than one correct answer)

A. Should be done after biliary anastomosis
B. Should be done at the level of the recipient's gastroduodenal artery or proximal to it
C. Should show a flow of approximately 200 ml/min
D. May be done before portal vein anastomoses
E. Is decisive for later graft function

3. Liver function after liver transplantation: (There may be more than one correct answer)

A. Can be predicted before transplantation
B. Has to be monitored repeatedly within the first 48 h after OLT
C. Should be checked by ultrasound
D. Is the most important factor for the decision whether PNF is present
E. Cannot be assessed in the presence of immunosuppressive drugs

Chapter 21

1. Liver transplantation in the presence of portal vein thrombosis may require: (More than one answer is possible)

A. Thrombectomy
B. Jump graft between donor portal vein and superior mesenteric vein
C. Hepaticojejunostomy
D. Cavocaval piggyback transplantation
E. Portocaval hemitransposition

2. Sufficient arterial reconstruction during liver transplantation: (More than one answer is possible)

A. Is only possible by anastomoses to the main hepatic artery
B. Can be done by infrarenal aortic conduit
C. May be feasible by supraceliac aortic conduit
D. Is possible on the splenic artery
E. Should be checked by intraoperative flow measurement

3. Dislocated vascular stents:

A. May require exposure of the superior mesenteric vein below the pancreas
B. May require dissection of the suprahepatic cava above the diaphragma
C. May require open cardiotomy
D. Can be impossible due to fragile vessel walls
E. Should be diagnosed before liver transplantation

Chapter 22

1. Which of the following statements is not correct about domino liver transplant?

A. Domino livers show no other abnormal functioning other than the underlying metabolic or biochemical dysfunction.
B. The anatomy of the domino liver is normal.
C. The domino donor is a relatively older individual.
D. It is assumed that in giving domino liver grafts to genetically unaffected patients, a long time will be needed for the development of symptoms or, at best, the disease may never manifest itself.
E. FAP patients are most often employed as domino donors.

2. Split-liver transplantation is an attractive alternative that can lessen waiting time for deceased-donor whole-organ transplantation because it is technically easy and does not require additional logistic as well as personnel support

A. First part is wrong, second part is wrong
B. First part is correct, second part is wrong
C. First part is wrong, second part is correct
D. First part is correct, second part is correct, "because" is incorrect
E. First part is correct, second part is correct, "because" is correct

3. Which of the following are criteria for selecting a donor for split-liver transplantation?

A. Young hemodynamically stable donors
B. Donor body weight ≤40 kg
C. Donors with normal liver function test results
D. Donors with short ICU stay (<5 d) and absent or fairly short down time

Chapter 23

1. Which of the followings is NOT the indication of living-donor liver transplantation?:

A. Acute liver failure
B. Acute-on-chronic liver failure
C. Colorectal liver metastasis
D. Hepatocellular carcinoma
E. Hepatitis B-related liver cirrhosis

2. All of the followings are types of liver graft in clinical practice EXCEPT:

A. Right liver graft with inclusion of middle hepatic vein
B. Right lateral sector liver graft
C. Left liver graft with inclusion of middle hepatic vein
D. Segment IV–VIII liver graft
E. Segment II/III liver graft

3. True or False? In the setting of living-donor liver transplantation, the recipient benefits should outweigh the donor safety

Chapter 24

1. Which phenomenon is not observed during the early reperfusion phase of the liver?(Choose one correct answer out of five)

A. Hypokalemia
B. Decreased arterial pressure
C. Metabolic acidosis
D. Arrhythmia
E. Increase of systemic inflammatory mediators

2. What belongs to a routine preoperative assessment regarding anesthesia for a patient undergoing liver transplantation? (More than one answer is possible)

A. Echocardiography
B. Lung function test
C. Blood electrolytes
D. Electroencephalogram
E. Coagulation factors

3. During liver transplantation a generous fluid therapy is recommended because maintenance of a normal arterial pressure is crucial for renal perfusion to avoid postoperative acute renal failure. (Sentences compounded with "because")

A. First part is wrong, second part is wrong
B. First part is correct, second part is wrong
C. First part is wrong, second part is correct
D. First part is correct, second part is correct, "because" is incorrect
E. First part is correct, second part is correct, "because" is correct

Chapter 25

1. During liver transplantation: (Choose one correct answer out of five)

A. Bleed patients abundantly if no coagulation abnormalities are corrected
B. Recombinant Factor VIIa is the drug of choice in severe bleeding
C. The risk of developing thromboembolic complications is almost nil
D. Drugs promoting coagulation should be cautiously used
E. The administration of fresh–frozen plasma to correct the PT and/or APTT is necessary

2. To avoid blood loss during liver transplantation: (More than one answer is possible)

A. It is important to keep the patient's temperature at 37°C
B. A high central venous pressure (CVP) is necessary
C. Is it always necessary to administer platelet concentrate
D. Thromboelastography/metry is helpful to guide therapy with FFP or procoagulant drugs
E. Serum ionic calcium (Ca^{++}) should be routinely monitored and corrected to maintain a serum Ca^{++} ≥1 mmol/L

3. Is this sentence correct?: "Patients with end-stage liver disease are believed to be in a hypocoagulable status because both pro- and antihemostatic pathways are compromised" (Sentences compounded with "because")

A. First part is wrong, second part is wrong
B. First part is correct, second part is wrong
C. First part is wrong, second part is correct
D. First part is correct, second part is correct, "because" is incorrect
E. First part is correct, second part is correct, "because" is correct

Chapter 26

1. Which one of the following clinical parameters is not routinely used to assess liver graft function after transplantation?

A. Bile production of the newly transplanted liver in the operating room
B. Level of transaminases after transplantation
C. INR and Factor V
D. Cholinesterase levels
E. Failure to correct metabolic acidosis

2. Hepatopulmonary syndrome is defined by the following triad:
   A. Elevated mean pulmonary arterial pressures, right heart failure, liver congestion
   B. PaO2/Fi02 ratio of <300, bilateral pulmonary infiltrates on chest radiogram, PCWP <18 mmHg
   C. Portal hypertension, abnormal gas exchange, evidence of pulmonary vascular shunts
   D. Need for prolonged intubation after liver transplantation, high oxygen requirements, normal chest radiogram
   E. Sudden deoxygenation after reperfusion of the liver graft, high ventilatory pressures, need for high PEEP

3. Which one of the following scores have not been validated as prediction models for survival *after* liver transplantation:
   A. Na-MELD
   B. SALT score
   C. D-MELD
   D. SOFT score
   E. BAR-score

Chapter 27

1. The most effective means to screen for acute cellular rejection is:
   A. Liver biopsy
   B. Liver function tests
   C. Hepatic Doppler ultrasonography
   D. Clinical symptoms
   E. Cholangiography

2. The most common regimen for prevention of rejection in liver recipients at the time of discharge from the hospital includes:
   A. Tacrolimus
   B. Sirolimus
   C. Corticosteroids
   D. Mycophenolate mofetil
   E. A,C,D
   F. B,C

3. True or False?: Sirolimus is administered to more than 10% of liver transplant recipients and therefore has an indication for use by the Food and Drug Administration

4. Tacrolimus is administered preferentially over cyclosporine, because:
   A. Cyclosporine is no longer available
   B. Tacrolimus is less expensive
   C. Tacrolimus is more efficacious
   D. Both drugs are equally efficacious

Chapter 28

1. Which of the following is an indication for placement of aortohepatic conduit during liver transplantation:
   A. Arcuate ligament syndrome
   B. Dissection of the recipient hepatic artery
   C. Hemodynamically unstable patient
   D. All of the above

2. Which of the following is the most specific for diagnosis of hepatic artery thrombosis:
   A. Doppler ultrasonography
   B. CT scan
   C. Magnetic resonance imaging
   D. Celiac angiogram

3. Splenic artery steal syndrome is associated with all the following except:
   A. Small spleen
   B. Enlarged splenic artery
   C. Liver biopsy showing ischemia
   D. Liver dysfunction

Chapter 29

1. The most therapy-resistant type of biliary complication after liver transplantation is: (Choose one correct answer out of five)
   A. Bacterial cholangitis
   B. Anastomotic biliary stricture
   C. Leakage at the T-tube entrance site
   D. Non-anastomotic biliary strictures
   E. Leakage from the parenchymal cut surface after split-liver transplantation

2. Which of the following statements are true? (More than one answer is possible)

A. Leakage from the bile duct anastomosis within 1 week after transplantation should be treated by careful observation as it usually heals spontaneously

B. The treatment of first choice for an anastomotic bile duct stricture that occurs 1 year after transplantation is surgical resection and construction of a Roux-Y hepatico-jejunostomy

C. Presence of a Roux-Y hepatico-jejunostomy is a risk factor for cholangitis after liver transplantation.

D. The use of ursodeoxycholic acid in the treatment of non-anastomotic bile duct strictures is supported by randomized, controlled trials.

E. The use of biliary T-drain in liver transplantation does not lead to a reduction in reinterventions for biliary complications.

3. Most cases of non-anastomotic biliary strictures can be prevented by a rapid surgical technique for organ procurement, because ischemia is considered the most important cause of this type of biliary complication (Sentences composed of two parts connected by the word "because")

A. First part is wrong, second part is wrong

B. First part is correct, second part is wrong

C. First part is wrong, second part is correct

D. First part is correct, second part is correct, "because" is incorrect

E. First part is correct, second part is correct, "because" is correct

Chapter 30

1. Which statement concerning the liver biopsy in the context of liver transplantation is correct? (Choose one correct answer out of five)

A. Lipopeliosis is a histologic finding characteristic for chronic rejection

B. Chronic viral hepatitis found in the biopsy of a potential donor organ is the most frequent condition leading to donor disqualification

C. Steatosis of 30% combined macro- and microsteatosis in a donor liver biopsy is the absolute threshold for accepting a donor liver

D. The portal inflammatory infiltrate characteristic for recurrent hepatitis C virus infection is a mixed infiltrate including a significant number of eosinophils and blastic cells

E. Widespread lobular necro-inflammatory activity and the lack of significant bile duct damage are histopathologic findings favoring recurrent hepatitis C virus infection over acute cellular rejection

2. Which of the following histologic findings are criteria for diagnosing and grading acute cellular rejection? (More than one answer is possible)

A. Ductopenia

B. Portal inflammation

C. Arteriopathy

D. Venous endothelitis

E. Bile duct damage and injury

3. Is this sentence correct?: Determination of the fat content of a donor liver is in some instances performed by frozen-section histology prior to transplantation because histopathologic assessment of the fat content of a donor liver provides a highly reproducible quantitative and qualitative measurement of the liver fat content (Sentences compounded with "because")

A. First part is wrong, second part is wrong

B. First part is correct, second part is wrong

C. First part is wrong, second part is correct

D. First part is correct, second part is correct, "because" is incorrect

E. First part is correct, second part is correct, "because" is correct

Chapter 31

1. Which of the following is NOT a component of metabolic syndrome?

A. HbA1c >6.5%
B. HDL in men <1.0 mmol/L
C. Waist circumference >88 cm in women
D. Triglycerides >1.7 mmol/L
E. Blood pressure >130/85

2. Which of the following are risk factors for the development of hypertension in the liver allograft recipient?

A. Use of calcineurin inhibitors
B. Use of mycophenolate mofetil
C. Hyperuricemia
D. Obesity
E. Renal dysfunction

3. Is this sentence correct?: "Certain calcium channel blockers interfere with calcineurin inhibitor metabolism and may lead to elevated cyclosporine and tacrolimus plasma levels because they inhibit CYP2A6"

A. First part is wrong, second part is wrong
B. First part is correct, second part is wrong
C. First part is wrong, second part is correct
D. First part is correct, second part is correct, "because" is incorrect
E. First part is correct, second part is correct, "because" is correct

Chapter 32

1. Which of the following is associated with rapid progression of fibrosis following transplantation for HCV cirrhosis? (Only one is possible)

A. HCV genotype
B. Liver allograft from live-related donor
C. Liver allograft from donor >50 years of age
D. Maintenance tacrolimus
E. Maintenance prednisone

2. Which of the following is associated with SVR following treatment of recurrent HCV infection with pegylated IFN plus ribavirin? (More than one is possible)

A. HCV genotype
B. Recipient IL-28 b genotype
C. Baseline fibrosis stage
D. Early (4 or 12 week) on-treatment virologic response
E. Maintenance prednisone

3. Is this sentence correct?: "Withdrawal of HBIG is feasible in some patients following transplantation for chronic hepatitis B because low HBV DNA levels prior to transplantation is associated with low rate of HBV recurrence"

A. First part is wrong, second part is wrong
B. First part is correct, second part is wrong
C. First part is wrong, second part is correct
D. First part is correct, second part is correct, "because" is incorrect
E. First part is correct, second part is correct, "because" is correct

Chapter 33

1. Which disease does not recur after transplantation

A. Autoimmune hepatitis
B. Wilson disease
C. Non-alcoholic steatohepatitis
D. Budd–Chiari syndrome
E. IgG4 autoimmune cholangitis

2. Which are true of recurrent PBC?

A. Always associated with cholestatic liver tests
B. Rarely causes graft failure
C. UDCA should be instituted immediately after transplantation
D. AMA titers predict recurrence
E. Is diagnosed on graft histology

3. Is this sentence correct?: "Liver transplantation is not indicated for porphyria because liver transplantation does not fully correct the underlying abnormality" (Sentence compounded with "because")

A. First part is wrong, second part is wrong
B. First part is correct, second part is wrong
C. First part is wrong, second part is correct
D. First part is correct, second part is correct, 'because' is wrong
E. First part is correct, second part is correct, 'because' is correct

Chapter 34

1. What is/are the most important steps in the work-up of the transplanted patient with suspected infection? (One correct answer out of five)

A. Aggressive microbiologic diagnosis
B. Rapid therapeutic intervention
C. Reduction of immunosuppression, if possible
D. Consideration of the net state of immunosuppression
E. All of the above

2. Prophylaxis with trimethoprim-sulfamethoxazole (TMP-SMX) has activity against: (More than one answer is possible)

A. *Isospora belli*
B. *Toxoplasma gondii*
C. Cytomegalovirus
D. *Nocardia* species
E. *Listeria* species

3. Is this sentence correct?: "Viremia should be assessed when cytomegalovirus disease is suspected, because a negative result always excludes cytomegalovirus disease" (Sentence compounded with "because")

A. First part is wrong, second part is wrong
B. First part is correct, second part is wrong
C. First part is wrong, second part is correct
D. First part is correct, second part is correct, "because" is incorrect
E. First part is correct, second part is correct, "because" is correct

Chapter 35

1. Which is the most frequent post-transplant cancer in liver transplant recipients? (One correct answer out of five)

A. Liver cancer
B. Squamous cell carcinoma
C. Basal cell carcinoma
D. Kaposi's sarcoma
E. Oral cancer

2. Tacrolimus-related alopecia may be improved by: (More than one answer is possible)

A. Dose reduction
B. Topical steroids
C. Switch to cyclosporine
D. Switch to mTOR inhibitors
E. Vitamin B6 supplementation

3. Skin cancers are more frequent in transplant patients under calcineurin inhibitors as compared to those under mTOR inhibitors because calcineurin inhibitors have oncogenic properties (Sentence compounded with "because")

A. First part is wrong, second part is wrong
B. First part is correct, second part is wrong
C. First part is wrong, second part is correct
D. First part is correct, second part is correct, "because" is incorrect
E. First part is correct, second part is correct, "because" is correct

Chapter 36

1. Which of the following is an established risk factor for post-transplant malignancy and which malignancy is it associated with?

A. Cytomegalovirus mismatch: colon cancer
B. Epstein–Barr virus: skin cancer
C. Epstein–Barr virus: PTLD
D. Hepatitis C virus: lung cancer
E. Herpes simplex virus: gastric cancer

2. What options exist to treat post-transplant lymphoproliferative disorder?

A. Acyclovir
B. Rituximab
C. CHOP therapy (cyclophosphamide, adriamycin, oncovin, and prednisone)
D. Minimization of immunosuppression
E. Options B to D

3. Compared to the general population, what is the overall risk for solid-organ malignancies in liver transplant recipients?

A. 10 times greater
B. 5 times greater
C. 2 to 4 times greater
D. 20% less
E. It is the same

Chapter 37

1. Which immunosuppressive agent should be completely avoided during pregnancy? (Choose one correct answer out of five)

A. Cyclosporine
B. Mycophenolate mofetil
C. Tacrolimus
D. Corticosteroids
E. Azathioprine

2. Which of the following statements are true? (More than one answer is possible)

A. Regular menstrual bleeding will reappear in the vast majority of women of child-bearing age within 1 year post transplant
B. Cyclosporine A is considered a class D drug in terms of its risk for pregnancy by the United States Food and Drug Administration (FDA)
C. Most data suggest better outcomes for mother and newborns with a transplant-to-conception interval >2 years
D. The fetal problems most commonly observed in children born to liver transplant recipients are fetal loss, prematurity (defined as birth occurring prior to 37 weeks' gestation) and low birth weight (<2500 g)
E. Medications that are frequently used in the treatment of patients with chronic liver disease such as beta-blockers (propranolol, nadolol) or diuretics (spironolactone, furosemide) do not affect sexual function

3. Is this sentence correct?: "The necessity of continued immunosuppressive drug therapy during pregnancy has been a major concern, because the commonly used immunosuppressive agents seem to carry a high risk of teratogenicity and fetal loss" (Sentences composed of two parts connected by the word "because")

A. First part is wrong, second part is wrong
B. First part is correct, second part is wrong
C. First part is wrong, second part is correct
D. First part is correct, second part is correct, "because" is incorrect
E. First part is correct, second part is correct, "because" is correct

Chapter 38

1. What is the most common cause of late (after 1 year) liver graft loss in pediatrics?

A. Chronic rejection
B. Hepatitis B
C. Hepatitis C
D. Hepatic artery thrombosis
E. Biliary atresia

2. Which are clinical findings in Alagille syndrome?

A. Paucity of interlobular bile ducts on liver biopsy
B. Occlusion of the extrahepatic duct on cholangiogram
C. Peripheral pulmonary branch artery stenosis
D. Butterfly vertebrae
E. Posterior embryotoxon

3. Is this sentence correct?: "Children are screened for Epstein–Barr virus prior to transplantation because children are at increased risk of developing rejection due to infection with Epstein–Barr virus" (Sentence compounded with "because")

A. First part is wrong, second part is wrong
B. First part is correct, second part is wrong
C. First part is wrong, second part is correct
D. First part is correct, second part is correct, "because" is incorrect
E. First part is correct, second part is correct, "because" is correct

Answers

Chapter 1

1. B. Active tuberculosis
2. A. Uncontrolled pruritus, D. Uncontrolled recurrent ascites, and E. Chronic encephalopathy
3. D. First part is correct, second part is correct, "because" incorrect

Chapter 2

1. A. Ciprofloxacin
2. A. Propranolol is indicated for the primary prophylaxis in patients with large varices and no previous bleeding episode, and D. Hepato-renal syndrome Type 1 can be treated with terlipressin and albumin
3. E. First part is correct, second part is correct, "because" is correct

Chapter 3

1. A. Patients without varices should be screened endoscopically for the appearance of varices every year
2. B. In acute variceal hemorrhage, the best approach is the combined use of a pharmacologic agent, started from admission and an endoscopic procedure, C. Patients surviving an episode of variceal bleeding are at a high risk of rebleeding; medical therapies, using beta-blockers +/– nitrates, endoscopic band ligation or both, are the recommended first-line treatments, and E. Volemia must be carefully replaced
3. E. First part is correct, second part is correct, "because" is correct

Chapter 4

1. A. First part is right, second part is wrong
2. True
3. C. Encephalopathy
4. B. Terlipressin with albumin
5. C. 42 days

Chapter 5

1. D. Pulse oximetry and contrast echocardiography
2. A. The presence of right ventricular hypertrophy on echocardiography warrants right-heart catheterization, and E. Almost 20% of transplant candidates have elevated RVSP on Doppler echocardiography
3. E. First part is correct, second part is correct, "because" is correct

Chapter 6

1. C. Alcohol abuse, defined as a tolerance or alcohol-related problems, but without clear evidence of the Loss of Control phenomenon, fails dependence criteria and therefore offers the best prognosis for abstinence
2. A. Social stability, B. Alcohol use diagnosis, D. Polysubstance use diagnosis, and E. Vaillant's factors. Pre-transplant abstinence >6 months has not been substantiated in carefully designed prospective study
3. B. First part is correct, second part is wrong. To present knowledge, alcohol-induced liver conditions and alcohol dependence overlap in only 70–80% of cases applying for liver transplant

Medical Care of the Liver Transplant Patient, Fourth Edition. Edited by Pierre-Alain Clavien, James F. Trotter.

Chapter 7

1. D. The difference between survival with and survival without a liver transplant
2. B. Different laboratory reagents for measuring pro-thrombin time
3. D. First part is correct, second part is correct, "because" is incorrect

Chapter 8

1. C. The presence of HBV DNA in serum at the time of transplantation
2. B. Donor age, C. Highest viral load at 3 months post transplantation, and E. Presence of F1 fibrosis in the year biopsy
3. E. Entecavir should not be used as an antiviral agent in the setting of lamivudine resistance because of the high rate of entecavir resistance in this setting

Chapter 9

1. D. All of the above
2. B. Protocol liver biopsies
3. A. Acute liver failure
4. A. Increased transferrin saturation >45%, ferritin >1000 ng/mL, and Hepatic iron index >1.9

Chapter 10

1. B. Ursodeoxycholic acid, 13–15 mg/kg/d
2. A. Colon carcinoma, B. Cholangiocarcinoma, D. Gallbladder carcinoma, E. Pancreatic carcinoma, and F. Hepatocellular carcinoma
3. B. First part is correct, second part is wrong

Chapter 11

1. C. Patients within Milan criteria
2. A. Patients with microvascular invasion and satelitosis in surgical sample
3. E. All of them are correct

Chapter 12

1. D. ERCP with brushings of the bile ducts for cytology
2. B. Extrahepatic CCA with bilateral involvement to the second-degree biliary radicals with no metastases, and D. Extrahepatic CCA with unilateral involvement in a patient with PSC with no metastases
3. A. First part is wrong, second part is wrong

Chapter 13

1. C. Myeloproliferative disease
2. D. First part is correct, second part is correct, "because" is incorrect
3. All are correct

Chapter 14

1. D. All these agents have anti-retroviral effects
2. D. Chronic cryptosporidiosis. Only opportunistic infections for which there is no reliable therapy post-transplant are contraindications to transplantation
3. C. Protease inhibitors. The protease inhibitors inhibit the cytochrome p450 system, thus CsA, tacrolimus, and sirolimus doses must be significantly reduced and carefully monitored

Chapter 15

1. D. Is associated with a mortality rate in the donor of 3–5%. It is associated with significantly higher rates of biliary complications than deceased donor transplantation
2. A. Allows earlier transplant at a lower MELD score, and E. Can be performed with a right or left lobe graft
3. A. First part is wrong, second part is wrong

Chapter 16

1. C. Encephalopathy
2. A. Pregnancy, B. Liver rupture, and C. Metastatic cancer
3. True
4. A. First part is true, second part is false

Chapter 17

1. A. First part is wrong, second part is wrong
2. A. Cold ischemia time >12 h, D. Split graft, and E. Nonwhite race
3. B. Graft survival

Chapter 18

1. D. Planned withdrawal of treatment and awaiting cardiac arrest
2. B. Time from post withdrawal hypotension/hypoxia to initiation of aortic perfusion, and D. Time from withdrawal of treatment to initiation of aortic perfusion
3. E. First part is correct, second part is correct, "because" is correct

Chapter 19

1. E. Crow
2. A. Prior surgery, B. Prior chemotherapy, C. Prior radiation therapy, and E. Ventriculoperitoneal shunt
3. A. First part is wrong, second part is wrong

Chapter 20

1. A. UW solution, C. IGL solution, D. Celsior solution, and E. HTK solution
2. B. Should be done at the level of the recipient's gastroduodenal artery or proximal to it, C. Should show a flow of approximately 200 ml/min, D. May be done before portal vein anastomoses, and E. Is decisive for later graft function
3. B. Has to be monitored repeatedly within the first 48 h after OLT, and D. Is the most important factor for the decision whether PNF is present

Chapter 21

1. A. Thrombectomy, B. Jump graft between donor portal vein and superior mesenteric vein, and E. Portocaval hemitransposition
2. B. Can be done by infrarenal aortic conduit, C. May be feasible by supraceliac aortic conduit, D. Is possible on the splenic artery, and E. Should be checked by intraoperative flow measurement
3. All answers are correct

Chapter 22

1. C. The domino donor is a relatively older individual
2. B. First part is correct, second part is wrong
3. A. Young hemodynamically stable donors, C. Donors with normal liver function test results, and D. Donors with short ICU stay (<5 d) and absent or fairly short down time

Chapter 23

1. C. Colorectal liver metastasis
2. D. Segment IV–VIII liver graft
3. False

Chapter 24

1. A. Hypokalemia
2. A. Echocardiography, B. Lung function test, C. Blood electrolytes, and E. Coagulation factors
3. C. First part is wrong, second part is correct

Chapter 25

1. D. Drugs promoting coagulation should be cautiously used
2. A. It is important to keep the patient's temperature at 37°C, D. Thromboelastography/metry is helpful to guide therapy with FFP or procoagulant drugs, and E. Serum ionic calcium (Ca^{++}) should be routinely monitored and corrected to maintain a serum $Ca^{++} \geq 1$ mmol/L
3. C. First part is wrong, second part is correct

Chapter 26

1. D. Cholinesterase levels (Cholinesterase levels are not routinely used to assess graft function after liver transplantation).
2. C. Portal hypertension, abnormal gas exchange, evidence of pulmonary vascular shunts
3. A. Na-MELD. NaMELD has only been validated for the endpoint mortality on the waiting list

Chapter 27

1. B. Liver function tests
2. A. Tacrolimus, C. Corticosteroids, and D. Mycophenolate mofetil
3. False
4. C. Tacrolimus is more efficacious

Chapter 28

1. D. All of the above
2. D. Celiac angiogram
3. A. Small spleen

Chapter 29

1. D. Non-anastomotic biliary strictures
2. C. Presence of a Roux-Y hepatico-jejunostomy is a risk factor for cholangitis after liver transplantation, and E. The use of biliary T-drain in liver transplantation does not lead to a reduction in reinterventions for biliary complications
3. C. First part is wrong, second part is correct

Chapter 30

1. E. Widespread lobular necro-inflammatory activity and the lack of significant bile duct damage are histopathologic findings favoring recurrent hepatitis C virus infection over acute cellular rejection
2. B. Portal inflammation, D. Venous endothelitis, and E. Bile duct damage and injury
3. B. First part is correct, second part is wrong

Chapter 31

1. A. HbA1c >6.5%
2. A. Use of calcineurin inhibitors, D. Obesity, and E. Renal dysfunction
3. B. First part is correct, second part is wrong

Chapter 32

1. C. Liver allograft from donor >50 years of age
2. A. HCV genotype, B. Recipient IL-28 b genotype, C. Baseline fibrosis stage, and D. Early (4 or 12 week) on-treatment virologic response
3. E. First part is correct, second part is correct, "because" is correct

Chapter 33

1. B. Wilson disease
2. B. Rarely causes graft failure, and E. Is diagnosed on graft histology
3. C. First part is wrong, second part is correct

Chapter 34

1. E. All of the above
2. A. *Isospora belli*, B. *Toxoplasma gondii*, D. *Nocardia* species, and E. *Listeria* species
3. B. First part is correct, second part is wrong

Chapter 35

1. B. Squamous cell carcinoma
2. A. Dose reduction, and C. Switch to cyclosporine
3. E. First part is correct, second part is correct, "because" is correct

Chapter 36

1. C. Epstein–Barr virus: PTLD
2. All are correct
3. C. 2 to 4 times greater

Chapter 37

1. B. Mycophenolate mofetil
2. A. Regular menstrual bleeding will reappear in the vast majority of women of child-bearing age within 1 year post transplant, C. Most data suggest better outcomes for mother and newborns with a transplant-to-conception interval >2 years, and D. The fetal problems most commonly observed in children born to liver transplant recipients are fetal loss, prematurity (defined as birth occurring prior to 37 weeks' gestation) and low birth weight (<2500 g)
3. B. First part is correct, second part is wrong

Chapter 38

1. A. Chronic rejection
2. A. Paucity of interlobular bile ducts on liver biopsy, C. Peripheral pulmonary branch artery stenosis, D. Butterfly vertebrae, and E. Posterior embryotoxon
3. B. First part is correct, second part is wrong

Index

Notes: Pages numbers in *italics* refer to Figures; those in **bold** to Tables

Medical Care of the Liver Transplant Patient, Fourth Edition. Edited by Pierre-Alain Clavien, James F. Trotter.